Emergency
Medical Guide
FOURTH EDITION

JOHN HENDERSON, M.D., F.A.C.S., F.A.A.P. (Hon.)
(Honorary Associate)
Corporate Director of Medical Affairs, Johnson & Johnson (Retired)
Consultant in Investigative Surgery, Middlesex General Hospital
New Brunswick, New Jersey

NEIL HARDY
Medical Illustrator

Emergency Birth Illustrations
by
Betty Jane Eager

McGRAW-HILL BOOK COMPANY
New York   St. Louis   San Francisco   Auckland   Bogotá
Düsseldorf   Johannesburg   London   Madrid   Mexico
Montreal   New Delhi   Panama   Paris   São Paulo
Singapore   Sydney   Tokyo   Toronto

Emergency Medical Guide

1 2 3 4 5 6 7 8 9 0   MUMU   7 8 3 2 1 0 9 8

Library of Congress Cataloging in Publication Data

Henderson, John, date
    Emergency medical guide.

    Bibliography: p.
    Includes index.
    1.   First aid in illness and injury.   I.   Title.
[DNLM: 1.   First aid.   WA292 H496e]
RC86.7.H46   1978   614.8′8   77-14433
ISBN 0-07-028168-8
ISBN 0-07-028169-6 pbk.

Notice

Medicine is an ever-changing science. As new research and clinical experience broaden our knowledge, changes in treatment and drug therapy are required. The editors and the publisher of this work have made every effort to ensure that the drug dosage schedules herein are accurate and in accord with the standards accepted at the time of publication. The reader is advised, however, to check the product information sheet included in the package of each drug he plans to administer to be certain that changes have not been made in the recommended dose or in the contraindications for administration. This recommendation is of particular importance in regard to new or infrequently used drugs.

Dedicated
to those devoted First-Aid and Rescue Squads
throughout America
and to those mothers who must often serve as
nurses, "extemporaneous doctors,"
and comforters to their families.

Contents

Appendix

Preface

This book was written to present a simple, straightforward discussion of a host of medical questions, many of them of an urgent or emergency nature. Many subjects are included which are not found in the usual texts on first aid, because we have tried to envision, as realistically as possible, the kinds of medical problems that arise in everyday life and to suggest procedures which are most likely to be effective until adequate medical assistance can be obtained. In a strict sense, this is not a first-aid book, nor is it intended to teach medicine; rather it is a review in some depth of many pressing medical problems any of which could face a person at some time in his life.

The matter of emergency care assumes great importance in the light of possible civil disaster—natural or military. As has been pointed out many times, even a major civil disaster may so sorely tax the medical resources of organized civil defense that effective first aid and self aid might in many cases mean the difference between life and death.

When any disaster strikes, the family group must be psychologically prepared to meet the emergency, without confusion or panic, and with the capability of handling immediate medical needs, possibly for extended periods of time, until professional aid becomes available.

Quite aside from the question of a civil or medical catastrophe, there arise many occasions when, for one reason or another, the services of a physician or a hospital are not immediately within reach and when an emergency, such as an accident, a sick child, or an acutely ill adult, must be met. In such a case, knowledge and proper technics quickly and correctly applied may, in fact, be life-saving tools.

Within the last few years, medical knowledge has increased amazingly, and new technics for saving life, which fall within the grasp of the layman, have become available. In addition to these, much new information with respect to medical developments in the prevention and treatment of various common illnesses, particularly in children, has been included.

This fourth edition has been amplified to cover several important areas of medical information of an emergency nature, including an expanded section on poisoning and new information relating to drug abuse.

It is our hope that, in this book, those who have had no special technical training, as well as those who have had basic first-aid instruction but who wish to acquaint themselves with more extended knowledge will find a helpful guide to the handling of such medical emergencies as they may be called upon to face and the answers to some medical questions which may have been puzzling them.

While indexed so that emergency information can be readily found, it is urged that the book be read in substance during leisure moments, so as to obtain a sound general background.

We are grateful to the American Medical Association, the American Heart Association, the American Academy of Pediatrics, and the American College of Surgeons for aid and cooperation in helping to procure much of the updated material incorporated in this Fourth Edition, as well as the many helpful suggestions made by Robert L. Beasley, Associate Professor of the University of South Florida, and William T. Brennan, Associate Professor of the University of Indiana.

We wish to acknowledge also the assistance of Miss Cathryne Davies in the arduous task of readying the manuscript for the printer, and the invaluable assistance of Miss Margaret Sutton in checking the accuracy of many new references. Without such help this book would not have been possible.

John Henderson

EMERGENCY
MEDICAL GUIDE

1 form and functions of the Body

The human body is so complicated and its structures so intricate that a general understanding of its form (anatomy) and the functions (physiology) of its more important parts is essential to rendering intelligent emergency aid.

THE SKELETON

The human skeleton is composed of approximately two hundred separate bones, so shaped and put together as to form the specific groups that make up the head, trunk, pelvis, arms, and legs (Fig. 1-1).

The Head

The head, composed of 22 bones, includes the skull, face, and jaw. The skull is the strong protective case for the brain and is made up of eight bones. The remainder of the bones form the face and jaw. The jaw is composed of two parts—the upper, which is immovable, is the maxilla and the lower, which is the only movable structure in the skull, is the mandible.

Although the skull provides a strong protective case for the brain, it is itself subject to several kinds of severe injury, particularly to fractures.

The Trunk

The trunk, which includes the vertebral column and ribs, totals 54 bones; it supports or encloses all the vital organs situated in the chest and abdomen.

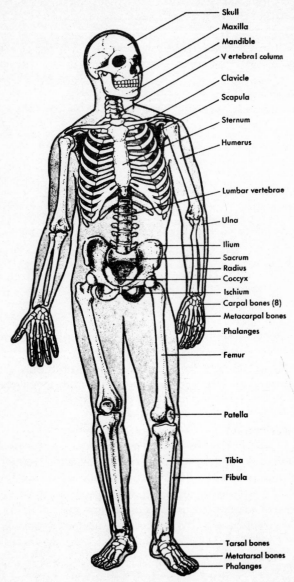

Fig. 1-1. The human skeleton, showing the principal bones of the body.

The Vertebral Column. The vertebral column, or backbone, is composed of 26 separate bones, known as *vertebrae*, so constructed as to surround and fully enclose the all-important spinal cord, which is the main distributing "cable" for almost all the nerves of the body. This protection is of extreme importance, since an injury, such as a fracture of the spine, may so seriously damage the spinal cord as to cause temporary or permanent paralysis of various muscle groups.

The vertebral column includes the neck, consisting of seven vertebrae, and the back itself. The vertebrae of the back are divided into the 12 of the chest portion, the five of the abdominal portion, and the five of the pelvic portion which are fused into what really amounts to one bone, the sacrum. Finally, below the sacrum there are four bones, forming the coccyx which would have been a tail if you had been a monkey.

All this is important in treating accident cases, because injuries of the various portions of the spinal column are not all treated alike nor are victims of spinal injuries transported alike. Therefore, it is important to understand its anatomy in order to evaluate the condition correctly and render the proper emergency care.

The Chest. The chest is composed of 12 pairs of ribs which are attached to and suspended from the 12 vertebrae of the chest portion of the backbone. The chest houses and protects such life-supporting structures as the lungs, heart, great vessels, trachea, and esophagus. Although the bony cage of the chest does a surprisingly good job of protecting these vital structures, when an injury to them does occur, it may be serious; therefore, it is of extreme importance to understand not only the anatomy but the physiology of the chest.

The upper seven pairs of ribs are attached to the breastbone by means of individual cartilages; the next three pairs are united by a common cartilage; and the last two, known as *floating ribs,* have no attachments in front at all. The points at which the ribs join the spinal column are true (or movable) joints which permit the ribs to be drawn in or out, a movement which is brought about by the various muscles attached to the ribs and which makes possible the mechanism of breathing.

This important function is accomplished by two basic actions: (1) As the muscles attached to the ribs contract, the ribs are pulled outward. (2) Simultaneously, the diaphragm (the dome-shaped muscle attached to the lower ribs and vertebral column) draws itself downward by contracting. The net effect is to increase the size of the chest and create suction, or negative pressure, between the chest wall and the lungs themselves. This vacuum sucks the lungs outward, and they expand in an attempt to fill the vacuum; and air, in turn, is sucked into the lungs. Then the rib muscles and diaphragm relax, like a rubber balloon, and the air which had previously been sucked into the lungs is expelled, thus completing the respiratory cycle.

Certain wounds of the chest can seriously interfere with these functions or cause them to cease altogether and, in this way, impede or halt the breathing process.

The Shoulder Girdle

Of special importance because of the frequency of injury is the collarbone, the inner end of which is fastened to the breastbone and the outer end to the shoulder blade. It lies just above the first rib and, together with the shoulder blade, forms the shoulder girdle.

The shoulder blade lies at the upper and outer part of the back of the chest and, since it provides the socket for the upper end of the arm, is an important and integral part of the shoulder joint.

Each arm is composed of the long bones and a collection of flat and irregular ones which make up the wrist, hand, and fingers, a total of 30 bones.

The Arms

The long bone of the arm, the humerus, fits into the shoulder joint and, at the elbow, forms a joint with the two bones of the lower arm—the radius and the ulna. These two join at their lower ends with the wrist, composed of eight bones. The wrist bones join with the five metacarpal bones forming the palm of the hand, and these in turn are joined with the bones of the fingers. Each finger has three bones, or phalanges, but the thumb has two.

The Pelvis

The pelvis forms the lowest part of the abdominal cavity. It surrounds and protects several important organs which lie in the pelvic cavity, including the bladder and rectum, which are particularly important from the standpoint of injury.

The pelvis consists of six bones (not counting those of the sacrum or coccyx). The two largest are the broad, wing-shaped bones, popularly referred to as the hipbones; technically they consist of three smaller bones (the pubis, ischium, and ilium) fused together. The pelvis also provides the sockets into which the upper ends of the thighbones fit to form the marvelous ball-and-socket joint of the hip.

The Legs

Each leg is composed of 30 bones, one of which is the biggest and strongest in the body—the thighbone, yet it is often subject to fracture. The thighbone fits into the socket in the hipbone to form the hip joint and, at its other end, joins at the knee with three bones (the kneecap, or patella; the tibia, the larger bone of the lower leg; and the fibula, the long secondary bone) to form the knee joint. At their lower ends, the tibia and fibula join with the ankle, which is composed of seven bones, and this is joined with the five metatarsal bones, which form the arch of the foot. The toes have the same number of bones as the fingers.

THE JOINTS AND MUSCLES

Wherever bones are connected with each other, there are joints. These may be movable, which is the type with which we shall be most concerned, or immovable, such as those of the skull or sacrum. Where bones come together to form a movable joint, their adjoining moving surfaces are covered with a highly lubricated, almost frictionless layer of cartilage, and the entire joint is held together by strong ligaments and encased in a fibrous tissue capsule. Dislocation of a joint may occur when the capsule is torn or stretched, thus allowing the bone to slip out of the joint. Sprains may occur because of undue stretching or actual tearing of the ligaments, without dislocation.

Bones are caused to move at their joints by muscles which exert their forces upon the bones through strong fibrous thongs, or tendons, by which they are attached to the bones at points of leverage. The muscles are composed of a highly specialized kind of tissue, which under stimulus from the nerves that supply them can contract, thus making it possible to move the various parts of the body.

When the nerve that stimulates a muscle is interrupted anywhere along its course between the cell in the central nervous system from which it originates and the muscle which it supplies, the muscle becomes paralyzed and will never again be under voluntary control unless the function of the nerve is restored.

In order to perform highly coordinated movements, opposing sets of muscles are required, and their actions are coordinated through the many delicate interrelationships of the nerve connections within the spinal cord and brain. When this co-ordination fails, one sees the manifestations of nerve disease in tremors, twitchings, and uncontrolled movements.

THE SOFT PARTS OF THE BODY

The body itself, as distinguished from its bony structure, is composed of various systems of organs to a large extent contained within the protective cavities provided by the skeleton. For simplification and convenience, these organs will be discussed by the systems of which they are a part.

The Skin

One of the most important organs of the body, in fact a system in itself, is the skin (Fig. 1-2). The prime function of the skin is to serve as a protecting envelope for all the underlying tissues. It is exposed to all kinds of weather—sun, cold, sleet, and rain; it is subject to an amazing number of infections; it may be bruised, cut, burned, and at times even torn to shreds, but fortunately, it possesses an amazing recuperative power.

The skin serves also as an organ of excretion and, through perspiration, helps to rid the body of a great deal of waste matter. It is largely responsible for the regulation of body temperature, a function which it accomplishes in two ways: (1) by the evaporation of so-called "insensible" water from the skin surface, which, under ordinary conditions, amounts to about a quart a day; and (2) by radiation of heat from the blood in the capillaries of the skin. This explains why a person who is overheated becomes reddened and flushed—the capillaries of the

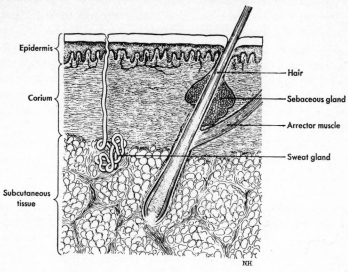

Fig. 1-2. The skin is composed of a number of layers and parts, each of which has a special function.

skin surface are dilated in an attempt to radiate larger quantities of heat and thus cool down the body.   There is a third factor which is relatively minor, and this is conveyance of heat from the skin surface itself.

If one doubts the importance of the skin as one of the major organs of the body, one has only to consider the plight of the person who has lost a large part of his skin surface, as by burns.   This will ultimately cause his death unless the loss can be replaced or repaired by some suitable means.

The Respiratory System

The respiratory system provides the means by which the blood is oxygenated and by which it is able to rid itself of the carbon dioxide it has absorbed as a waste product from the tissues, to which it simultaneously gives up its oxygen.

The blood gives off carbon dioxide and absorbs oxygen in the minute air spaces of the lungs, known as *alveoli*.   The supply of fresh air required for this interchange is brought to the lungs by the windpipe, or trachea, from the upper respiratory passages: the nose, the nasopharynx, and the larynx.   Since there are two lungs, the windpipe, which is a large firm tube supported by strong cartilaginous rings, divides into two main smaller tubes known as *bronchial tubes (bronchi),* one going to each lung. Within each lung, these large bronchial tubes divide and redivide until they get down in size to the smallest bronchioles, which bring air to each little alveolus. The alveoli form the substance of the lungs in very much the same way that a honeycomb is constructed (Fig. 1-3). These tiny air spaces are formed by exceedingly delicate tissue which is thin enough to permit the diffusion of oxygen and carbon dioxide between the very small blood vessels in their walls and the air in the alveoli.

Each lung is surrounded by a glistening, smooth, airtight sac known as the *pleura,* which is also carried over onto the inside of the chest wall. As has already been indicated, there is normally no air in this sac, so that as the chest cavity is expanded

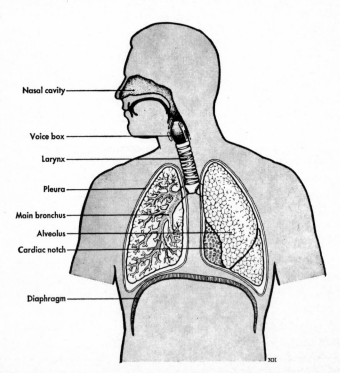

Nasal cavity

Voice box

Larynx

Pleura

Main bronchus

Alveolus

Cardiac notch

Diaphragm

Fig. 1-3. General structure of the respiratory system, showing relation of pleural sac to the lungs.

by the ribs moving outward and the diaphragm downward, there tends to be created a negative pressure within the pleural sac.   This causes the lungs to expand, and air is sucked into the alveoli.   Then, the need for oxygen and the need to dispose of carbon dioxide having been satisfied, the rib muscles and diaphragm relax, the chest cavity diminishes in size, the lung tissue contracts, and the air is expelled from the lungs, taking its waste products with it.   A new cycle is then ready to begin.

If for any reason a leak is produced in the pleural sac from the outside, as may occur in certain chest injuries, a sucking wound is created; this is a very serious condition, since, no matter how hard the person tries to breathe, he cannot expand his lung on the affected side, for air is simply sucked into the pleural space and further collapses the lung on that side.   A similar condition, known as *spontaneous pneumothorax*, is created from the inside when, due to some disease process, a connection develops between a lung and the pleural sac, thus creating an internal leak.

Respiration is under the control of a center in the brain which automatically regulates breathing in a wholly unconscious manner, although, of course, breathing is partially under voluntary control.   But you can make yourself breathe faster or slower for only just so long before you have initiated a series of chemical changes in the blood that force the respiratory center to take over in an attempt to regulate things.   Similarly, you can hold your breath for only just so long before you *have* to breathe.

In certain types of respiratory paralysis, the normal nervous activation of the muscles of respiration is interrupted by disease, as in certain types of infantile paralysis, and breathing must be done for the patient in an iron lung, or some other type of forced respiration system.

The respiratory function automatically maintains a delicate chemical balance between carbon dioxide and oxygen in the blood and is closely related to other mechanisms which control the transportation and excretion of other waste products.

The respiratory rate may be increased by a need for oxygen or by an accumulation of carbon dioxide in the blood, resulting in a demand for more rapid excretion.   This can occur as the result of a number of disease conditions not necessarily directly related to the respiratory system.   Knowledge of this physiologic fact is used advantageously in anesthetics, for instance, and in oxygen tanks for resuscitation which may contain a small percentage of carbon dioxide to stimulate the person to breath deeper and at a more rapid rate, thus taking in more oxygen.

The Cardiovascular (Circulatory) System

Intimately associated with the respiratory system and indeed an integral part of it is the cardiovascular system. Its main function is to circulate blood to the most minute cells of the body, to which it brings life-giving oxygen from the lungs and from which it absorbs waste to be excreted by the lungs and kidneys.

The Heart. The organ which makes this circulation possible is the heart, and it is one of the most efficient pumping mechanisms known. In spite of all kinds of abuse, it has been known to function without a breakdown and with no repairs for well over a hundred years—and there is no standby replacement within the body; sometimes it goes on for years with leaky valves, wrong connections, or defective cylinder walls. That it keeps going so long and so dependably is one of the most wonderful facts in nature.

This remarkable mechanism is located in the chest cavity between the two lungs, in a compartment, called the *mediastinum,* which is completely walled off anatomically from each lung. In the mediastinum are the great blood vessels, many important nerves, the thoracic duct, the windpipe, and the esophagus.

The heart is divided into two halves, right and left, each of which is further subdivided into two compartments, the upper one called the *auricle,* and the lower one the *ventricle* (Fig. 1-4). Normally, there is no direct connection between the two sides of the heart, but each auricle connects directly with its ventricle through an ingenious flutter valve which prevents backflow when the ventricle on that side contracts to force the blood from it out into the circulation.

Arterial blood is distributed to the body by means of many arteries stemming from the aorta, which divide and subdivide until they terminate in tiny arterial capillaries in the tissue themselves. Here they join, at the point of smallest subdivision, with the venous capillaries which empty into veins of

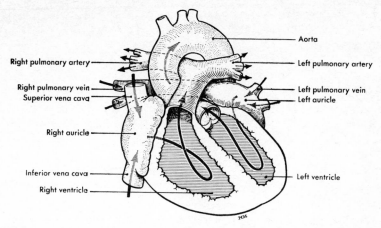

Fig. 1-4. Main components of the heart, showing the course of the blood flow through the two sides.

ever-increasing size which finally return it to the great vein known as the *vena cava,* and then into the right auricle of the heart. It is important to know and understand the course of the main vessels, because one of the most common emergencies is the control of hemorrhage.

The right half of the heart carries blood to the lungs and the left half to the rest of the body. The way it works is, very simply, as follows: Since one has to start at some particular point, let us start with the blood being returned to the heart from the rest of the body. This is venous, or "impure," blood, carrying too much carbon dioxide. It enters the right auricle of the heart through the vena cava and is pumped at low pressure into the right ventricle. From there it is pumped at higher pressure through the pulmonary artery to the lungs, from where the "freshened" blood is carried by means of the pulmonary veins to the left auricle. (Note that, paradoxically, the pulmonary veins are carrying arterial blood.) From the left auricle the bright-red, fresh arterial blood goes into the left ventricle, from which it is pumped at high pressure through the aorta to all parts of the body, whence it returns to repeat the cycle (Fig. 1-5). Normally, the circulation time is about 21 seconds, which means that a hypothetical drop of blood completes the entire course in that space of time.

The rate of heartbeat varies tremendously, of course, ac-

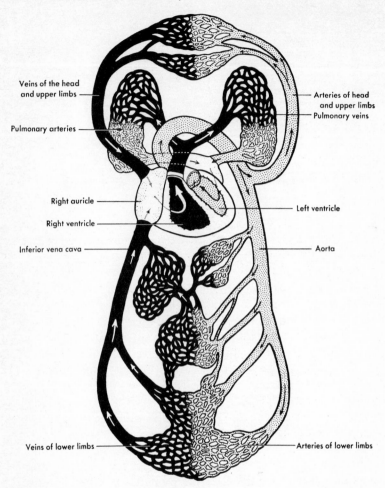

Veins of the head and upper limbs

Pulmonary arteries

Arteries of head and upper limbs

Pulmonary veins

Right auricle

Right ventricle

Left ventricle

Inferior vena cava

Aorta

Veins of lower limbs

Arteries of lower limbs

Fig. 1-5. Schematic representation of the relationship of the systemic and pulmonary circulations to the heart.

cording to age, circumstances, and an individual's emotional or physical condition, but normally it is about 70 to 80 beats per minute. This can be counted by the pulse.

Arteries of the Upper Portion of the Body. The general scheme of blood circulation can be discussed in terms of the larger vessels and the areas which they serve (Fig. 1-6). Within the chest cavity the aorta branches at its arch (just above where it comes out of the heart) into the large arteries which supply

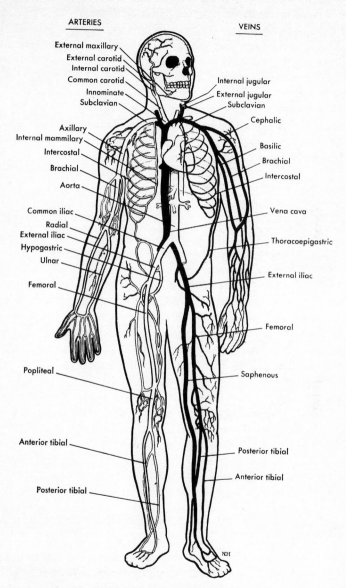

ARTERIES

VEINS

External maxillary
External carotid
Internal carotid
Common carotid
Innominate
Subclavian

Internal jugular
External jugular
Subclavian
Cephalic

Axillary
Internal mammilary
Intercostal
Brachial
Aorta

Basilic
Brachial
Intercostal

Common iliac
Radial
External iliac
Hypogastric
Ulnar

Vena cava

Thoracoepigastric

External iliac

Femoral

Femoral

Popliteal

Saphenous

Anterior tibial

Posterior tibial
Anterior tibial

Posterior tibial

Fig. 1-6. General arrangement of the major arteries shown on right side and veins shown on left side of the body.

the head and arms. These vessels are the innominate artery, a very large artery which comes from the aorta and divides into the right common carotid artery (going to the right side of the neck and head) and the right subclavian artery (going to the upper part of the chest and arm). The left subclavian and left common carotid arteries branch off the arch of the aorta directly.

The common carotid arteries divide into the internal carotids which supply the brain and the external carotids which supply the face and scalp. The external carotid arteries are important in case of hemorrhage of the face or neck.

The subclavian artery becomes the axillary artery in the armpit, giving off a number of important branches, then passes into the upper arm as the brachial artery, and divides at the elbow into the radial and ulnar arteries, which pass down the forearm, branching out to the various muscles, and finally into the hand as the deep and the superficial volar arteries.

Arteries of the Lower Portion of the Body. After rounding its arch, the aorta passes downward through the chest cavity, where the intercostal arteries branch off and, with branches of the internal mammary artery, go to the muscles controlling the ribs. Branches also go to other organs of the chest cavity, and the aorta then passes into the abdominal cavity, where it supplies blood to all the organs therein.

At about the point where the pelvic cavity joins the abdominal cavity, the aorta divides into two very large vessels, the right and left common iliac arteries, which again divide into the external iliac and hypogastric arteries. The hypogastric arteries supply the organs of the pelvis, and the external iliac arteries continue downward to the legs.

As the external iliac enters the thigh under the ligament in the groin, it becomes the femoral artery, its branches supplying the various muscles of the thigh, and passes down the thigh along the inner side of the femur. At the knee, where it lies behind the joint, it becomes the popliteal artery, and just below this point, it divides into the anterior (front) and the posterior (rear) tibial arteries. The peroneal artery also rises at this point. These pass downward, supplying the muscles of the leg, and then into the various muscles of the foot. The pulsation of the anterior tibial artery can be felt on the top of the foot just below the ankle joint, alongside the heavy tendon that leads to the big toe.   The pulsations of the posterior tibial can be felt by pressing gently behind the leg bone of the ankle joint on the inner side of the leg.

Important Veins of the Body.   For the most part, the veins bringing the blood back to the heart follow the arterial system quite closely and have comparable names, but there are a few exceptions that are important from the standpoint of emergency care.

One of these exceptions is the internal saphenous, a vein close to the surface which runs up the inner part of the leg and empties into the femoral vein just below the inguinal ligament in the groin.   It is the vein which is commonly tied off in an operation for varicose veins, or which often is used in those whose arteries have become occluded by disease to replace or bypass the obstructed segment.   The other, the external saphenous vein, is also close to the surface, running up the outer part of the foot and the back of the calf; it empties into the popliteal vein, back of the knee.

In the arm, the basilic vein is important, since it is the one from which blood is commonly taken or into which fluids or transfusions are given.   It lies quite close to the surface in the bend of the elbow.

Also of importance is the cephalic vein, quite close to the forward surface of the shoulder.   This is a large vein, and, because of its nearness to the surface, it can be injured easily.

There are several large veins, the jugular veins in the neck which lie relatively near the surface, and hence are easily cut, either accidentally or by suicidal intent.   Bleeding from these may be profuse, but usually is not very difficult to control.

In this discussion of the circulatory system, certain important anatomical relations have been omitted, but where these parts are relevant to emergency care, they are discussed as required.

The Urinary System

Closely integrated with the circulatory and respiratory systems for the excretion of waste substances is the urinary system. This system, in conjunction with the respiratory system, is principally responsible for the control and regulation of the general body chemistry. Together with the respiratory system, skin, and, to some degree, the digestive tract, the urinary system controls the water balance, or water metabolism, of the body. In certain diseases, because the kidneys cease to function, the body retains excessive water, a situation which may become serious enough to cause death. Among the principal waste products eliminated by the urinary tract are substances containing nitrogen which, if not eliminated at a reasonable rate, accumulate alarmingly and become exceedingly toxic. On the other hand, in certain conditions, as in severe burns, there is a lack of nitrogen (protein) in the blood, which is very difficult to correct. If such a condition is severe over a prolonged period, the patient will die.

The basic components of the urinary system are the two kidneys, which lie in the abdominal cavity, on either side of the vertebral column, well up beneath the arch of the diaphragm, at about the level of the second and third lumbar vertebrae (Fig. 1-7). Perched on the upper pole of each kidney are two of the most important glands in the body. These are the adrenal glands. They perform many important functions, since they not only secrete epinephrine and many other important hormones, but have much to do with the reactions of the body to stress.

Blood is brought to the kidneys by the renal arteries, which branch off on either side of the aorta. The blood, purified of waste matter, leaves the kidneys by way of veins that empty into the abdominal vena cava, the large vein going to the heart. The waste products extracted from the blood by the kidneys, together with water, are excreted as urine.

Urine contains many substances, since, to maintain proper health, the body must excrete about 2 ounces of chemical wastes every 24 hours. These materials are contained in the urine in the form of soluble compounds, the average total urine volume for a 24-hour period being a little more than a quart. This varies with circumstances and may be increased or decreased in a number of disease conditions.

The urine is collected from each kidney by a ureter which runs downward along the muscles covering the vertebral column, dips over the brim of the pelvis, and empties into the urinary bladder. The ureters are thick fibrous tubes which are not readily injured, except under severe conditions.

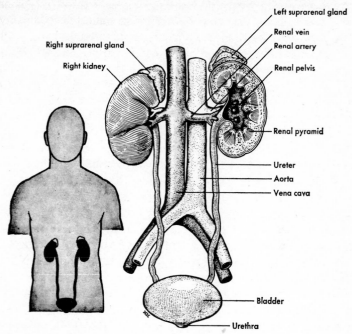

Left suprarenal gland
Renal vein
Renal artery
Renal pelvis

Right suprarenal gland

Right kidney

Renal pyramid

Ureter
Aorta
Vena cava

Bladder

Urethra

Fig. 1-7. General relationships of the various parts of the urinary system.

The urinary bladder is a thick muscular organ situated deep in the pelvis, in men lying between the rectum and pubic bone; when full, it rises above the pelvic bone. In women, the uterus, ovaries, fallopian tubes, and broad ligaments lie behind the bladder, between it and the rectum. The capacity of the bladder, of course, varies greatly, depending on many conditions, but in part upon the rapidity with which urine is secreted.

The bladder empties through the urethra. In women this is a short and fairly straight tube and opens in the vulva between the vaginal orifice and the clitoris, but in men it is a long, rather winding tube divided into two parts—the internal urethra, the part embedded in the prostate gland, and the external urethra, the part going through the penis to the external urinary meatus.

Various portions of the urinary tract may be subject to illnesses from injury or otherwise, most of them of a serious nature and beyond the scope of emergency care, except for preliminary supportive measures. In general, injury to the kidneys is relatively infrequent, except as the result of strong bruising forces such as occur in prizefights and football, but serious injury to the bladder, such as rupture, occurs frequently enough, especially in automobile accidents, for one to be on the alert for this possibility.

The Reproductive System

Male.   The male reproductive system is comprised of the testicles (testes), which are contained in a pendulous sac (the scrotum), and the penis.   These constitute the external sex organs, or genitalia.   The testicles, which are the counterpart of the female ovaries, not only supply the sperm that make fertilization possible, but are also organs of internal or endocrine secretion and are the principal source of the male hormone androgen.   Like the ovaries, the testicles develop within the abdominal cavity, but, as the fetus grows, they descend through the inguinal canal (groin) into the scrotum, where they are at about the time of birth.   Their presence in the inguinal canal leaves an anatomically weak area, which accounts for the high incidence in men of hernia or rupture in that region.

Within the pelvic cavity are found the internal reproductive organs, consisting of the prostate gland, the seminal vesicles, and the ducts (ductus deferens) connecting the testicles with these organs.   The prostate envelops the internal urethra near the base of the bladder and discharges its secretion through a series of ducts opening into the floor of the urethra.   Its enlargement in later life may produce a partial obstruction of the urethra where it passes through the gland, causing difficulty in urinating and sometimes urinary retention.   This condition is so severe as to require relief by catheterization, a procedure requiring professional medical aid.

The seminal vesicles are located just behind the prostate at the base of the bladder and serve as reservoirs for the storage of sperm and semen.

Female.   The female reproductive organs are situated wholly within the pelvis.   The only external genitalia consist of the vulva with its labia majora and minora (the counterpart of the male scrotum), the clitoris (the counterpart of the male penis), and the external opening of the vagina in front of and just above the anus (Fig. 1-8).

erally, on the body, but in some abnormal conditions, there may be serious blood loss or very severe pain and prostration. Such conditions require special medical attention.

The Digestive System

With the exception of the mouth and esophagus, the organs of digestion lie in the abdominal cavity, although technically the lower end of the large intestine and the anus lie in the pelvic cavity (Fig. 1-9).

The stomach is a large, hollow, muscular organ located high in the abdominal cavity just below the diaphragm. It is subject to many diseases requiring professional medical and surgical treatment, the gravest and most dramatic of which is perforated gastric ulcer.

The stomach empties into the upper portion of the small intestine known as the *duodenum,* which itself may be subject to ulcers. Within the curve of the duodenum and emptying into it through a small duct is the pancreas, which supplies

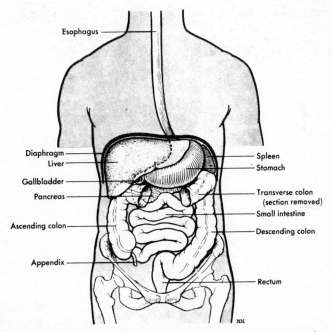

Fig. 1-9. The various organs forming the digestive tract, showing the relationships of the contents of the abdominal cavity.

digestive enzymes to the intestinal tract and also secretes the hormone, known as *insulin,* that regulates carbohydrate metabolism. Failure of the pancreas to function properly produces diabetes. The pancreas is also subject to acute inflammation and infection (even mumps!) and may thus give rise to a serious condition requiring surgical or medical intervention.

The succeeding portions of the small intestine are known as the *jejunum* and *ileum,* and it is in these portions that much of the digestive process takes place. The ileum empties into the cecum, the first portion of the large intestine. The cecum often gives rise to acute abdominal symptoms through its small appendage, the appendix, which is of no known use, but which can cause a great deal of trouble.

The next portion of the large intestine is the ascending colon, which passes into the transverse colon as it crosses the upper portion of the abdominal cavity, and then turns downward as the descending colon to enter an S-shaped part, known as the *sigmoid,* as it passes over the brim of the pelvis. The sigmoid passes into the rectum, which finally terminates in the anus, with its set of internal and external muscles, the sphincters.

Another important organ of digestion found in the abdominal cavity is the liver. This large organ, composed of solid glandular tissue, contains many blood vessels and lies high up in the abdominal cavity under the diaphragm on the right side.

The liver has many functions, including the conversion of carbohydrate and its storage as glycogen and the manufacture of bile and other digestive juices. This organ and its functions are so important that the absence or total nonfunctioning of the liver will cause death. In recent years there has been an increasing incidence of hepatitis, a liver infection caused by viruses. This condition is one of our most important public-health problems at the present time.

On the under side of the liver is the gallbladder, which is connected to the duodenum by a Y-shaped duct leading from the liver. It serves to store concentrated bile until it is needed to participate in the various digestive functions; at such times it is released into the intestinal tract. Of interest to the first-aider is that the gallbladder is prone to form stones, which may give rise to excruciating pain and require prompt medical assistance (see page 557).

One other organ, the spleen, lying in the abdominal cavity, although probably not directly concerned with digestion, requires mention because of its importance in abdominal injury. It is situated near the ribs on the left side, and it is commonly ruptured as the result of a severe bruising or crushing force to the abdominal area.   Possible rupture of the spleen should always be suspected in this type of injury and the symptoms of internal bleeding (q.v.) carefully watched for.   Rupture is especially likely to occur in young people suffering from mononucleosis, a condition in which the spleen may become greatly enlarged and easily subject to injury even as the result of some very minor (sometimes unnoticed) blow.

Although the functions of the spleen are not well understood, it appears to have much to do with the formation and destruction of the blood cells.   However, because a person can live without it, if the spleen ruptures, it is easier and quicker to remove it than to try to repair it.

The entire abdominal contents, or at least a good portion of them, are draped in front with a thick apron of fat, the omentum, which hangs down from the lower border of the transverse colon and serves the very useful purpose of walling off infection or other disease conditions, since it is surprisingly free to move about.

The walls of the abdominal cavity and almost all the organs which it contains are covered by a glistening, pearly white fibrous tissue sac, the peritoneum.   In men it is completely closed, but in women it is perforated by the free ends of the fallopian tubes, which open directly into the peritoneal cavity; hence, the sac is not completely closed and there is a potential opening to the outside through the uterine and vaginal canals —an important fact from the standpoint of infection.   The peritoneum is one of the largest and most important membranes in the body, and plays a vital protective role against infection.   Inflammation of this membrane, which may be incidental to many conditions, is known as *peritonitis* and is extremely serious.

The Nervous System

The nervous system is the most complicated and highly integrated of all of the body systems.   Man is distinguished from other animals by the superior development of his nervous system, which confers upon him the gift of intellect and the ability to think, to create, and to talk. It also confers the power of conscious control of his bodily functions, allowing him to exist as an individual rather than a vegetative organism. A general understanding of the nervous system means a better understanding of the general functioning of the body.

The nervous system as a whole may be divided into the several units of is component parts: the central (cerebrospinal or voluntary) nervous system and the autonomic (involuntary) nervous system (Fig. 1-10).

The central, or cerebrospinal, nervous system consists of the brain and the spinal cord. The spinal cord is continuous with the brain and is composed of nerve tracts leading to and · from the brain, controlling all parts and functions of the body with the exception of those areas activated by the 12 cranial nerves that arise in the brain itself. Both the brain and spinal cord are bathed in a clear colorless fluid, known as the *cerebrospinal fluid,* which is important as a protective agent for the delicate tissues of the nervous system. Leakage of this fluid as the result of accident is very serious. Blockage of the circulation and absorption of this fluid in the cavities in the brain are responsible for the overgrowth of the skull, known as *hydrocephalus.*

Altogether, there are 43 pairs of cerebrospinal nerves. Of these, 12 pairs come from the brain itself and are responsible for the sense of smell (I); nerves of the eyes (IV) and the face (II); the senses of hearing and balancing (I); nerves of the tongue and its sense of taste (II); a special nerve to the heart, lungs, and gastrointestinal tract which controls a great many of our physiologic functions (I); and a nerve to one of the large muscles of the back (I). Most of the voluntary muscles and the skin are controlled by 31 pairs of spinal nerves.

Injury to any one of the spinal nerves or injury directly to or above their origin in the spinal cord will produce paralysis of the muscle group they control or will produce a change or loss of sensation in the skin over the area they control. These areas have been thoroughly mapped out so that it is possible to tell exactly which part of the spinal cord is involved or whether only a single nerve is involved. Such conditions, however, call for a trained neurologist rather than for emergency-care measures.

CRANIAL NERVES
(viewed from below)

CROSS SECTION OF BRAIN

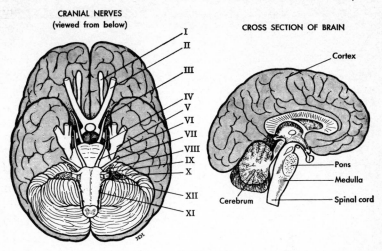

I
II
III
IV
V
VI
VII
VIII
IX
X
XII
XI

Cortex

Pons
Medulla
Spinal cord
Cerebrum

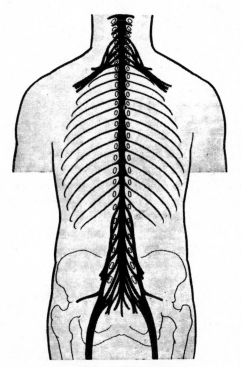

CENTRAL NERVOUS SYSTEM

A

Fig. 1-10. See legend on next page.

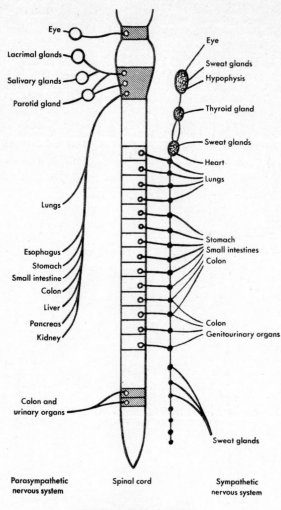

Fig. 1-10. Diagrammatic representation of the parts of the human (A) central nervous system, and (B) autonomic nervous system.

The importance of observing whether or not certain muscle groups, as of the legs or arms, are functioning properly is pointed out in the discussion of fractures of the spine.

The autonomic nervous system controls all the *involuntary* muscles and glands of the body, the muscles of the heart, and the blood vessels. It is not under conscious control, but often mediates secondarily many conscious or subconscious psychic forces. Although its nerves have their origin in certain cells of the spinal cord, it is a more or less independent system, forming a chain of groups, or nodules, of nerve cells that runs along each side of the spinal cord, whence nerves run to the various organs of the body.

Although the autonomic nervous system is of utmost importance, it has little direct bearing upon emergency care, except insofar as it controls the various responses to shock and injury.

The Ear

The ear is an amazingly complex device which depends for proper function upon many tiny, intricately related parts (Fig. 1-11). The normal ear receives sound as vibrations in the air which set up matching vibrations in the hearer's eardrum. The vibrations are transmitted via three tiny bones called the malleus (hammer), incus (anvil), stapes (stirrup), through the cochlea to the auditory nerve, which then passes them along as electrical impulses to the brain, where they are recognized as

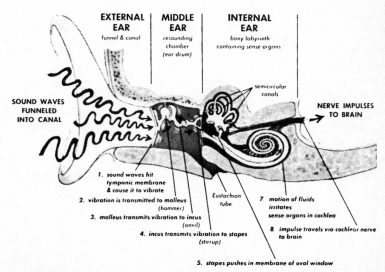

Fig. 1-11. Cutaway drawing showing the many complex parts of the ear serving the dual functions of hearing and balance.

noise or meaningful sounds. Malfunction in any one part of this system adversely affects its overall efficiency.

Because of the very delicate nature of the ear's many working parts, several types of injury and disease can affect their function, causing deafness, which can be of two main types—conductive and perceptive.

Conductive deafness occurs when any part of the ear that transmits physical sound waves loses its ability to function. For example, a simple and temporary form of conductive deafness can be caused by an excessive accumulation of wax in the auditory canal. Conductive deafness can also result from such things as perforation or inflammation of the eardrum, or inflammation within the middle ear. Its onset may be abrupt, but it is usually quite insidious, with hearing loss so gradual that the victim often does not realize that he is becoming deaf in one or both ears.

The most common cause of conductive deafness in children is large, infected adenoids, which block the opening of the eustachian tube which connects the throat and the middle ear, thus creating an imbalance of pressure within the ear itself and interfering with the conduction of sound waves.

In adults, otosclerosis is the most common cause of conductive deafness, especially in women. This disease usually begins between the ages of 18 and 40 and is caused by fixation of the tiny bone known as the stapes, as the result of hardening of the tissues which surround it. Thus the stapes, which is shaped like a tiny stirrup, cannot move freely in response to sound waves striking the eardrum, and with which it is in contact. When the stapes cannot move, it cannot transmit the sound waves onward to the inner part of the ear. Why this hardening process occurs is unknown, but there does seem to be some hereditary predisposition.

Formerly these cases were considered hopeless, but modern surgery has devised ways of operating on the minute structures involved under specially developed surgical microscopes and inserting a tiny wire or plastic tube to conduct the sound waves. This technic is highly successful in many cases.

Perceptive deafness, the other principal type, is caused by disorders of the inner ear, the auditory nerve itself, or the various hearing pathways within the brain. Such impairment may be commonly brought about by any one of many infectious diseases, including laryngitis, mumps, measles, and several other kinds of infection.

The importance of congenital deafness, as well as its frequency, has been demonstrated by Borton and Stark, who found that 77 mothers of 80 children with hearing losses had suffered from rubella (German measles) during the first three months of pregnancy. Three-fourths of the infections occurred during the second or third month, and three cases occurred during the fourth month. In 55 of these children, audiograms showed that the loss was moderately severe to profound.

Toxic substances, such as quinine, arsenic, alcohol, salicylates, or mercury, also can cause injury, as can continuous excessive noise.

A thorough physical examination, including special hearing tests, is needed to substantiate a diagnosis of perceptive deafness and determine, if possible, its underlying cause. Anyone who has ever had a hearing test probably has noticed that the doctor uses a tuning fork during part of his examination and wondered what was going on. The doctor usually uses two methods. First, he places the stem of the tuning fork on the bone just behind the ear. When the sound gradually disappears, he then holds the vibrating prongs alongside the ear itself. This is known as the Rinne test. In people whose hearing is normal, the sound is heard by means of air conduction about twice as long as it is by bone conduction.

He then performs the Weber test by holding the stem of the vibrating fork on the top of the forehead. The sound is heard more clearly on one side than the other when conduction deafness is present, because the bone-conducted sound seems to be directed toward the deaf side. When true nerve deafness is present, the sound seems to appear loudest on the healthy side.

Treatment of perceptive deafness is based on eradication of the underlying cause and the proper fitting of a hearing aid if a usable level of natural hearing cannot be restored without mechanical means. Victims of this type of deafness often become expert lip readers as well.

Hearing loss is the number one physical impairment in this country, affecting between 15 and 18 million people, or about one out of every ten Americans. Many of these are simply hard of hearing to a degree which even they themselves may not suspect. Often children so affected are considered to be either mentally ill or retarded. Some, but not all, can be helped by hearing aids.

An editorial in the *Journal of the American Medical Association* points out: "Noise pollution is rapidly joining air and water pollution as an environmental problem of major concern. The diverse effects of noise range from deafness caused by years of exposure to very loud industrial noise to the mere annoyance caused by a dripping faucet or a squawking automobile horn.

"It is well established that substantial hearing losses are found among experienced chippers, drop forge and paper machine operators, and boiler makers—all operators of machines that produce very loud noises. It has been conclusively demonstrated by hearing tests and measurement of noise levels and duration of exposure that employees exposed to such noises will sustain hearing impairment, unless protected by wearing well-fitting ear protectors."

However, studies published in the *Archives of Environmental Health* indicate that if continuous high-level noise is interrupted about 40 times daily for brief periods, the noise level can be 20 db more intense than if it were continuous without producing the same degree of damage as defined by standard criteria.

It is a fact of life that noise pollution is an inescapable concomitant of the highly industrialized society in which we live, and, when excessive, it must be curbed or otherwise controlled in order to avoid serious deleterious effects on the individual.

The Eye

The eye is composed of some of the most delicate and amazing structures in the body (Fig. 1-12). Through the integrated functions of its various parts, the eye transforms images formed by light rays into impulses that are transmitted to the brain by the optic nerve to be recognized and interpreted in our consciousness, thus providing us with the priceless function of vision.

It is important to understand the construction of the eye because it so often is injured and improper care could lead to partial or total blindness, either of which may be permanent.

Basically, the eye is like a camera, which, within limits, can

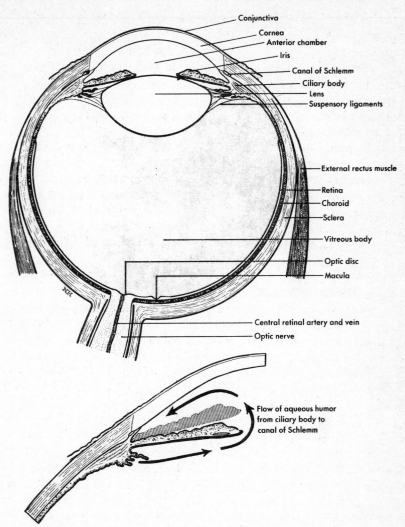

Fig. 1-12. Cross section showing the principal structures of the human eye.

be moved so as to focus on any object within range. The six muscles that control the movement of each eye are so coordinated with the muscles of the opposite eye through the cranial nerves which activate them that normally the eyes always move and focus together. If they fail to move and focus together, two separate images are perceived by the brain—a condition commonly referred to as *cross-eyes*, since the eyes are turned inward or outward and seem to be looking at two different things.

The crystalline lens of the eye corresponds to the lens of the camera. The lens of the eye helps to focus the light rays to form an image on the retina and is constructed in such a way as to permit small changes in focusing power which enable the eye to accommodate itself to near or distant objects as required, almost exactly as one would focus a camera or moving picture projector. The actual focusing is accomplished by changes in the thickness of the lens itself, brought about by the delicate ciliary muscles, which are located in a ring around the lens and tighten or relax the ligament in which the lens is suspended, thus increasing or diminishing its focusing power.

Throughout a person's life, the lens grows by creating new fibers. Simultaneously, there is a shrinkage of its central nucleus, thus keeping the lens from becoming so large as to fill up the entire eyeball.

At the same time the lens capsule thickens, and this thickening, together with hardening and drying of the central nucleus, may progress to the point where the nucleus is too hard and dry to transmit light efficiently and it becomes opaque. Technically speaking, every lens opacity is a cataract, the most commonly feared eye disease. But surgery is not required to remove the opacity in order to improve sight in the affected eye until the opacity becomes so dense as to seriously affect usable vision.

The decision as to whether to remove a cataract is not always an easy one, for many reasons. For instance, the patient may have some other concomitant eye disease. The question then arises as to whether removal of the cataract will give him sufficiently improved vision to warrant the procedure. There is often the question also as to whether an advanced cataract in one eye should be removed when the patient has useful vision in the other. This is because an eye from which the lens has been removed cannot coordinate with the other eye simply by using ordinary spectacles. True, effective binocular vision can be obtained by the use of a contact lens in the operated eye, but older people have difficulty in learning how to use contact lenses and are very apprehensive about trying.

In any event, the only treatment for advanced cataracts is surgery. Fortunately, the technics for cataract removal are so perfected that the results obtained, particularly when contact lenses can be used, usually offer a vast improvement over the blurred and ineffective vision under which the cataract victim had previously been laboring.

In front of the lens is the iris, the structure that gives a characteristic color to the eyes. By means of delicate muscles, the size of its central opening, known as the *pupil,* is varied to control the amount of light entering the eye. This corresponds to, and fulfills the same function as, the diaphragm of a camera, which controls the amount of light entering the camera (the exposure) when the stop opening is changed.

The iris is protected in front by a tough transparent tissue, the cornea, which is separated from the lens by the aqueous humor, a clear fluid. The cornea functions in conjuction with the crystalline lens to focus light and is responsible for about two-thirds of the focusing power of the eye.

Except for the part in front of the iris, the tough outer wall of the eye is not transparent, but is densely opaque; this opaque portion is the sclera, the white portion of the eye.

Just beneath the cornea are two tiny but very important chambers—one between the iris and the cornea, technically known as the anterior (or front) chamber, and the other between the iris and the lens, technically known as the posterior (or back) chamber. Both are filled with the so-called aqueous humor.

The aqueous humor is manufactured at the rate of about two or three drops per minute by a bit of tissue known as the ciliary body, located in the posterior chamber. After filling the posterior chamber, the fluid flows through to the anterior chamber between the iris and cornea, from which it empties into the tiny veins in the sclera. As long as the outflow exactly equals the rate of production of the fluid—a relationship which is extremely delicately balanced, there is no difficulty. Just how this is done still remains a mystery. But when, for some reason, fluid is excreted from the anterior chamber at a slower rate than it is formed, a pressure imbalance develops which eventually leads to the common and serious disease, glaucoma (see page 531).

The cornea, sclera, and under surface of the eyelids are

covered with a very thin delicate membrane known as the *conjunctiva*. This tissue is easily irritated by dust, foreign bodies, and other causes, its tiny blood vessels easily becoming swollen with blood and thus producing a bloodshot appearance of the eyes. In the case of conjunctivitis this membrane becomes inflamed, causing the redness of the eyes which one usually associates with this condition.

The inner surface of the sclera is covered with a dense, black, pigmented membrane, the choroid, which lines the entire inner surface of the eyeball, except for the pupil. The function of the choroid is to keep light out of the eye except where it should come in through the pupil, or lens opening— just as in a camera.

Overlying the choroid membrane at the rear of the eyeball is an almost transparent membrane, covering the inner surface in such a position that images transmitted through the cornea and lens are projected upon its surface. This is the retina, and it corresponds in a general way to the film in a camera. Although the retina is only about 1/100 of an inch in thickness, it is composed of an exceedingly complicated system of cells, the rods and cones; these cells differ from any others in the body in that they are capable of transmitting nerve impulses when stimulated by light.

The eyeball itself is filled with a clear jelly-like liquid, the vitreous humor, and is under sufficient pressure (intraocular tension) to give the eyeball its shape—like that of a distended balloon. The vitreous humor serves also to hold the delicate retina firmly in place against the choroid. However, as the result of injury, shock, or other causes, the retina may become detached from the choroid. This is a serious condition, for it impairs the vision of the affected eye to the point of total blindness. Sometimes, with proper care, natural healing processes may repair the damage; sometimes surgery is required.

In close vision, light rays passing through the vitreous humor from the lens converge upon a central spot, the fovea. This is the most sensitive part of the retina and, when one wishes to observe fine details, as in close vision, the eyes automatially move so as to focus the image on this spot.

The optic nerves, which carry the impulses set up in the retina to the brain, arise in cells in the front layers of the retina, known as *ganglion* cells, and are so arranged that the nerve fibers coming from the right half of each retina go to the right side of the brain, and those from the left half of each retina to the left side of the brain. This is a fact of great importance in determining the location of a growth or an injury which may be affecting the normal extent of the visual fields.

2 Principles of Emergency Care

One of the most important aspects of understanding medical problems of an urgent or emergency nature is a thorough familiarity with the basic principles of first aid. First aid is the art of giving quick and correct emergency care to those who are sick or hurt. Although certain basic knowledge is essential, it is not necessary to be a medical expert, for in any injury or illness there is often much that can be done to ease the pain or discomfort of the victim until medical aid arrives. Also, when medical assistance is not quickly available, measures taken by someone trained in rendering emergency care can save a life.

In its barest essentials, first aid seeks to offer emergency care to the ill or injured, to prevent further injury, to lessen pain, and to prevent shock. However, in its fullest concept, much more is involved than the rendering of assistance at the time of accident or illness. One of the basic principles of first aid is the *prevention* of accidents and their complications. Through safety campaigns, basic instruction in first-aid procedure, and an understanding of the predisposing factors that may cause accidents, we can go far in cutting down the terrible toll in lives and injuries exacted from our population every minute of every day.

Injury is the leading cause of death in this country between the ages of 1 and 44. The economic cost of injury and traumatic death approximates 27 billion dollars a year.

PREVENTION OF ACCIDENTS ABOUT THE HOME

Almost 51 million people are injured each year, and of these, about 21 million are injured in the home. Many of these injuries would have been preventable had a few simple precautions been followed. Good accident prevention technics about the home include:

1 Good housekeeping. Neatness—keeping things where they belong—is one of the most important ways to prevent household accidents. Tripping over articles, such as toys, chairs, or utensils, is a frequent cause of falling, a type of home injury which kills about 10,000 people a year.

2 Keep such things as cutlery and sharp tools in their regular places. This will lessen the chances of an accidental cut.

3 Keep medicines in properly labeled containers, *out of the reach of children.*

4 Don't put a poisonous substance in any container of a type usually used for foods or beverages.

5 Don't store poisons where food is kept.

6 Don't be impatient. Shortcuts may result in permanent injury. Play it safe—do it the *right* way.

7 When working in the kitchen, be careful that an interruption does not divert your attention so that liquids are inadvertently left on the stove to boil over and put out the gas flame or grease is allowed to get so hot as to splatter or explode and cause a fire.

8 If you are not skilled at do-it-yourself jobs, get someone who is. You may thus prevent a smashed finger or more serious injury.

9 Don't let your household appliances and equipment get into a run-down condition. It's cheaper and safer to keep such things as oil burners and lamps in good repair. There are about 149,000 fires a year caused by faulty electrical wiring or equipment; about 5,600 people die every year as a result of fires in dwellings alone.

10 Have your vision checked regularly. Poor vision, combined with poor lighting, is a major cause of accidents.

11 Have your hearing checked to make sure you will not miss sounds that may warn of an impending accident. For instance, you should be able to hear the bubbling of boiling water, the cry of a child, or the crackling of a fire. Get a hearing aid if you need one.

12 Keep your medicine cabinet well stocked with fresh first-aid and other essential medical supplies. .

13 Maintain an up-to-date list of emergency telephone numbers so that you can summon help quickly in case of necessity. Use the form in the back of this book.

It is a truism that accidents don't just happen; most often, someone—maybe you yourself—causes them. There is no immunity to accidents except through alertness and a fundamental understanding of factors which cause them.

ACCIDENT PRONENESS

More than 40 years ago it became apparent that the person who had one, two, or three accidents was more likely to have another than the person who had no accidents at all; from this the concept of an accident-prone personality gradually evolved and now is generally accepted as designating an individual who has a predisposition to accidental injury. This idea of an accident-prone personality is a part of the larger concept of "accident liability," which embraces not only personality factors, but the physical factors of environment. The fundamental factors involved in the cause of accidents may be divided roughly into three groups: (1) the external environmental factor, (2) circumstantial factors, and (3) the personality factor of the hapless victim.

Everyone has accidents, but some people have more than their share and have come to be recognized as accident-prone. They present a most difficult problem, since conventional mechanical safeguards do not work effectively in such cases. These individuals, unconsciously, may even create their own hazards; for example, they fall on clean floors; they stumble against well-lighted, familiar objects; and when driving, they pass a car on a hill, even if their view is obstructed. One study showed that nearly one-sixth of those involved in fatal accidents in their homes fell while merely walking around in a room or from one room to another on the same floor.

But perhaps even worse than the danger they cause to themselves and to their families is the danger they cause to the innocent bystander who unwittingly puts himself in the path of the accident-prone. Nearly one-fifth of serious or fatal accidents could probably be prevented if the deep underlying psychologic drives of the perpetrators could have been recognized and corrected before the accident. When a group of 95,000 work accidents was carefully studied, it became evident that 90 percent of them were caused by a combination of external and personal factors. Recognizing this, when a large transportation company took the accident-proneness factor into consideration in an accident-prevention program, its accident rate was reduced by 42 percent and over $300,000 was saved.

Many studies have indicated that the accident-prone person is emotionally unstable and that he may have physiologic imbalances which disturb his reactions to stress. An understanding of these problems is essential to the prevention of accidents and the treatment of an accident-prone personality, since an individual's patterns of reaction to stress, consciously or unconsciously, are of major significance in vehicular, industrial, farm, or home accidents.

In order to understand the many underlying factors which play such an important part in the makeup of the individual, it must be realized that the most significant part of the personality, and hence the most important cause of action, is that part of the mind which works at the "unconscious" level. In other words, most of an individual's actions are conditioned by the experiences of babyhood and the very early years of life. Conscious awareness of these experiences is lost, but they are forever impressed on the subconscious mind, and to a very large extent, they govern what the individual is and does in later life.

Two subconscious drives are basic: the aggressive drive gives us "push," and the constructive drive gives us creativity and the ability to love and to grow. When these two drives work together, they are complementary and result in achievement. However, when aggressiveness takes the upper hand, feelings of hate, physical violence, and accidents result. The accident becomes the means of either self-punishment or revenge.

A group of people who had more bone fractures than usual was studied and found to possess many psychopathologic factors in common. These included aggressiveness, impulsiveness, impetuousness, a high degree of independence and self-reliance, and feelings of rebellion and of guilt, particularly after injury. At the time of their accidents, most of these people were angry with a parent or their boss. Many resented authority because they had been brought up under very strict discipline. The victim of the accident he himself causes not only expresses his resentment and revenge by way of the accident, but he also atones for his rebellion by his own physical suffering. All this is substantiated by fact. Accidents happen in particularly stressful situations: the adult victim is on his way to a job he doesn't like or to an interview relating to a new job, or the child is doing something which was forbidden by his parents. By having an accident, either the victim avoids a dreaded situation, or he punishes himself for something he thinks or feels he should not do.

Early Factors Contributing to the Accident-prone Personality

According to experts in this field, it is apparent that anti-social behavior in the adult has its roots in childhood rebellion against authority. The child who is insecure, unsettled, or unhappy is suspicious, shows bravado, and is apt to test a dangerous situation, such as an oncoming car (which to him may represent a parent) to see whether or not it will respect him. The child may confuse the motorist with his fussy mother or a policeman and react by annoying, defying, or attacking the motorist, or he may harbor a deep desire to be hurt, for some children invite punishment just as others attract bullying.

When driving a car, adults seem to react in much the same way as they do to other aspects of life. The well-balanced, mature individual is aware of driving hazards and knows how to cope with them just as he is aware of the other hazards of daily living and how to meet them. The reaction of the unstable and the immature individual involves not only driving situations, but his own fantasies of fear, violence, power, and aggression as symbolized by the traffic and, as a result, he may meet the potentially hazardous situation psychopathically and cause an accident. A secure, happy home life in childhood seems to be a basic factor in the prevention of traffic accidents in later years.

Psychiatric Aspects of Accident Proneness

Psychoses and mental deficiencies are true mental diseases and should disqualify anyone from driving a car or from operating other complex machinery.

Depression and the desire to punish someone, expressed by "After I'm dead and gone they'll miss me and then they'll be sorry," or the desire to punish oneself may lead to the suicide crash and the involvement of whoever may inadvertently be in the way.

There is also the person who feels misused and who unconsciously shows the effects of murderous fantasies. He is driven to atone for his own sake. He may become an alcoholic or a drug addict, or he may ask for unnecessary surgery. Thus he seeks atonement in self-administered punishment.

Some individuals who tend to have both an exaggerated self-esteem and a decreased sense of responsibility may, at times, become excited and end up rebelling against restraint. This type of experience may become manifest in some degree during festive occasions—particularly during the Christmas season—when previously restrained rebellion against the mores may be released because of social condonement. This is the time that the death phrase *one for the road* is construed to mean: *Have a few extra—everyone is celebrating, all bets are off—it's every man for himself and have fun!*

Neurotic conflict is responsible for most criminal and antisocial behavior, and it is the individuals in this group who are responsible for the highest accident statistics. They misunderstand the present and see it as the past repeating itself. Apparently, they transfer childhood feelings and attitudes to the present without understanding or even being aware of what they are doing. Their behavior seems to be an unconscious attempt to act out old impulses for present gratification and to relieve inner tension. Thus, the environment becomes a stage on which old conflicts are enacted and reenacted, sometimes against the individual's best interests.

The maladjusted (sociopathic) individual simulates emotion, but feels deprived and has a faulty sense of conscience and timing. He must gratify an impulse immediately. His outstanding characteristic is that, while no neurologic or psychologic defect may be detected by testing, he fails to meet adequately the exigencies of everyday life. In the hands of such a person, the automobile or any other piece of machinery is potentially a lethal weapon.

Drinking and Accidents

The more alcohol consumed, the greater the danger of traffic accidents, but drinking on isolated social or festive occasions is not necessarily linked to accident proneness. Drinking is well known to be a false refuge for the depressed and unhappy and a source of "whiskey courage." Many people need only a drink or two to become aggressive and unduly brave, and this, added to the serious impairment of perception, vision, motor-reflex activity, neuromuscular coordination, and recognition, makes the operation of any kind of machinery, be it stationary or mobile, extremely hazardous. Alcohol is involved in from 25 to 50 percent of all automobile fatalities (Fig. 2-1). As little as two drinks (or two beers) may seriously impair driving ability or judgment, usually without the realization of the driver.

Other Factors Contributing to Accidents

There are many other factors which may be taken into consideration, but which are not necessarily linked directly with accident proneness in the strict sense of the term. These in-

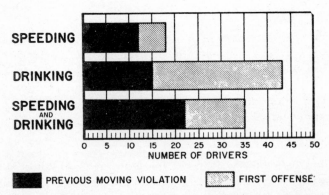

Fig. 2-1. A breakdown of statistics based on 96 drivers involved in fatal accidents over one fourth of July holiday emphasizes the significant relationship of drinking to accidents and the high percentage of repeaters.

clude side effects of drugs, temperature extremes, seasonal trends, and medical factors (such as visual acuity or sudden illness).

As a matter of fact, Waller has shown that impairment to drivers or pedestrians from chronic medical problems, frequently acting at a subclinical level, is believed to be a contributing factor in 15 to 25 percent of crashes.

Of particular importance in older drivers, as emphasized by Foley, McGinn, and Lindenauer, is cerebral vascular deficiency. This condition, which is so common in older age groups, can cause transient neurologic dysfunction without warning, often with bizarre effects. As a result, the ability of a person to drive an automobile can be suddenly and seriously impaired. This is an important cause of transient driver disability.

Many drugs which may be obtained without a doctor's prescription and are widely used for motion sickness, allergy, colds, and the prevention of sleepiness may have potent side effects including drowsiness and marked hallucinations—all of which are obvious predisposing causes of accident.

All these dangers may be included and become additive in any one situation. For instance, the effect of exposure to carbon monoxide from running motors, inhalation of exhaust fumes in bumper-to-bumper driving, and excessive smoking are cumulative and may be quite dangerous.

In addition, as M. L. Schulzinger (*Industrial Medicine and Surgery*, Vol. 25, 1957) points out:

> The additive impairing effect of fatigue, low blood sugar, carbon monoxide, sedative drugs, alcohol, high altitude, poor illumination, and emotional stress must be considered catastrophic. Many of these additive impairing factors, and sometimes all of them, are concurrently present in holiday traffic and during rush-hour homebound traffic. The combination of a tired driver, a few aspirins or a sedative drug, several cigarettes, and a shot of whiskey are common enough. Add a bit of twilight and/or an exciting experience and the driver is now virtually a keg of dynamite with the fuse lit.

Interestingly enough, there is a marked seasonal trend, the incidence generally being lower in winter and higher in summer. Children under 15 years of age have three times more accidents in summer than in winter, but in the age groups above 60 there is little if any seasonal difference. The cycle for all groups is lowest in February and reaches a high peak in June, July, and August, gradually decreasing thereafter.

The time of day also has significance. The accident rate increases from a low at 5 A.M. to a high at 5 P.M. and then begins to fall off slowly. However, in the older age groups the range is from 3 A.M. to about 6 P.M., which may possibly be due to the increased fatigue factors in older persons.

Many other factors also must be taken into consideration. The matter of visual acuity—a factor which is related to both age (falling off rather rapidly after age 50) and illumination—shows a definite relationship to all types of accident occurrence.

Such factors as excessive fatigue, worry, preoccupation (as with one's job or a difficult problem), and acute or chronic illness are so obvious as to require little more than mention.

The case of the driver who falls asleep at the wheel and crashes can be found in almost any daily newspaper. Perhaps less well known is the accident caused by the driver who takes "pep" pills to stay awake and suffers from hallucinations caused by the drug—usually amphetamine or a related compound, or a form of caffeine. Because of hallucinations, the driver may think he sees another vehicle heading for him or, perhaps, a pedestrian in the road and swerves sharply to avoid an accident, but causes one instead.

Many accidents, including airplane crashes, have been caused by sudden illness, such as coronary thrombosis, striking the person in control of the vehicle at a critical moment. Various forms of stroke, particularly in older people, have a similar effect; vertigo, from various causes, may also be implicated. In particular, individuals known to be suffering from disturbances of the vestibular apparatus, such as Ménière's disease, or convulsive disorders, such as epilepsy, should not be permitted to drive or to be near hazardous machinery. The incidence of accidents due to such causes can, of course, be reduced by frequent medical examination and more stringent medical controls.

Finally, there are a host of physical, environmental, or situational hazards which contribute to the extent that a certain number of accidents will occur, without relation to human motivation, as the result of relatively rare equipment failure (aside from careless operation) or some wholly unforeseeable and uncontrollable circumstance. Some industries and occupations are naturally more hazardous than others, and it seems inescapable that a certain small accident rate, resulting from inherent situational or environmental hazards, is inevitable.

Recognizing the Accident-prone Personality

The sorting out of individuals who are more likely to have accidents than the rest of the population is a hard job, but personnel studies in industry have come up with a number of psychophysical tests to be used along with medical examinations in order to identify these individals. In the study mentioned previously, it was found that the operators who successfully passed both the "motorability" and the psychologic tests had the lowest number of accidents, while those who were employed without taking both of these tests had a far higher number of accidents; furthermore, those who were given only the "motorability" test had a lower accident rate than those not tested. It was concluded, on a statistically significant basis, that psychologic testing is a finer discriminant than "motorability" testing and that both together are better than either one alone.

In a study of 50 accident-prone motormen, the six factors which showed up with the greatest regularity were faulty attitude, failure to recognize a potential hazard, faulty judgment of speed and distance, impulsiveness, irresponsibility, and failure to pay constant attention.

Gass, in an extensive and detailed study of the relationship between hardcore personality and industrial illness and accidents, found that in most cases these represent an attempted solution to a difficult life or emotional problem. Without deep personal insight into an individual's emotional makeup and conflicts, these problems are exceedingly hard to handle and prevent.

Hirschfeld and Behan also found in a study of more than 300 cases that physical injury was the result of a psychological process in almost every instance; many of these patients anticipated that "something was going to happen"—a clear cry for help!

Treating the Accident-prone Person

Through proper psychometric and psychologic testing methods, combined with psychiatric and medical counselling when necessary, accident proneness can be detected. Such detection programs should be established by responsible social, civic, and medical agencies, as well as by the family physician, on as wide a scale as possible, for economic, not to mention humanitarian, reasons.

Organizations dealing with young people and various church and welfare groups have opportunities to contribute their counselling and instruction at levels at which such efforts can be most effective. Once found, the accident-prone person should be removed from environments containing potential dangers and helped to make the necessary psychologic adjustments.

It should be recognized further that accident prevention really begins during childhood, by providing the love, care, understanding, and security which the child must have if he is to become a responsible well-adjusted adult. It is never too early to inculcate a child with an understanding of the hazards and the safeguards of life, even as he takes his first faltering steps.

A secure and happy childhood, with its later rewards of a stable, serene and constructive adulthood, can be thought of in terms of a simple mnemonic, based on the word SAFE, which all parents would do well to remember and practice.

S = Safeguard—protect your child from harm until he is old enough to protect himself.

A = Affection—a child who is loved and given a sense of security and protection is a happy child without fears and frustrations.

F = Facts—explain the difference between right and wrong, between safety and danger. A child's mind is an inquiring one and partial explanations lead to fruitless questioning and anxiety in adult life.

E = Emulation—a child learns by example, by doing what you do and wanting to be like you. If he sees you run through a red light often enough, he will do the same thing when he is older.

Finally, every adult should be aware of the signs that indicate an accident-prone personality so that he may be able to recognize them in himself. If he does find such signs, with proper help he may gain insight into his personal problems and be able to make a better adjustment to life, thus becoming a more stable individual.

HOW TO HANDLE AN EMERGENCY

When you are faced with the necessity of caring for an accident victim or an acutely ill person, take a few seconds to ascertain whether he may be a laryngectomee (neck breather). Individuals who have had their vocal cords removed require special resuscitation methods and therefore usually have a warning sticker affixed to the windshield of their car, or a similar card in a wallet or elsewhere on their person (Fig. 2-2). (*Vide infra.*)

Also determine whether the victim is wearing the emergency medical identification symbol designed by the American Medical Association to be a universal sign that information important to the life and health of the wearer is being carried on his person (Fig. 2-3). This alerting device may be found as a "dog tag" around a wrist, ankle or neck. The essential information will be found on a medical identification card which applies specifically to the victim's particular health problem (Fig. 2-4).

For example, diabetics must be identified so that a person in a diabetic coma will receive proper treatment and needed doses of insulin will not be overlooked during treatment for injury. Identification as a diabetic also protects a person in coma from being mistaken for a drunk.

In other instances, the need for certain medicines must be known. Heart patients taking drugs to prevent clots may bleed profusely, if injured, unless they receive special care. For some patients, failure to provide anti-inflammation drugs, such as a corticosteroid like hydrocortisone, may endanger life. Other people are sensitive to certain drugs and must never take them. All such information is noted on the record card.

In addition, certain allergies can pose a serious problem. For example, people allergic to horse serum should not have tetanus *antitoxin* (q.v.) prepared from horse serum. The emergency identification card should mention the allergy to horse serum and indicate when the last immunization against tetanus was given in the form of tetanus *toxoid* (q.v.).

Penicillin sensitization is common; a warning against the use of penicillin or other drugs to which a person is sensitized should be noted on the card.

Epileptics could be saved much trouble and unnecessary hospitalization if they carried a card indicating that they may have seizures, which as a rule do not require hospitalization once the individual is over the attack.

These and a host of other problems may be so serious that it is essential for those attempting to render first aid or medical assistance to know about them in an emergency. It is the purpose of the emergency medical identification symbol to alert those attempting to render assistance that emergency medical

EMERGENCY!

I am a laryngectomee (no vocal cords).

I breathe through an opening in the neck, not through the nose or mouth.

If artificial respiration is necessary:

1. Keep neck opening clear of all matter.

2. Don't twist head sidewise.

3. Apply oxygen only to neck opening.

4. Don't throw water on head.

5. Mouth-to-opening breathing is effective.

Fig. 2-2. Facsimile of warning card carried by those who have had their vocal cords removed.

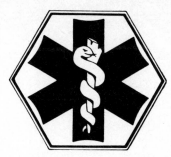

Fig. 2-3. The universal emergency medical identification symbol devised by the American Medical Association. The person who displays it carries upon his person information which should be known to anyone helping him during an accident or sudden illness. The symbol means: "Look for medical information that can protect life."

information is being carried on a record card by the person being assisted.

Emergency medical identification cards, as well as information concerning alerting devices, can be obtained by writing directly to Emergency Medical Identification, American Medical Association, 535 North Dearborn Street, Chicago, Illinois 60610.

In handling any emergency, it is important to do the *right* things in the *right order*. Remember the axiom: First things first. Above all, don't panic (many people tend to), and reassure the patient that he will be given every possible care.

Clues to Look For

One of the most important "firsts" is to consider the immediate surroundings and circumstances for a clue to the kind of emergency with which you are dealing. Then direct a specific person to call a doctor or an ambulance. Be sure that he can tell the doctor the general nature of the emergency, where it took place, and how many people are involved.

If you are alone, decide whether immediate aid is necessary to save life, or whether the victim is not in immediate danger and you can simply make him comfortable and go for help yourself.

If immediate aid is indicated, several things should be done as quickly as possible in the following order:

1   If the victim is not breathing, start artificial respiration at once. (See page 123 for methods.)

EMERGENCY MEDICAL IDENTIFICATION

prepared by the
AMERICAN
MEDICAL ASSOCIATION
535 N. Dearborn St.
Chicago, Illinois 60610

ATTENTION

In an emergency where I am unconscious or unable to communicate, please read the other side to know the special care I must have.

PERSONAL IDENTIFICATION

Name_____

Address_____

_____

_____

Religion_____

NOTIFY IN EMERGENCY

Name_____

Address_____

_____

Phone_____

Name_____

Address_____

_____

Phone_____

My Doctor is_____

_____

Address_____

_____ _____

Phone_____

MEDICAL INFORMATION
(with date of notation)

Present Medical Problems_____

_____

_____

Medicines Taken Regularly_____

_____

_____

_____

_____

Dangerous Allergies_____

_____

_____

Other Important Information_____

_____

_____

Last Immunization Date

Tetanus Toxoid_____	Polio: Salk_____
Diptheria_____	Sabin_____
Smallpox_____	Typhoid_____
Measles_____	Others_____

REMEMBER: This is the minimum medical and personal information needed by those who help you in an emergency. It is not designed to be a complete medical record. Check its accuracy with your doctor.

Fig. 2-4. Facsimile of emergency medical information card (front and back) which should be carried by all persons having serious medical problems.

2 When respiration is reestablished, if there is profuse bleeding take control measures *before doing anything else.*

3 When bleeding is controlled and breathing is satisfactory, cover the victim with blankets or anything else available (coats, tarpaulin, car rug) to conserve his body warmth. Be sure that something warm is placed *under* the person as well as over him. Do not use so many blankets that he becomes overheated. It is necessary simply to create an environment which will be conducive to maintaining normal body temperature. Keeping an ill or injured person warm is one of the most important steps in preventing shock, but overheating may precipitate shock.

4 Prevent vomited matter from being aspirated (sucked) into the lungs by turning the victim's head gently to one side so that he will not choke. If he chokes on his own vomitus, aspiration pneumonia probably will result.

5 While doing these things, notice the victim's skin. Does it feel hot? cold? dry? clammy? Does it look red? blue? mottled? white? These observations are important in evaluating the victim's condition and the nature and extent of his injury or illness. In a nonwhite individual, the changes may not be as obvious as in those of light complexion. However, the telltale changes can usually be observed in the nail beds and the lips, which will tend to become blanched or turgid as the case may be.

6 If circumstances indicate, make a careful search for fractures, bruises, and abrasions. The presence of such injuries, if severe, should alert you to the possibility of the victim's going into shock. In addition, the type of injuries will influence the method and position of transportation.

7 Do not move an injured person until adequate transportation facilities become available unless he is in danger of further injury, or unless he must be moved in order to receive emergency care. Never urge a sick or injured person to sit up, stand up, or walk until you are sure that his condition warrants it. Attempts to transport an accident victim in a sedan or squad car can cause permanent damage in cases involving spinal injury (see page 210). A station wagon can be used in place of an ambulance, if the latter is not available, by carefully laying the person out on the rear deck and padding him so that he will not be thrown around during the ride to the hospital.

Clues in the Absence of Visible Injuries

If there are no visible injuries and no signs of an accident, the person probably has been seized with a sudden illness. There are many clues to the person's condition and the immediate measures to be taken in order to alleviate his suffering or improve his medical situation.

If the person is unconscious, he may be suffering from any one of many conditions.

Classification of Unconsciousness.

An easily remembered classification of unconsciousness is based upon the appearance of the person. For example, ask yourself: Is his face red (flushed)? white (pale)? blue (cyanotic)? Any one of these signs is a clue to one or more possible conditions.

Red unconsciousness usually indicates a condition (such as a stroke) due to high blood pressure or to sunstroke. But there are other conditions that also may produce such an appearance, as, for instance, chronic alcoholism or diabetes.

White unconsciousness usually indicates a state of shock as a result of hemorrhage, injury, a severe heart attack, or even a massive stroke (see pages 511 and 505).

Blue unconsciousness usually indicates respiratory obstruction (such as a foreign body in the windpipe), drowning, or acute heart attack. Certain poisons (cyanide) or gases (carbon monoxide) also can produce this appearance.

Alcoholic intoxication, which commonly complicates an accident situation, may be a cause of red, white, or blue unconsciousness. It must be remembered, however, that the odor of alcohol on the breath, a staggering gait, or incoherent speech is not necessarily evidence of alcoholism. If a person appears drunk but no odor of alcohol is detected, he may be the victim of barbiturate intoxication (q.v.).

Not uncommonly, a person mistakenly suspected of drunkenness has later been found to be suffering from diabetic coma, a head injury, or some other medical condition. In such cases, the outcome can be fatal as the result of improper treatment; with better evaluation and adequate aid, death might have been averted.

The respiration and pulse also give valuable clues to a person's condition. For example, the *rate of breathing* may be rapid and shallow in shock; gasping and labored in respiratory obstruction or heart disease; irregular in brain injury, apoplexy, uremia, or diabetic coma.   In any of these conditions, particularly severe head injury, a type of breathing known as Cheyne-Stokes respiration occurs.   This is a serious sign and consists of regular periods of variation in the *depth* of respiration interspersed with regular periods of apnea (no respiratory movement) (Fig. 2-5).

The *pulse* often is full, bounding, and racing in states of fright or in early stages of hemorrhage.   However, in the later stages of hemorrhage and in states of shock, it is thin, thready, rapid, and weak; and in severe injury or illness, it may be very irregular or imperceptible.

The fact that you cannot feel a pulse beat does not necessarily mean that the patient is *in extremis,* since the pulse is often difficult to find quickly under emergency conditions, even for a physician.   Often it is easier to feel the temporal pulse, or the femoral pulse just below the groin, than it is to feel the radial pulse (Fig. 2-6).

Paralysis of any portion of the body, though alarming, is a useful clue to the nature, extent, and location of an injury or to the occurrence of a stroke (Chap. 15).

Bleeding or the discharge of a *thin watery fluid* from the ears is an almost certain sign of a tearing fracture of the skull. In the presence of this sign, the injured person must be treated as if he had, in fact, sustained a skull fracture (see page 198) until the condition is known to be of less serious nature.

Vomiting may accompany many conditions, from shock to simply an overloaded stomach.   The nature of the vomitus is significant; bright-red blood suggests a fresh, acute hemorrhage from the stomach or esophagus, or it may be seen when much blood has been swallowed from a nosebleed or following a

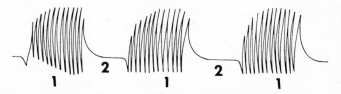

Fig. 2-5. Cheyne-Stokes respiration, a serious sign, is characterized by periods of rhythmic breathing alternating with periods of apnea. 1—Hyperpneic period. 2—Apneic period.

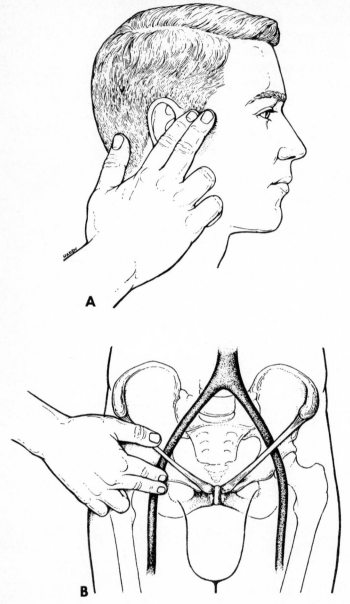

Fig. 2-6. Method of feeling for temporal pulse (A) or femoral pulse (B).

tonsil operation; it is also seen in hemorrhage from a bleeding stomach ulcer or ruptured esophageal varices.   Vomitus having the appearance of coffee grounds suggests a slow, long-lasting gastrointestinal hemorrhage, usually due to disease rather than to injury. It is often associated with gastric neoplasm.

Coughing up blood (hemoptysis) indicates a direct injury to the lungs, to some other part of the respiratory tract, or to some medical condition causing pulmonary hemorrhage.   In handling this problem under emergency conditions, unless there is an obvious chest injury which can be given emergency care, the patient should simply be made as comfortable as possible in a sitting or semireclining position, reassured, and kept as quiet as possible.   Medical treatment should be procured as soon as proper transportation becomes available.

Convulsions, though fairly common, are a frightening experience for most people, but convulsions are not necessarily serious.   They can be, but usually are not, due to injury.   Many medical conditions may produce convulsions; perhaps the most common are a high fever in children and epilepsy in children and adults (Chap. 15).   The determination of a convulsive disorder under emergency conditions is not uncommonly complicated by the fact that several of the phenothiazine class of tranquilizer drugs may produce symptoms in some individuals, within a day or two after starting the drug, which may closely simulate convulsions, especially if the dose has been excessive.

Usually, all that need be done is to protect the victim from injuring himself by clearing the surrounding area of articles which might cause burns, bruises or other injuries.   Don't put him on a bed; he may fall to the floor as the result of thrashing about and injure himself.   Do not try to restrain the patient or interfere with him in any way.   *Don't* force anything between his teeth. If his mouth is already open, a soft object such as a handkerchief can be placed between the teeth.   An epileptic attack ordinarily does not require calling a physician unless the seizure is prolonged (more than 10 minutes) or is immediately repeated.

Multiple Emergencies

What has been said so far has necessarily been directed toward the handling of an individual casualty or emergency. Often one is faced with an emergency involving several people;

it then becomes the responsibility of those seeking to give assistance to decide which ones are the most critical and should receive aid first, which ones are not severly enough injured to require immediate care, which ones are so severely injured as to be beyond help, and which ones are probably dead.

The object in such a situation is to provide the greatest amount of help for the most people in the shortest period of time. The decisions involved require great judgment and, on a purely technical basis, would often be beyond the capabilities of a lay person. Nevertheless, some effort must be made in this direction, and those who are alive, but either not breathing or are hemorrhaging badly, obviously demand immediate attention as a life-preserving measure.

A more detailed discussion of multiple-injury victims will be found in Chapter 10.

Determination of Death

The decision as to whether a person is alive or not cannot, of course, be made with finality by anyone except a physician. On the other hand, in an emergency situation when a physician is not yet present, it becomes of somewhat more than academic interest to determine whether an individual in a group of injured people is alive or dead, so that time will not be wasted in bringing aid to those for whom it can do no good.

Even for a physician, the determination of death is not always an easy matter. As a general consideration, the earliest sign of death is the absolute loss of movement of any part of the body, but this is by no means a sure criterion since there are several conditions which can simulate death and have on occasion led to an erroneous conclusion. As an example, one of the most likely conditions to simulate death under an unfavorable emergency situation is profound shock, or reversible cardiac arrest.

Because of these considerations, one should not jump to the conclusion that a person is dead simply because no visible movement is apparent. For practical purposes, complete stoppage of the heart and all respiratory movement, in the vast majority of cases, indicates that death has occurred. However, there are occasions when people who have, to all intents and purposes, been "dead," perhaps as the result of an acute heart attack, have been revived by an alert ambulance squad and, upon reaching a hospital, have been fully resuscitated through electrical stimulation of the heart and other sophisticated means based on our modern understanding of cardio-respiratory physiology.

In truth, the exact moment of death, from a legal as well as a medical standpoint, is sometimes extremely difficult to determine and, in the final analysis, can only be done by a physician after all means of resuscitation have failed.

For practical purposes, where there are many casualties, if a victim appears to have been dead for several minutes, on the basis of the criteria mentioned, the time that would be spent on efforts at revival can probably best be allocated to those for whom there is a better chance.

Psychologic Reactions to Disaster

There is another type of injury which may occur as the result of any major catastrophe and is not necessarily related to a nuclear disaster, although the overwhelming catastrophic nature of such an episode might be expected to produce correspondingly greater effects.   That type of injury is psychologic injury.

The American Psychiatric Association, which has studied this question in great depth, points out that knowledge of a few basic surgical principles enables many nonmedical people to give first aid for physical injuries, and that, similarly, awareness of certain psychologic facts would greatly simplify the handling of terrified, depressed disaster victims, regardless of what the disaster might be.

To understand what might happen, it is important to realize that there are more or less typical reactions to disaster in general.

Normal Reaction.   Some people remain calm, even under extraordinary circumstances, although the majority of us react in one way or another without necessarily losing our heads. We may perspire profusely, even tremble or feel weak and nauseated, and some people react so strongly that they may actually be nauseated to the point of vomiting.   These reactions are not uncommon, and it is important to understand this, since nausea and vomiting are not only signs of radiation sickness, but of several other conditions discussed in this book. One must realize, therefore, that, under the overwhelming impact of a disaster, a person who is nauseated or who is actually vomiting may simply be reacting psychologically in a more or less normal manner. However, they recover quite promptly, become entirely stable emotionally, and serve very usefully in doing their part in the emergency.

Blind Panic. A less desirable type of reaction is individual blind panic. Although this occurs less frequently than might be expected, it is potentially dangerous, because all the individual's judgment seems to disappear completely, and he may very easily, as a result of his hysterical reaction, precipitate an exceedingly difficult-to-handle mass panic.

Depression. A third type of reaction is depression, in which the individual may simply stand or sit about in a numbed condition. Such an individual may be completely useless until he can be more or less brought back to reality, which usually can be done rather quickly, and put to some useful task.

Overreaction. Then there is the individual who becomes overly active, talks too much, jokes inappropriately, flits about from one task to another without accomplishing anything useful, simply getting in other people's way and making the carrying out of organized assignments difficult.

Conversion Hysteria. Finally, there is the common reaction, known technicaly as *conversion hysteria,* in which the individual subconsciously converts his tremendous anxiety into a belief that some part of his body has ceased to function. He may be unable to see, to hear, or to speak, or he may appear to have lost all power to move one or more of his limbs. It is important to realize that such an individual is not deliberately malingering, but that he is completely unaware that there is no physical basis for his apparent disability, and that he is, in fact, just as disabled as if he had sustained a physical injury.

Any and all of the reactions described may appear in a given individual in some degree and in some individuals may be considerably more transient or far less intense than in others. It is therefore important to recognize the situation and attempt to salvage whatever you can in order to avail yourself of such abilities as the afflicted person may be able to offer; this in itself is a definite step in the right direction in the treatment of his condition.

○ TREATMENT

From the standpoint of the layman, the American Psychiatric Association enumerates four main principles of treatment:

1 As a basic tenet, you must accept every person's right to have his own feelings, since everybody's background and emotional experience is different and, therefore, everyone must react differently, each in his own way, to any given specific situation. Don't try to tell him how he should feel; try to understand how he feels and let him recognize that you are trying to understand his reaction, in order to be able to help him. Don't, however, try to overwhelm him with pity; just do enough to establish as much contact as you can with him.

2 Accept a casualty's limitations as real. If a man had a shattered leg, you would not expect him to get up and run about; an individual's shattered feelings are just as real, and nothing will be gained by attempting to browbeat or goad him into the way you think he ought to be acting. Actually, the casualties, for the most part, do not want to feel as they do and want to be as effective as possible, but under the particular circumstances they are unable to control their feelings in this direction.

3 To help them regain as much effectiveness as you can as quickly as possible, it is necessary simply to accept the handicaps which these individuals present and try to help them rediscover a few abilities which they can put to good use at once.

The biggest mistake is to resent the casualty's reaction and compare it in a derogatory manner with the fine job which you think you yourself are doing on the grounds of "Why can't he do the same thing?"

It is obviously, then, very important to size up the casualty's potentialities as accurately and as quickly as possible and, while making allowance for his limitations, to be on the lookout for such skills as he has that you can revive and put to good use.

4 Accept your own limitations in a relief role. You cannot be all things to all people, and there will be much to be done which will be beyond your physical strength, your knowledge, and your skill. Rate yourself objectively and undertake to do those things which you know that you can do and which lie well within your personal capabilities. Do not push yourself beyond these limits, lest you yourself become ill and require help, thus putting an additional burden on the already strained facilities.

From a general point of view, in dealing with emotionally disturbed individuals, be calm and sympathetic, and make it obvious that you recognize and understand their difficulties and are trying to help them. With most, it will not be difficult to establish contact and return them to active usefulness fairly promptly.

On the other hand, there will be a few who will remain unresponsive to your best effort, and the more panicky casualties may need to be brought under trained medical care as promptly as is feasible. Immediate care for the depressed and those with severe conversion hysteria is less urgent than for victims of severe physical injuries, but they should be gotten to mass care centers as soon as it is possible. In the meantime, basic physical needs can be taken care of as the situation permits.

One important point to emphasize is that sedatives should be used as a last resort in handling psychologic casualties. In these cases, even though a sedative may be initially calming, it inevitably adds to the individual's confusion in the long run and makes him more difficult to treat. Also, an individual who is seriously disorganized requires an inordinately large dose to be put to sleep, and he may show a dangerous type of reaction in which he becomes much more excited, rather than calmed, as would be expected.

If you feel that a sedative must be given, properly tag the casualty, showing the time and the amount of the medication that was given, in order to prevent someone else from giving him a second dose later on, which, in combination with the first, could well prove fatal.

Finally, the importance of handling this type of casualty deftly, quickly, and quietly cannot be overemphasized because of the ever-present danger of mass panic, which can easily be precipitated by the reactions of a single disturbed individual. The application of the principles of sound psychologic emergency care will contribute tremendously to the prevention of mass panic, which, once it has gotten under way, is extremely difficult and, unfortunately, often impossible to control.

No matter how overwhelming the calamity, never be deterred from effectively applying the principles of psychologic emergency care as determinedly as you would the principles of physical emergency care.

SUMMARY AND CHECK LIST OF IMMEDIATE MEASURES

Always treat the most dangerous and urgent condition first. Remember the four B's: *breathing, bleeding, broken bones,* and *burns.*

A summary and check list of the fundamental general procedures follow:

Whether or not the injured person is conscious:

1 Make sure that he is breathing. If he is not, begin artificial respiration immediately.

2 If breathing is satisfactory, see whether he is bleeding. If the bleeding is profuse, take measures to control it immediately.

3 When breathing is satisfactory and there is no evidence of bleeding, look for signs of shock and fractured bones.

4 Obtain medical aid quickly—phone a doctor, get someone else to phone him, or get the injured person to a doctor or hospital.

5 Work quickly, but carefully.

6 Loosen tight clothing—collar, waistband, or belt.

7 If the victim vomits, lower his head and turn it gently to one side so that the vomitus will not be aspirated.

8 Remove any loose objects, such as artificial dentures, from the mouth of an unconscious person.

9 Keep the victim quiet and warm. Do not overheat.

10 Don't give an unconscious person anything to drink.

11 Don't aggravate an injury by unnecessary movements.

12 Don't allow a person with a fracture or suspected fracture to be moved until splints have been applied or he has been fixed to an adequate backboard in the case of possible spinal injury.

13 Never urge an injured person to sit up, stand up, or walk until you are *sure* he can safely do so.

FIRST-AID SUPPLIES

The majority of those who are called upon to render emergency care rarely have all the necessary materials at hand until a well-equipped ambulance arrives. Hence, it is necessary to use common sense and ingenuity in making the most effective use of whatever may be available. For the most part, the requirements are simple, since specific treatment almost always must await the arrival of expert medical aid, or transportation to a hospital or a physician's office.

However, when an emergency arises at home or in a place of business, hopefully there is a well-stocked first-aid kit on hand. Many required articles come packaged in the proper sizes and amounts, in already made-up first-aid kits. These can be obtained in various sizes to meet the needs of the traveler, the home, or the industrial plant, the size depending on the amount of each item supplied, but all good kits contain the various items in handy and accessible form.

A list of essential items for general household purposes follows:

6 roller bandages (1 in.)	36 adhesive bandages
6 roller bandages (2 in.)	6 sterile eye pads
6 roller bandages (3 in.)	3 triangular bandages
2 muslin bandages (6 in.)	1 tourniquet
6 large gauze dressings	1 bottle of antiseptic solution
1 25-yd roll sterile gauze (4½ in., 8 ply)	2 oz aromatic spirits of ammonia
2 oz sterile absorbent cotton	3 ammonia inhalant ampuls
2 waterproof adhesive tape (1 in.)	6 oz syrup of ipecac
12 sterile gauze pads (2 in. x 2 in.)	1 tube of water-soluble burn ointment
12 sterile gauze pads (3 in. x 3 in.)	1 box sterile cotton-tipped applicators
1 measuring cup	2 wood splints
1 package of paper drinking cups	1 pair tweezers
1 pair scissors	12 tongue depressors
	12 large safety pins
	1 S-type airway

In addition to these items, the following will be found useful to have on hand and will help to meet many of the basic needs of first-aid and nursing care at home:

sterile gauze (5-yd roll)	rubbing (isopropyl) alcohol
disposable masks	antiseptic soap

hydrogen peroxide solution

baby oil

Epsom salts (1 lb.)

1 box table salt

aspirin tablets (or equivalent)

milk of magnesia

antihistamine tablets
(prescribed by your doctor)

boric acid solution (for an
eye wash)

eye cup

hand basin

sanitary napkins

seasickness tablets (of the

type prescribed by your
doctor)

phenylephrine hydrochloride
(0.5%) or ephedrine nose
drops

sharp needle for removing
splinters

oral thermometer

rectal thermometer

enema bag

hot-water bottle

icebag or ice collar

chemical heat pack

chemical cold pack

bedpan

Keep these items in a convenient cabinet large enough to permit a readily accessible arrangement. The cabinet should not be within reach of children, nor should it be used as a repository for nonmedical items, such as toiletries and other household articles. Check supplies regularly and replace them as they are used up.

MEDICAL SELF-AID DURING DISASTER

It is obvious that in times of general disaster our civil defense forces must be prepared to care for victims of every kind of human injury and illness, often in unprecedented numbers.

In such situations it is a certainty that self-aid is important to a great extent in individual and group survival; therefore, for each individual a sound knowledge of the principles of emergency care may spell the difference between life and death for himself or his family. The delivery of such knowledge is a prime objective of this volume.

But while knowledge is of prime importance, facilities are essential to implement this knowledge; in other words, while one may know how to treat a wound or an illness, one's capabilities are seriously limited if the necessary tools are not available.

Although quantities of essential goods have been stock-piled at various strategic points about the country, no one can guarantee that these materials would be accessible to family units or small groups at a time when they would be most needed.

It seems clear, then, that each family unit should maintain a reasonable supply of basic medical essentials at least as a stopgap, realizing that hopefully they may never be required. The important point is that if a family were isolated from medical services over any extended period of time as the result of a catastrophe, anyone in the family could succumb to an acute illness, and that the illness might be amenable to the proper medication if it were on hand. Obviously, if one had diabetes or some other condition requiring maintenance medication, treatment would have to go on—often as an essential to life, regardless of wars, earthquakes, or hurricanes.

This situation is a far cry, in our opinion, from the practice of self-medication, properly deplored by medical organizations as potentially dangerous; it is simply a means to survival under conditions of great stress and hardship at a time when previously accepted ground rules are no longer practical.

The following recommendations will probably prove controversial, but, since many of the items suggested can be obtained only on prescription, follow a physician's advice and stock only those items which he thinks you should have to meet special needs, or none at all, as you and he see fit:

1 The basic first-aid, sickroom, and nursing items listed on pages 62, 63, 65, and 580.

2 A complete emergency medical manual, together with the most recent guides and bulletins from the Department of Health, Education, and Welfare, local and state civil defense agencies, and similar responsible organizations.

3 Water for drinking, medicinal use, and minimal washing— at least 1 gallon per day per person; more if practicable.

4 Table salt for soaks and for fluid replacement.

5 Sugar for use in conjunction with fluid replacement.

6 Baking soda for treatment of burns (see page 242) and as an indigestion remedy.

7 Cold remedies:

   a   Analgesic tablets (as recommended by your doctor or obtained on his prescription).
   b   Nose drops: 0.5 percent phenylephrine in saline or 1 percent ephedrine in saline.
   c   Cough mixture—nonnarcotic, available over the counter.

8   Gastrointestinal remedies:
   a   Milk of magnesia for constipation and as an antacid.
   b   Gastrointestinal sedative and antidiarrheal preparation (as recommended by a physician).
   c   Rectal suppositories or disposable enema units.
   d   Specific intestinal antibacterial sulfonamide, antibiotic, or other medication for specific or nonspecific intestinal disease, such as dysentery (as recommended by a physician).

9   Miscellaneous medications:
   a   Ear drops for relieving pain in ear inflammation, in conjunction with other remedies.
   b   Preparation to temporarily replace dental fillings and relieve toothache.
   c   Lubricating jelly.
   d   Antibiotic ointment for treating minor wounds.
   e   Aromatic spirits of ammonia for inhalation and internal use in case of fainting.
   f   Antihistamine preparation for allergy (as recommended by a physician).
   g   Detergent germicide for washing wounds and hands.
   h   Antiseptic soap.
   i   Household bleach solution for general sanitation and, diluted, for preparing wet dressings.
   j   Water purification tablets.
   k   Special baby needs as required.

10   Special medications (obtainable only on prescription; check with your physician):
   a   Tranquilizer tablets.
   b   Sedative and sleeping tablets, such as phenobarbital or equivalent.
   c   Epinephrine for injection.
   d   Atropine sulfate: oral tablets and/or solution for injection.
   e   Disposable syringes for hypodermic injection.
   f   Broad-spectrum oral antibiotic.
   g   Such special maintenance medication as may be specifically required, as for diabetes and epilepsy.

Taken all together, this seems to be a rather imposing list, but actually the items can be stored quite compactly. It is strongly recommended that they be accumulated and packed as units, in easily transportable boxes or suitcases, and stored where they are accessible to a responsible adult, but where they cannot be reached by children. Everything, of course, should be clearly marked with the name of the product, instructions for use, and all necessary warnings, such as "for external use only"; those items which may be considered poisons should be so labeled in large print. Keep all units in a clean, dry place not subject to freezing or overheating.

The reason for emphasizing portability of your medical supplies is an obvious one: In the event of a disaster, it may be necessary for you to move to an undamaged portion of your house, to a shelter, or even out of the vicinity. If this should happen, your supplies are packed and ready to go at a moment's notice.

We have not attempted to suggest quantities of any given item, since this, of course, will be determined by the size of the group which the supplies are intended to service. As a general guide, a minimum time for which one should be prepared to operate on a self-sufficient basis would be 2 weeks.

It should be emphasized also that some of the supplies are of such nature that they should be replaced with fresh materials periodically. Since many of the items listed are used more or less frequently in everyday life, there is no objection to using the emergency supply as a base source, providing the items are replaced conscientiously as rapidly as they are used up.

In any catastrophe, the individual's outcome is largely conditioned by his ability effectively to apply self-aid and mutual aid within a group. While there is no question that the medical and civil defense facilities of this country are highly organized, it is possible they could not be brought to the aid of the individual within a short period of time in many instances. It is of paramount importance, therefore, that individuals and small groups have the knowledge and facilities available to tide them over any particular situation until help can arrive.

3

Basic Technics of Emergency Care

WOUNDS

Regardless of the nature of an accident, only certain types of wounds can occur. It is important to be able to recognize these in order to render proper emergency care.

Bleeding

In caring for most wounds, the first consideration is the control of excessive bleeding. Although a little bleeding helps wash out the germs that contaminate every wound, excessive bleeding (hemorrhage) can be dangerous and must be controlled promptly, by whichever one of the special methods, described in Chapter 5, seems most applicable to the case.

Prevention of Infection

If the wound is relatively superficial and bleeding is not a problem, the next consideration is to minimize the likelihood of the wound becoming infected.

The signs of infection, to use the old Latin terminology, are *rubor, dolor, calor,* and *tumor*—redness, pain, heat, and swelling. Red streaks up an arm or a leg are a sign of spreading infection and make it mandatory to obtain medical aid as soon as possible so that a suitable antibiotic may be administered, and other necessary measures taken.

Often a wound fails to heal and remains infected, or becomes worse, because of an embedded foreign body, which can be extremely irritating, such as a piece of glass, gravel, or a thorn.

If left alone, the foreign body will sometimes extrude itself from the wound after a period of time; but waiting can be a dangerous practice, since the infection may worsen in the meantime. The best procedure is to clean the wound of all foreign material as soon as practicable. In the meantime, warm soaks of either saline or Epsom salts will help ease the pain and bring the infection to a "head."

But the first treatment, if the wound is only superficial, is to clean it and the surrounding area with mild antiseptic soap and water. Be careful to wash dirt *away* from the wound and not into it, and be gentle so as not to irritate or injure the exposed tissues further. Soap or detergents, especially those containing one of the long-acting antiseptic agents, are effective for this purpose, but any soap, so long as it is nonirritating, is better than nothing.

Before treating any wound, assemble dressings, bandages, scissors, and such other articles as you will need. Thoroughly wash your hands and prepare a place to work as clean and uncluttered as possible. Where this cannot be properly done (as under emergency field conditions), be especially careful not to touch the wound with your fingers, and keep dressings and other articles from becoming directly contaminated by the surroundings.

Do not do anything to a wound until you have removed dirty objects (such as clothing) from its immediate vicinity, gotten rid of the loose dirt on the surrounding skin, and cleansed the area near the wound as well as possible.

Dressings for direct application to a wound come in especially sealed envelopes which have been sterilized so as to be free of germs. Open the envelopes in such a way as not to touch the part of the dressing that will go on the wound. The best type of sterile dressing comes in an envelope with a "peelable" seal which can be opened by simply pulling the corner marked with an arrow. The dressing can then be removed without being touched.

Do not use a bandage as a dressing for a wound. Bandages are intended to hold dressings in place and should only be used as a dressing if nothing else is available. In such a case, be careful not to touch the part that will go on the wound.

If you intend to use a "first-aid cream," put it on the dressing and then apply the dressing to the wound instead of applying the cream directly. This prevents direct contamination of the cream in the tube and the tube itself.

By gentle cleansing of the wound and the surrounding area, a great many germs, as well as dirt and debris, are removed, and there will be less interference with the natural defenses of the tissues themselves. If superficial wounds are treated in this manner, infections are much less likely to develop than when treated with strong "antiseptics," which only cause further tissue damage.

Deep wounds should not be washed out except under proper conditions and by competent medical personnel, since these wounds require special technics for their effective treatment. Their emergency care consists in applying a thick, protective, sterile dressing and a firm bandage which will keep the injured part at rest and help control bleeding.

Under no circumstances attempt to close the wound or to put anything into it. Leave everything, except the application of a sterile pressure dressing and the control of hemorrhage, for professional definitive care.

In all but the most minor cuts or scrapes, and especially in street and farm injuries, the possibility of a serious specific infection, such as tetanus, must be considered in the case of *all* wounds. The likelihood of tetanus is minimized by the injection of tetanus antiserum or tetanus toxoid. All wounds caused by animals must be suspect as to tetanus as well as rabies (q.v.).

While the incidence of tetanus had declined in the last 20 years, due largely to the use of tetanus toxoid, there is no really effective treatment. Once the disease has occurred, the mortality rate runs between 50 to 60 percent. Any deep wound must be considered a potential source of this infection and treated accordingly.

Tetanus Antiserum versus Tetanus Toxoid. It is important to understand the difference between tetanus antiserum (antitoxin) and tetanus toxoid. *Tetanus antiserum* formerly was prepared from the serum of horses or cows hyperimmunized against tetanus (lockjaw) and contained a high concentration of protective substances, known as *antibodies,* against this disease. When injected into a person who may have been infected with tetanus organisms, these antibodies react with the tetanus bacteria to prevent the development of the disease—

provided the dose is large enough to fight all the bacteria which may have been present or may have developed in the wound. This process by which immunity to a disease is acquired by injection of antibodies (an antiserum or antitoxin) is known as *passive immunization.* It is effective only for the injury for which it was given, since the antibodies are lost from the body quite readily.

It is important to realize that a person can become sensitized to either horse (equine) or cow (bovine) serum and that the next time an antiserum prepared from either of these sources is given for any reason he may experience a severe reaction unless special precautions are taken.

A much safer type of product, which is widely available and now is used almost exclusively, is human Tetanus Immune Globulin. It is prepared from the blood of adult humans who have been hyperimmunized with tetanus toxoid and contains a very high level of antibodies in the form of 16.5 percent $\pm$ 1.5 percent gamma globulin.

This material has three important advantages over the older types of antisera, the use of which is now largely obsolete. First, Tetanus Immune Globulin (Human) can be injected immediately without previous testing, since there is little, if any, risk of immediate or delayed reaction; second, a smaller dose will produce a concentration of circulating antibodies well above the accepted protective level (0.01 unit of tetanus antitoxin per milliliter of serum); and third, the level of circulating antitoxin is more predictable and longer lasting than when heterologous sera are used.

Tetanus Immune Globulin (Human), in adequate amounts governed by the types of wound and the degree of likelihood of exposure to tetanus infection, should always be given *unless* the person has previously been immunized against tetanus toxoid. The usual prophylactic dose of Tetanus Immune Globulin (Human) for routine wounds in adults is 250 units intramuscularly. For simple wounds in children, the dose is calculated on the basis of 4 units per kilogram of body weight. In severe extensive or highly contaminated wounds, or in severe animal or human bites, the dose should be increased accord-

Should Tetanus Immune Globulin (Human) not be available within 24 hours and the person not have been previously immunized, then the older type antitoxin must be utilized.

Tetanus toxoid is prepared from tetanus toxin (the poison secreted by tetanus bacteria). When the tetanus toxoid is injected, it stimulates the body to produce its own antibodies against the disease. The process by which immunity to a disease is acquired by injection of a toxin (or a toxoid) of the causative organism is known as *active immunization* and is one of the most effective means we have in controlling and fighting many of our common diseases such as whooping cough, diphtheria, and many others.

During World War II, all our troops, for the first time, were given injections of tetanus toxoid with the result that the incidence of tetanus was so low as to be almost nonexistent compared with the very high incidence during World War I. After the war, it became the general practice to immunize children against tetanus, along with other immunization shots (see page 613), as well as adults in industry and in the armed forces, so that an ever-increasing portion of the population has now received tetanus toxoid. The result is that tetanus, instead of being a common disease as it was formerly, is now relatively rare.

If a person with either a puncture or a deep wound has, in the past, received an injection of tetanus toxoid, he will only require, at the time of injury, a *booster* shot to restimulate antibody production and to give him almost certain protection against this infection. This is one great advantage of tetanus toxoid. The others are that, with booster shots, protection is essentially permanent, and the toxoid, unlike heterologous antiserum, rarely causes sensitization, although it may produce a local reaction.

Classes of Wounds

Contusions (Bruises). Contused wounds, more commonly called *bruises,* result when tiny blood vessels in the tissues are broken by a hard blow. They are simple to treat unless they are extremely extensive or there is a fracture or possible involvement of the internal organs. A massive contusion, such as may occur in the buttocks as the result of a fall, presents a problem in that the huge pool of blood which collects as the result of the severe blow may become infected, with resultant abscess formation. Cases of this type should be treated conservatively with ice packs and antibiotics by mouth, in the hope that the contusion will resolve without becoming infected and thus avoid the necessity for surgical incision and drainage. Even aspiration should be avoided if possible in order not to take a chance on introducing infection.

○ TREATMENT

1   Use *cold wet* compresses, an ice bag, or pack in fresh water ice, to prevent the further leakage of blood into the tissues from the broken blood vessels. Do *not* use salt water ice, as the temperature of the slush will be too low and cause further damage to the tissues.

2   Put the injured part at rest in order to further diminish blood flow.

3   After 24 hours or so, apply heat in the form of comfortably *hot wet* dressings or a heating pad.

If a contusion does not begin to improve within 24 hours or increases in size, it should be seen by a physician.

If the injured person is a hemophiliac or if he has another blood disorder characterized by an excessive tendency to bleed, medical aid is imperative, regardless of the degree of injury. This is important, as an individual whose blood fails to clot because of some inherent or artificial defect in the clotting system, may literally bleed to death within his own tissues. Hemophiliacs and those on anticoagulants require particular attention in this regard.

Severe Contusions.   There are, of course, much more serious types of contused wounds, which are of a specialized nature and will be discussed separately.   For example, a blow to the head, resulting in a concussion of the brain or a fractured skull, is a type of contusion, as are certain crushing fractures. Severe blows also may cause bruising of internal organs, which may throw an injured person into profound shock, and falls, as has already been noted, often produce such large bruises deep within a muscle that, if such a wound is handled ineptly, a severe infection may develop.

Black Eye.   A black eye is a type of contusion which should be treated by the immediate application of cold, wet compresses, preferably prepared from saline solution or alternatively, plain ice water.   If there is a possibility of injury to the eye itself, an ophthalmologist should be consulted immediately. It should be borne in mind that it takes a certain amount of time for the black-and-blue mark to be absorbed. To avoid embarrassment, use one of the cosmetic preparations especially designed to cover up skin discolorations.

Bruised Fingertip. A common and painful example of a contusion results from hitting the fingertip with a hammer or catching it in an automobile door. Here, the bruise occurs under the fingernail, since the nail bed contains many tiny blood vessels which break easily. A little pool of blood accumulates under the nail and, in the course of a few days, the blood turns black, and the finger becomes extremely painful. As a result of the pressure and the direct injury caused by the blow to the growing part of the nail, it may loosen and come off. However, there is a chance to save the nail by promptly draining the accumulated blood from beneath it, but prompt treatment by a doctor is necessary (Fig. 3-1). Recently a cordless nail drill has become available from Concept, Inc., of St. Petersburg, Florida, which should prove very useful. If the nail later starts to shed, do not try to remove it, but keep it fastened in place with a small adhesive bandage until the new nail pushes the old nail off as it grows. In this way, the new nail will have a better appearance, and the nail bed will be less tender.

Abrasions (Scrapes). An abrasion is an irregular, superficial open wound of the skin, in which the outer layers are scraped off; there usually is little bleeding unless the abrasion

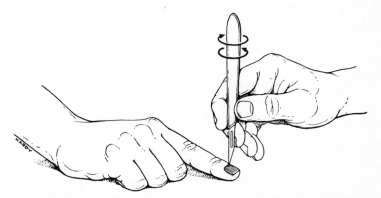

Fig. 3-1. Method of trephining for the evacuation of blood beneath nail. A dental bur also works well. Specially designed trephines are also available for this purpose.

is very deep. A skinned knee is an example of this type of wound.

Abrasions, particularly those which occur as the result of street or highway accidents, frequently contain bits of grease, gravel, or other foreign matter, which are often ground into the skin. If such dirt is not removed, not only may a serious infection develop, but a permanent tattoo-like scar may result. If the wound is not deep, the foreign matter can be loosened and flushed away with fresh hydrogen peroxide solution followed by gentle washing with antiseptic soap and water or a detergent. Careful cleansing is important, since deep abrasions are very prone to infection.

After cleaning the wound, cover it with a single layer of *nonadhering* gauze, or place a small amount of an antiseptic first-aid cream or antibiotic ointment on the dressing before covering the wound; this will help to prevent sticking and prove soothing, especially to children. Over this, either bandage a sterile gauze pad in place or hold it with adhesive tape. Should the gauze tend to stick when redressing the wound, soak it for a few minutes with fresh hydrogen peroxide solution or with a solution of 1 teaspoonful of salt to a quart of boiled water.

Lacerated Wounds. A lacerated wound (*laceration*) is one in which there is a jagged, ragged tearing of the tissues. This type of wound frequently is combined with contusions, in which case the wound is spoken of technically as a *contused lacerated wound*. Going through a windshield in an automobile accident usually produces this type of wound.

O TREATMENT

Like abrasions, lacerated wounds may contain foreign matter which must be cleaned out in order to prevent infection and ensure proper healing. Soak the wound with fresh hydrogen peroxide to help mechanically loosen and flush away foreign matter, and then gently wash it with antiseptic soap and water, first cleansing the surrounding area thoroughly; make sure to wash dirt away from the wound, not into it!

When lacerations are extensive (as from automobile accidents), no attempt should be made to treat them at the site of the accident, since definitive treatment often is a complicated procedure, requiring hospital facilities. Simply cover the injured area with a thick sterile dressing, bandage it firmly in place, and get the victim to a hospital as quickly as possible.

If the wound is not too large or deep, the edges can be gently drawn together and held in place with so-called "butterfly" strips, which can be made by the very simple procedure shown in Fig. 3-2. These are applied in such a way as to draw the edges of the wound together, thus helping to control bleeding and aiding the skin edges to grow together without the use of sutures (stitches). This technic is timesaving and painless and is particularly useful with children and apprehensive adults or when the size or type of the wound does not require sutures (Fig. 3-3). In many wounds treated in this way, the healing is as good as if sutures were used. "Butterfly" strips are available in any drugstore, ready-made and sterilized. A supply should be kept on hand in case of emergency.

If, however, the wound is large or there is extensive bruising of the tissues about the wound or persistent bleeding, a physician should, of course, be consulted.

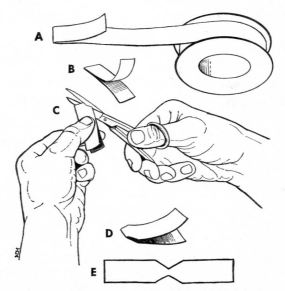

Fig. 3-2. To make a butterfly strip, fold a strip of ½-inch-wide adhesive tape back on itself (A) and (B), and cut off the corners evenly at the folded end to form broad nicks (C) and (D) when the strip is unfolded (E).

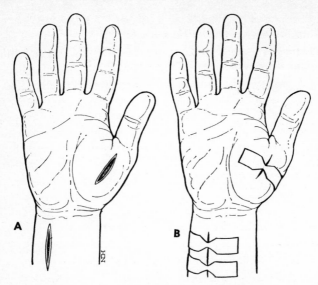

Fig. 3-3. Butterfly strips are convenient for closing minor lacerations of the hand or arm and avoid the use of sutures.

Incised Wounds (Cuts). An incised wound is usually a single clean cut, such as is made by a surgeon in performing an operation. Cuts on the fingers or hands from broken glasses while washing dishes, for instance, or on the feet from broken bottles or pieces of glass, which sometimes occur when walking on a beach, are often of this type.

One of the major dangers of deep incised wounds is injury to underlying structures such as tendons, nerves, or blood vessels. Such injury can only be repaired under surgical conditions.

○ TREATMENT

Deep incised wounds may bleed profusely, since an artery or vein may also have been cut. Deep incised wounds should be covered with a sterile pressure dressing, and medical aid sought immediately. However, many superficial cuts of this type are everyday occurrences in any household and can be easily treated by washing them thoroughly with soap and water and applying a dry nonsticking dressing. If the wound edges gape, they may easily be drawn together by using the butterfly strip technic.

If healing does not progress rapidly or there is any evidence of swelling, increased tenderness or redness, or streaks extending outward from the wound, it is probable that infection has occurred, and a physician should be consulted immediately.

Puncture Wounds.   A puncture wound is, as the name implies, a perforation of the skin and tissues made by a sharp object.   A wound resulting from stepping on a rusty nail is an example of a puncture wound.   Such a wound can have serious consequences, if not properly cared for, because of infection.   (Dog bites and beestings also are puncture wounds.)

If a puncture wound has been acquired on a farm, it must be assumed that the wound is contaminated with tetanus germs; immediate tetanus prophylaxis is a must (see page 69).

○ TREATMENT

A superficial puncture wound sustained under conditions where tetanus germs are unlikely to exist (as at the seashore or on a boat) should be encouraged to bleed freely, scrubbed thoroughly but gently with soap and water, and covered with a dry dressing.

Do not use an ointment on this type of wound, since this might prevent drainage by sealing the wound off and encourage infection instead of preventing it.   If swelling, pain, redness, or tenderness occurs, see a physician immediately.

Animal Bites.   A special form of puncture wound is caused by the bite of an animal.   Such wounds are often torn, lacerated, and bruised as well.   Bite wounds are always dangerous because serious infection may follow, and the possibility of rabies must always be kept in mind.

○ TREATMENT

1   If it is not possible to get a doctor or go to a hospital quickly, clean the wound thoroughy with an antiseptic soap or detergent solution; then rinse it well with running water or a salt solution as warm as the victim can comfortably bear.

2   Cover the bitten part with a thick sterile dressing, and bandage the part so as to immobilize it at rest; in the case of an arm or hand, use a sling.

3   Take the victim to a doctor or hospital as quickly as possible.

4   Report the bite to the police or to the local health authorities immediately.

Rabies

Since bites by dogs, cats, or any wild animal always present the danger of infection with rabies, *a biting animal should never be killed* unless unavoidable as a matter of safety, but should be caught and held for observation for at least 15 days, in order to determine whether it develops rabies.

If it is necessary to kill the animal at the time of the biting, the carcass should be sent to the state public health laboratory for an examination of its brain. If the laboratory finds that the animal was rabid, it is essential that treatment be initiated at once.

Human rabies is no longer very common in this country, thanks to greatly improved methods of control, but it is still one of our most dangerous diseases since without preventive treatment rendered before symptoms are manifest, it is invariably fatal. Understandably, therefore, rabies is a disease fraught with great emotionalism; almost everyone even remotely associated with the victim of a dog bite fears the possibility of this dread condition.

But what many people do not realize is the existence of a vast potential reservoir among many common wild animals closely associated with man's environment. The most important among these include bats, cats, raccoons, rabbits, rats, mice, skunks, and squirrels. Any wild animal that allows itself to be petted is probably sick and therefore suspect. Even pet "tamed" animals, such as raccoons, will bite unexpectedly and have been the cause of several near fatal cases of rabies.

Rabies is essentially an infection of the brain that affects all age groups, although it seems to have a special predilection for the very young; approximately one-fourth of all cases reported in the United States involve children. For some reason there seems to be a greater incidence among males than females.

The disease may be transmitted by any warm-blooded animal; more than half of the cases are the result of bites by various wild animals. Recent evidence suggests that about one-third of human cases cannot be associated with the bite of any animal—a fact which raises the suspicion that rabies may be transmitted in ways other than by a direct bite.

Most bites occur on the extremities, but it has long been supposed that bites around the face, head, and neck may be more dangerous and have a shorter incubation period. It would appear that, with wide variations, the average incubation period between infection and the appearance of symptoms is in the neighborhood of 57 days. However, in cases of extensive tissue destruction or severe bites about the face, head, and neck, the incubation period may be as short as 17 days.

Not all rabid animals go berserk and foam at the mouth. There is a *paralytic* form of the disease in which the saliva is infectious without other obvious symptoms of rabies. When this occurs with a family pet, for instance, rabies may quite unwittingly be contracted by one or more members of the family who accidentally get the animal's saliva into a minor wound and thus contract the disease.

Symptoms. Once symptoms have appeared, the disease runs its course in a little over 7 days. The total course from the time of the bite to the time of death, in one series of cases, averaged a little over 65 days, with the shortest period being 24 days and the longest 155 days. Fortunately, the time between the bite and the appearance of symptoms is long enough in the majority of cases for effective vaccine therapy to have been started and to build up protective antibodies to ward off the disease before the patient succumbs.

While the symptoms of hydrophobia (rabies) are well known, the prodromal symptoms of the disease, before air hunger and pharyngeal spasm on the sight or thought of water (hence the name hydrophobia) have set in, may be very confusing unless it is definitely known that the patient has received a bite from a potentially rabid animal. The diagnosis of rabies is supported by the history of an animal bite and by laboratory studies, which usually must be carried out by the state department of health.

O TREATMENT

Within the last few years, new and safer vaccines and the use of hyperimmune (antirabies) serum have done much to prevent the disease in those who have been exposed, but to be effective, treatment must be administered before symptoms of the disease appear, or it will be of no avail.

The preferred vaccine consists of embryonic duck tissue containing killed virus and suspended in an especially formulated liquid for injection. This vaccine was developed to circumvent the use of the older brain tissue vaccines and has the advantage that it contains little or none of the so-called "paralytic factor" present in the older vaccines. Myelin, contained in conventional vaccines of brain origin, has been implicated as the causative factor in rabies treatment paralysis. The incidence of minor reactions from the use of the newer vaccines appears to be in the order of one in two thousand, or less.

Two vaccines currently are approved for use: Duck Embryo Vaccine (DEV, Lilly) and Nervous Tissue Vaccine (NTV, National Drug). Rates of treatment failures with the two vaccines are not significantly different, but the incidence of central nervous system reactions seems to be somewhat less with Duck Embryo Vaccine than with Nervous Tissue Vaccine.

Of prime importance in rabies treatment is the earliest possible development of protective antibodies. Vaccine of duck embryo origin produces antibodies in most patients by the tenth day, and in almost all subjects by the fifteenth day after beginning a course of at least 14 daily doses. Thus the patient is able to develop his protective antibodies before symptoms of the disease appear in most cases.

The question of whether to give rabies vaccine or not is not an easy one. In favor of giving the vaccine is the fact that if rabies develops, it will almost certainly prove fatal. Against giving it is the danger of developing severe side effects involving the central nervous system, particularly if the vaccine used contains brain tissue.

Also entering into the decision is the fact that only approximately 20 percent of persons untreated with vaccine who are bitten by animals *known* to be rabid have developed rabies if not treated with rabies vaccine, and secondly, rabies is not likely unless the individual actually has been bitten.

The recommendations of the World Health Organization Expert Committee on Rabies may be summarized, as a general guide, as follows:

If contact with a rabid animal has been indirect or if there has been only a lick on unabraded skin, vaccine treatment is not recommended.

For a lick on abraded skin or on mucous membranes, or for single bites *not* on the head, neck, face, or arm, vaccine may be withheld if the animal is healthy at the time of exposure. But the animal should be observed for 10 to 15 days.   If during the observation period the animal is proved to have rabies or becomes clinically suspicious, the vaccine should be started immediately.   If the animal has signs suspicious of rabies at the time of exposure, the vaccine should be given but stopped if the animal is normal on the fifth day after exposure.   If the animal is rabid, if it escapes or is killed, or if its condition is unknown, a complete course of vaccine is required.   If the biting animal is wild, rabies antiserum also should be used. Conventional antiserum is of equine origin, but serum of human origin has been under study for some time and offers promise since it is not sensitizing. Human-cell vaccines are also being studied with some optimism.

In the event of multiple bites or single bites on the head, neck, face, or arm, the same principles are followed but, in addition, rabies antiserum should be administered.

An additional problem arises in connection with evidence that serum administered concurrently with vaccine may interfere with the development of active immunity.   If serum is used, supplementary doses of vaccine should be given at 10 and 20 days after the last dose given in accordance with the conventional vaccine schedule.

Local treatment of the bite wound is extremely important. Such wounds should be thoroughly scrubbed with soap and water, and some form of quaternary ammonium antiseptic, such as benzalkonium chloride (Zephiran®), should be applied liberally.   All soap must be flushed from the wound before applying the benzalkonium chloride solution, which is neutralized by soap.   Bite wounds should not be immediately closed surgically but left open to drain for several days until local infection has been cleared up.

If antirabies serum is used, a portion of the total dose should be thoroughly infiltrated around the wound.   Since ordinary antirabies serum is composed of horse serum, tests should be made for hypersensitivity to horse serum.   If these tests are positive, desensitization must be attempted before administering the required dose.   Human hyperimmune serum, which avoids the dangers and inconvenience of horse serum, is now under clinical study but at this writing has not yet been licensed for commercial distribution.

Hyperimmune serum in combination with vaccine is considered the best possible post exposure prophylaxis. Lederle Laboratories offer the only *equine* antirabies serum available in the United States. In spite of a 20 percent incidence of allergic reactions, hyperimmune serum is recommended for most exposures classified as severe, and for all bites by rabid animals, wild carnivores, and bats. Antirabies serum should be used regardless of the interval between exposure and treatment, but every effort should be made to give it as soon as possible after exposure. The recommended dose is 1,000 units (one vial) intramuscularly per 40-pound body weight. A portion of antiserum is used to infiltrate the wound, and the remainder is given intramuscularly.

The table on page 83 provides a guide for post exposure antirabies prophylaxis and is based on recommendations of the Public Health Service Advisory Committee on Immunization Practices, published in the *Morbidity and Mortality Weekly Report,* Vol. 16, No. 19, week ending May 13, 1967.

The preventive treatment of rabies is a complicated therapeutic process, but fortunately time is in the favor of the victim if the biting animal can be observed in confinement over a period of 15 days. Because of the long incubation period of the disease, there will still be time to administer preventive treatment in the event that the animal develops symptoms of rabies within the 15-day period. If it does not, the animal did not have rabies in the first place and there is no need to subject the bite victim to a possibly hazardous series of inoculations.

If a victim undergoes preventive treatment as a matter of safety, the chances of contracting rabies from the bite of even a proven rabid animal are now considered to be only one in six.

MAJOR INJURIES

Lawn-Mower Injuries in Children. Some of the most devastating and deforming injuries occur among children as the result of power-lawn-mower accidents. The children may be injured simply as bystanders who come too close to the machine and are struck by flying debris, or who slip and fall under the mower; as operators who are allowed to use the equipment at too early an age before sufficient mechanical

GUIDE FOR POSTEXPOSURE ANTIRABIES PROPHYLAXIS

			Treatment	
			Exposure	
Species	Status at Time of Attack	No Lesion	Mild	Severe
Healthy		None	None. Begin vaccine at first sign of rabies in biting dog or cat during holding period	Antirabies serum. Begin vaccine at first sign of rabies in biting dog or cat during holding period
Dog or cat	Signs suggestive of rabbies	None	Rabies vaccine. Discontinue vaccine if biting dog or cat is healthy 5 days after exposure	Antirabies serum and rabies vaccine. Discontinue vaccine if biting dog or cat is healthy 5 days after exposure
	Escaped or unknown	None	Rabies vaccine	Antirabies serum and rabies vaccine
	Rabid	None	Antirabies serum and rabies vaccine	Antirabies serum and rabies vaccine
Skunk, fox, raccoon, coyote, bat	Regarded as rabid in unprovoked attack	None	Antirabies serum and rabies vaccine	Antirabies serum and rabies vaccine

knowledge and judgment have been gained (sad, but true—their fathers often make this mistake); and as passengers riding on the seat with the operator (usually the father or older brother) and fall off, either getting hit by the rapidly revolving blades and sustaining extensive soft tissue and bone damage or at best suffering minor injury as the result of the fall.

Even a push-type mower is dangerous, since it is very easy to unwittingly pull it backward onto a foot, while mowing back and forth in a confined area. Most injuries involve preteenage youngsters.

All types of injuries result from such accidents—fractured skulls, fractured and dislocated hips, penetration of vital structures by foreign bodies which have been converted to high velocity missiles by the revolving blades; severance of important nerves, blood vessels, and bones; and extensive lacerations and avulsions resulting in excessive tissue loss which requires prolonged major (sometimes multiple) surgical procedures to correct.

The sad part of all this is, as stressed by Grosfeld, Morse, and Eyring, that all these maiming and often permanently damaging injuries are preventable. No child should ever be permitted to ride as a passenger on a power mower or get near one while it is operating. No child should be permitted to operate a power mower of any type until after he is 13 years of age, and then only if he shows good mechanical sense and judgment and has no emotional "hang-ups."

The emergency first-aid treatment of these injuries follows the lines previously outlined for the specific types of injuries concerned.

Crush Injuries. A crush injury is usually the result of a person being buried or pinned beneath a pile of dirt or falling debris, as from houses collapsing during an earthquake or an explosion. (One frequently reads of this kind of injury to workers caught in a cave-in while excavating.) Crushing injuries are considered to be generalized contusions, internal as well as external, of a major portion of the body. As the result of such overwhelming bruising, all kinds of secondary injuries may occur including multiple fractures and the rupture of internal organs.

○ TREATMENT

Because this type of injury usually leads to severe shock (Chap. 6), it is of great importance that all possible steps be taken to minimize this possibility by treating the case as one of severe shock, even though at first the victim may show no signs of being in this condition. Multiple injuries should always be suspected and looked for.

Splinting of fractures of the extremities and major soft tissue injuries is particularly important to combat hypotension. It is extremely important to keep the victim as quiet as possible to minimize the release of toxic substances, especially potassium, from the crushed tissues into the system.

While awaiting the arrival of expert medical aid, treatment of the victim includes:

1 Putting him in the shock position (see page 175).
2 Doing whatever is possible to minimize pain.
3 Keeping him comfortably warm and supplying him with fluids by mouth, if he is conscious.
4 Moving him *as little as possible* once he has been removed from danger.

● PRECAUTION

Crush injuries commonly involve the extremities. In attempting to keep the victim warm, *never apply heat to an injured arm or leg.* Heat would increase the absorption by the bloodstream of toxic substances from the injured part and would further tend to throw the victim into shock. If the injury is limited principally to an extremity, recent evidence suggests that refrigeration of the part with fresh water ice or some equivalent means may be helpful in reducing toxic absorption and minimizing shock.

Do not transport the victim until the injured parts have been splinted or immobilized and until sufficient help is available to transport him with a minimum of body movement. Do not use excessive dressings, as these simply serve to increase warmth of the part and facilitate absorption of the toxic products of tissue destruction.

Wringer Injuries of the Upper Extremity. A special, but not uncommon, variety of crush injury is caused when the hand or arm is caught between the rollers of the wringer of an electric washing machine or even between the rollers of a hand-cranked wringer. Most of the newer machines are equipped with automatic release mechanisms, but they often do not trip quickly enough to prevent a small hand or arm from being drawn into the machine and sustaining extensive damage.

As might be suspected, except for industrial accidents, young mothers and children are the principal victims, and boys seem to outnumber girls by a considerable margin—probably because of their greater mechanical inquisitiveness.

As the hand and arm are drawn in between the rollers a crushing effect is exerted, the degree of which depends on the tension of the roller springs, the size of the arm, and the churning effects produced by the desperate efforts of the victim to extricate his arm from the machine before the release trips and the motor shuts off. As a result, any combination of lacerations of the skin, broken bones, and crushing of the muscles of the forearm may be produced. Very often, however, the injuries are not unduly extensive and one may simply see lacerations and brush burns of the arm, with few, if any, other immediate symptoms or signs. The danger is that upon first examination the injury may be erroneously dismissed as a trivial one and that no adequate initial treatment will be provided.

Similar injuries may occur to young children left unattended on escalators and require the most meticulous surgical care.

○ TREATMENT

Without proper treatment within a few hours, the arm will begin to swell badly as a result of bruising of the deep tissues and, if improperly treated, the swelling will become so severe as to result in serious complications later on. The importance of early treatment, therefore, cannot be overemphasized and cases of this type should, of course, be taken to a hospital as quickly as possible.

The case should be treated as a potentially serious injury and the victim should be hospitalized for observation for at least 48 hours.

1 In case medical aid is not immediately available, gently clean the arm with antiseptic soap and water, cover the abrasions

with sterile dressings, and wrap the entire arm in a heavy compression dressing from the fingers to the armpit. This dressing should be made of a soft, springy material; if surgical dressings especially designed for this purpose are not available, clean cotton waste or clean, soft bath towels may be used.

2 Apply an elastic bandage, making certain that the arm is wrapped firmly but not so tight as to constrict the circulation or cause pain. If the victim complains of severe pain after the bandage has been applied, the wrapping probably has been applied too tightly and should be loosened.

3 Suspend the arm straight upward above the body, by some suitable arrangement, in order to decrease the blood flow to the extremity and thus help to prevent further swelling.

Blast Injuries. A blast injury is also in a sense a crushing injury, caused by the strong "shock wave" transmitted by the atmosphere following an explosion. This results in internal hemorrhage, especially in the lungs and other important organs, including the brain. Hemorrhage in the adrenal glands increases the likelihood of shock. This type of injury would be common and take a major toll of life in a nuclear war.

Blast injuries result from many different types of explosions. For example, gas stoves may explode; boats blow up all too often because some boatmen fail to take the elementary precautions essential for safe boating. And then there are the civil disasters—gas-tank explosions, ammunition explosions, and, in wartime, bomb and shell explosions.

At first there may be little external evidence of injury, unless the victim has been burned or has sustained injury from falling debris. But a person suffering from blast injuries may go into shock very easily and, therefore, must be treated promptly to prevent this. Stimulants, such as tea, coffee, or aromatic spirits of ammonia should be given, and the victim should be kept warm in the shock position. Where accessible crush injuries have occurred, refrigeration of the part, as previously outlined, is helpful in minimizing shock.

Even though a victim's condition appears good, he should be under observation in a hospital for several days, as shock and collapse may develop some time after injury.

Injection Injuries of the Hand. A very common industrial injury, similar in some respects to some blast injuries, is the accidental high pressure injection of various materials into the hand such as paint, fuel oil, grease, and various plastics used in injection guns.   Such injuries can become extremely disabling and demand immediate radical surgery to rid the hand of all foreign materials, according to Apfelberg et al. of the Palo Alto Medical Clinic.

Obviously, such accidents should not be neglected; the hand should be swathed in sterile dressings, splinted if necessary, and the victim taken to the nearest hospital.

FOREIGN BODIES

All kinds of substances or objects, such as pins, food, insects, splinters, and soot can become accidentally lodged in an organ or in a part of the human body where they do not belong.   Such *foreign bodies* sometimes cause only discomfort to the person, but they can be harmful and often create an emergency.

Eye.   A foreign body in the eye, such as a speck of soot, is very common.   If the speck cannot be seen or easily removed, an ophthalmologist should be consulted promptly.

○ TREATMENT
If the foreign body is under the upper lid, it can sometimes be removed by drawing the upper lid down over the lower lid; the flushing and wetting effect of the tears which the irritation produces will tend to make the foreign body stick to the lower lid.   If the foreign body is not flushed out, turn back the upper lid for inspection in this way:

1   Grasp the eyelashes gently.
2   With the patient looking down, turn the lid back over a cotton swab, a clean matchstick, or a pencil (Fig. 3-4).
3   If the speck is seen, wipe it off very gently with a bit of moistened sterile gauze or a wisp of moistened, twisted absorbent cotton.

A foreign body under the *lower lid* usually is easily seen and is fairly easy to remove with moistened gauze or cotton.

Quite frequently, a foreign body may be lodged on the cornea of the eye, over the iris, and be overlooked because of its dark, matching color.   Extreme care should be taken with

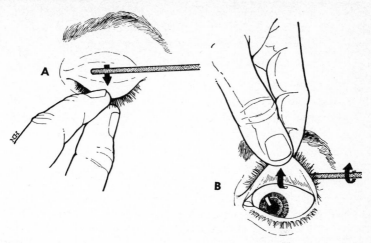

Fig. 3-4. The upper eyelid can be easily turned back over a cotton-tipped applicator or stem of a smooth wooden kitchen match.

any particle in this location because of the danger of damaging the cornea; let a doctor handle such a situation. In the meantime, place a sterile compress (eye pad), held in place by a light bandage or adhesive tape over the eye to help avoid painful and irritating movements.

It should be mentioned that the National Society for the Prevention of Blindness believes that specks in the eye that cannot be washed out with tears (or by pulling the upper lid down over the lower) should have medical attention. However, circumstances do occur when it is not possible to obtain medical aid promptly, and on such occasions the above mentioned steps may prove useful.

Ear. Foreign bodies, such as beads, are often put in ears by children, but sometimes foreign bodies, such as insects, fly into ears by accident.

Never try to dig anything out of an ear—you may only push it in further and may actually perforate the delicate eardrum.

Drop some warm olive oil, mineral oil, or baby oil in the ear and let it remain there for a few minutes, while the head is turned to the opposite side.

When putting drops into the ear canal, pull backward a little on the lobe of the ear; this straightens the canal and lets it fill more easily (Fig. 3-5). Then let the oil run out and the drowned insect or other foreign body may come out with it. Gently wipe the canal with a cotton-tipped applicator.

If these measures do not dislodge the object, see a physician.

Nose. Foreign bodies in the nose, such as peas (which children often put there) or insects, can usually be removed by sneezing, which can be induced by tickling the opposite nostril or by sniffing pepper. If the object is not expelled, consult a nose and throat specialist.

Do not attempt to hook out objects in the nose with hairpins or similar instruments, as damage to the tissues may result, or the foreign body may be pushed to an inaccessible position.

Stomach. Foreign bodies in the stomach are common in children, who like to swallow strange things or who do so by mistake. Except for pins or other sharp objects, no great harm

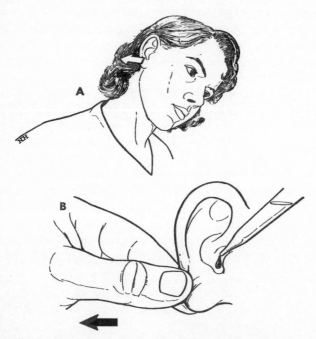

Fig. 3-5. To put drops in an ear, pull back the lobe so as to straighten the external canal.

usually results, as nature eventually takes its course and the object is removed.

However, a doctor should be consulted, since examination of the digestive tract through a fluoroscope may be desirable in order to determine what form of treatment, if any, is indicated.   Surgery is rarely necessary except when pins or similar objects have been swallowed.

Do not give a cathartic or an emetic.

Splinters.   Generally, splinters lie close to the surface and are easily removed.

○ TREATMENT

A splinter that can be seen just underneath the skin can be removed by using a needle which has been sterilized by passing it through a flame until it glows.   (Let it cool before using!)

1 Clean the skin overlying the splinter with soap and water.
2 With the sterile needle, split along the length of the splinter until the end can easily be grasped with a pair of tweezers and gently pulled out (Fig. 3-6).   Go slowly in order to avoid breaking the splinter, which would be much more troublesome.
3 After the splinter is out, wash the wound with soap and water and cover it with an adhesive bandage.

A splinter under a fingernail is very painful, and its removal is best left to a doctor.   If the splinter is large and lies deep, it should be considered a deep puncture wound and treated accordingly.

Fish Hooks.   Fish hooks provide another rather unusual type of foreign body when they become embedded in some portion of the anatomy, usually a finger, sometimes in the back or scalp as the result of a wild cast by an over-eager fisherman. Usually the hook becomes only partially embedded but, if the cast has been made hard enough, it will occasionally tear away a portion of flesh.

When the hook is embedded with the point still buried in the tissues, one is faced with the problem of getting it out, since fish hooks generally are designed with a barb which is intended to keep them from being pulled out while playing a fish.   Under ordinary circumstances, removal should be at-

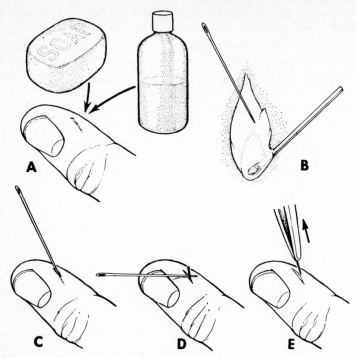

Fig. 3-6. A sterile sharp cutting-type needle is used to slit skin at a sharp angle over splinter so that it may be lifted out gently without breaking. (A) Cleanse area around splinter with soap or antiseptic. (B) Heat needle in flame. Hold until it cools. (C) Break skin over splinter. (D) Elevate exposed splinter. (E) With tweezers withdraw splinter.

tempted only by a physician, using a local anesthetic, but there are occasions, for instance when one is at sea, when a physician is not available and something must be done.

As a rule, the simplest way of accomplishing this is to force the point of the hook on through the flesh until the barb itself emerges so that it can be grasped.   Then, using a pair of nipper pliers, the shank can be cut off very close to where it enters the skin and the barb portion then pulled out with very little difficulty, as shown in the illustration (Fig. 3-7).

An alternative method is simply to back the hook out once the barb has been cut off.   This method, in our opinion, is often the simpler of the two and has the advantage of not dragging a piece of the shank which has not already entered the flesh, through the tissues, thus adding further to the already existing contamination.

After removal of the hook, the wound should be cleansed as thoroughly as possible with antiseptic soap or a detergent and a dry dressing applied.   A physician should be seen, if he has not already performed the removal, and the patient should receive a tetanus toxoid booster shot or a dose of tetanus anti-serum, as the circumstances may indicate.   In most cases an antibiotic should be administered, since used fish hooks are contaminated with potentially highly pathogenic organisms and infection can readily result.   The wound should be watched for redness, swelling, pain, and possibly red streaks radiating

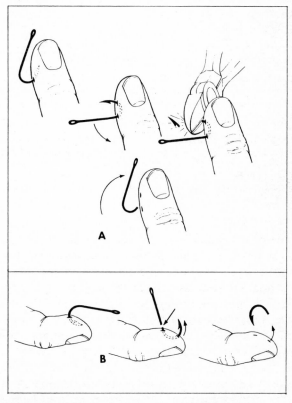

Fig. 3-7. Two methods of removing an embedded fish hook by cutting either the barb (A) or the shank (B), whichever is easier in a given case.

from the area; these signs would indicate the presence of infection, and in such an event a physician should be consulted immediately.

BANDAGES AND BANDAGING TECHNICS

Types of Bandages

Although there are several kinds of bandages used in emergency care of the injured, those most often used are roller bandages (strips of ordinary gauze or specially woven guaze that conforms to a part, rolled into cylinders), triangular bandages (triangles of muslin which can be folded to make a cravat bandage or a tourniquet), adhesive bandages (ready-to-use sterile adhesive dressings, including butterfly strips).

Functions of a Bandage

The functions of a bandage may include one or all of the following:

To hold dressings or splints firmly in place.

To supplement a dressing by providing a clean protective covering for the affected part.

To minimize further contamination of the wound.

To partially immobilize and rest the injured part and, at the same time, to help maintain body warmth.

To apply and maintain pressure for the control of bleeding.

Applying Bandages

A bandage should *not* be applied directly to an open wound; the wound should first be covered with a sterile gauze compress.

Special care must be taken to put a bandage on firmly enough to do the job, but not so tight as to cause constriction. It should be remembered that some types of gauze tend to shrink when they are wet; therefore, if a wet dressing is to be used, allow for shrinkage when applying the bandage.

After a bandage is applied, it may be fastened with adhesive tape (but not satisfactorily if wet dressings are used) or by splitting the free end of the bandage to form two tails and then bringing one around the bandaged part and tying the two ends with a square knot (Fig. 3-8).

When bandaging has been completed, check to make sure

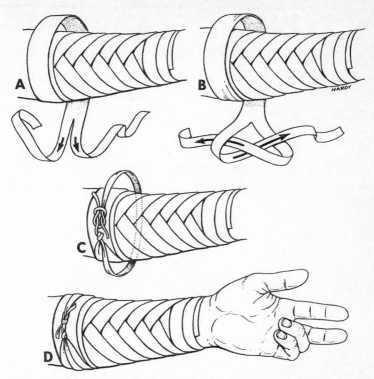

Fig. 3-8. Simple method for securing a gauze bandage without using adhesive tape. After bandage is in place, the end is split down the center for about 8 inches and tied at the base to prevent raveling. The two new ends are then used as ties.

that it is not too tight, because injury frequently causes swelling. If you have not allowed for this and the patient complains of the bandage being too tight or painful, reapply the bandage. It is better to do this than to take a chance on stopping the blood supply to the part and possibly causing discomfort, or even gangrene.

Bandaging is a technic requiring a dexterity that comes only with much practice, but an effective bandage doesn't necessarily have to be a pretty one. A description of the types of bandages and a few of the bandaging technics used most frequently will serve to illustrate the general principles involved.

Roller Bandage. Most commonly used is the roller bandage, which can be of muslin or gauze or a new specially woven and treated gauze that greatly improves conformability and ease of application. These bandages are usually sterilized (and are so marked) and are available in several widths. Using the proper width for a particular part makes bandaging easier. For example:

To bandage fingers or toes, use 1-inch bandage.

To bandage head, hands, or limbs of children, use 2-inch bandage.

To bandage arms or legs of adults, use 2- or 3-inch bandage.

To bandage thigh, groin, or trunk, use 3-inch bandage.

For Fingers or Toes. Fingers or toes are best bandaged as follows (Fig. 3-9):

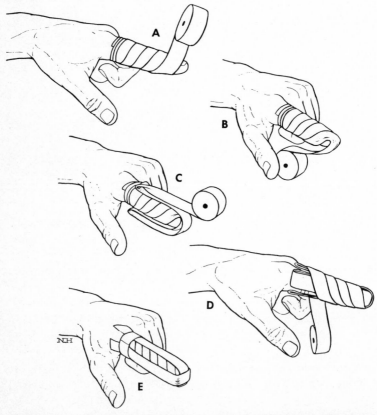

Fig. 3-9. The spiral and recurrent loop technic for bandaging a finger, and the manner of finishing off the dressing with narrow strips of adhesive tape.

1   Starting at the base of the finger, secure the bandage with one or two turns.

2   Then wind the bandage toward the tip of the finger in such a way that each turn overlaps the previous one about a quarter of the width.

3   Cover the tip of the finger by making one or two loopbacks from the base of the finger up over the tip and back down the other side, anchoring these loops by winding an additional layer around them.

4   Finish off neatly with narrow strips of adhesive tape run over the tip of the finger from each side and with one or two strips circled around the vertical ones to hold them in place. This provides a firm dressing which will not easily come off.

If the wound is near the base of the finger or in the web between the fingers, run several successive layers of the bandage back over the wrist and up around the finger in a figure eight, to anchor the dressing firmly in place (Fig. 3-10).

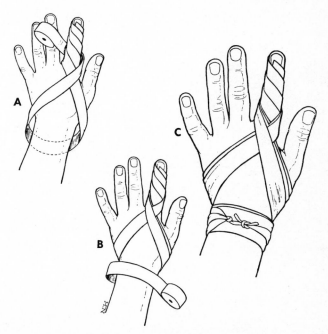

Fig. 3-10. The spirals of a finger bandage may be brought back over the wrist, utilizing the figure-eight technic to secure the dressing firmly near the base of the fingers.

For a Limb. If a limb or a part of a limb is to be bandaged, the *spiral reverse technic* is very useful. This technic keeps the bandage from bunching up because of the variations in the contour of a limb, and it helps to keep the bandage firm and in place. The technic is quite simple.

1 Start by anchoring the bandage with one or two turns at the smallest part of the extremity, such as the ankle or wrist.

2 Then reverse the bandage at each turn or when required to keep the bandage smooth. To do this, twist the top of the roll *away* from the direction in which you are bandaging (Fig. 3-11).

If the new, conforming type of bandage is used, the reverse spiral technic is not often required, since the bandage automatically conforms to the contours of the part. This kind of bandage is much easier to use and generally stays in place better than the regular roller bandage.

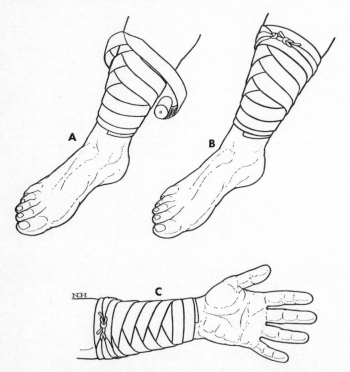

Fig. 3-11. The spiral reverse technic for bandaging a leg or forearm.

For the Jaw.   A roller bandage may also be used to hold in place a dressing applied to the jaw or to support the jaw.   The technic is as follows:

1   Start the bandage with two or three turns about the forehead.

2   After the third turn, as it reaches a point just behind the ear, turn the bandage and pass it up over the head and down beneath the jaw, just forward of the angle of the lower jaw, and up over the head again (Fig. 3-12).   Three or four such turns are usually ample to give the desired support.

Roller bandages are, of course, used to bandage other parts of the body, but the examples illustrate the general principles employed.

Triangular Bandage.   A triangular bandage, usually made of bleached muslin and, as generally supplied, measuring 54 inches in length at the base, is particularly useful in all kinds of emergency situations, especially as a quick dressing for a part.   It can be folded to make a cravat bandage or a tourniquet.

For the Head.   To bandage the head quickly with a triangular bandage for holding dressings in place in the case of extensive head injury (Fig. 3-13):

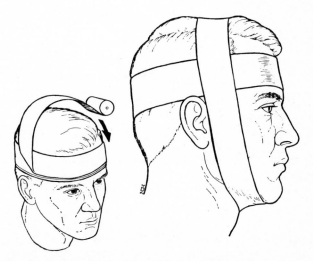

Fig. 3-12. A simple method of immobilizing the jaw, using a roller bandage.

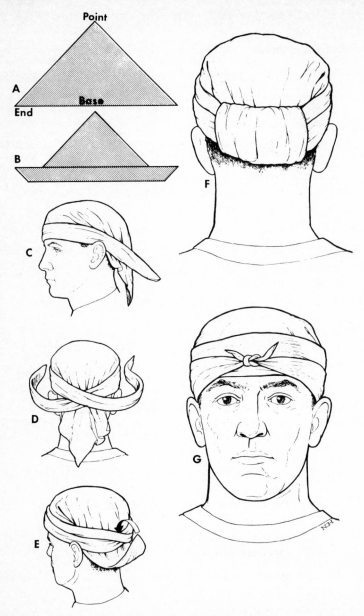

Fig. 3-13.   The steps in making a head dressing, using a triangular bandage.   This type of bandage is particularly useful for large scalp wounds and burns.

1 Fold a hem, about 2 inches wide, along the base of the triangle.

2 Grasp the ends of the bandage and apply it to the forehead so that it is centered, with the fold on the outside, and just above the eyebrows.

3 Bring the ends back behind the head, cross them under the back of the skull, bring them around to the front, and tie them over the forehead.

4 Then pull on the apex of the triangle, which is hanging down in back, so as to draw the bandage firmly and evenly over the top of the head.

5 Keeping the bandage taut, tuck the point in where the bandage crosses behind the head.

For a Hand or Foot. To bandage or wrap a hand or foot:

1 Place the injured part on the spread-out triangular bandage so that it is pointed toward the apex of the triangle.

2 Bring the apex of the bandage over the injured part.

3 Bring the other two points of the bandage up and over, and tie them behind the hand or foot.

For the Chest and Back. A triangular bandage can be applied quickly to make an excellent chest bandage. (In case of an open wound, a thick, sterile compress must be placed over the wound before it is bandaged.)

1 Place the apex of the bandage over the shoulder nearest to the injured side, and let the bandage fall over the chest or back so that the center of its base is below the point which has been placed over the shoulder (Fig. 3-14).

2 Carry the ends around the body and tie them directly below the shoulder.

3 Bring the longer end up to the shoulder and tie it to the original starting point of the bandage.

4 The same type of application is made when a triangular bandage is used for a back dressing.

For an Arm Sling. To make an arm sling:

1 Hang one point of the bandage over the shoulder opposite to the injured arm and let the bandage hang down in front.

2 Then place the injured arm in the desired position, bring the lower point up over the arm and around the neck, and tie the points at the shoulder (Fig. 3-15).

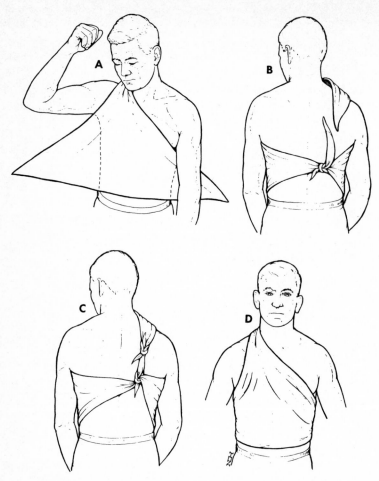

Fig. 3-14.   Using a triangular bandage for a chest or back dressing.

3   Bring the third point over the elbow, and fasten the bandage with a safety pin.

4   Adjust the bandage so as to elevate the arm 2–4 inches.

Cravat Bandage.   A triangular bandage can also be used for a number of purposes when folded as a "cravat." This is done by bringing the apex of the bandage to the center of its base and then folding the bandage lengthwise one or more times until the desired width is obtained (Fig. 3-16).

For the Jaw, Face, or an Ear.   A cravat can be used to bandage the jaw, a side of the face, or an ear in the following way:

1   Pass the cravat under the midpoint of the jaw and bring one end up and over the head to meet the other end just above the ear.

2   Then cross the ends, bring them around the head, and tie them on the opposite side.

For the Head.   To bandage the head quickly:

1   Center the cravat at the center of the forehead.

2   Bring the ends behind the head, cross them and bring them to the front.

3   Tie the ends over the forehead (Fig. 3-17).

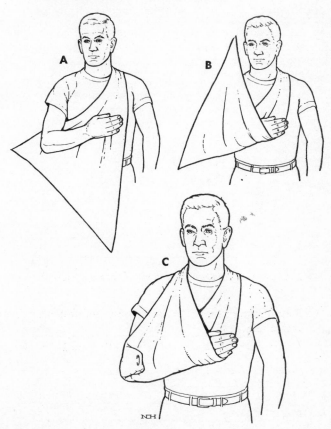

Fig. 3-15.   Using a triangular bandage as a comfortable arm sling.

For Fractured Ribs. One or more cravats also may be used as a temporary bandage for fractured ribs.

1 Place the center of the cravat over the side of the chest which is fractured, bring the ends of the cravat around to the opposite side, and gently snug down over a suitable padding the first throw of a square knot.

2 When the injured person expels his breath, pull on the ends of the cravat just enough to take up the slack and to apply gentle pressure to the chest.

3 While the breath is still expelled, tie the second throw of the knot, thus securing the bandage.

Several cravats may be applied in this manner in the event that several ribs are fractured (Fig. 3-18).

Tourniquet. To use a cravat bandage as a tourniquet:

1 Tie the ends of the cravat to form a large loop around the place that is bleeding.

2 Place a soft thick compress over the blood vessel.

3 Insert a short stick or a similar object through the loop, and turn it until the bandage tightens sufficiently on the compress to exert the proper amount of pressure (Fig. 3-19).

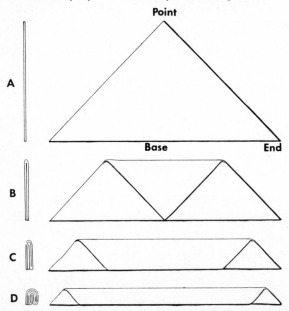

Fig. 3-16. Folding a triangular bandage to make a cravat bandage.

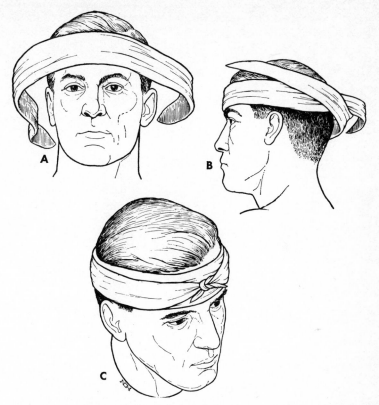

Fig. 3-17. A cravat bandage makes a good, quickly and easily applied head dressing.

Adhesive Tape. In addition to holding dressings in place, adhesive tape is often used as strapping to rest an injured part in order to permit more rapid healing and to alleviate discomfort by supporting the soft tissues. It is also used to protect injured joints by providing rest and gentle compression. Relief from pain is often immediate when an adhesive strapping is properly applied. If there is no relief or if the pain is aggravated, it may mean that the strapping has been applied too tightly; in this case, it should be reapplied.

Applying Adhesive Strappings. Much of the success in the use of adhesive tape depends upon the proper technic in applying it. The comfort of the victim is not only the chief aim but a good indication of the efficiency with which the adhesive strapping was applied.

Consider carefully the nature of the injury or defect before deciding whether or not to apply adhesive tape. If adhesive tape is to be used, these procedures should be followed:

1 If the skin where adhesive is to be applied is hairy, it should be shaved, clean and dry, and free from oily contamination, but *do not* use preparations containing solvents which remove all the natural oils.

2 If protective padding is required, use gauze, stockinet, sponge rubber, felt, or a similar material.

3 The injured part must be placed and held in a slightly *overcorrected* position while applying the strapping, so as to give the greatest relaxation and support to the injured structures. Strapping should give firm support but avoid constriction.

After the part is strapped, if movement causes undue tension or pain, the strapping was incorrectly applied. Do not hesitate to restrap correctly. When strapping is finished, *check the circulation!*

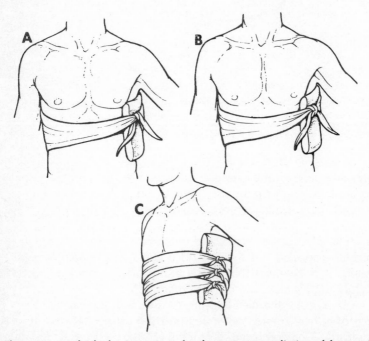

Fig. 3-18. Method of using cravats for the temporary splinting of fractured ribs. Note the padding provided for protection under knots which are tied on side opposite injury.

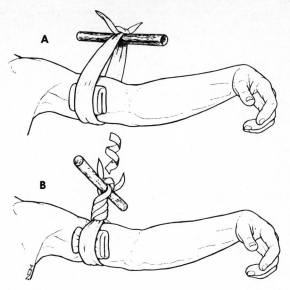

Fig. 3-19. Using a cravat as a tourniquet. Protective padding over the artery to be compressed is important.

Tearing Adhesive Tape. Tearing tape into strips is readily accomplished by holding the end between the thumbnails and forefingers of both hands, and the tearing is started by a quick rotary twist of the hands in opposite directions. Being able to tear adhesive tape does not depend on strength, but on getting the knack of it so as to apply a shearing force in the correct direction (Fig. 3-20).

For home use, special packages of adhesive tape now are available which provide means for cutting the tape to any desired length as it is drawn from the package.

Removing Adhesive Tape. When it is necessary to remove adhesive tape, as much care should be exercised as when applying it.

1 *Be gentle;* do not rip or tear the tape off.

2 The edges, which are sometimes difficult to loosen, can be easily peeled back by holding the *skin taut and pulling it away* from the tape, rather than by pulling the tape away from the skin. New types of adhesives which do not stick so hard to skin and hair and do not cause irritation are available and can be used where special firmness is not required.

3   To remove strips of adhesive tape which hold a dressing in place, cut across the strips at the gauze edge and then remove the strips by pulling *away* from the line of cutting.

4   To remove tape near a wound, pull *toward* the wound.

5   To remove a bulky strapping, as from an ankle, cut the tape horizontally and vertically with bandage scissors.

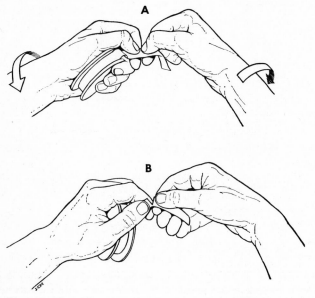

Fig. 3-20. Tearing of adhesive tape is readily accomplished by holding the edge of the strip between the thumbnails and forefingers. The tearing is started by a quick rotary twist of the hands in opposite directions in order to apply the proper shearing force.

4 Respiratory Emergencies and Resuscitation

Respiratory emergencies may be divided into three general categories: those associated with respiratory obstruction; those associated with cessation of breathing; and those associated with mechanical interference with respiration. Quite commonly, cessation of breathing is a complication of respiratory obstruction, as in cases of drowning. But whatever the respiratory difficulty, it will produce signs and symptoms characteristic of conditions that are caused by lack of oxygen. Generally speaking, these are

Early stages:
Mild dizziness
Shortness of breath
Chest pain
Rapid pulse

Later stages:
Dusky discoloration of the fingernail beds
Bluish-purple skin color
Dilated pupils
Increasingly irregular breathing
Loss of consciousness

RESPIRATORY OBSTRUCTION

Respiratory obstruction is one of the commonest respiratory emergencies, and the cause must quickly be removed or alleviated before any further measures, such as artificial respiration, can be undertaken.

Respiratory obstruction may be caused by foreign objects such as chunks of food or trinkets (especially dangerous are the opening tabs of soda pop cans which may be swallowed by children, or such substances as vomited matter, mucus, or even water, which, by entering the windpipe instead of the esophagus, can block the air passages or cause reflex closing of the epiglottis. Swelling of the vocal cords or "swallowing" of the tongue by an unconscious person may also cause obstruction. Acute epiglottitis in adults or children can cause acute obstruction and even prove fatal.

A not uncommon type of respiratory obstruction has been brought to light by a study of sudden deaths in restaurants, which shows that many such deaths result from blockage of the nasopharynx or trachea by a chunk of food. Such attacks have been given the very apt descriptive name of "café coronary" or "backyard barbecue syndrome."

What happens is that the victim simply chokes on too large a piece of food which he could not swallow and which partially or completely blocks his air intake. It is noteworthy that in all of the cases reported, the piece of food found to be blocking the pharynx was of large size. Gastroesophageal reflux may also cause choking.

In many cases, the amount of alcohol found in the patient's bloodstream is substantial, in addition to which the victim is usually in a high state of enjoyment so that he does not realize how much food he actually has put into his mouth. On the other hand, in older people with dentures, it is often very hard for them to chew properly, so that too large a chunk can easily get down into the throat and stick there.

However, the odd part of the "café coronary" syndrome is that the classical symptoms of respiratory obstruction are often not present. The individual may just suddenly cease to eat and talk; this, for the moment, does not particularly alarm anyone because there is no other evidence of acute distress. Shortly, however, he collapses and is presumed by those present to have suffered a "heart attack."

Since in these cases the bolus of food is firmly lodged in a position where it can be neither seen nor felt and would be almost impossible to remove by any immediately available mechanical means, the only means of saving life in a situation like this is to make an opening into the windpipe surgically, a procedure which is known as tracheotomy. This has been done on occasion under the most dramatic circumstances, using a penknife or similar instrument for the purpose. It is a relatively simple procedure, but the important point is to know when it is indicated and to have the technical competence and courage to carry it out, even under the most adverse circumstances.

Some physicians carry on their persons at all times a large intravenous needle, or trocar. Under emergency conditions, this can be very easily and with little or no danger inserted into the trachea just below the larynx or "voice box." This simple and effective method, known as a *medical tracheotomy*, provides enough air to support survival without the necessity of performing a "surgical tracheotomy" on the spot.

Unfortunately, "café coronaries" are not medical rarities either in restaurants or in the home. It has been said that the condition is the sixth largest cause of accidental death in the United States. Sudden collapse of the middle-aged or older person who grasps his throat while eating should alert one to the possibility of a chunk of food being stuck in the larynx.

The difficulty is especially likely to occur in those with poor, incomplete, or ill-fitting dentures, or in those in whom a number of teeth are missing, thus making chewing difficult. In addition, there would appear to be a degree of correlation with the frequency with which intoxicating quantities of alcohol are found in "café coronary" victims. However it is important to note that at least one-quarter of choking victims are children, who have swallowed toys or other objects.

In a Special Communication to the Journal of the American Medical Association, Dr. Henry J. Heimlich has described a maneuver which will frequently disgorge the offending object within the fatal 4 minutes before the patient sustains permanent brain damage from lack of oxygen. It requires no instruments. The procedure as described by Heimlich is as follows:

A person is observed to be in distress, which he signals with hand to neck, meaning "I am choking" (Fig. 4-1A). The rescuer grasps him from behind, making a fist with one hand and clasping it with the other hand so that the fist lies thumb side against the victim's upper abdomen. The fist is then pressed sharply into the abdomen just below the sternum (Fig. 4-1B), with a quick upward thrust. This maneuver can be repeated several times if necessary. If the victim is sitting, the rescuer simply stands or kneels behind his chair and follows the same procedure.

Sometimes the victim will be found lying on his back. In that case, the rescuer faces the victim, astride his hips, again

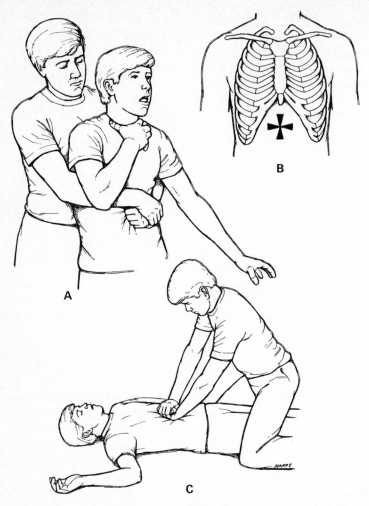

Fig. 4-1. The Heimlich maneuver. (A) As quickly as the victim signals distress, the rescuer grasps him from behind. (B) the rescuer's fist should be pressed into the upper abdomen at the spot marked by the cross. (C) Correct position of rescuer when patient is found lying face up. Note the placement of the hand, which permits a quick upward thrust.

following essentially the same procedure outlined above, pressing with a quick upward thrust on the upper part of the abdomen with the heel of one hand, instead of a fist, but using both hands to exert adequate pressure (Fig. 4-1C). This position is also valuable for the small or weak rescuer, who can use the weight of his torso to apply the thrust of the Heimlich maneuver.

The Heimlich maneuver has proved successful in saving many lives. Rarely, injuries to the abdominal viscera have been reported but were the result of improper application of the various steps.

One other problem is that the maneuver might be used inadvertently by the untutored in emergencies that may simulate choking, such as epileptic seizures, heart attacks, including angina pectoris, or simple fainting. In each of these situations, however, the victim can breathe; therefore, the differential diagnosis is obvious.

At any rate, there is little question at this point that, in spite of potential hazards, many people are alive because of this simple procedure.

Symptoms of Respiratory Obstruction

Signs of acute respiratory obstruction are usually easily recognized: There is a great effort on the part of the victim to breathe in, his head is thrown back, his eyes bulge, and his face becomes a mottled bluish red. If there is only partial obstruction, some air may be felt or heard coming from the victim's mouth, but, if there is complete obstruction, no air can be felt entering or leaving. In the attempt to breathe, the abdomen bulges out as the diaphragm contracts downward, but the lower chest and the depression above the collarbone, instead of expanding, are sucked in by the vacuum created by the great effort. When this occurs, *the person is in the gravest danger.* Try quickly to determine what is causing the difficulty in breathing, so that the proper corrective measures can be taken.

General Procedures

Respiratory obstruction must be relieved at once and followed immediately with artificial respiration if breathing has ceased or is so irregular as to be ineffectual. General procedures for immediate measures and emergency care follow.

Foreign Bodies. No attempt should be made to remove pieces of food or other objects with the fingers unless it is certain that they can be reached and hooked out *without pushing them further into the air passages* (see page 111).

In many instances the victim himself can be encouraged to expel the foreign substance by an explosive expiratory effort, with the head lower than the rest of the body, assisted, if necessary, by the Heimlich maneuver. If this effort is not immediately successful, the jaw should be extended so as to provide maximum freedom of the airway in an attempt to at least partially relieve the obstruction. The victim may then be able to expel the foreign material. At the same time the mouth should be freed of mucus or other secretions by wiping with a handkerchief- or gauze-covered finger, and other foreign objects such as false teeth removed.

If obstruction still persists, mouth-to-mouth *aspiration*, the reverse of mouth-to-mouth resuscitation, should be tried. This is a new concept which seeks to supplement the victim's expiratory forces, if any, by the rather strong negative pressure or suction that the rescuer can himself create by strongly sucking in on direct mouth-to-mouth contact, rather than breathing out as in conventional resuscitation. This may be just enough to dislodge the obstruction.

These steps can all be covered in about 30 seconds or less

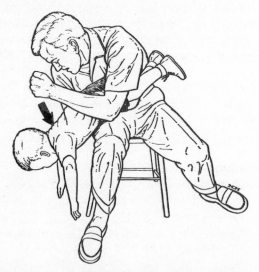

Fig. 4-2. Ejecting a foreign body stuck in child's windpipe by a sharp blow between the shoulder blades.

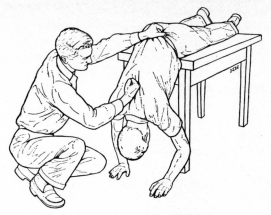

Fig. 4-3. Ejecting a foreign body from windpipe of an adult too heavy to hold. Place him on a table and strike very sharply between the shoulder blades with the fist.

but, if they obviously do not prove fruitful and the Heimlich maneuver has not been attempted or has failed, more drastic steps must be taken. Efforts should, of course, have been made in the meantime to procure medical assistance, but until this becomes available there is one time-honored step (short of tracheotomy still available:

If the victim is a child, hold him upside down by his legs and strike one or more hard, sharp blows on his back between the shoulder blades. This often will tend to cause the air trapped in the lungs to act as a ram and force the object out (Fig. 4-2).

If the victim is an adult or is too heavy to hold, place him on a bed or table, face down, with his entire body above the waist hanging over the side, and strike sharply between his shoulder blades. In most cases this will dislodge the obstruction (Fig. 4-3). Some objection has been raised to this procedure on the grounds that a sharp blow may create a negative pressure in the lungs, which might suck the obstructing object further into the windpipe. The important point is, however, that the victim is already *in extremis*—other measures having thus far failed—and this next most drastic step must now be taken regardless of the possibility of what probably is a small risk.

If the object is not dislodged, start mouth-to-mouth respiration (see page 123), making sure that the jaw and the head are in the maximally extended position, in the hope of getting some air past the obstruction. If these measures fail, the only recourse is to make an opening in the windpipe (tracheotomy), so that air can get into the lungs until the object can be extracted. Hopefully a physician will have arrived or the victim can be gotten to a hospital in time.

Vomited Matter and Mucus. Respiratory obstruction may occur in an unconscious person who cannot properly expel vomited matter or in whom a large amount of mucus has accumulated in the respiratory tract. Such obstructions can be greatly relieved or prevented by turning the patient on his side, with his head lower than his body, and with the fingers at the angle of the jaw, jutting it forward, so that the tongue cannot block the opening of the windpipe and the most maximally patent airway is obtained. If aspirating equipment is available, as it usually is if a first-aid or ambulance squad is in attendance, every effort should be made to remove the obstructing fluids or food particles from the accessible parts of the respiratory tract.

Swelling of Vocal Cords (Laryngeal edema). Obstruction caused by swelling of the vocal cords can be treated only by competent medical personnel. Get the victim to a hospital or doctor immediately, as this is a very dangerous situation. That it may occur in severely allergic persons, particularly those sensitive to beestings or to certain foods, should be realized. *Do not wait for the condition to develop to the danger point, but obtain medical aid quickly. Medical measures are available to counteract extreme sensitivity reactions, but treatment should be started promptly.*

Many individuals who know that they are highly sensitive to insect stings carry kits containing special drugs with them at all times in case of emergency. An ounce of prevention is worth a pound of cure!

Drowning. Drowning ranks as the fourth most common cause of accidental death in the United States—about 7,000 cases per year; the number of survivors from near drowning is not known.

Most people think that a victim dies of drowning because his lungs are full of water and it makes little difference whether he has drowned in salt water or fresh water. Neither of these beliefs is entirely correct.

Studies have shown that when an individual can no longer

keep himself afloat and begins to submerge, the urge to breathe becomes so great that he can no longer hold his breath, and there occurs a series of involuntary spasmodic swallowing movements and a certain amount of water is drawn down his "Sunday throat," so to speak; this causes a spasm of the larynx and he chokes and gasps.   As the victim becomes unconscious due to lack of oxygen, this spasm relaxes as he loses consciousness, and he is unable to prevent further intake of substantial quantities of water into his lungs and into his stomach.   In addition to efforts at cardiopulmonary resuscitation, the Heimlich maneuver may aid substantially in emptying the stomach of water.

But in about 10 to 15 percent of the cases, spasm of the larynx prevents any large intake of water into the lungs, and these individuals die of true asphyxia without any significant quantity of water being present in the lungs.   In the remainder of victims, the asphyxia ultimately causes the laryngospasm to relax and the lungs do, in fact, become partially flooded with water.

Subsequent events depend upon whether the water taken into the lungs is fresh or salt.   In the case of fresh water drowning, there is an enormous absorption of water directly through the thin capillary walls of the lungs into the bloodstream.   The dilution of the blood can quickly become so great that the red blood cells themselves are destroyed and the delicate and critical relationships between vital chemical elements in the blood are thrown into imbalance.   This disturbance of chemical balance is so great that the heart itself is affected and goes into ventricular fibrillation, a state in which it can no longer contract properly and therefore pump blood effectively. It is now believed that ventricular fibrillation is probably the most frequent cause of death in fresh water drowning.

In salt water drowning, on the other hand, the salt content of the water is in such excess in comparison to that of the blood as to attract fluid from the bloodstream into the lungs. This reverse flow may be so great that as much as one quarter of the victim's total blood volume may be lost into his lungs. In effect, the patient drowns in his own fluids as much as in the sea water itself.   Death in cases of salt water drowning, when it occurs immediately, may be the result of either severe shock or actual blocking of the alveoli of the lungs with water. Delayed deaths after apparent survival are not infrequent.

They are due either to the continued water-logged condition of the lungs—a situation which is known technically as pulmonary edema—or to some intervening complication such as bronchopneumonia.

While pulmonary edema and anoxia (insufficient oxygen in the blood) occur in both fresh and salt water drowning and may take place anywhere from 1 to 2 minutes after rescue, or up to 48 hours after restoration of apparently normal respiration, the severity of pulmonary edema is much greater in salt, than in fresh water drowning.

Nevertheless, the immediate critical factor is not the amount of water in the lungs at the time of rescue; the prime factor is the absolute necessity of restoring oxygen to the bloodstream to survival levels and reestablishing adequate cardiac circulation.

○ TREATMENT

As soon as a drowning victim is removed from the water, he should be prepared to receive artificial respiration, preferably by the mouth-to-mouth or mouth-to-airway method (see pages 123 and 128).   If it is possible to begin mouth-to-mouth resuscitation even before the victim has been removed from the water, this should be done.   The objective is to get air into the victim's lungs with the least possible delay.

As soon as a rescue squad arrives, resuscitation should be switched to artificial ventilation with oxygen in order to achieve a more favorable respiratory exchange.   If no heart beat or pulse can be discerned, supplemental cardiac massage should be initiated.

In any case in which the victim shows some signs of spontaneous breathing at the time of rescue and there is an adequate heart beat, survival is likely, irrespective of immediate resuscitative efforts.   However, when respiratory movement is absent, efforts to remove water from the lungs are only a waste of time.   Mouth-to-mouth resuscitation should be started immediately.

The long-held idea that the older methods of artificial respiration are of value in expelling water from the lungs, as an essential feature of resuscitating a drowning victim, is erroneous.   Compared to the ability of the mouth-to-mouth method to increase the oxygen level of the blood quickly, they are inadequate, and there is little point in trying to empty the lungs (or stomach) until respiration and circulation have been restored.

Any drowning victim should be hospitalized regardless of his apparent recovery at the scene of rescue. Delayed complications are common, and complicated medical procedures, including the use of 100 percent oxygen for considerable periods, corticosteroids to reduce pulmonary inflammation, and other supportive measures may be necessary to prevent delayed death.

Caution. At this point a word of caution is in order to even the most expert swimmers. A person swimming under water may lose consciousness without any warning that anything is going wrong or that he may be in trouble. Often he will have gone through a series of deep breathing exercises prior to diving in, in order to increase the oxygen content of his blood and prolong the time he can stay under water. A number of instances of well-trained individuals attempting to cover considerable distances under water have been observed in distress in swimming pools where prompt rescue was possible. Almost without exception the victims said they felt wonderful and as if they could have gone on "forever," with no hint they were going to black out. Upon recovery, there was complete amnesia for events immediately preceding their blacking out. If a rescuer had not been present, they would invariably have drowned.

Never swim alone under water or try to stretch the distance or time under water to the point where any undue strain is put upon your physical limitations or capabilities.

CESSATION OF BREATHING

Many conditions, such as the bulbar type of poliomyelitis, concussion of the brain, fracture of the skull, or certain types of neck fractures, may entirely stop respiration. Described briefly are other important agents and conditions which may cause cessation of breathing and which should be considered when the cause is not otherwise obvious.

Drugs. Certain drugs produce extremely slow or faint breathing or cessation of breathing. These drugs include almost *all* the sleeping pills, the principal offenders being the barbiturates, heroin, morphine, and other narcotics.

Electric Shock. Electric shock, as a result of contact with powerful electric circuits or of being struck by lightning, is an important cause of respiratory paralysis. Reestablishment of breathing by artificial respiration is most urgent if the victim's life is to be saved (see page 121 for methods).

Lack of Oxygen in Air. Respiratory paralysis may be caused by too low a concentration of oxygen in the environmental air, such as is found in deep wells, long-unused tanks, or any confined space where the atmosphere has been stagnant for long periods of time. The respiratory failure produced under these conditions comes on so quickly that a person simply suddenly stops breathing.

This type of accident can be avoided by taking the time and precaution to ventilate such places thoroughly before entering, and to have a rope about the person entering the area so that he may be quickly rescued.

For similar reasons, plastic bags should not be left within the reach of small children, nor should refrigerators be discarded with the doors left on their hinges, since these are frequently implicated in accidents to children who become trapped inside and die because of lack of air.

If an accident resulting in cessation of breathing should occur from any cause, the victim should be given *artificial respiration at once.*

Heart Disease. Certain forms of heart disease, particularly acute heart failure as well as other conditions such as emphysema or severe asthma, bring about a serious impairment of respiratory exchange. Such a situation is best handled by the administration of oxygen by a resuscitator or by placing the victim in an oxygen tent. However, if such equipment is not available, and the impairment is such as to jeopardize life, proceed with artificial respiration, preferably the mouth-to-mouth or mouth-to-airway method; if the heart has stopped, apply external cardiac massage (see page 135).

Toxic Gases. About 1,500 deaths occur each year as the result of gas poisoning which produces cessation of breathing by a direct poisoning effect on the respiratory center or by preventing the red blood cells from picking up oxygen. Such gases are not only encountered in mining, oil drilling, and similar industries, but also, occasionally, in the home. Among the common toxic gases are sulfur dioxide, methane, the oxides of nitrogen, ammonia, hydrogen sulfide, and hydrogen cyanide; and (most commonly) carbon monoxide.

Mechanical Interference with Respiration. Interference with respiration may occur when a person is buried beneath a pile of debris in such a way as to make it impossible for him to use the muscles of his chest or abdomen effectively enough to maintain an adequate amount of oxygen in his blood. As a result, there will be an insufficient supply of oxygen to the brain, and respiratory effort will cease within a few minutes.

A similar situation may arise when an adult, in seeking to protect a child from injury, throws his body across the child's. Because of the weight of the adult's body the child may be prevented from breathing. Under the stress of excitement, the child's condition could go unrecognized until too late.

In either case, *immediate treatment consists of artificial respiration.*

ARTIFICIAL RESPIRATION

Artificial respiration, or the restoration of breathing, encompasses several methods, but, basically, it is accomplished by forcing air in and out of a person's lungs and thus stimulating as nearly as possible the action of the respiratory muscles. This is done either by manual compression of the chest wall or by breathing directly into the person's mouth, with his nose held shut, or into the nose itself.

When to Use Artificial Respiration

Artificial respiration should be used when breathing has stopped or is so irregular and shallow as to be ineffective. Often the heart will continue to beat, however feebly, for many minutes after there is no apparent breathing. But it is important to remember that during this brief period of time it is often possible to save a life. Seconds count, and nothing must delay or interfere with getting air into the victim's lungs as quickly as possible. Therefore, *no more than 10 seconds* should be spent in preparing the person for artificial respiration.

General Procedures

Place the victim with his head slightly lower than the rest of his body, and start artificial respiration. An assistant should perform the following steps, working as quickly as possible, in the order listed:

1 Free the victim's mouth and upper respiratory tract of all foreign material, such as chewing gum and false teeth.

2 Delegate someone to call a doctor and first-aid squad.

3 Keep the victim's jaw and head fully extended so as to keep the air passages as free and clear as possible. If there is a discharge of water, stomach contents, or mucus from the nose or mouth, turn head to one side and clean mouth with a finger wrapped in gauze or a handkerchief.

4 Loosen tight clothing; if the victim's clothes are wet, remove as many of them as can be done without delaying artificial respiration.

5 Cover the victim with blankets or with anything else at hand, to conserve body warmth. Get a blanket *under* him if possible; even newspapers are better than nothing.

6 Look at the victim's neck to see if there is a surgically made opening into his windpipe. If there is such an opening, the victim is a laryngectomee, or a "neck breather," and treatment should proceed as directed on page 148.

7 Begin resuscitation immediately and continue, *without interruption for any reason whatsoever* except to switch to oxygen when this becomes available, until the victim is again breathing normally or until he has been pronounced dead by a physician.

Recovery Period

The onset of breathing is often preceded by slight twitching movements of the fingers, followed by a sigh-like catching of the breath. This is a good sign, but continue with artificial respiration until regular breathing has been reestablished. Then stand by and be ready to start again at a second's notice, as sometimes the victim will stop breathing and must again receive aid.

When breathing is well established and it is certain that the person is *fully conscious,* give him a teaspoonful of aromatic spirits of ammonia in a glass of cool water, some hot coffee, or tea. Do not allow the victim to stand or sit up, but his head may be raised a little to help in taking liquids. As he may not yet be able to swallow well, he should be fed with a teaspoon until he is able to drink by himself without choking.

Until recovery is complete, the case should be handled as one of potential shock, as delayed pulmonary edema may occur; the victim should be seen by a physician and removed to a hospital, where adequate facilities for observation and further treatment are available.

METHODS OF ARTIFICIAL RESPIRATION

There are several methods of artificial respiration, each of which has advantages and disadvantages. Three, which have been found to be particularly useful and effective, are the mouth-to-mouth or mouth-to-airway method, the modified Silvester method, and the Holger Nielsen method.

Of these three methods, the first is the most effective from the standpoint of getting air into the victim's lungs and reestablishing normal respiration and has therefore widely been accepted as the method of choice. It should not be used, however, in cases of fractured jaw or acute contagious disease. It is, therefore, important to know how to use either the modified Silvester method, if the injuries are such that the victim *cannot* be turned face down or if there is a severe back injury, or the Holger Nielsen method if the victim's arms are not injured and he *can* be turned face down. For these reasons and because of the various conditions that might be encountered in the event of a mass disaster, detailed instructions follow for each of these methods. Use the method which will be most effective under the circumstances.

Mouth-to-mouth Method

Mouth-to-mouth resuscitation is a method of artificial ventilation by which the *rescuer's breath* is forced directly into the victim's lungs. It is by far the most quickly applied and effective method for reviving a person who is breathing poorly or not at all, and best of all, no equipment is needed. It is the most practical and efficient emergency method for getting oxygen into an individual *of any age* and is more effective than manual methods because the rescuer can (1) keep the victim's air passage open and easily detect and correct an obstruction (the tongue or foreign matter); (2) provide pressure to inflate the victim's lungs *immediately;* (3) move a much greater amount of air into the victim's lungs than with other methods of artificial respiration; (4) watch the victim's chest to see if it rises and falls properly; (5) listen at the victim's nose and mouth to hear if air exchange is actually taking place; and (6) breathe for the victim during transportation to a hospital or physician's office.

The key to obtaining successful results from the mouth-to-mouth method is an open air passage. The best way to do this is by keeping the victim's head tilted back and his jaw pulled upward. For those who have not had advanced training, the easiest method of obtaining neck extension is to put a thick support under the victim's shoulders and let his head drop gently backwards to the ground. However, the latest recommended method is as follows:

1 Keep air passage open by tilting the victim's head back and pulling his jaw up. The best position is with your right or left hand under the neck and your other hand on the forehead, ready to pinch the nostrils closed and force the neck into extension so as to aid in opening the airway. Further extension can be obtained by placing a support under the victim's shoulders.

2 Get air into victim's lungs without delay.

3 Be sure the air you are blowing in does not leak out of the victim's nose or from around his mouth instead of actually getting into victim's lungs.

4 Blow vigorously into adults, *gently into children.*

Do These Things Step by Step:

Step 1: Prepare victim for mouth-to-mouth resuscitation.

a Place victim on his back (face up).

b If foreign matter is visible at his mouth, turn his head to one side, force his mouth open and wipe mouth and throat with your fingers covered with handkerchief, cloth, or gauze if available. Remove false teeth, chewing gum, or any other foreign object from the victim's mouth (Fig. 4-4). (If it is tightly closed, insert your index finger between his cheek and teeth; wedge it behind the *back teeth* and pry his jaw open.)

Step 2: Tilt victim's head way back—pull jaw up.

a With both hands just in front of the victim's ear lobes, tilt his head back as far as you can and pull jaw upward so that it juts out and the lower teeth are in front of upper ones (Fig. 4-5).

b (If it is easier for you, use this alternative method.) Tilt the

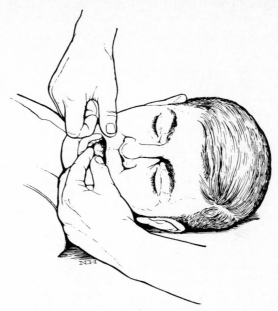

Fig. 4-4. Before starting artificial respiration, take time to clear the mouth and throat. To do this turn the victim's head to one side, force his mouth open, wipe it clean with your fingers or a piece of cloth, and remove his false teeth or other foreign bodies.

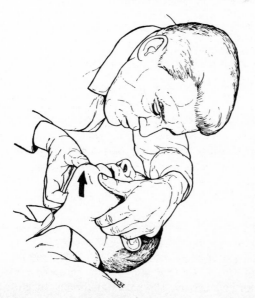

Fig. 4-5. To keep the windpipe straight and assure a free airway, pull up on the victim's jaws so as to pull the head backward as far as possible; at the same time, force the jaw open with your thumbs. Place yourself behind or to one side, ready for the next step.

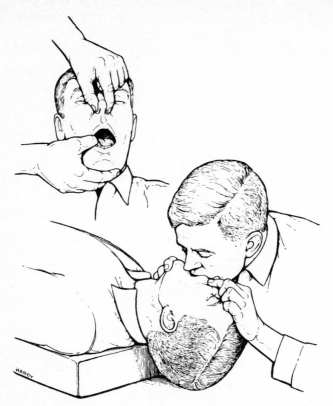

Fig. 4-6. For direct mouth-to-mouth resuscitation in adults, insert the thumb of one hand between the victim's teeth. Hold his jaw upward so that the head is tilted backward. Close his nostrils with your other hand; take a deep breath and place your mouth tightly over victim's mouth and your own thumb; blow forcefully enough to make his chest move; then take your mouth away to let him exhale passively. Repeat inflations about 12 times a minute.

victim's head way back, insert your left thumb into corner of his mouth and between his teeth, grasp his lower jaw firmly, lift it upward, and pinch his nostrils together with your right hand (Fig. 4-6).

Step 3: Prevent air leakage.

a   Open the victim's mouth or push lower lip down with your thumbs.

b   Take a deep breath.

c   Open *your* mouth wide and place it tightly over the victim's mouth, while pressing firmly with your cheek against the victim's nostrils to prevent air leakage (Fig. 4-7A). If

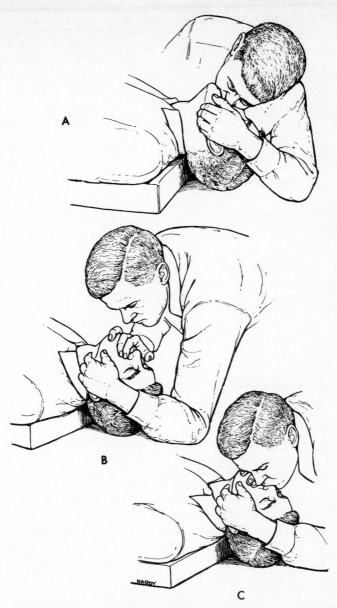

Fig. 4-7. (A) When the two-handed jaw lift is used, place your mouth tightly against the victim's; at the same time press his lower lip downward and close his nostrils with your cheek. In this way adequate air can be blown through the clenched teeth. (B) Correct position for mouth-to-nose resuscitation, used when injuries make mouth-to-mouth resuscitation impractical. (C) Mouth is clasped tightly over victim's nose and air forced in by rescuer.

necessary you can blow your breath through the victim's clenched teeth, or you can close victim's mouth and blow into his nose.

Step 4: Blow your breath into the victim's mouth.

a   Blow *forcefully* into the mouth or nose of an adult (Fig. 4-7*B* and *C*), but *gently* into the mouth *and* nose of an infant or small child.

b   Use puffs from your cheeks for children under 3 years of age.

c   Force breath 4 times very quickly in order to get at least a little oxygen into the victim's lungs. When you see his chest rise, take your mouth off his and let the victim exhale by the natural contraction of his own chest muscles. (If the chest does not rise, increase the head-back, chin-up position and blow into his mouth again, deeply.) Listen for the return rush of his breath.

d   When the victim's exhalation is complete, blow in the next deep breath. Repeat inhalations every 4 or 5 seconds, or 12 times a minute.

Breaths twice as large as normal should be blown into the victim. Start rapidly at first, then slow down to roughly 12 times a minute. To avoid becoming fatigued because of nervous tension, keep the muscles of your hands and back relaxed. Don't be fooled by the "apparent" breathing of the victim. Movements of the victim's chest and abdomen may occur even though no air is actually getting into his lungs. This is usually due to complete blockage of the air passage, either by inadequate head tilt or by the presence of foreign matter. Listen closely or feel for breath with your fingers to ascertain that the victim is really breathing. Inflation of the stomach may occur if the air passage is blocked by improper support of the head or if the blowing is too forceful. If the victim's stomach is seen to bulge, stop blowing momentarily, and press on the area, between the naval and breastbone, with your hand. This causes the air to be expelled, or burped. If this makes the victim vomit, his mouth and throat should be cleaned at once.

Remain at the victim's head during transportation to a hospital, in order to resume mouth-to-mouth resuscitation if the victim stops breathing.

Mouth-to-airway Modification. There is available a specially designed airway made of plastic (known as the approved Safar or "S" airway), which overcomes the distasteful features of the direct mouth-to-mouth method. It is designed to make mouth-to-mouth resuscitation easier and even more effective. The airway provides a mouthpiece for the rescuer and a breathing tube for the victim that helps to keep his air passage open.

It is easily carried in a pocket, glove compartment, or bag and is now available in most first-aid kits. This type of airway is effective for use by trained personnel especially in (1) reviving unconscious, *nonbreathing* victims of drowning; electric shock; smoke or gas inhalation; drug or chemical poisoning; and cardiac arrest; and (2) helping to prevent asphyxia by maintaining an open air passage in victims who are unconscious but still *breathing*. The airway is helpful also when administering external cardiac massage (see page 138).

This type of device is used as follows:

Step 1: Clean the victim's throat of foreign matter only if necessary (otherwise, start with Step 2).
   a Place the victim on his back.
   b If foreign matter is visible at his mouth, turn his head to one side, force his mouth open, and wipe clean.

Step 2: Insert the airway.
   a Take a position behind the victim's head.
   b With his head tilted back, insert the airway over the victim's tongue until the flange rests upon his lips (Fig. 4-8A).
   c If his mouth is tightly closed, wedge it open by inserting your index finger between the cheek and teeth, behind the wisdom teeth.
   d Make certain the tongue is not pushed back into the victim's throat. If necessary, hold it forward with your fingers while inserting the tube.
   e If the victim is an adult, insert the long end of the tube. But if the victim is a child over 3 years of age, insert the tube with the flange inverted toward the short end, to cup the child's mouth snugly.

Do not use this tube in children under 3 years of age. Use direct mouth-to-mouth breathing or the pediatric airway designed especially for infants and children.

Step 3: Hold the victim's chin upward, keep his head tilted back so that the front of the neck is stretched, and prevent air leakage.
Pinch the victim's nose with your thumbs and press the flange over his lips with your index fingers, to prevent air leakage. Hold his chin upward and toward the rescuer with the rest of the fingers (Fig. 4-8B).
Never let the chin sag.

Step 4: Take a deep breath and blow into the mouthpiece of the tube (Fig. 4-8C).

If the victim is an adult, blow forcefully; if a child blow gently.

a   When the victim's chest moves, take your mouth off the tube and let the victim exhale by himself.

b   When his exhalation is complete, blow in the next deep breath. The first few breaths you blow must be deep and at a rapid rate; thereafter, about one breath every 4 or 5 seconds is adequate.

c   If the victim's chest does not move, increase the angle of chin-up position, improve the position of your fingers, and blow into the tube more forcefully. If the chest still does not move, readjust the position of the tube, which may have been inserted too deeply or not deeply enough. Make sure the flange is resting firmly against the victim's lips so that there is no air leak and so that the nostrils are held firmly closed.

To assist shallow, natural breathing, blow in at the moment when the victim inhales and take your mouth off quickly when he exhales.

Modified Silvester Method

The Silvester, or chest pressure–arm lift method (with the victim on his back and some support under his shoulders), allows for a slightly better air exchange than the push-pull methods (with the victim in the face-down, or prone, position). However, with the victim lying on his back, there is danger of his choking on vomitus, blood, or mucus. This hazard can be reduced by keeping his head tilted backward, turned to one side, and a little lower than his body.

The Silvester method is particularly useful in contaminated

Fig. 4-8.   (A) Take a position at the top of the victim's head. With his head tilted back insert the airway over his tongue until the flange rests upon his lips. If the victim is an adult, insert the long end of the tube; if he is a child over 3 years of age, insert the short end. (For children, the flange should be inverted toward the short end to cup the child's mouth snugly.)   (B) Pinch victim's nose with your thumbs and press the flange over his lips with your index fingers to prevent air leakage. Hold his chin upward and toward you with your remaining fingers. *Never let his chin sag.*   (C) Take a deep breath and blow into the mouthpiece of the tube. *For an adult blow forcefully; for a child blow gently.* Watch the victim's chest. When it moves, take your mouth off the tube and let the victim exhale passively. When his exhalation is finished, blow in the next deep breath. The first few breaths you blow must be deep and at a rapid rate; thereafter, about one breath every 4 or 5 seconds is adequate.

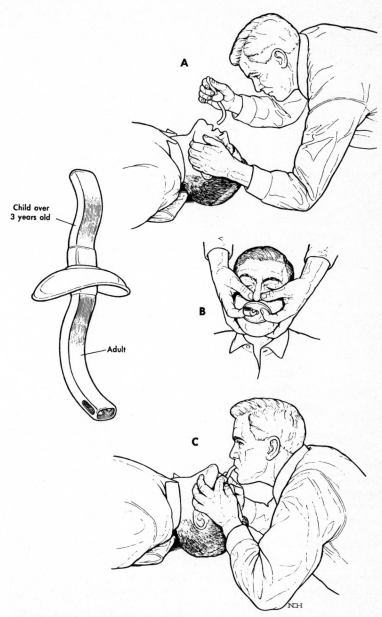

Child over
3 years old

Adult

A

B

C

Fig. 4-8.   See facing page for caption.

atmospheres such as would occur in the event of a nuclear or gas attack, or in a mine disaster, since the victim's mask could be kept on him during resuscitation.

1 Place the victim on his back with his arms folded across his chest.

2 Quickly clear his mouth by running your fingers behind his lower teeth and over the back of his tongue. If necessary and the victim is not already masked, put one on him. (If he is wearing a mask, quickly remove it, wipe away any fluids that may have collected in his mouth or in his mask, and replace the mask.)

3 Place a rolled blanket or a similar support under his shoulders so that his head will fall backward, but do not waste time looking for these materials. Tilt his head back so that the neck is stretched and the head is in the chin-up position with the jaw fully extended so as to gain the best possible airway. Keep his head in this position, so that the air passages do not become blocked by "kinking" or pressure.

4 Kneel behind the victim's head, placing your knee at one side of it and the opposite foot on the other side.

5 Take the victim's arms just above his wrists and place them over his lower ribs (Fig. 4-9A). Rock forward and exert steady, uniform pressure almost directly downward until you meet firm resistance (Fig. 4-9B). This pressure forces air out of his lungs.

6 Move his arms slowly outward, away from his body, and upward above his head. Continue this motion of his arms and sweep them above his head and backward as far as possible (Fig. 4-9C). Be sure to keep his arms straight throughout this maneuver as you raise them first vertically upward and then above his head. This expands his chest and draws air into his lungs.

7 Slowly bring his arms back to his chest, and repeat the complete cycle, starting with procedure 5.

8 Repeat the cycle 10 to 12 times per minute, at a steady, uniform rate, to the rhythm: Press, lift, stretch, release. Give longer and equal counts to "press," "lift," and "stretch" and make the count for "release" as short as possible.

When one knee becomes tired or uncomfortable, quickly switch to the other one. If it is more comfortable for you, kneel on both knees, although the forward and backward motion is easiest to obtain while kneeling on one knee only.

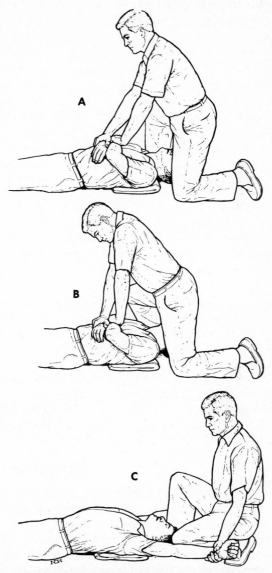

Fig. 4-9. Basic steps in chest pressure-arm lift method of artificial respiration (modified Silvester). (A) Proper position. (B) Pressure exerted on chest (exhalation phase). (C) Pressure released and arms extended (inhalation phase). Repeat cycle (B) and (C) 12 times per minute.

When a relief operator is available, he may take over with practically no break in the rhythm. This can be done by the first operator moving to one side while the second one comes in from the other side. When the second operator is ready, the victim's arms are released to him during the "stretch" count, and he continues in the same rhythm.

Be sure to keep the air passages clear of fluid and other obstructions. If this method is being used under conditions requiring a mask, remove the mask for a moment to empty fluid from the facepiece as necessary. While the mask is off, quickly wipe out the mouth to clear it of fluids that might interfere with breathing, and replace the mask as quickly as possible. Keep the head tilted backward so that the neck is stretched and the head is fully extended in the chin-up position.

Holger Nielsen Method

1 Place the victim face down, with his head lower than his feet (as on a slanting beach), elbows bent, hands one on top of the other under his head, and head turned to one side so that his cheek rests on his hand (Fig. 4-10A).

2 Kneel on one or both knees, facing the victim and close enough to be comfortable when your hands are placed on his back just below his shoulder blades, with the tips of your thumbs touching and four fingers spread downward and outward (Fig. 4-10 inset).

3 *Compression phase:* Rock forward until your arms are almost vertical, so that the weight of the upper part of your body exerts slow, steady pressure on your hands and directly downward on the victim's back. This forces the air out of his lungs (Fig. 4-10B).

4 *Expansion phase:* Release the downward pressure without giving a final thrust, and rock backward slowly. As you come backward, grasp the victim's arms just above the elbows (Fig. 4-10C). Draw them toward you, applying just enough force to feel the tension of his arm, shoulder, and back muscles. During this maneuver, keep his elbows straight until the arms have been pulled as far *forward and upward* as reasonable tension will permit (Fig. 4-10D). His arms are then gently lowered to the ground, completing the expansion phase and the full respiratory cycle. Then swing back so that your hands are again on the victim's back, ready to start a new compression phase.

5 Repeat the cycle, starting with procedure 3, at a steady rate

(12 to 15 times per minute) taking about the same amount of time with each phase.

To change rescuers, the relief operator kneels on one knee beside the rescuer and the victim, facing the operator. He swings sideways in unison with the operator, picking up the rhythm. This should be done for three or four cycles.

Then, at a prearranged signal and at the end of a phase (which, with the Holger Nielsen method, is when the arms of the victim are lowered to the ground), the rescuer swings to one side and out of the way, and the relief operator, resting on one knee, swings into place, with his hands in the proper position on the back of the victim. He is now ready to swing forward in the compression phase of the cycle and to continue the treatment.

EXTERNAL CARDIAC MASSAGE

A famous surgeon once said: "Death occurs in hearts too good to die . . . often the heart needs only a second chance to beat."

Between 7,500 and 9,000 people die in the United States each year from cardiac arrest (standstill of the heart) which need only have been temporary had the proper resuscitative measures been applied quickly.

The beating of the heart may stop because of any one of many conditions which temporarily bring about a blocking of the impulses generated within the heart itself that cause it to beat. In other words, the heart stalls—much as a car stalls. Without some means of "cranking it up" again quickly, since it won't start by itself, permanent damage results and a person will die from lack of oxygen to the brain and in other tissues.

There are many causes of cardiac arrest, including pulmonary asphyxiation caused by food stuck in the throat, drowning, electrocution, pulmonary embolus, drug toxicity—particularly quinidine and digitalis—and trauma to the region of the heart. Cardiac arrest must be considered whenever a person suddenly collapses and loses consciousness, making sure that a grand mal seizure (see page 000) may not have occurred. On the spot confirmation of cardiac arrest depends on the absence of all pulses, particularly the carotid, no heart sounds, and the absence of breathing.

It used to be thought that to restart the heart it was necessary to open the chest surgically, grasp the heart with one hand, and squeeze it rhythmically to start it pumping again.

We now know that the same result can often be obtained (by any person familiar with external cardiac massage) simply by squeezing the heart rhythmically between the breastbone (sternum) and the backbone (spinal column) (Fig. 4-11*A* and *B*). This compresses the heart and forces blood into the arteries (Fig. 4-11*C*). When pressure is released, the chest expands and the heart fills with oxygenated blood, which is circulated to the tissues. To be successful, it is also essential to begin mouth-to-mouth or some other form of artificial resuscitation immediately or within 4 to 6 minutes after the heart has stopped beating. Failure to circulate oxygenated blood for a longer period of time will cause permanent damage to the brain; although the individual might survive slightly longer periods of anoxia, he would do so only in a purely vegetative state. If for any reason mouth-to-mouth or mouth-to-airway resuscitation cannot be

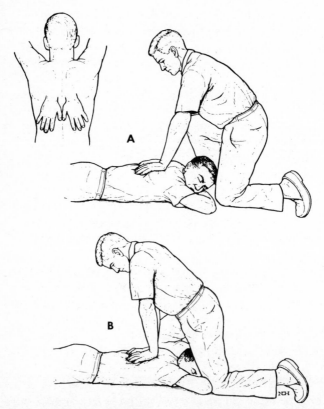

Fig. 4-10. See legend on facing page.

used, the modified Silvester method (page 130) is the one of choice, because both the rescuer and the victim are in a position to render and receive aid without wasting time.

Indications for External Cardiac Massage

By far the majority of cases of unconsciousness or cessation of breathing will not require cardiac massage. Only for those in whom the heart has stopped altogether, or is beating so faintly or so rapidly that it cannot maintain the circulation, should cardiac massage be undertaken. The best indication

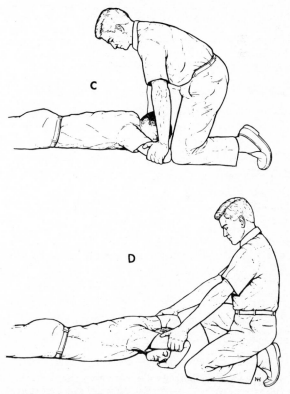

Fig. 4-10. Holger Nielsen method. (A) Correct position for starting the Holger Nielsen method of artificial respiration; insert, correct position of hands on victim's back. (B) Downward pressure starts compression phase and expels stale air from lungs. (C) End compression phase and begin expansion phase by grasping victim's elbows preparatory to pulling forward and upward. (D) The elbows are pulled firmly forward and upward to expand his chest fully and pull fresh air into his lungs. Expansion phase ends by lowering the victim's arms and returning to original position (A).

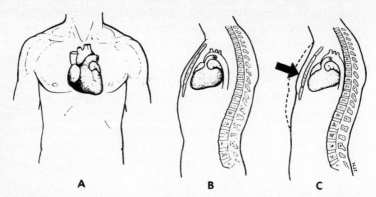

Fig. 4-11. (A) and (B) Front and side views showing position of heart in relation to breastbone. (C) Pressure on breastbone moves it inward and compresses the heart against the spinal column, forcing blood out of the heart into circulation. When pressure is released, breastbone springs back to normal position, and heart again fills with blood.

for this procedure is the absence of a carotid pulse. This is most easily located in the groove immediately to one side of the larynx. If a viable carotid pulse is present, cardiac massage should not be undertaken.

The signs and symptoms are unconsciousness, lack of breathing, no carotid, femoral or radial pulse, no heart beat, and enlarged pupils.

Procedures

To prepare for external cardiac massage, follow these procedures: (1) lay the victim down on his back on the floor or on some other firm surface; (2) stand or kneel at right angles to his chest; (3) tilt his head back and make certain that his mouth is clear and that his air passage is open; (4) blow into his lungs three times, using the mouth-to-mouth method.

For Adults. Start cardiac massage by doing the following:

1 Place the heel of one hand with the heel of the other hand on top of it, fingers parallel, on the lower third of the victim's breastbone, just above the xiphoid cartilage where the ribs join the sternum, and apply firm pressure downward about 80 times a minute so that the breastbone moves approximately 1 to 2 inches toward the spine (Fig. 4-12). A downward pressure of between 70 to 90 pounds must be exerted with the average adult. Your arms should be in a straight up and down position and you should be as close

to the victim as is compatible. Do *not* let your hands become crossed. Sometimes a "thump" with the heel of the hand, starting 8 to 10 inches above the chest, may start the heart going again.

2   After each downward pressure, relax hands completely, to permit the chest to expand. Although the chest is subjected to considerable pressure, the danger of fracturing ribs is minimized when only the heel of the hand is used, but *do not* put pressure on the ribs with your fingers. However,

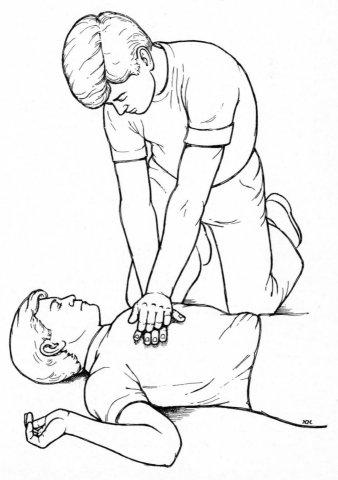

Fig. 4-12. Correct position of hands for external cardiac massage, using the heel of the hand to exert pressure on the breastbone.

don't get excited and use too much pressure, as you *can* break the ribs or actually bruise the heart muscle.

3 While you are massaging the heart, have someone give mouth-to-mouth or mouth-to-airway resuscitation (Fig. 4-13). If no one else is available, do 15 chest compressions, then stop, and give mouth-to-mouth resuscitation yourself, for 2 deep breaths.

As soon as possible, have someone notify a hospital to expect a victim of cardiac arrest, and get the patient to the hospital as quickly as possible in a vehicle such as ambulance, truck, or station wagon, so that massage and mouth-to-mouth breathing can be continued on the way. Resuscitation methods *must* be carried on until the patient is pronounced dead by a physician or until the physician has determined that the pulse

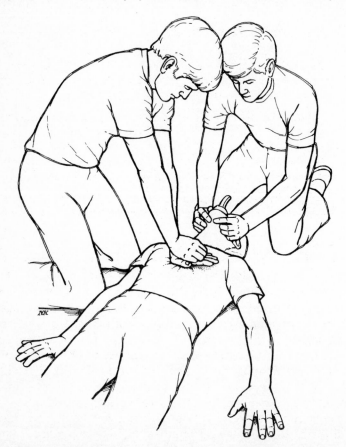

Fig. 4-13. Mouth-to-mouth or mouth-to-airway breathing should be administered along with external cardiac massage.

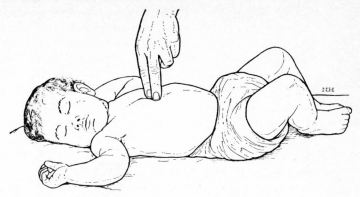

Fig. 4-14. For external cardiac massage in children, gentle pressure is exerted with tips of fingers rather than with the heel of hand.

and blood pressure are normal and that emergency resuscitation is no longer required.

For Children. The procedures for external cardiac massage are the same for children as for adults. However, much *less* pressure should be applied to the chest of a child.

1 *On babies,* apply moderate pressure, with the *tips* of the fingers only, to the center of the breastbone (Fig. 4-14). *Don't press* too hard, as in babies or young children it is easy to bruise the heart muscle.

2 *In children* 9 to 10 years old, use the force of the heel of one hand only.

3 Use mouth-to-mouth, mouth-to-nose, or mouth-to-airway resuscitation.

Signs that the method is being carried out properly are the ability to feel the carotid pulse or one in the patient's arm, wrist, or groin, with each compression of the heart, and the beginning of gasping breaths. Do not stop resuscitation, however, until released by a physician or until the patient has been admitted to the emergency room of a hospital and other treatment begun.

Remember: Mouth-to-mouth breathing is as important as external cardiac massage—one won't work without the other. But, when properly carried out, external cardiac massage has proved its effectiveness in many cases of cardiac arrest, since it provides enough circulation to maintain the heart and brain until the heart itself can resume beating. For condensed summaries of general cardiopulmonary resuscitation procedures (CPR), see Tables 4-1–4-3 and Fig. 4-15.

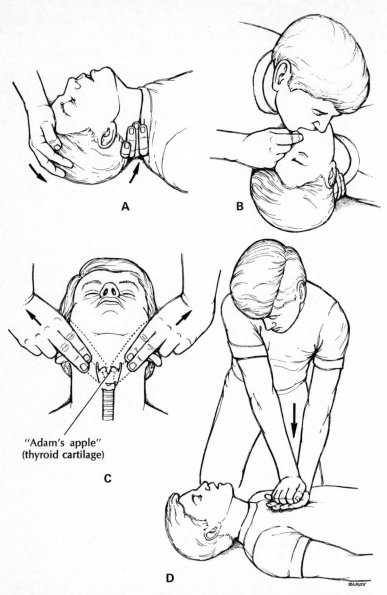

"Adam's apple"
(thyroid cartilage)

Fig. 4-15. Major steps in cardiopulmonary resuscitation. (A) Make certain
the victim has an open airway. (B) Start respiratory resuscitation immediately. (C) Feel for the carotid pulse in the groove alongside the "Adam's
apple" or thyroid cartilage. (D) If pulse is absent, begin cardiac massage.
Use 60 compressions a minute with one lung inflation after each group of
5 chest compressions.

TABLE 4-1

BASIC LIFE SUPPORT PROCEDURES INCLUDING UNWITNESSED CARDIAC ARREST (ONE OR TWO RESCUERS)*

Time Required for Preparation	What to Do First	General Procedures	Remarks
4–10 seconds	Make sure victim is unconscious and not breathing.	Turn victim face up. Shout at him to see if he responds.	Make sure victim is not suffering from some disease that does not require resuscitation (simple fainting, diabetes, coma, etc.).
7–15 seconds	Establish patent airway (Fig. 4-15A).	Place one hand under neck, other hand on forehead in order to tilt head back and extend neck.	In this way, neck can be extended and nostrils closed, and jaw jutted forward for mouth-to-mouth inflation.
10–20 seconds	Give 4 quick inflations (Fig. 4-15B).	Make sure nostrils are pinched off, neck is extended, mouth seal is tight.	Volume of each inflation should be about 800 milliliters—enough to give a quick supply of oxygen. Check chest for expansion.
15–20 seconds	Check for presence or absence of carotid pulse on each side (Fig. 4-15C).	This is most easily found in the groove just to one side of the larynx.	Time is of the essence and sometimes pulse may be weak and difficult to find.
75–90 seconds	Start cardiac pulmonary resuscitation in the ratio of 15 compressions to 2 inflations (Fig. 4-15D).	Make sure you and the victim are properly positioned and in trying to do two things at once there is no air leakage.	During compression it is particularly important that both hands and arms be correctly positioned. When there is a single rescuer, try to give 80 compressions/minute; with two rescuers, use 60.† Two very fast lung inflations are given after each 15 chest compressions.
80–100 seconds	Determine if breathing and pulse have returned.	Continue efforts, if necessary, until a satisfactory CPR function is established.	The pupil size (beginning contraction) will give a good hint of returning function.

* This material is reproduced in condensed form from the *Instructors' Manual of Basic Cardiac Life Support*, by permission of the American Heart Association.
† When two rescuers are available, one should do inflation and the other cardiac compression. Functions may be switched as fatigue requires; it is important not to get in each other's way or interfere with either rhythm. When a second rescuer arrives on the scene, the change in rhythm to 60 compressions/minute is accomplished as follows: Rescuer No. 1 says: "One-one thousand, two-one thousand, three-one thousand, four-one thousand, five-one thousand," and so on until the second person is ready. Then Rescuer No. 1 says "We switch on next breath." The inflator takes over at the count of three-one thousand and the new compressor begins and picks up the count without pause. Rescuer No. 1 then quickly checks for pulse and pupils.

TABLE 4-2

WITNESSED CARDIAC ARREST*

Time Required for Preparation	What to Do First	General Procedures	Remarks
4–10 seconds	Make sure victim is unconscious.	Turn victim gently, if necessary, face up.	If you have seen victim collapse, he may still be breathing, but be sure his airway is unobstructed.
5–12 seconds	Make sure of an open airway.	Get neck extended with right hand under neck, left hand on forehead.	Be sure you cannot feel carotid or other pulse.
11–24 seconds	If no pulse, try cardiac "thump."	Place fleshy part of fist on his chest. Raise other fist with sharp blow from 8–10 inches.	Sometimes a "thump" alone will restore cardiac function.
14–29 seconds	Give 4 quick inflations.	Be sure mouth seal is tight.	If still no pulse, begin cardiac compression.
34–55 seconds	Give 15 compressions to 2 inflations in span of 15–16 seconds.	Continue making sure to keep mouth and nose seal tight.	Even though the cardiac "thump" may not have accomplished anything [its use is discouraged by some authorities], persistent CPR may eventually restore life.

* This material is reproduced in condensed form from the *Instructors' Manual of Basic Cardiac Life Support,* by permission of the American Heart Association.

RESUSCITATING THE LARYNGECTOMEE

In the United States and throughout much of the rest of the world, there are between 40,000 to 50,000 people who, because of cancer or other disease of the vocal cords or of the surrounding area, have had to undergo surgery to save their lives. The specific operation is called *laryngectomy* and means *the surgical removal of the larynx* which is at the uppermost part of the trachea (windpipe). People who have had this operation are called *laryngectomees.* Their number increases each day.

In a laryngectomee there is no longer a connection between the mouth and the lungs (Fig. 4-16A and B), but, to enable the person to breathe, a surgical opening (stoma) is created in the lower front part of the neck and is joined to the trachea. Hence, a laryngectomee breathes, coughs, sneezes,

TABLE 4-3

INFANT RESUSCITATION*

Time Required for Preparation	What to Do First	General Procedures	Remarks
3–5 seconds	Make sure infant is unconscious.	Place infant in horizontal position.	Make sure that cardiac arrest has taken place.
6–10 seconds	Establish patent airway.	Do not overextend the neck.	Simply tilt head gently backward.
9–15 seconds	Give 4 gentle puffs into mouth.	In infants do not breathe forcefully as in adults.	Horizontal position facilitates cardiac massage, if necessary.
14–25 seconds	Determine lack of pulse.	Use carotid or precordial pulse.	Overextension of head may block airway (collapsed trachea) rather than help it.
44–55 seconds	If cardiac arrest is present, begin cycles of 5 compressions to 1 inflation.	Use 2 fingers for compression—gently—as sternum is very flexible (Fig. 4-15). Pressure is exerted about mid-sternum as in infants the heart lies higher than in adults. Danger to liver is also greater for the same reason.	In infants, rate should be 80–100 compressions per minute with rapid inflation after every 5 compressions. (This equals about 5 compressions every 3 seconds with 1 inflation every 3 seconds, i.e., 5 to 1 ratio.)

* This material is reproduced in condensed form from the *Instructors' Manual of Basic Cardiac Life Support,* by permission of the American Heart Association.

and "blows his nose" through the opening in his neck. However, food and liquid can be taken by mouth as usual.

In general, a laryngectomee can do almost everything he did before the operation; there are, however, a few exceptions. For example, because of the opening in his neck, he cannot go swimming, since there is no way to prevent water from entering his lungs, and he cannot strain to lift heavy loads, since he cannot "lock" his breath in.

His greatest loss is, of course, the ability to speak, laugh aloud, sing, or whistle, although some laryngectomees make very good efforts at doing so, especially after learning a new way of speaking; and, because he cannot breathe through his nose, he has lost the ability to smell and taste.

It is dangerous for the laryngectomee to be out in a small,

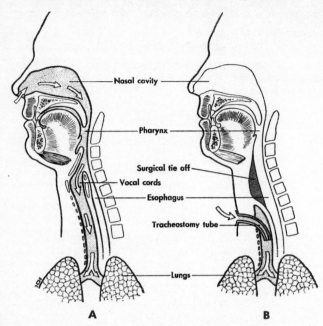

Fig. 4-16. Diagrammatic representation of normal anatomy of breathing apparatus (A), and as it is changed in the laryngectomees through loss of the larynx and the created a new opening to the outside for breathing (B).

light boat and he must always be careful when bathing. He must be extremely cautious while shaving or having a haircut. For even though he usually uses a small gauze pad or a filter of some sort to guard the stoma from dust, dirt particles, lint, hair, and small insects, foreign bodies inhaled through the stoma can be a most serious threat to his life. Because of the opening in his neck, he must be constantly aware of the risk he creates for himself, as well as the problem he poses for his rescuer, in the event of an accident which requires emergency treatment.

Most laryngectomees dress well and usually try to conceal their stoma. Hence, the possibility of an injured person being a laryngectomee—a fact which at first may not be obvious— must always be borne in mind. Laryngectomees wear bibs, often the same color as their shirts or flesh-colored, which defy detection except upon very close examination. Female laryngectomees often wear jewelry, scarves, or high-collared dresses to conceal the stoma.

As a safety precaution, prominent red stickers are available for use on the window of a car in which one or more laryngectomees may be riding, in order to alert anyone rendering first aid in the event of accident. Always check to see whether the casualty is a laryngectomee.

In some laryngectomees a *tracheostomy tube* is inserted into the opening. It is made of silver, plastic, or nylon and is kept in place by a ribbon, cord, tape, or chain which goes around the neck. The tube itself is in two parts—an outer tube and an inner tube (Fig. 4-17).

The important thing to remember is that in the event of an emergency, the tube can be removed from the stoma, pried apart, and reinserted without harm. However, timidity or delay in removing the tube *can* result in harm. Since the victim must be kept breathing to maintain life, infection or slight damage to the neck opening is of small consequence and can be attended to by a surgeon or physician later. Therefore, if the victim is not breathing or has difficulty in breathing, *remove the tube first*.

Before administering resuscitation *in any manner,* the tube *must* be taken out of the neck for two reasons: first, there may

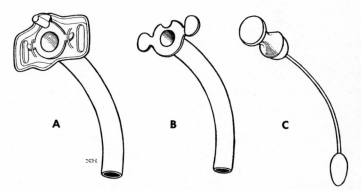

Fig. 4-17. The parts of a tracheostomy tube: (A) Outer tube. (B) Inner tube. (C) Obturator. The obturator is left inside the outer tube while it is being inserted and removed after insertion has been completed. The inner tube is then inserted in the outer tube. It is left in place for routine use except to remove periodically for cleaning.

be a blockage in the tube and there is no use wasting time looking for it; secondly, it is easier to get an airtight seal with the lips directly on the stoma than on the tube flange itself.

The tube can be cleaned with anything at hand and easily slipped back into the neck. Lubricate it, if necessary, by rolling the tube on the victim's tongue. Since the inner tube may become stuck to the other one, *remove the complete set* to avoid delay, and break or untie the tape or chain around the victim's neck. However, be certain that the tube is securely tied again after cleaning and slipping it back into the neck, for a reflex-action cough may blow it out.

○ TREATMENT

To render emergency care to a laryngectomee who is *conscious,* follow these rules:

1 Keep the victim in a seated position. If he indicates to the rescuer that he would prefer to clean out mucous secretions himself, he should be permitted to do so. He has been taught this procedure at the hospital as part of his recovery program and will probably do a much better job of it, for he will know just where the trouble spot is in the windpipe.

2 If he removes a tracheostomy tube, clean it for him. The outside of the tube can be wiped clean and the inner portion can be cleaned by forcing a twig or any other implement into it or even by blowing air through it. However, make certain that the stoma and the trachea are both free of obstruction before replacing the tube.

3 If the victim is nervous, ill at ease, or frightened, remember that an attitude of confidence will be of great assistance in treating him. Any apparent indecision on your part will only worry him all the more and make it more difficult to treat him.

4 It is a common occurrence for laryngectomees to cough up blood mixed with mucus. Unless there is excessive bleeding (not merely a smear mixed with mucus), there is no cause for immediate alarm. Keep the victim quiet and calm, and take him to a hospital emergency room or to his physician in a *seated* position. Do *not* encourage him to cough because of the mistaken belief that this will eliminate the trouble. Coughing may cause irritation of the stoma or the trachea and add to the trouble.

To render emergency care to a laryngectomee who is *unconscious,* follow these rules:

1   Keep the victim warm and on his back, with a folded blanket, coat, or similar item placed beneath his shoulders (Fig. 4-18). This will expand the chest, and in this position, the stoma is readily accessible for mouth-to-stoma resuscitation.

2   Aspirate, if necessary, by use of mechanical means or, if not obtainable, suck, by the mouth-to-stoma method. The necessity to aspirate can be ascertained by the rescuer placing his ear next to the stoma and listening for the sound of breathing.

3   After aspiration, proceed with mouth-to-stoma resuscitation. Place your mouth tightly over the stoma and blow into it (Fig. 4-19). Turn your head to the side and listen for the return of air, which will indicate exchange. Repeat the blowing and listening for as long as necessary, at the rate of about 12 times per minute.

4   In instances where mouth-to-stoma resuscitation is not feasible, either the Silvester or the Holger Nielsen method is useful and, in fact, provides the only means, short of mechanical equipment, by which one laryngectomee can aid another in the event of an accident when no one else is with them. The procedures used in both methods are the same as those for normal individuals except for the precautions which must be taken to assure that the victim does not inhale particles or other foreign matter into the stoma. One means of safeguarding against this is shown in Fig. 4-20.

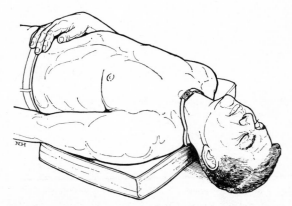

Fig. 4-18.   Correct position of laryngectomees for mouth-to-stoma resuscitation, with tracheostomy tube still in place prior to removal.

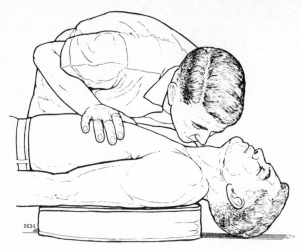

Fig. 4-19. The victim in position with tube removed, and rescuer prepared to begin direct mouth-to-stoma resuscitation.

5 As soon as possible have someone summon an ambulance, and transport the victim to a hospital while continuing artificial respiration. Mechanical resuscitation and oxygen should be substituted if the necessary equipment is available in the ambulance.

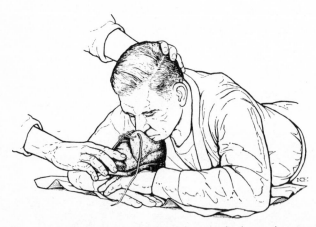

Fig. 4-20. In carrying out the Holger Nielsen method on a laryngectomee, he must be protected from sucking dust into his stoma. Place clean paper under his chest and use a shoe, as shown, to make certain his head and neck will not rotate during the procedure.

The mouth-to-stoma method has many advantages over the conventional mouth-to-mouth approach when administering artificial respiration because the victim's teeth, tongue, or nose are no hindrance, nor will the contents of the victim's stomach ever enter the mouth of the rescuer.   However, the rescuer must be sure always to keep the victim's head straight to avoid the danger of elongating or twisting the stoma.

INJURIES OF CHEST WALL WHICH MAY AFFECT BREATHING

Certain wounds of the chest, such as contusions, abrasions, and similar injuries, may affect breathing, but are not in themselves necessarily indications for artificial respiration.

Puncture Wounds

A puncture wound made by a knife, bullet, or some other sharp object often tends to close itself on the surface.   But swelling of the chest wall or the neck that is crepitant (crackling to the touch) indicates that air is leaking into the subcutaneous tissues as the result of the injury.   This is known technically as subcutaneous emphysema.

Tension Pneumothorax

When the lung becomes collapsed as the result of air leaking into the pleural space, the condition is known as tension pneumothorax, a situation which may be serious or even fatal (Fig. 4-21).

Technically, tension pneumothorax exists when the pressure in the pleural cavity equals or exceeds atmospheric pressure.   It may readily be produced by the sharp ends of fractured or crushed ribs tearing the surface of a lung and thus permitting alveolar air to enter the pleural space, or by penetrating wounds from the outside such as caused by a knife, bullet, or other missile.

The pressure within the pleural sac increases as the result of a one-way ball-type valvular mechanism created by the injury which lets air in during each inspiration but permits little or no escape during expiration.

Minor degrees of tension pneumothorax are not serious; marked tension, however, requires prompt aid, since the pressure within the pleural cavity must be relieved by surgical or other suitable means.

Symptoms. The diagnosis of tension pneumothorax is predicated upon the presence of severe chest pain, shallow rapid respiration, rapid heart rate (tachycardia), cyanosis, and extreme apprehension and anxiety. Confusingly, reflex abdominal pain also may occur.

Often the victim will be in shock, and upon inspection it will be seen that one-half of the chest shows little movement as the patient strains to breathe.

The condition may not require emergency treatment outside the hospital, but when intervention is necessary, entry to the pleural space in order to relieve the excessive pressure must be gained by whatever means are at hand. The simplest is to insert a large-caliber intravenous needle into the pleural space, which in essence creates an open pneumothorax and relieves intrapleural pressure. Even though the lung may not expand under these conditions, the dangers of mediastinal shift are largely avoided and the patient can be safely transported to a hospital.

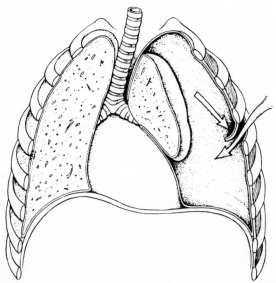

Fig. 4-21. Mechanism of tension pneumothorax. Air can enter the pleural cavity but cannot escape; pressure thus builds up and displaces the heart and great vessels to the opposite side.

Sucking Wounds

Jagged fragments, as from a high explosive shell or some other explosive source may cause a ragged, tearing type of wound which does not close or seal itself off. This creates the so-called "sucking" type of wound; it is an injury that undoubtedly would be common in the event of nuclear attack or some other kind of civil disaster, and it is frequently seen on the battlefield.

A sucking wound is probably the most serious type of chest wound because air is admitted from the outside to the space between the lungs and the chest wall (Fig. 4-22). This causes the lung on the injured side to collapse and interferes with the efficiency of the opposite lung. Air entering or being expelled from the wound creates a characteristic sucking sound which may be accompanied by a loud grunt due to closure of the glottis as the victim makes a desperate effort to breathe. All penetrating wounds of the chest wall must be considered to be sucking wounds until proved otherwise and should be treated as such.

○ TREATMENT

Apply a large thick compression dressing (saturated, if possible, with petroleum jelly to assure a tight seal) over the wound and fix it firmly in place with a cravat or heavy wide elastic bandage (Fig. 4-23). The dressing should be applied during the exhalation phase. Sucking wounds of the chest are serious emergencies; the victim should be taken to a hospital as quickly as possible. In time of civil disaster he would be given a high priority rating for further treatment.

Flail Chest. The mechanism of paradoxical movement of the chest wall (flail chest) is described and illustrated in Fig. 4-24. This condition results when there are multiple rib fractures or badly fractured sternum. It can be handled temporarily by having the victim lie on the affected side and holding him in position with sand bags or some suitable substitute. More effective, however, is the application of a wide elastic type bandage completely around the chest wall to keep it from ballooning outward and to help stabilize the diaphragm so that it can function more efficiently.

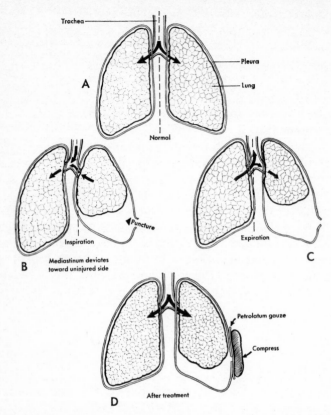

Fig. 4-22. Mechanism of sucking wound of chest. (A) Diagram showing normal relationship of lung and pleural sacs. (B) Pleura opened by missile, admitting outside air into pleural cavity. Lung collapses and is pushed over toward uninjured lung as patient breathes in. (C) When he breathes out there is a shift in the opposite direction; the pressure within the pleural cavity increases, often to the extent that the heart is unable to fill completely. (D) Covering of opening with a sturdy dressing minimizes air being sucked in through wound during inhalation and pushed out of wound during exhalation. Respiration is thus partially stabilized. Dressing should be applied, if possible, during forced expiration.

Penetrating Foreign Bodies. Foreign bodies such as a knife, stick or other object which has penetrated the chest wall should not be touched, nor should any attempt at removal be made until the victim is in the operating room, ready for surgery. If the object has penetrated the lung or is near a large blood vessel, any movement may initiate internal bleeding or fatal hemorrhage.

Secure a bulk-type dressing over the wound but around the protruding object in much the same way as for a sucking wound, but at the same time securing the missile from movement during transportation of the victim to the hospital.

The importance of careful transportation of any victim of a severe chest injury cannot be overemphasized.   A slow ride is far safer than a fast one, since a rough, bumpy road can very well throw the patient into shock or cause penetration of a major blood vessel.

Fractured Ribs.   Another common type of injury, frequently caused by falls about the home or in auto accidents, is fracture of the ribs.   It is characterized by severe pain at the site of the fracture when the victim breathes deeply and by acute pain and tenderness over the fracture.   Sometimes the break is serious, but more often it may be just a hairline split through part of the bone.   Because of the pain the victim will breathe as shallowly as possible and will go to great lengths to avoid coughing.   Sometimes the break itself is so severe that one end of the rib pierces a lung.   When this happens the victim will cough up bright-red frothy blood.

○ TREATMENT

    1   Immobilize the fractured rib by means of cravat bandages or a suitable substitute, to relieve pain.

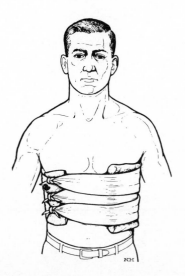

Fig. 4-23. Applying a large firm dressing to a sucking wound of chest; using cravat bandages or any suitable substitute.

2 Take care to apply the bandage tight enough to provide support, but not so tight as to cause the rib to pierce the lung.

3 If there is reason to believe that the lung already has been pierced, *no bandage* should be applied, and the victim should be taken to a hospital immediately.

Procedures for Strapping. If such an accident should occur in an isolated spot or one where there is no doctor, treatment must be given by someone—even if he has no medical training. Provided there is no evidence of lung puncture, such a person could do an excellent job of treating a fractured rib, as a doctor would, by using adhesive tape in the following manner:

For an adult, strips of adhesive tape 3 inches wide are applied horizontally from below upward, and from the midline of the body in front to the midline in back (Fig. 4-25).

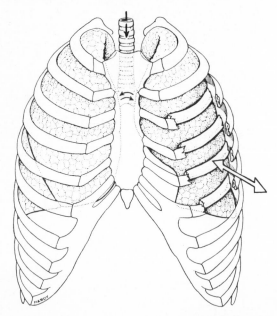

Fig. 4-24. In flail chest, the fixation of the rib cage on the injured side is destroyed so that during inspiration the flailing segment moves inward, and the lung on the injured side cannot be expanded, thus diminishing the volume of fresh air to the affected lung. On expiration, the flail segment moves outward and some of the air from the uninvolved side is forced out the trachea, but some is also forced into the involved lung, so that to some extent the victim is forced to rebreathe his own air. Fixation and tracheotomy are important steps in alleviating this condition.

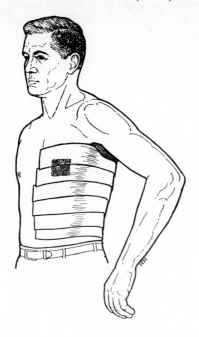

Fig. 4-25. A standard method for strapping the chest, using strips of adhesive tape 2 to 3 inches wide.

1 Begin the strapping low to immobilize the eleventh and twelfth ribs first, and then proceed upward.

2 Apply each strip during exhalation, or with the victim breathing short, shallow breaths.

3 Protect the nipples with gauze even in males. It may be difficult to strap the chests of women with large breasts; rather than compressing the breast tissue to a point of discomfort, run the strips of tape above and below the breasts, being sure not to constrict them.

Guard against strapping every case of fractured ribs without regard for the type of injury. When a fracture of the ribs occurs with overlapping or overriding of the broken ends, as can be seen from the "silver fork" appearance of the rib, further compression will tend to aggravate the overlapping (Fig. 4-26). This increases the pain and the danger of injuring the pleura or the lung itself. Where there is much overlapping, do not strap the chest, but apply strips of tape over each side of the site of the fracture so as to pull the bone ends away from the fracture site and thus reduce the overlapping.

Another method utilizes a wide piece of tape secured over

the lowest two or three ribs so as to immobilize the diaphragm firmly on the affected side. Thus, movement of the chest on that side is limited, since breathing is initiated by the diaphragm, the movements of which are largely restricted by this method of strapping.

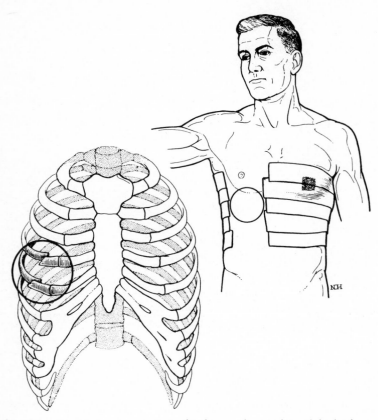

Fig. 4-26. Strapping may accentuate the degree of overriding of the broken ends (left); therefore, strapping must be applied as in smaller drawing (right) in order to prevent this.

5 Control of Hemorrhage

Second only in importance to the proper handling of respiratory emergencies is the control of hemorrhage. It is one of the most urgent conditions requiring emergency care.

TYPES OF BLEEDING

Bleeding may be classified according to the three main sources from which it can occur: arterial, venous, and capillary; it can be superficial, external, or internal. For all practical purposes, general control measures are employed for the first three types without regard to the exact nature or source of the bleeding. It is valuable to understand the basic differences in order to be able to assess more accurately the seriousness and extent of the injury.

Arterial Bleeding

Arterial bleeding is characterized by a flow of bright-red blood, which comes from the wound in *spurts* and which, at times, is alarmingly profuse. But unless a very large artery has been severed, it is unlikely that a person will bleed to death before control measures can be put into effect.

However, there are certain large arteries which are vulnerable to injury, and bleeding from these could be so profuse that the person might bleed to death in 3 minutes or less. These arteries include the aorta (ruptured as the result of an aneurysm or severe trauma—either penetrating or nonpenetrating) or any of its main branches such as the carotid, in the neck; the axillary, in the armpit; the brachial, in the arm; and the femoral (or one of its large branches), in the leg.

In arterial bleeding, the nature of the damage to the artery is important. For example, an artery which is only partially severed is liable to bleed more profusely than one which has been completely severed. This is due to the fact that the walls of an artery are elastic so that, when they are partially severed, the walls around the cut pull away from each other, thus making the opening larger. On the other hand, when an artery is completely severed, the elasticity of the walls causes the ends to pucker, thus making the opening smaller and minimizing the flow; therefore, the blood loss may be less alarming than from an artery which has been only partially severed.

Unlike bleeding from other vessels, arterial bleeding, unless it is from only a small artery, will not clot, for a blood clot can form only when there is a slow flow or no flow at all. It is for this reason that *arterial bleeding is dangerous,* and that some external means of control must be used to bring about cessation of the flow.

Some vessels are so large and carry such pressure that, even if a clot did form, it would be forced out. This might happen, too, if inept handling of a wound disturbed a clot or if pressure, such as exerted by a tourniquet, were released too soon. Therefore, once arterial bleeding is stopped control must be maintained long enough for the injured person to be safely transported to an adequate medical facility.

Venous Bleeding

Bleeding from a vein is characterized by a *steady* flow of dark-red blood, which may be profuse, but is easier to control than arterial bleeding.

There is one danger associated with venous bleeding, particularly from a large vein, which should not be overlooked— the danger of an air bubble, or air embolism. This can happen because the blood in the larger veins is being sucked back *toward* the heart; hence, when a large vein is cut, air may actually be sucked into the opening in the vein. If the air bubble is large enough, there is interference with the ability of the heart to pump the blood, because of the air block which is formed. This is one reason for controlling venous bleeding quickly.

Varicose Veins. One form of venous bleeding which may be profuse arises from the rupture of large varicose veins, particularly in the esophagus, either spontaneously or as the result of injury. Esophageal bleeding may be dangerous and difficult to control; bleeding from varicosities of the lower extremities is quite easily controlled simply by elevating the extremity and by applying a sterile compress over the bleeding area and elastic bandage above and below the point, just tight enough to compress the vein.

Sometimes the vein ruptures into the surrounding tissues without bleeding externally. This is very painful and produces a large black-and-blue mark. Treatment is the same as for external bleeding, with the addition of an ice bag for 24 hours or so, followed by heat to hasten absorption of the old blood.

Capillary Bleeding

Capillary bleeding is usually not serious and is easily controlled. It is characterized by a general ooze from the tissues, the blood dripping steadily from the wound or gradually forming a puddle in it. This type of bleeding is not immediately dangerous. If there is some more pressing requirement, capillary bleeding may be given secondary consideration insofar as emergency treatment is concerned. Quite frequently, this type of bleeding will more or less control itself by clotting spontaneously.

INTERNAL BLEEDING

Since, in cases of hemorrhage, a person's life may depend upon the speed with which he can be brought to the operating table, it is important to be able to recognize the signs that indicate severe hemorrhage, *even though the actual bleeding may not be visible.* These signs and symptoms are restlessness; thirst; faintness; dizziness; cold, clammy skin; dilated pupils; shallow or irregular breathing; thin, rapid, weak, and irregular pulse beat; and a vague feeling of great anxiety. These symptoms are very similar to those of shock.

Internal bleeding is always an extremely serious condition and requires medical attention as quickly as possible. As the term is generally used, it refers to bleeding into the chest or into the abdominal or pelvic cavities or into any of the organs which they contain, such as a bleeding stomach ulcer. Internal bleeding may be from an artery, a vein, or capillaries, or it may be from a combination of any or all three sources.

Internal bleeding usually is brought about by a tearing or bruising force which actually ruptures or tears apart one of the internal organs, such as the liver or spleen, or by a hole cut in a blood vessel, as when a bullet passes through the abdominal wall and pierces a large artery or vein. A person may bleed to death internally, without a drop of blood ever leaving the body.

Severe internal bleeding can only be controlled by adequate surgery. Until surgery is available, the victim can be kept alive by blood transfusion in adequate amounts or by whatever fluids (glucose in saline; plasma; plasma expanders) are available which can be used as expedients until whole blood is procured. In situations where definitive medical aid is not immediately available, it is imperative that the victim be kept at complete rest, in a slightly reclining position, with as little movement as possible. If available, a sedative should be given by injection (*not* by mouth in any case where abdominal bleeding is suspected) to control restlessness. Even if internal bleeding is only *suspected,* the victim must receive expert medical attention as soon as possible.

Symptoms. The signs and symptoms indicating internal hemorrhage are the same as those of hemorrhage in general, except that there is a greater tendency toward early onset of shock, and there is, of course, no externally visible bleeding.

The early onset of profound shock may be the only factor to alert one to internal bleeding, although this possibility in the case of any severe injury should always be kept in mind.

Bleeding from the lungs or stomach may, of course, be apparent because of the blood that is coughed up, vomited, or excreted. For example:

1 If bleeding is from the lungs, the coughed-up blood will be bright red and frothy.

2 If bleeding into the stomach is recent, the vomited blood will be bright red; if bleeding into the stomach is chronic (occurring slowly over a long period of time), the blood is quite liable to resemble coffee grounds.

3 Slow bleeding in the intestinal tract above the sigmoid colon will cause the stools to be jet black (the color of tar).

4 If bleeding is low down in the intestinal tract and fresh, the stools will be streaked with bright-red blood and, in severe cases, may consist almost wholly of blood.

Intra-abdominal Bleeding

If the bleeding is within the abdomen, the common signs of acute abdominal illness may or may not be present: vomiting, abdominal tenderness, and rigidity of the abdominal muscles. It must also be borne in mind that if injuries are of such nature as to produce internal bleeding, there may also be rupture of one or more hollow organs, such as the intestines or urinary bladder, so that the condition may be further complicated.

In the case of any person who has sustained a crush injury or been severely injured in an automotive accident, the possibility of severe internal bleeding from rupture of the spleen, the liver, or the kidneys should be kept in mind and the patient observed in the hospital over a period of at least 24 hours for evidence that this type of injury has, in fact, occurred.

As has been mentioned previously, rupture of the spleen should be suspected in any accident involving a contusive force to the abdomen or lower chest. While the symptoms of acute rupture of the spleen (85 percent) are well recognized, the importance of recognizing occult rupture has been stressed by Drapanas, Yates, Brickman, and Wholey. The principal factors common to all cases studied included dull, lower thoracic, upper abdominal, or back pain; left upper quadrant space-occupying mass; medial displacement of stomach; pathognomonic angiographic pattern. If these factors are borne in mind, the diagnosis of occult rupture of the spleen is less likely to be missed.

Rupture of the bladder is common in severe pelvic fractures or crush injuries of the lower part of the abdomen, and also is one of the first things to be kept in mind in this type of injury. A telltale sign of injury to the bladder or, in fact, any part of the urinary tract, is blood in the urine. When blood is found in the urine in any substantial quantity, diagnostic procedures must be undertaken promptly to determine the source of the bleeding in order to take corrective measures. While such procedures are highly technical and, of course, can only be carried out in a hospital, it is important for anyone attempting to render assistance to any seriously injured person to realize the various medical contingencies which may exist.

Aneurysmal Bleeding

A special example of an extremely dangerous type of internal bleeding is leakage from, or rupture of, an aneurysm of the aorta. An aneurysm is a localized or diffuse enlargement of an artery which results from weakening of the arterial wall, much as a weak spot in the wall of a tire tube will lead to its bulging out and eventually blowing out.

Once an aneurysm has formed, its continued enlargement is a medical certainty, leading eventually to leakage or actual rupture.

Most aortic aneurysms appear in people 40 years of age and over, most commonly as the result of extensive arteriosclerotic disease; because our older age groups are increasing, the incidence of aortic aneurysmal rupture is increasing.

Prompt suspicion of such a possibility is becoming more important, since with better diagnosis and improved and more widely utilized vascular surgical technics, lives are being saved which but a few years ago would have been lost, the cause of death never suspected in some cases until disclosed by autopsy.

Many aortic aneurysms can exist for long periods of time without any symptoms except those which may be caused by the pressure of the growing aneurysm on structures surrounding it. However, when the aneurysm is in the thoracic aorta and begins to leak slowly into the surrounding tissues, a severe chest pain radiates to both shoulders and may also radiate into the back and neck.

Leaking or ruptured aneurysms of the abdominal aorta often herald their presence by acute back pain in the lumbar region, and may be misdiagnosed as "back strain." Fortunately most of these patients are x-rayed, and the aneurysm often is apparent because of calcium deposition in its walls. Later, signs of hemorrhage, such as increased pulse rate, falling blood pressure, and the other characteristic signs of a failing circulatory system, occur. In addition, there may be the development of a pulsating and slowly enlarging mass in the abdomen, which is sometimes first noted by the patient himself.

In many of these patients, the leakage of blood is not immediately catastrophic, and in untreated cases, death, as a result of the hemorrhage, may be delayed for several hours or days. For this reason if the possibility of ruptured aneurysm is borne in mind and the diagnosis is made promptly, surgical intervention, particularly if undertaken within 48 hours of the initiation of the bleeding, offers the patient a reasonable hope, even though the mortality rate in this type of case is high.

Traumatic Rupture of Aorta

Traumatic rupture of the aorta, if not immediately lethal at the scene of injury as the result of exsanguinating hemorrhage before the patient reaches the operating room, may result in a traumatic aneurysm with slow leakage of blood into the mediastinum or other tissue spaces, which is not immediately fatal. This type of injury, as emphasized by Meyer, Neville, and Hansen, is coming to be recognized more and more frequently and is often subject to prompt surgical correction. While most common among adult age groups, it has been reported on several occasions in children. Wilentz et al., who reported nine cases of ruptured aorta during a 3-month period in a single county in New Jersey, noted that the majority of these occurred in auto accidents, and they stressed the fact that waist-type safety belts alone do not prevent this kind of injury. Aortic rupture must be suspected in all cases of chest trauma in which x-ray discloses widening of the mediastinum. In some cases, surgical correction has been carried out at considerable periods after injury.

In the light of today's high speed auto crashes, the possibility of aortic rupture of a type subject to successful surgical correction always should be borne in mind.

BLOOD CLOTTING

The only way that nature, unaided, has of controlling hemorrhage is by the process known as *clotting*. Emergency efforts to control hemorrhage are directed toward helping nature to form a clot. Where temporary stoppage of the flow has been achieved by any of various means or spontaneously, as in the small-sized veins or capillaries, the blood, by a series of chemical changes initiated by the injury, forms a clot which acts as a cork in the opening of the bleeding vessel.

To describe what happens very simply, the changes leading

to clot formation are brought about by the release of *thromboplastin* from the injured tissues and the blood platelets. This acts upon a substance present in the blood, known as *prothrombin,* in such a way as to convert it, with the help of calcium, to *thrombin.* Another substance in the blood, known as *fibrinogen,* is converted by the thrombin into a sticky network of *fibrin,* which forms the basic network of a blood clot. Any interference with any part of this clotting system will diminish the ability of the blood to clot.

In some diseases, such as *hemophilia,* the tendency to bleed, as well as the inability of the blood to clot, may be so great as to be a hazard to life. Bleeding, in a person with this condition, is a particularly difficult type of hemorrhage to control, since the problem is in the failure of the blood-clotting mechanism itself, and there is as yet no known specific curative measure. In most cases hospitalization will be required, since often transfusions and the use of special types of plasma fractions are necessary to bring the bleeding under control. However, as an emergency measure, an effort should be made to stop the hemorrhage by firm compression on the bleeding site.

In childhood hemophilia, it is of primary importance for the family to understand the potential dangers of the situation so the child will be protected from injury and the proper precautions taken if an operation, such as an appendectomy, or a tooth extraction is unavoidable. As the child grows older, he should be made aware of the nature of his condition so that he will be able to guard himself against injury and will know what to do should bleeding occur. Newly isolated blood fractions are now becoming available which greatly aid in the alleviation of this condition.

TREATMENT OF HEMORRHAGE

There are four basic methods of controlling hemorrhage from any wound, but always, as a first step, elevate the bleeding part as high above the level of the heart as possible; this tends to lessen the hydrostatic pressure of the blood flowing to the wound area.

Direct Pressure on Wound

The simplest, and often most effective method of control is direct pressure on the bleeding vessel, if it is visible, or, more often, by direct pressure on the wound.   This may be achieved by using a heavy, sterile gauze compress over the wound, if this is available, or by using a pressure dressing and applying finger pressure (Fig. 5-1).

Applying a Pressure Dressing.   A pressure dressing is most effective for the control of capillary hemorrhage or of relatively mild venous bleeding, as well as for maintaining control of arterial hemorrhage after the bleeding has been stopped by other means.   Pressure dressings are particularly helpful in controlling scalp bleeding.   In applying a pressure dressing, care should be taken to cover the wound in such a way that its edges are not forced apart, but are actually brought together by the pressure of the dressing.   To do this:

1   Hold the edges of the wound together with the fingers if necessary (one or more strips of clean adhesive or prepared butterfly strips can be used to draw the wound edges together), and cover the wound with a thick sterile gauze compress.

2   If sterile gauze is not available, use any clean fabric, such as a freshly laundered handkerchief, a piece of bed sheet, or a sanitary napkin, which, incidentally, serves very well.   Whatever the compress may be, bandage it firmly in place, using a roller bandage, conforming bandage, cravat (see page 102), or, if necessary, a belt.

3   If the injury is to a leg or an arm, it is vital that enough pressure be applied to control the bleeding, but not so much as to obstruct the flow of blood to the rest of the limb.   The

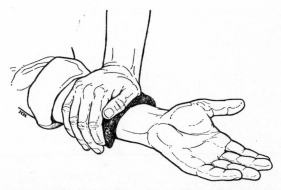

Fig. 5-1.   Proper method of applying direct pressure to a wound to control bleeding.

best way to avoid exerting too much pressure is to apply as much pressure as necessary to control the bleeding and then to determine whether a pulse can be felt below the point where the dressing was applied. If not, loosen the dressing until a pulse can be felt.

4 If the wound starts to bleed again, it should be recognized that the bleeding may be of such character that it cannot be controlled by a pressure dressing and that other means will be required.

5 Another important point must be taken into consideration: the constriction produced in applying a pressure dressing may increase the bleeding, particularly if it is from an artery, since the degree of constriction exerted may be sufficient to cut off the venous return flow without cutting off the arterial supply. This same consideration is equally applicable to the use of a tourniquet.

It goes without saying that certain areas of the body are *not* adaptable to the use of pressure dressings; one of these, for obvious reasons, is the neck.

Use of Pressure Points

In the event that a pressure dressing is ineffective or that necessary materials are not available, the bleeding can usually be controlled by strong finger pressure on the main artery of supply to the wounded part. Such pressure can be applied most effectively at the point where an artery is relatively near the surface and where it passes close to a bony structure against which it can be compressed. These points are known as pressure points. There are 22 such points, 11 on each side, and of these about six are usually used to control most cases of external hemorrhage (Fig. 5-2). Of these six the easiest and most commonly used are the brachial point in the arm and the femoral point in the groin (see Fig. 5-2 *E* and *G*).

Pressure points are particularly useful where the application of a tourniquet would be dangerous or impossible, but it must be pointed out that with the exception of the two just mentioned, they are not always completely effective and do little more than slow down the flow.

For Scalp Bleeding. Bleeding from the scalp, which is almost always profuse, can often be controlled by pressure on the temporal artery (Fig. 5-2*A*) at a point just in front of the ear.

However, because there is extensive circulation of blood to the scalp, finger pressure may have to be applied on *both* sides of the head. This method is cumbersome, and, except for some special circumstance, a pressure dressing is likely to do a better job. Scalp hemorrhage is often more frightening than serious.

For Head and Neck Bleeding. Bleeding from the head and neck can often be controlled by exerting pressure on the common carotid artery (Fig. 5-2*B*) and by pressing on it sufficiently to cause it to constrict against the vertebrae of the neck. To constrict the common carotid artery, locate the windpipe in the midline of the neck, slide the fingers around to the side of the neck (on the side from which the bleeding is coming), and feel for the pulsation of the large artery. Place three fingers over the artery and the thumb behind the neck, and exert pressure between the fingers and thumb so as to squeeze the artery against the vertebrae.

Care must be taken in carrying out this procedure, as it may produce unconsciousness by restricting the flow of blood to the brain. In addition, some people faint readily as the result of pressure exerted on a little bundle of nerve tissue, known as the *carotid body,* in close contact with the carotid artery in the neck, which in certain individuals is very sensitive, even to slight pressure. Also be careful not to constrict the windpipe in this procedure.

For Bleeding from the Face. Bleeding from the front of the face can often be controlled by compressing the facial artery (Fig. 5-2*C*) against the jawbone. This may not be wholly effective because of the extensive circulation to the face, and both sides may require compression; the procedure often is not very effective.

For Armpit and Chest Wall. Bleeding from the armpit and, incidentally, from the side of the chest and from the entire arm, can be controlled by pressure on the subclavian artery (Fig. 5-2*D*) as it passes behind and beneath the collarbone. Pressure should be exerted downward with the thumb so as to press the artery against the first rib.

For an Arm. Bleeding from the arm can be controlled quite easily by pressure on the brachial artery (Fig. 5-2*E*). This artery is easily felt as it passes along the inner side of the arm between the large muscles on the inner surface. It is easily compressed against the bone at a point about halfway between the shoulder and the elbow. Pressure applied below this point will *not* be very effective if the bleeding is farther down the arm, as there are a number of branches from the brachial artery.

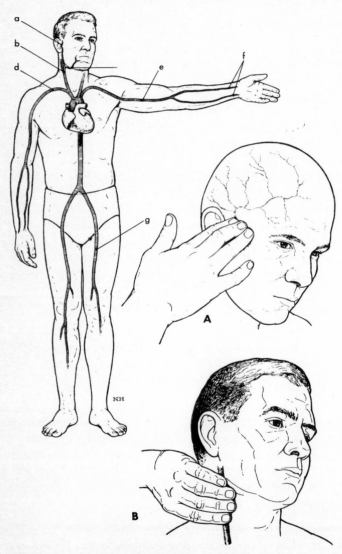

Fig. 5-2. See legend on facing page.

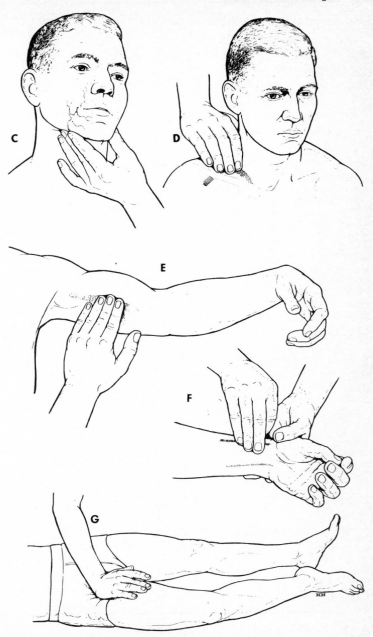

Fig. 5-2. Diagram of available pressure points for control of arterial bleeding. (See text for areas controlled by pressure on the various points indicated.)

The only way to stop such bleeding is to use a tourniquet in the event that coaptation of the wound edges and a pressure dressing doesn't work.

Pressure can sometimes be effectively exerted on the brachial artery just below the bend of the elbow, at the point where it divides into the two main arteries of the forearm. In case the bleeding is from the hand, these two arteries may be compressed at the wrist—the radial artery on the thumb side and the ulna artery (Fig. 5-2F) on the side of the little finger. Again, because there is extensive circulation, pressure on one artery or the other may not be wholly effective; pressure may have to be exerted on *both*.

For a Leg. Bleeding from the leg can be controlled by deep pressure on the femoral artery (Fig. 5-2G) in the groin, the pulsations of which are readily felt. Pressure is achieved by placing the heel of the hand or the fist high up in the groin, at a point just below where the thigh joins the torso. If the victim is very muscular, this is sometimes difficult for the inexperienced person to do and requires considerable force.

Bleeding from the lower leg and foot can sometimes be partially controlled by pressure on the popliteal artery at a point just above the back of the knee joint before it divides into the posterior and anterior tibial and peroneal arteries.

Tourniquets

If the measures to control bleeding discussed above are not effective, a tourniquet may be used as a last resort. A tourniquet must be used intelligently, with a full understanding of its functions, and certain precautions heeded. If used improperly, it may prove *worse than ineffective* by endangering the part to which it was applied.

It was formerly taught that a tourniquet should never be left on for more than 20 minutes without loosening it. It is now known that a tourniquet, once applied, should be left in place until it is loosened under conditions where immediate definitive surgical and supportive measures can be carried out.

There are two reasons for this: First, frequent loosening of a tourniquet may dislodge clots and result in sufficient bleeding to produce shock or death. Second, so-called "tourniquet shock" is now recognized as a very real cause of shock in cases to which tourniquets have been applied. This type of shock is thought to be caused by harmful substances released by the injured tissue, which are held back by a tourniquet, and then are allowed to enter the general circulation in large concentration when the tourniquet is released. Unless adequate measures are available to combat shock, loosening of the tourniquet may prove fatal. Extensive study has proved that, by leaving the tourniquet in place, although more *limbs* may possibly be lost, more *lives* will be saved. To apply a tourniquet properly, follow these steps:

1 Place the tourniquet as close to the wound as possible, between it and the heart, but not right at the wound edges.

2 Tighten it just enough to control bleeding. If it is too loose, it will increase bleeding; if unnecessarily tight, it will cause further damage.

3 If a regular tourniquet is not available, use some kind of flat article, such as a cravat bandage, stocking, or belt, and be sure to place an adequate pad over the artery to be compressed.

Never use rope, wire, or anything else that will cut, and be certain that you use adequate padding of some sort.

Always make a notation, on the victim, of the time the tourniquet was applied. If a tag is not available for this, mark the information on the victim's forehead with iodine, indelible pencil, or lipstick.

A tourniquet should be used *only as a last resort* to control a *life-threatening* hemorrhage which cannot be stopped by any other means.

Supportive Treatment

In addition to the control of bleeding, care is directed toward the *prevention* of shock, or its control if it has actually set in.

With few exceptions, the bleeding person should be in a reclining position, although his head may be raised slightly on a small pillow. If the bleeding is from an arm or leg, it is sometimes helpful to raise it above the rest of the body, thus lowering the blood pressure in the affected limb and slowing the bleeding.

Keep the patient comfortably warm, but not overheated. A

bleeding person is often restless and apprehensive; therefore, every effort should be made to keep him quiet and reassured. It is particularly important to keep the victim as quiet as possible in order to encourage clotting. Because of his great need for oxygen, a bleeding person should be given as much fresh air as possible, but, at the same time, sheltered from drafts.

Unless the case is one of abdominal injury or the victim is unconscious, *encourage* him to take water or other liquids by mouth. Do *not* give him alcohol, hot coffee, or any stimulant, at least until after the bleeding his been controlled. Stimulants increase both the rate and fullness of the heartbeat and raise the blood pressure, thus increasing the rate of blood flow to control restlessness and apprehension. A sedative may be used and should be given by injection if materials and medically qualified personnel are available.

In controlling bleeding, never put anything into or on the wound except a sterile compress or some clean, suitable substitute. The use of any such substance as mud, cobwebs, and tobacco, which are popular in old wives' tales, is not only ineffective but dangerous.

Sometimes heat, in the form of hot sterile compresses, or cold, in the form of an ice bag or similar application, is helpful in controlling capillary or venous bleeding. Heat is used in an attempt to accelerate clot formation, but cold may be more helpful in causing contraction of the blood vessels, thus slowing the bleeding so that a clot is better able to form.

Refrigeration for controlling hemorrhage, particularly of the capillary type, is being used more and more for this purpose as well as for the treatment of other forms of injury.

NASAL BLEEDING

Nosebleed

Nosebleeds are very common in childhood, especially in young girls during their early menstrual periods, and in older people with such conditions as hardening of the arteries and high blood pressure. Injury, excessive nose picking, and certain diseases may also be causes.

The bleeding usually begins suddenly and without warning except, perhaps, a preliminary feeling of fullness in the nose. Although in most cases the flow is not really very great, it may seem to be dangerously profuse. Sometimes an attack may occur during sleep, and the blood will be swallowed and later vomited.

The bleeding most frequently comes from the network of veins lying very near the surface of the membrane just inside the nose.

○ TREATMENT

Sometimes the bleeding can be controlled by simply applying firm pressure with the thumbs against the upper lip just below the nose (Fig. 5-3). A more effective method is to gently insert into each nostril a small wad of sterile absorbent cotton so that a little cotton still protrudes from the openings. Then gently but firmly compress the nostrils between your thumb and fingers steadily for at least 6 minutes *by the clock* (Fig. 5-4). Keep the patient in a sitting position—*not* lying down. Keep him calm and reassured; anxiety and emotional tension can easily make the bleeding worse by raising the blood pressure.

After the 6 minutes are up, gradually release the pressure on the nose and watch for further bleeding. Do *not* remove

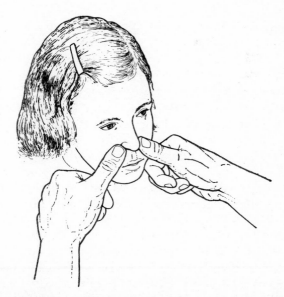

Fig. 5-3. Controlling nosebleed with thumb pressure, which is effective in some, but not all, cases.

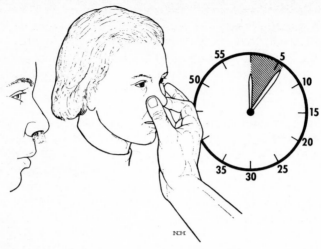

Fig. 5-4. Pack the nose with absorbent cotton or gauze, and hold packing firmly in place with gentle pressure for at least 6 minutes.

the inserted cotton for several hours, as the bleeding may start up again. When you do remove the cotton, work it out very gently.

A much more effective material to use than plain absorbent cotton is a specially treated gauze known as *oxidized regenerated cellulose* (Surgicel®), which possesses strong inherent hemostatic properties. This material is also slowly soluble in blood so that it gradually loosens itself after the bleeding has stopped. Otherwise, it is used the same way as absorbent cotton. It is particularly useful in hemophilia and other bleeding dyscrasias of the blood; the product can be obtained only on a physician's prescription, and it is important to follow directions carefully.

If a nosebleed cannot be controlled by these simple measures in a short period of time or if episodes of bleeding recur frequently, the cause may be of a more serious nature and a physician should be consulted. The bleeding may be coming from areas far back in the nose to which packing can be applied only through the use of special technics. This type of bleeding may be very profuse, especially in older people or in those with high blood pressure.

Postoperative Nasal Bleeding

Nosebleeds which occur a few days to a week following a tonsillectomy or adenoidectomy cannot be stopped by simple means, and the surgeon who operated should be called promptly.

○ TREATMENT

In the meantime, keep the patient calm, in a sitting position; apply an ice bag to the back of his neck; and encourage him to spit out the blood from the back of his throat and not to swallow it. Do not attempt to pack the nose with cotton, as this might do more harm than good, since the blood is probably coming from the raw adenoidal bed behind the nose, where only a doctor can take the special steps required to stop it.

6

∫hock—
Type∫ and Treatment

SHOCK DUE TO INJURY (TRAUMATIC SHOCK)

Shock is a serious depression of vital functions that often accompanies or follows many kinds of injuries. Shock is characterized by circulatory insufficiency without accompanying congestive heart failure per se.

The term "shock" does not indicate a single entity but, rather, a complex physiologic state which may be brought about by a great many different factors, any one of which may alter the clinical picture considerably, both in character and degree.

Traumatic Shock. While our understanding of the mechanisms of shock is not wholly complete, there is general agreement that in traumatic shock loss of plasma through the capillary walls into the extravascular tissues spaces is constant, with a decrease in blood volume and an increase in blood concentration. The decrease in blood volume causes the fall in blood pressure which is characteristic of shock, with resultant failure of circulation of the red blood cells and ultimate anoxemia.

Along with the loss of plasma through the capillary walls, dilatation of the capillary bed also takes place, thus immobilizing large quantities of blood, principally in the splanchnic zone. The circulating blood volume is greatly diminished, causing hemoconcentration, which causes a sharp increase in the number of red blood cells per cubic millimeter of blood.

Berdjis and Vick have emphasized the role of endotoxin secreted by various bacteria, particularly *Escherichia coli,* as being a major factor in producing injury, particularly vesiculation, to the capillary walls.

The venous pressure becomes greatly reduced because of the diminished blood volume; this results in incomplete filling of the heart, diminished cardiac output, and a further lowering of blood pressure. The fall in pressure within the aorta itself stimulates accelerator nerve endings, thus speeding up the heart rate. Ultimately, the decreased blood pressure and blood volume, plus deficient oxygenation, leads to cerebral anoxia. The pulse becomes rapid and weak, the peripheral blood pressure drops, and, because of the decreased cardiac output, varying degrees of stasis occur in the pulmonary circulation, leading to congestive pulmonary failure.

Hemorrhagic Shock. In shock resulting from severe hemorrhage, both internal and external, the circulating blood volume is diminished by direct loss of both plasma and cellular elements. Therefore, at first, the number of red cells per cubic millimeter is unchanged. As tissue fluids tend to be drawn into the bloodstream, however, blood dilution and tissue dehydration result. Due to the decreased blood volume and possible vasodilatation, arterial and venous pressure fall. Impaired cardiac filling develops because of inadequate blood volume and lowered venous pressure, resulting in decreased cardiac output. Again, the lowered pressure in the aorta causes a greatly accelerated heart rate.

Oxygenation of the tissues may be maintained with as few as 2 million red corpuscles per cubic millimeter, providing there exists sufficient blood pressure and volume to circulate them. But if blood pressure and volume fall too low, anoxia of the brain and other tissues develops. Ultimately the pulse becomes rapid and thready, and there is a marked fall in the peripheral blood pressure.

Burn Shock. In burn shock there is extensive transudation of plasma from capillaries into the tissues of the burned area. There also takes place a loss of plasma from capillaries into tissue spaces in other parts of the body, as the result of toxic absorption. Capillary dilatation may also immoblize large quantities of blood. The circulating blood volume is diminished, thus causing hemoconcentration and an increase in the number of red blood cells per cubic millimeter. The venous pressure is reduced because of diminished blood volume, and incomplete filling of the heart and diminished cardiac output result, causing a further lowering of blood pressure, with a concomitant acceleration of the heart rate. The peripheral blood pressure may fall because of decreased blood volume and diminished cardiac output, and the pulse may become very rapid and thready.

Bacterial Shock. Bacterial shock has come to be recognized as an important clinical entity. Barnett and Sanford state that "As a cause of clinical shock, sepsis is surpassed in frequency only by hemorrhage and myocardial infarction."

The overwhelming infection which produces the shock syndrome is most commonly caused by gram-negative organisms, although many other types are less frequently implicated, with urinary tract infection being the most common underlying clinical condition. These authors found in a large series that the mortality of gram-negative bacteremia approximated 40 percent, but that in patients in whom shock developed the mortality ranged from 50 percent to 80 percent.

Shubin and Weil point out that the most common causative organisms are *Escherichia coli, Klebsiella pneumoniae, Enterobacter* spp., *Proteus, Pseudomonas, Serratia marcescens,* and several other less common organisms. Gram-positive bacteria, viruses, *Rickettsia,* and fungi may also occasionally play a part.

Many sites, including the biliary tract, uterus, cervix (septic abortions), colon, and lungs, also may seed infectious organisms into the bloodstream following surgery or some other manipulative procedure, particularly in individuals debilitated by some chronic illness such as diabetes, cirrhosis, or blood disease.

It seems probable that the basic mechanisms which produce shock are contingent upon a complex endotoxin present in the cell wall of gram-negative bacteria which, to quote Barnett and Sanford, "effects a redistribution of blood within the vascular bed in a manner precluding the maintenance of an adequate circulating blood volume."

The physiologic results of such pooling, aside from the question of infection, are similar to those in other types of shock.

Symptoms.   In *nonseptic shock* any or all of the signs and symptoms of shock may be present, or they may develop gradually and become apparent after an hour or more.   They are weakness, faintness, mental sluggishness, collapse; face pale, skin cold and moist (clammy); eyelids drooping, eyes vacant and dull, pupils dilated; breathing rapid and shallow, irregular, or deep; nausea with or without vomiting; thirst and restlessness (sometimes indifference and unawareness); pulse weak, fast, irregular, or too weak to feel; and unconsciousness.

In *septic shock* the first sign is frequently a severe shaking chill accompanied or shortly followed by a sharp rise in temperature.   In very profound septic shock the temperature may be subnormal.   The respiratory and cardiac rates are greatly increased, resulting in alkalosis, and the urine output is either greatly diminished or, in severe cases, absent.

Early laboratory findings do not, as a rule, indicate the potential gravity of the situation.

General Procedures

The essential aims in the treatment of shock, regardless of its origin, are the restoration of the circulating blood volume by the administration of suitable fluids, by vein and, when possible, by mouth, and to correct the underlying cause.   The choice of fluid used to restore the circulating blood volume depends partly on expediency and what is immediately at hand and, ultimately, upon the physiologic needs of the patient as indicated by laboratory tests.   It is often possible to administer glucose or saline solutions immediately, since some ambulance squads now carry these as part of their equipment and qualified personnel are available for their administration.   In the hospital, plasma or some form of plasma expander such as dextran, or whole blood, is used in sufficient amounts to reverse the adverse physiologic changes which have occurred, as part of the shock picture, and bring the patient out of shock.

The important point is that the sooner the treatment begins, the less profound the state of shock is liable to become, and the better the patient's chances of recovery.

If not recognized and allowed to progress, shock may become severe enough to be fatal (although the injury itself or underlying cause may not have been). All apparently severely injured persons must receive emergency preventive care for shock; do not wait for shock to develop.

As simple first-aid measures, keep the victim lying down; conserve his body heat; and give him fluids by mouth if he is conscious and his injuries offer no contraindication. If materials and personnel are available to administer fluid intravenously, this should be done.

The sooner shock is treated definitely, the more likely is survival. Therefore, as soon as circumstances permit get the victim to a hospital, where effective resuscitation and surgical facilities are available. In the meantime, follow these procedures:

Be sure that the victim is, in fact, suffering from shock, and *not* from some other condition, such as acute myocardial infarction (q.v.), for which the corrective measures for shock per se, might do actual harm.

Unless shock is the result of an acute heart attack, place the victim in the reclining position, with his feet higher than his head, and loosen his clothing to aid circulation (Fig. 6-1). If the shock is cardiac in origin, treatment depends essentially on measures directed specifically to the heart. (For preliminary first-aid measures, see pages 512 and 513.) If the victim must be treated on the ground, his feet and legs may be elevated on rolled-up blankets, pillows, a box, or whatever else may be available. If he is in bed, "shock blocks" are placed under the foot of the bed so as to raise it about 12 to 16 inches higher than the head.

The so-called "shock position" is used in those cases in which true shock is present and is uncomplicated by other factors such as head injury, and which is severe enough to require fairly extreme measures. As a general rule, it is best to keep the average case in a flat position, particularly if one is not sure what other injuries may be present, or whether the case is one of uncomplicated shock.

If the victim is suffering from a head injury, keep him *flat*, and turn his head *away* from the injured side to relieve pressure. If the victim is suffering from a chest injury or a respiratory difficulty, or both, *raise* his head and shoulders.

If hemorrhage is present, control it (see page 166).

Keep the victim warm by supplying gentle, *not excessive*, heat.   This is done by placing a blanket or whatever is available *under* him as well as *over* him.   If the outside temperature is cold, hot-water bottles or other sources of heat may be used, *provided two dangers are recognized:* (1) an unconscious or semiconscious person is very easily burned; (2) too much heat causes a general dilation of the blood vessels of the skin; the victim may look better, but actually he will be worse as the result of further loss of circulating blood volume.   *Do not overheat; merely prevent undue body cooling.*   Do not apply heat to an injured limb, as this may only serve to increase absorption of toxic substances formed as a result of the injury and worsen the degree of shock.

Since shock is caused or made worse by pain, take whatever measures may be possible to relieve the pain.   In the case

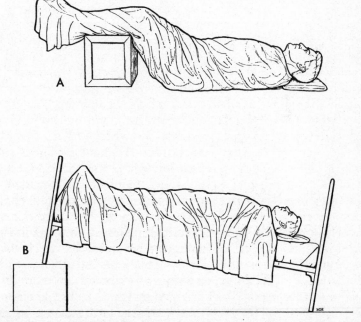

Fig. 6-1. Two methods of placing a victim in the shock position.   (A) Under emergency conditions, use a box or other device to elevate the legs. (B) Under hospital or home conditions, use "shock blocks" under foot of bed.

of a fracture, this means suitable splinting (see page 197). Although the pain may be so severe as to require a strong medication, such as a narcotic, except under the most unusual circumstances, such as on shipboard where no physician is immediately available or under disaster conditions, its administration must be considered outside the scope of anyone not medically trained.

There are several conditions for which a narcotic, such as morphine, should not be administered. The most important of these are a fractured skull or concussion of the brain, since morphine increases intracranial pressure.

If fluids can be given by mouth, urge the patient to take as much as he can comfortably tolerate. If possible, the fluid should contain sugar or salt. Orange juice is excellent, as are ginger ale and other "sparkling" beverages. If a salt solution is given, it should have a concentration of about 1 teaspoonful of salt to a quart of cool water.

If medical aid is to be long delayed and the victim is unable to take fluids by mouth, a retention enema of a sugar or salt solution, at body temperature, should be administered slowly. The solution is allowed to run into the rectum very slowly through a tube inserted about 6 inches into the rectum. In this way a large amount of fluid can be absorbed by the body. While this is a procedure which could readily be carried out in the home, using ordinary enema equipment, it is unlikely that suitable equipment could be found quickly at the scene of an automobile accident. However, first-aid squads should have proper equipment available, so that the administration of fluids may be started on the way to the hospital.

The treatment of *bacterial shock* requires additional specific measures which, except for some very unusual situation, must be carried out as hospital procedures. Basic measures consist of determining the infecting organism and administering that antibiotic or chemotherapeutic agent to which the organism is most sensitive, maintenance of blood volume with whole blood and plasma expanders as indicated, prompt correction of alkalosis and acidosis, and the maintenance of blood pressure and blood flow through the use of a suitable vasoactive agent—either vasopressor or vasodilating agent as indicated.

The handling of septic shock is obviously a highly complicated procedure and requires the most sophisticated monitoring and therapeutic methods available.

FAINTING

Fainting may result from many different causes, the most common being a psychic disturbance of an unpleasant nature, which sets off a chain of effects not unlike those seen in shock. Lack of oxygen to the brain brings about the characteristic loss of consciousness seen in fainting.

Some persons faint from merely seeing blood or from seeing or hearing unpleasant things. Also, there is a type of fainting which occurs in those who are required to spend a long time in an upright position with little movement, as, for instance, a soldier who is being held at attention for a considerable period. In such a case there is a loss of circulating blood volume, due to accumulation of blood in the legs. This results from the loss of tone in the blood vessels of the legs and of the massaging effect that would occur if the muscles were active, a necessary help in returning the blood to the heart for recirculation. When enough blood is thus lost from the circulation to affect oxygenation, the person faints because the brain is not getting enough oxygen to maintain consciousness.

It is probable that, in most cases of fainting, stagnation of the blood in the legs is of greater importance than the accumulation in the vessels of the abdominal area. For this reason, wherever possible, fainting can better be prevented or more quickly cured by laying the victim flat, with his head lower than his legs, instead of by the time-honored method of putting his head down between his knees (Fig. 6-2).

ANAPHYLACTIC SHOCK

Anaphylactic shock is the *reaction of the body* to overwhelming sensitization by a foreign protein. An example of anaphylactic shock is the serious illness (or even profound collapse) experienced by some people when stung by a bee, after taking certain medications, after eating certain foods, or as the result of an injection of a therapeutic or prophylactic agent containing horse serum.

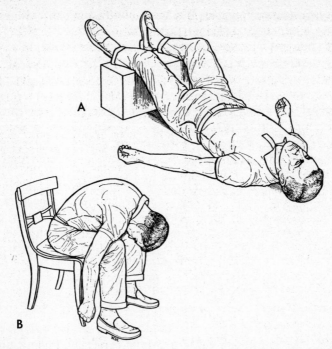

Fig. 6-2. (A) Most effective position for the treatment of a person who is about to faint or has actually done so. (B) If, for some reason, the person cannot be laid down, the head-in-between-the-knees position may help.

Anaphylaxis can produce death if counter measures are not taken immediately.

It is for that reason that desensitization to some substance to which an individual may be sensitive must be carried out very carefully and in such small doses that a severe reaction is not provoked. Gradually, over a long series of such desensitizing injections, the individual's immunity is built up to the point where he no longer reacts violently to the offending substance or substances in his environment. However, if desensitization is too rapid, too large a dose is given, or the individual's current or recent exposure to the offending substance has been too great, a reaction will occur. In most instances a doctor would be present, since such reactions are most commonly seen very shortly after the person receives a desensitizing injection of the offending substance.

As an example, anaphylactic shock can occur in an individual who, for instance, has had a hay fever injection, the dosage of which is near, or slightly exceeds, his level of tolerance.   If such an individual is subsequently environmentally exposed too heavily to the substance to which he is sensitive— as pollen or house dust—he may quickly experience collapse, akin, in degree, to profound shock.

Another important manifestation of anaphylaxis in very sensitive individuals is the severe type of generalized reaction (sometimes death-producing) to insect stings.   Such reactions are on the increase.   This is another example of the body's reaction to overwhelming sensitization, where the whole process is set off by the venom injected by the insect.   Usually, death results from respiratory obstruction due to swelling of the vocal cords or to severe bronchial constriction and congestion.

The victim of this type of reaction is *in extremis*.   As the result of anoxemia he is restless, with congestion of the lungs, and swelling (edema) of the vocal cords gives rise to mottled, livid, blue skin, severe coughing, difficulty in getting breath, and severe headache.   Unconsciousness and death follow rapidly if urgent corrective measures are not taken.

Even if there is no difficulty in breathing, the appearance of the victim may be similar to one who is in profound shock; in addition to the general collapse, there may be swelling of the abdomen and intestinal distress, such as severe nausea, vomiting, and diarrhea.

O TREATMENT

   1 Obtain medical aid as quickly as possible.

   2 If the victim has difficulty in breathing, he should be in a sitting position.

In the event that medical aid is not immediately available, as in a disaster or similar situation, and the necessary supplies are on hand, give the victim an injection of 0.5 milliliter (cubic centimeter) epinephrine (1:1000) subcutaneously immediately—and every 10 minutes thereafter if there is no immediate response.   If the victim is alive 15 to 20 minutes after initial onset of acute symptoms, he will probably survive the attack, but he should be watched very carefully for the next 3 to 4 hours, as partial relapses are common.   He should also receive a corticosteroid, such as hydrocortisone 100 milligrams, intravenously.   Oxygen should be administered by inhalator to relieve the anoxia and make breathing more comfortable.

If the anaphylaxis is the result of an insect sting on an extremity of a known highly sensitive individual, a constricting band should be placed between the sting and the base of the extremity.   The stinger should be scraped out gently with fingernail, needle, or knife blade, and treatment continued as above.

Laryngeal obstruction due to edema usually responds rapidly to the administration of epinephrine and the intravenous administration of a corticosteroid such as hydrocortisone (Solu-Cortef®); therefore, tracheotomy is rarely required. If, however, epinephrine fails to act quickly enough, tracheotomy is the last resort and offers the only chance of saving the person's life.

After the acute-reaction phase is over, antihistamines and one of the cortisone-like drugs (prednisone or similar preparation) may be given by mouth to hasten complete recovery, but these drugs are of little emergency use, except possibly when they can be given by intravenous injection.

It is true, of course, that anaphylaxis can best be treated by a physician in a hospital where oxygen and all other facilities are available, but under conditions where medical aid is not and would not be expected to be available, adequate foresight in the provision of supplies and in the training of personnel will save a life that might otherwise be lost.

ELECTRIC SHOCK

Properly used, electricity is our cleanest and safest source of power.   Abused, its unleashed energies can wreak havoc and death.   One has only to witness the devastating destruction caused by a bolt of lightning, or witness its paralyzing and sometimes killing effects on animals and man, to understand and appreciate the enormous energies which may be involved.

Electricity takes many forms, from the enormous static discharges represented by a lightning bolt to the conventional house current.   Many people think it takes a large amount of electricity to prove dangerous.   This is far from the truth; the amount, in fact, depends upon the conditions under which the shock is sustained.

The two basic units for measuring electricity, to put it very simply, are the volt, which is analogous to the pressure in a water system, and the ampere, which is roughly analogous to the amount of water flowing in the system. Under certain conditions which can exist in the average household, electricity at relatively low voltage but fairly high amperage can produce serious injury or death. It has been estimated that the amount of current that it takes to be dangerous is in the neighborhood of about 1/20 of an ampere at average household voltages.

While deaths from electrical accidents or from being struck by lightning are, fortunately, not high in relation to other types of accidents, there is really no way of knowing how many people sustain severe shocks or are knocked unconscious by accidentally coming in contact with an electric current.

What happens is that an electric shock may paralyze the breathing center in the brain and, in addition, so affect the beating mechanism of the heart as to either stop it completely or throw it into a state of twitching (fibrillation), so that pumping action becomes ineffective, and circulation fails.

The amount of electric power required to produce these effects varies in accordance with how good a contact is formed between the victim, the source of electric current, and the ground, electrically speaking. Under dry conditions, for instance, when the humidity is low and one is standing on a dry wooden floor, the contact would be less efficient than under humid conditions or when the floor, one's skin, or one's clothing is wet. Cement or terrazzo floors are particularly dangerous.

In the case of circuits carrying large amounts of electric power, it is not necessary even to come into actual contact in order to receive a shock, since an arc of electricity may jump from the power line to a person's body. Being struck by lightning, the result of being in the path of a heavy charge of electricity seeking an electrical ground, is a good example of severe shock.

Certain precautions regarding the use of electricity cannot be emphasized too strongly. Given the right circumstance, the ordinary 110-volt house current can be fatal. For this reason one should be especially careful about coming in contact with any home electrical circuit, such as a radio or television set, when any portion of the body is in water, as when taking a bath or washing one's hands, or even standing on a wet bathroom floor.

Of very particular everyday importance is the safeguarding of little children from electrocution. Children love to stick things into things! Inserting a metal object such as a hairpin or small screwdriver into a standard electric service outlet is all that is needed to bring about a tragedy. Where small children are in a household, use the foolproof capped type of outlet to avoid such danger.

Frequently an electrical appliance becomes defective and develops a partial short circuit or electrical leak. Often this is noticed only when one happens to touch the appliance while the current is on and gets a mild shock; some type of failure may produce a dangerous shock if the device is connected even though the current is not actually turned on. In such a case, the appliance should not be used again until it is repaired. The defect will only get worse, and if neglected might become serious enough to produce a dangerous or even fatal shock.

Television sets can be particularly dangerous because of the high voltages required to energize the picture tube, and no one who does not have special training and the proper equipment to make the necessary repairs should ever tamper with a television set.

Never use a radio or telephone while taking a bath or otherwise in contact with water.

Another very common source of danger is frayed extension or electric light cords, particularly in fixtures employing the old-fashioned type of metal socket.

Occasionally during a severe storm, a high tension power line will be blown down across a road or actually on top of an automobile. Under no circumstances should the occupants attempt to leave the car until the power has been shut off, since while in the car they are protected by the metal body and frame which, as a rule, will safely conduct the current to the ground. A number of fatalities have resulted when individuals have attempted to leave a car in contact with a power line; whereas, if they had stayed put until help arrived, they would not have jeopardized their own safety.

For safety's sake, some good general rules to remember are

that the combination of water and electricity can be dangerous. Respect the power of electricity, and keep equipment in good repair. Do not use defective equipment even temporarily.

In any event, the patient who has sustained a strong electric shock is often rendered unconscious, and both breathing and the heartbeat may be absent. Electrical burns may or may not be present; often they are not. Remember that in the case of electrical accident artificial respiration and cardiac massage promptly applied may spell the difference between life and death.

Rescue Procedures

1 Remove the victim from contact with the electrical current, or shut it off, *immediately!* Every second during which he is acting as a conductor lessens his chance of survival. Make sure *not* to make contact with the victim, since to do so would mean exposure to the same degree of shock.

2 If there is no way to shut off the current quickly, stand on a dry board or on a *dry nonconducting material,* such as rubber-soled shoes or rubbers, and drag the victim from the contact with one hand that has been thickly insulated in a nonconducting material, such as rubber, dry cloth, or several layers of heavy paper or newspaper.

Another method is to make a loop of dry rope on a dry stick and, by looping this over the victim's foot or hand, drag him away from the contact. Sometimes the electric wire can be pulled away from the victim in this way, or even cut, if a dry tool, such as an ax, is available (Fig. 6-3).

O TREATMENT

1 Break the contact between victim and the source of electricity.

2 Start artificial respiration (see page 123) and external cardiac massage if the heart is not beating or is fibrillating (see page 135). Continue until the victim is breathing normally or a doctor pronounces him dead. Continue resuscitation while en route to a hospital to avoid damage to the brain from lack of oxygen.

3 After the victim has resumed normal breathing, keep him warm, quiet, in a semirecumbent position. If it is required,

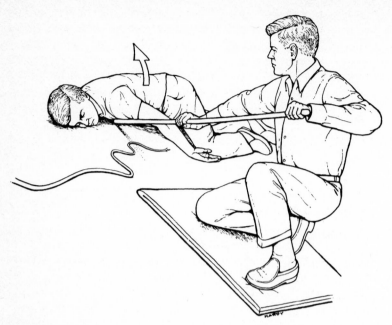

Fig. 6-3. Method of rescuing a victim in contact with a high tension power line, using a piece of dry rope or stick to pull victim from live wire, or vice versa.

administer oxygen and watch for signs of secondary shock which not uncommonly sets in.

4 At *this* point, competent medical aid is of the utmost importance. Electric shock victims, upon recovery, are prone to hysterical outbursts and may attempt to run about or act in a completely disoriented fashion. The person must, of course, be guarded against himself.

7 Fractures

Emergency care of fractures is of great importance in order to prevent or minimize the occurrence of shock, relieve pain, and prevent further injury because of improper handling and help in obtaining a good functional result.

CLOSED AND OPEN FRACTURES

A fracture is a break in a bone and is classified according to the nature of the break, but any fracture may be closed or open.

A *closed fracture* is any break in a bone which is not associated with an open wound. A fracture is referred to as an *open fracture* when an open wound exists. Any fracture may be associated with bruising or tearing of adjacent nerves, blood vessels, and other soft tissues.

In cases of *open fractures*, bleeding should be controlled before moving the injured part or applying splints. This is usually best done by applying a heavy pressure dressing or by using a suitable pressure point.

Never attempt to set a fracture—that is a job for a doctor. Simply cover the open wound with thick sterile gauze compresses or similar dressings and bandage them firmly in place, being sure that in open fractures the broken ends of bone are covered by thick padding. No fracture case should be moved before adequate splinting has been applied. The old adage of "splint 'em where they lie" is still the best advice.

Closed (simple) fractures are further subdivided to describe the way the ends of the bones have broken. This is usually determined by x-ray and is important for the doctor to know in order to set the bones properly. The principal types are described here.

Greenstick Fracture. A greenstick fracture is one in which the bone is not broken completely through. This type of fracture occurs particularly in young children, because their bones are soft and relatively pliable. Fractures of the wrist in young children very commonly are greenstick fractures and hence are not very difficult to treat.

Fissure Fracture. Fissure fractures are those in which there is little or no separation of the broken ends; they usually require only suitable immobilization for their proper healing.

Oblique and Transverse Fractures. An oblique fracture is one in which the break extends *diagonally* across the bone. A transverse fracture is one in which the break extends across the bone at approximately a *right angle* to its long axis. These types of breaks are important, since a nerve or blood vessel may be caught between the jagged ends and injured. Therefore, in setting such fractures, it is necessary to be sure that nothing is interposed between the broken ends of the bone.

Impacted Fracture. An impacted fracture is one in which the broken ends of a bone are not separated, but are actually jammed together. They may or may not require restriction.

Causes and Prevention of Fractures

A break in a bone may be produced by a direct blow; by opposing forces brought to bear on opposite ends of a bone, tending to bend it beyond the breaking point; by crushing forces; and, in rare instances, by muscular action alone, which may twist or tear a bone to the breaking point.

The vast majority of all fractures is the result of falls or automobile accidents; a small proportion occurs as the result of various sporting and industrial accidents; and fractures of all types are common in any major disaster.

The majority of falls occurs in the very young and the older age groups; the mortality in the later group is high because of the other infirmities which are so often present. With the increasing number of automobile accidents at excessive speeds, there is a very high incidence of severe and complicated fractures.

Falls, responsible for many fractures, result largely from unsafe practices and poor housekeeping; most of them are preventable. They are caused by such conditions as improper lighting, wet or slippery floors, unsafe or insecure ladders, makeshift substitutes for ladders (as barrels, boxes, and chairs), and objects left lying about (as shoes, roller skates, tools, or bundles). Children fall off things (as a swing, trapeze, high chair, or porch) or fall down stairs. These falls can be prevented by more careful supervision of the child, the use of well-constructed sturdy equipment, and the use of suitable barriers, such as gates at the top (or bottom) of stairs.

Indications That a Fracture Exists

In some cases there are no clear indications that a fracture has actually occurred, even though a serious one may be present. However, if any one or more of the following signs or symptoms are present, a fracture should be suspected and the victim handled accordingly: the injured person hearing or feeling something "pop"; acute tenderness at the site of the break; considerable pain and swelling (occurs in most cases, but not always); a deformity of the broken part (grotesque position); partial or complete loss of function (not a certain diagnostic sign); grating sensation in the affected area; shortening of the broken limb; and any wound with bone visible or projecting through it.

A simple closed fracture, carelessly handled, may easily become a much more serious injury. Avoid moving the victim without first splinting, as the grating of the broken bone sections is extremely painful and may cause faintness or shock. Rough handling greatly increases pain and shock and may endanger the victim's life.

Fractures, even though not necessarily severe or extensive, may readily lead to a train of serious medical consequences: *Shock* should always be considered as an imminent possibility, and measures should be taken to prevent shock in handling any fracture case. The more severe the fracture, particularly open fractures, the greater likelihood is there of shock. *Infection*, needless to say, poses a definite hazard in any open-type fracture, against which the patient must be given every possible protection.

Fat embolism is another serious danger which is more frequent than commonly supposed. As emphasized by Scudese, Hamada, and Awitan, this is a problem of increasing importance, especially in fractures of the long bones, and particularly in fractures of the tibia and femur.

Fat embolism is most frequent in individuals between 20 and 40 years of age. Symptoms may develop up to the fourth day following injury; they include sudden acute respiratory distress, fever, tachycardia, restlessness, and headache, followed in severe cases by delirium, paralysis of one side of the body, and coma. In about half the cases, petechiae develop over the chest, axilla, and conjunctivae. Fat droplets may be found in the urine. The low level of oxygen characteristically found in the arterial blood in the presence of fat embolism is of diagnostic significance.

Wertzberger and Peltier, as well as many others, emphasize that fat embolism is a relatively self-limited pulmonary process and that the administration of high oxygen tensions is the specific therapy of choice.

In assisting any fracture case, follow these general rules:

1 Do not attempt to change the position of the injured person until the exact nature of his injuries is known.

2 Do not permit him to sit up or move around until it is certain that no harm will result.

3 Except under the most dire emergency, never move an injured person unless fractures have been immobilized.

4 *Never under any circumstances* attempt to transport a victim in any but a reclining or semireclining position. Extensive anatomical damage can, and has, resulted from jamming a seriously injured person into the back seat of an automobile in order to rush him to a hospital, whereas he would have been far better off to have waited for proper ambulance or, at least, station-wagon transportation. Never try to force a victim of *any accident* into the back seat of an automobile.

FRACTURES OF THE EXTREMITIES

In dealing with fractures of the extremities, the injured limb should be placed very gently in as natural a position as possible before proceeding with padding and splinting. To do this with a minimum of discomfort, the break should be supported on each side while the limb is gently straightened and held until the splints are firmly in place.

Types of Splints

In this connection, it should be mentioned that there are many types of splints used to immobilize the upper and lower extremities; many of these are too complicated, or otherwise contraindicated, for emergency aid work, where whatever apparatus used must be simple and easily and quickly applied. The most common type for this purpose is the ordinary wooden splint of suitable dimensions. Wooden splints have the advantage of simplicity, effectiveness, and ready availability, and they can be easily applied by anyone with a minimum of training. Incidentally, rolled-up newspapers or magazines make usable substitutes when regular splints are not available.

Many ambulances carry upper and lower extremity Thomas-type splints which can be slipped over the injured extremity and traction applied so as to provide immobilization of the limb. In our opinion, this type of splint should be used only by especially trained or professional personnel, since improper application may not only cause severe pain, but may do further damage.

Recently there has been developed a new type of splint utilizing pneumatic principles, which offers certain advantages for use in immobilizing extremity fractures under emergency conditions. This type of device consists essentially of a double-walled sack made of transparent vinyl plastic, fitted with a zipper so that it may be slipped over an injured extremity, zipped closed, and then simply inflated by lung pressure through a valve provided for this purpose.

These splints are useful for quick temporary application in the emergency handling of fractures of the extremities, severe burns, crushing injuries, or avulsions, where bleeding is otherwise difficult to control. Certain manufacturers supply these splints in sterile form so that where indicated, as in the control of bleeding in a crush injury, they may be applied against an open wound; being plastic, they do not tend to adhere seriously to the wound upon removal.

Their use is not without hazard except under direct professional observation. They should never be inflated to a pressure greater than 30 millimeters mercury (about as much pressure as can be obtained by lung power) and should be considered only a temporary measure until the victim can be gotten to a hospital. If the interval between application and definitive care is prolonged, the circulation in the extremity should be carefully watched, and the pressure within the split decreased if any sign of impairment is noted or the victim complains of undue constriction or discomfort.

This type of splint also has a place in the definitive care of certain types of injury, particularly those of the hand, but only under the most carefully controlled conditions.

The Upper Extremities

The Upper Arm.   If the bone of an upper arm is fractured, there will be tenderness, pain, swelling, and lack of function of the arm.

○ TREATMENT

If the fracture is open, control any serious bleeding and cover the wound with heavy sterile gauze dressing. Minimize, by proper splinting, the possibility of damage to nerves or blood vessels which run close to the bone and may be caught between the broken ends.

Procedure for Splinting.   Immobilize the arm *against* the *chest,* with the forearm across the chest and suspended by a sling from the neck (Fig. 7-1).

1 Have an assistant hold forearm.
2 Pad two short wooden splints (or boards or newspapers) and place them on inner and outer surfaces of the arm (A).
3 Bring the arm against chest and secure it with two cravat bandages (B).
4 Place the *forearm* comfortably in a cravat sling suspended from around the neck (B).

The Elbow Joint.   Fractures about the elbow joint are common, particularly in children, and may cause extensive damage to the surrounding tissues, nerves, and blood vessels; hence, if not expertly cared for, such fractures may result in varying degrees of permanent disability.

Signs and Symptoms.   One or all of the signs and symptoms may be present. Extensive black-and-blue areas may

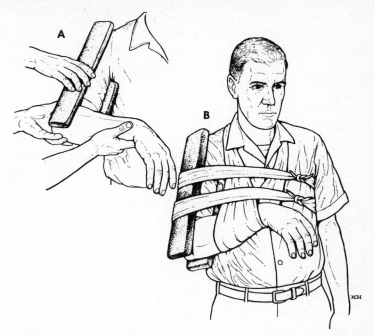

Fig. 7-1. Temporary splinting for broken arm, using splints and three cravats.

develop around the elbow shortly after injury; usually, the arm is in almost a straight-out position; bone may be visible or projecting at the site of the wound.

Do not attempt to straighten, bend, or twist the arm in *any* direction.

Beware of possible further damage to the bone and surrounding blood vessels, nerves, tissues, and large (brachial) artery of the arm by rough handling or movement of the injured part.

If not cared for properly, this type of fracture may easily result in permanent disability.

Procedure for Splinting

1 Apply *extremely well-padded*, protective splints (extending from armpit to fingers) to the arm so that it will be maintained in the position in which it was found.

2 If the fracture is open, *gently* cover the wound with a sterile dressing *before* applying splints. No attempt should be made to clean or otherwise treat the wound.

3 *Only if bleeding is very severe,* apply a tourniquet around the upper one-third of the arm (near the shoulder), over a heavy padding.

4 Get the victim to a hospital as quickly as possible. Do not move the injured arm when transporting him.

The Wrist and Forearm. The most common type of forearm fracture occurs at the lower end of the radius near the wrist, producing a characteristic "silver fork" deformity. This type of fracture usually is caused by falling onto the extended hand, thus snapping the bone; it is known as a "Colles" fracture.

Breaks of one or both bones of the forearm also may occur higher up, either as the result of falls or from direct blows to the forearm.

These fractures should be splinted with padded splints, with the hand in the normal, palm-downward position. The injured person should receive medical attention promptly, since immediate setting of the bones and immobilization of the part in the correct position greatly facilitates healing and recovery.

The Bones of the Hand. The *metacarpal bones* of the hand may be broken as the result of a direct blow or an impact (such as commonly occurs to the hand of a prize fighter when striking a blow).

Signs and Symptoms. There is acute pain, tenderness, and swelling, and the knuckle of the injured bone is much larger than the other knuckles.

○ TREATMENT

This injury should, of course, be seen by a physician, but in the meantime the hand should be immobilized by bandaging it firmly, but not too tightly, with a roller bandage.

The *finger* bones are often broken by striking a hard object in such a way as to bend the finger sharply backward. This is a common injury in baseball, occurring when the ball hits the tips of the fingers during a miscalculated catch.

It is not always easy to be sure of the diagnosis, but a break certainly should be suspected, and may be confirmed by an x-ray picture. In the meantime, the finger should be immobilized in a straightened position on a splint. (Fig. 7-2).

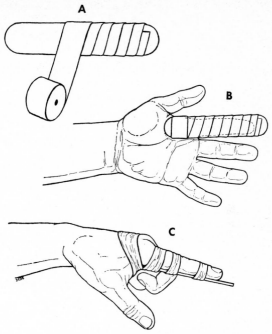

Fig. 7-2. Using a tongue depressor to make a finger splint.

The Lower Extremities

The Hip.   A broken hip is very often the result of a fall and is especially serious in elderly people, in whom complications such as pneumonia frequently occur.   It is sometimes difficult to diagnose a fracture of the hip, because, at the time of injury, the broken ends may jam together, or become impacted, and the victim will continue to use the leg, even though he has considerable pain.   Sometimes it is assumed that the victim has a bad bruise or sprain, and he hobbles about for a while.   However, healing does not take place, the impaction breaks up, and the bone ends come apart, which is likely to mean another fall.   Any bad bruise of the hip region, *particularly in an older person,* should be handled as if a fracture existed until proved otherwise by x-ray pictures.

Signs and Symptoms.   When the hip is fractured, there will be pain in the region of the hip following a fall; signs of a bad bruise or strain; inability of the injured person to lift his leg when he is lying on his back; and a characteristic turning outward of his leg and foot.

O TREATMENT

Make the victim comfortable; treat him for shock if onset is suspected; and immobilize the fractured hip.

Procedures for Splinting.

1 Procure a board about 6 inches wide and long enough to reach from the victim's shoulders to his feet.

2 Pad the board with a blanket, newspaper, or cotton, using a gauze bandage to keep the padding in place.

3 Slide the padded board under the victim, *on the injured side.*

4 Secure the board firmly to the body in such a way as to immobilize the entire leg, the pelvis, and the spine.

5 Transport the victim to a hospital as soon as possible.

If a board cannot be procured, place a blanket between the victim's legs and bandage them firmly together, from the pelvis (abdominal region) to the ankles (Fig. 7-3).

The Knee. The most common fracture of the knee occurs at the kneecap, as the result of a crushing blow. The majority of such injuries are sustained in automobile accidents when the person riding next to the driver ("suicide seat") is thrown forward against the dashboard. Many such accidents are preventable by using a safety belt. Occasionally, a kneecap may be actually torn apart by the force of the great muscles which are attached to it, as during a strenuous athletic effort.

Signs and Symptoms. A diagnosis can be made on the basis of the pain, tenderness, and swelling of the knee joint and the inability of the victim to straighten his knee. Usually, the separated fragments of the kneecap itself can easily be felt.

A fractured knee (if uncomplicated) should simply be immobilized on a padded splint which runs from the thigh to the foot, with the leg fully straightened out. The victim should be transported to the hospital in this position, where surgery will be required to repair the kneecap.

The Lower Leg. Of the two bones of the lower leg, a break in the shinbone (the tibia), which is the main weight-bearing bone, is more serious and produces more pain than a break in the smaller bone (the fibula).

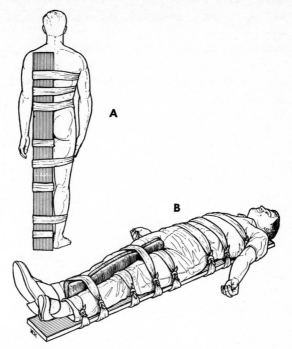

Fig. 7-3. Using a board to splint a broken hip so that the victim can be transported safely.

A fracture of the shinbone is usually apparent if there is any displacement at all, since the bone is so near to the surface; also, it may be quite easy to feel the break in the bone. In addition, the foot will usually be turned outward, as in fractures of the hip.

Quite often fractures will occur simultaneously in both bones just above the ankle joint, particularly in skiing injuries which now occur at the rate of about 225,000 a year. Serious ankle sprains may accompany the fracture; 89 percent of all ski fractures involve a leg, according to Ellison. This type of injury is not only very painful, but is sometimes very difficult to heal.

○ TREATMENT

To treat fractures of the lower leg:

    1 Grasp the foot by taking the toes in one hand and the heel in the other (Fig. 7-4).

2   Pull gently while raising the leg enough to apply padded
    wooden splints so as to immobilize the extremity from well
    above the knee joint to below the ankle joint.

If no other material is available for padding, rolled-up
newspapers or pillows will do.   Fractures of the smaller bone
often require no special splinting.   However, no person suspected of having a leg fracture should be permitted to use his
leg until an accurate diagnosis can be made.

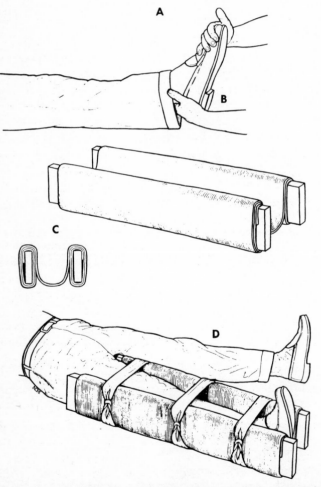

Fig. 7-4. Improvised splinting of a fractured leg. Hold the foot and apply
gentle traction while splints are being applied.

The Foot and Toes.   Fractures of the foot and toes usually are caused by falling heavy objects and result in a type of crushing injury.

Remove the shoe, cutting it away if necessary, and apply a large thick compress and bandage it firmly in place.   The victim should be taken to a hospital or a doctor for proper medical attention.

FRACTURES OF THE SKULL AND FACE

The Skull

Any injury to the skull must be considered serious because of the potential damage to the delicate structures of the brain itself or to the blood vessels which supply it.   A fracture may occur to any portion of the skull, some being potentially more serious than others; those near the back of the head are particularly dangerous.   There may be a severe skull fracture without visible injury to the overlying scalp.   Any unconscious or semiconscious person who has sustained an injury to the head should be treated as though he had sustained a skull fracture.

Signs and Symptoms.   One or all of the following may be present: The victim may or may not be conscious; there may be bleeding or oozing of watery fluid from one or both ears, from the nose and mouth, or from all; and the pupils of the eyes may be of unequal size.

Head injury, whether the skull is fractured or not, may be the cause of epidural or subdural hemorrhage, and it is exceedingly important to watch the patient closely in order to deal with such a development.   The cardinal signs to watch for include an initial period of unconsciousness (as a rule) preceding a period of lucidity, gradually developing intense headache followed by general deterioration of the patient's condition, and ultimate lapse into coma.   The pupil of the eye on the injured side will be dilated, while there is a gradually developing spastic paralysis of the muscles on the opposite side of the body.   Immediate neurosurgical intervention is essential.

In uncomplicated skull fractures, if the victim is conscious, his degree of lucidity and recall of immediate events leading up to the injury are important in judging the amount of brain damage which may have been incurred. Total recall indicates the probability of relatively little brain damage, but excessive motor activity is a bad prognostic sign.

Rubsamen has emphasized that cervical fractures may often accompany head injuries and should always be searched for by both x-ray and neurological examination.

○ TREATMENT

Gentle handling is essential.

The most important first step in caring for a victim of head injury, particularly if he is unconscious, is to make certain that he has a clear airway. There is always a tendency for the tongue to fall back into the pharynx and produce at least partial obstruction, or aspiration of blood or vomitus may have occurred. As a most important step in preventing irreversible coma, an open airway must be maintained and oxygen administered as promptly as possible in order to prevent carbon dioxide buildup.

Bouzarth, in discussing the management of industrial head injuries, condemns the usual procedure of placing the patient on his back, largely because of the possible enhancement of airway obstruction. He recommends, instead, that the patient be placed and transported in the semiprone position. A folded blanket is placed under the torso, with the chin supported on a smaller blanket or some other soft material. This position is preferred for the reasons mentioned, unless it is contraindicated by the nature of the injuries.

Turn the head and body slightly away from the injured side so as to relieve pressure.

Keep the victim absolutely quiet; *never* permit or urge him to get up or move around.

Control bleeding from the scalp by simple compression dressings, or by digital pressure on the temporal artery (q.v.), being as gentle as possible and avoiding any unnecessary movement.

Convulsions occur in a small percentage of head injury cases; the patient should be restrained as gently as possible to avoid injury to himself or others until such time as the proper medication can be administered. It is permissible to place a padded tongue depressor between his teeth to prevent biting of the tongue, but no anticonvulsant medication should be given except under the direction of the neurosurgeon.

If the patient is conscious, he may be extremely apprehensive, and sheer fright may initiate unruly conduct or an actual convulsion.

Except for position, consider the case one of shock and treat it accordingly. Keep the victim as warm and comfortable as possible, since shock in these cases may become profound.

Never give stimulants or any analgesic agent (including narcotics) as these tend to raise intracranial pressure, increase the degree of unconsciousness, and depress respiration.

Evacuate the victim, firmly immobilized, to a hospital as quickly as possible under the supervision of a trained person such as a nurse or a qualified ambulance crew.

Do not give anything to drink, as vomiting is likely; fluid requirements can be taken care of at the hospital. It may, in fact, be necessary to *withdraw* blood in fairly sizable quantities, or utilize some other means of cerebral dehydration such as hypertonic mannitol or urea, in order to lessen the hemorrhage and intracranial pressure.

The Bones of the Face

The bones of the face are often fractured as the result of automobile accidents; of severe blows, such as are received in boxing; or of falls when the face strikes against a hard object.

The Nose. This type of fracture is very common and may result from any hard blow to the nose. It has been known to be caused by such a simple thing as a baby's jerking its head against the mother's nose. Many fractures of the nose are unrecognized, but a good general rule is that any blow to the nose sufficient to produce nosebleed warrants an x-ray. If a broken nose is not repaired soon after injury, particularly in children, serious deformity may result, producing an obstruction to the nasal passages, which will not be easy to repair as the person grows older.

O TREATMENT

1 Do not attempt to splint the fracture itself; internal splinting may be carried out later by the surgeon.
2 If an external wound is present, clean it gently with soap and water.
3 Apply a soft protective compress.

4 Try to control nasal bleeding, if it should occur using extreme gentleness (see page 175).

5 Take the victim to a physician or hospital.

The Upper Jaw. Fractures of the upper jaw or cheekbone require the services of an oral surgeon. There is little that can be done from a first-aid standpoint other than to follow the general procedures for all fractures, with the realization that other extensive injuries (perhaps a fracture of the skull) also may have occurred.

The Lower Jaw. This type of injury is not infrequent, particularly in athletes and in victims of auto accidents. Severe fractures are obvious because of the deformity produced; however, it must be noted that, when there is little displacement of the broken parts, the injury may not be apparent.

Signs and Symptoms. The indications of a fracture of the lower jaw are: open mouth; drooling of saliva and blood; difficult and painful movement of the jaw; teeth unevenly lined up —some often broken or missing.

○ TREATMENT

1 Gently close the jaw so that the lower row of teeth rests against the upper one.

2 Secure the jaw in this position with a four-tailed bandage or two cravat bandages (Fig. 7-5).

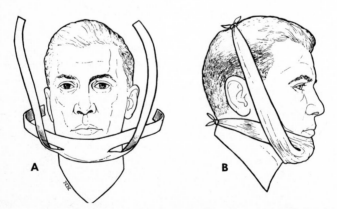

Fig. 7-5. Four-tailed bandage for temporarily immobilizing a fractured jaw.

3 If the victim vomits, loosen the jaw bandage and turn his head to one side; support his jaw gently with your hand until vomiting is over.

FRACTURED COLLARBONE

This is a very common type of fracture, particularly in children and athletes. It may also be caused by auto accidents or by falls from fairly great heights. Ordinarily, it is not a very serious kind of fracture and, with proper care, mends readily.

Signs and Symptoms. The victim usually is aware that he has broken his collarbone; the shoulder on the affected side drops down (tending to bend broken ends of bone upward so that they are noticeable); the arm on the injured side cannot be raised. (The person usually supports his arm on the injured side by holding it at the elbow.)

○ TREATMENT

Immobilize the injured arm and shoulder in the following manner:

1 Place soft padding between the arm and the chest wall.

2 Hold the arm against the side of the body with a triangular bandage, a cravat bandage, or a towel (Fig. 7-6).

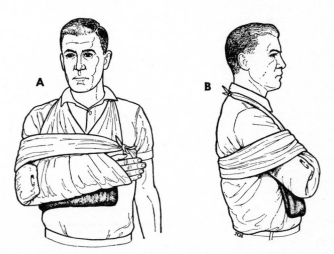

Fig. 7-6. Method of temporary immobilization for broken collarbone, using two triangular bandages—one of which is folded as a cravat.

The fingers should be carefully watched to be sure that the circulation has not been cut off; if so, loosen the bandage, making sure that the hand becomes warm and there is a pulse.

FRACTURED SPINE

There is no injury in which correct handling and emergency care are more important than in fractures of the spine. This is a relatively common type of fracture in these days of high-speed transportation. It occurs as the result of a great compressive force such as is encountered in automobile accidents; train and airplane wrecks; falls from great heights and very often, especially in summertime, from diving into shallow water or into empty swimming pools.

Great good or great harm can be done by the *first person to reach the victim*. The danger arises not from the fracture itself, but from the damage it causes to the delicate tissues of the spinal cord or, if the fracture is very high up in the neck, also to the spinal nerves. Sometimes, the injury is merely a compression or twisting, without actually cutting or tearing the bundles of nerves that make up the spinal cord, which, if relieved promptly enough, will cause only temporary paralysis. However, if the cord is actually cut, all the muscles supplied by the nerves leaving the spinal cord *below* the injury become paralyzed. Paralysis is permanent, as the injured nerves are incapable of growing together again and of restoring the function of the muscles.

The manner in which the injured person is handled, from the time of injury until he is brought under hospital care, can accomplish one of two things: (1) if properly handled, no *further* damage to the cord will be caused, and the nature of the injury may be such that the person has a good chance of escaping permanent paralysis; (2) if improperly handled, the broken fragments of the vertebrae could further grind, bruise, or cut the spinal cord, thus condemning the person to lifelong paralysis, if not death.

To illustrate this point is the often-cited case of the victim of a diving accident making his way to shore unaided, whereupon incompetent handling of the victim, who had an unrecognized fracture of the neck, brought about permanent paralysis. A similar situation may arise when the victim of an automobile accident is bundled into the back seat of another car and rushed to the hospital. With such handling, if he did not have an irreparable injury of the spinal cord when he started for the hospital, it is quite likely that he will have one before he gets there.

Steckler, Epstein, and Epstein have stressed that an auto accident victim (or airplane accident victim—ed.) who has been wearing a seat belt must be suspected of also having sustained both abdominal and spinal injury. Seat-belt injuries to the spine almost always involve the second and third lumbar vertebrae, together with the interspinous and other supporting ligaments.

It cannot be too strongly emphasized that evacuation of any vehicular accident victim, especially one in which seat belts were used, must be accomplished with the possibility in mind that a spinal fracture may have occurred, and the victim transported with an absolute minimum of spinal column movement.

That is why an accident victim should never be moved until you know two things: (1) whether or not he has a fractured spine; (2) if so, where?

Signs and Symptoms. If the victim is conscious, he can be of great assistance in helping to diagnose his condition. He can tell the rescuer whether he has severe pain at any point along the spinal column, since there may or may not be tangible evidence of injury, such as deep tenderness or deformity, at the painful spot. He can also cooperate with the rescuer in trying to move some part of his body so that the seriousness and the site of the fracture can be better determined. For example, if the victim has a broken neck, he will not move his fingers or hands, and, when asked to grasp your hand, his grip will be weak; if he has a broken back, he will not move his feet or toes.

If the victim is *not* conscious, possible damage to the spinal cord may be determined by pricking the sole of his foot (using a pin or sharp-pointed knife). If the muscles of the leg are *not* paralyzed, the foot will be pulled quickly away. If the leg muscles *are* paralyzed, the foot will not move. Prick the victim's hands in the same way; if the hand "jumps" upon being pricked, the injury is below the neck (broken back). If there is no reflex (jump) when the hand is pricked, the victim probably has a broken neck.

O TREATMENT

Emergency treatment of fracture of the spine centers largely on how carefully the victim is moved to a hospital and on preventing his being moved improperly by others. Transportation is a very grave problem and should not be undertaken until you are sure just how you are going to do it and until there are at least three strong persons available to help you by doing exactly what you tell them to do, in the way you want them to do it.

Fractured Neck (Fracture of Cervical Vertebrae). If the victim has a broken neck, he must be transported on a rigid support, flat on his back (*face up*). If he is not already lying on his back, he must be turned to that position. This must be done as a coordinated effort by at least three persons so that his head and neck are kept at all times in line with the rest of his body, without twisting. It is better to wait to turn the injured person until the rigid support on which he will be transported is ready; then he can be turned and placed on the support in one operation.

An ordinary stretcher is not suitable for transporting a person with a broken neck, as even the firmest ones are too flexible.

1　Procure a board or boards, at least 7 feet long and wide enough to amply accommodate the victim. If two boards are used, leave a space of at least 2 inches down the center.

2　Unless the boards are very heavy, they must be reinforced with cross pieces, nailed or tied crosswise at points corresponding approximately to where the person's shoulders, hips, and heels will be.

3　Pad the boards with blankets, and arrange ties in such a way that they may be tied over the victim at frequent intervals so as to hold him absolutely firm and immobile during transportation (Fig. 7-7).

4　Next, place the improvised stretcher as close as possible to the victim.

5　Assign one person to do nothing but hold the victim's head in order to keep it line with the rest of the body at all times, or do this job yourself.

6 Assign one person to hold his shoulders; one, to his hips; and another, if available, to his legs and feet; if not, the one assigned to the hips will have to be responsible for the legs as well.

7 At a prearranged signal, gently lift the victim just enough so that the stretcher can be slid under him or, if there is insufficient help, so that he can be lifted onto it.

8 Be sure that the entire body is moved as a unit, without any twisting of, or pushing or pulling on, the spine.

9 When the victim is on the stretcher, secure him firmly with the ties and cover him with blankets.

10 Do *not* use a pillow of any kind under the head, but *do* use sandbags, rolled-up newspapers, sweaters, or coats on each side of the head to keep it from moving during transit.

11 Someone should guard the victim's head during the trip to the hospital and until released by a doctor, to be sure that it does not move.

Fractured Back. The procedures for caring for a victim of a broken back are the same as those listed for one with a

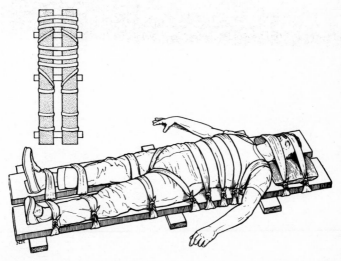

Fig. 7-7. Properly improvised splint for the transportation, in the face-up position, of a person with a fractured neck.

broken neck, *with this important exception:* the victim must be transported in the *face-down position.*

The injury which produces a broken back often occurs when the victim is bent forward so that he is often found lying on his abdomen. In that case:

1 Gently straighten the victim's body with the same care and in the same way as for broken neck, but place him *face down* on a rigid stretcher.

2 If the victim should be found lying wholly or partially on his back, apply the splint *before* turning him.

3 After the splint is firmly secured along *the front* of the victim's body, he may then be safely and easily turned.

4 If it is not possible to do this, turn and place him on the stretcher as described for a broken neck, except that he must be placed in the face-down position (Fig. 7-8).

5 If nothing is available with which to make a rigid support, a blanket may be used to make a carry, but at least *four helpers* are needed if the victim is to be lifted in this way (Fig. 7-9).

If sufficient help or materials are not available to move the victim, cover him with a blanket and wait for adequate help. *It is better to do nothing than to do harm.*

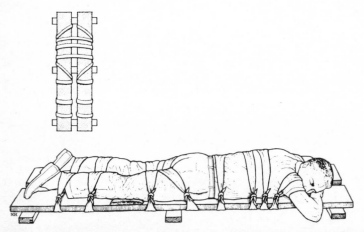

Fig. 7-8. Properly improvised splint for transportation, in the face-down position, of a person with a broken back.

FRACTURE OF THE PELVIS

This injury is a common one, but, while it would always be suspected in severe accident cases, it is not always easily recognized immediately. Probably more than 75 percent of fractures of the pelvis are sustained in auto accidents; falls and other accidents which cause a severe crushing force to be brought to bear on the pelvis account for the remainder.

Fractures of the pelvis may be dangerous for several reasons: (1) There are usually other associated injuries which may be severe, and these victims are very prone to go into shock. (2) Fragments of the pelvic bones may pierce the bladder or tear the ureters, causing leakage of urine into the abdominal cavity, which is extremely serious. For this reason, if there is reason to suspect a fracture of the pelvis, the victim's urine should be examined for blood. (3) These fractures tend to cause intestinal obstruction because of the intense traumatic peritoneal inflammation which they provoke so that the victim must be watched very carefully for this complication, which often can be relieved by medical means without surgery.

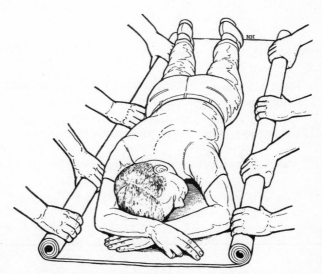

Fig. 7-9. Proper method of using a blanket as a stretcher to carry a person with a broken back.

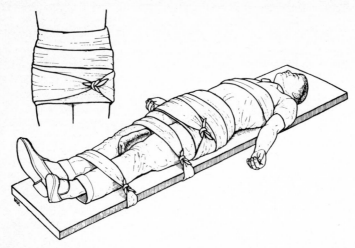

Fig. 7-10. Improvised splinting of a pelvic fracture, using one or more cravats depending upon the size of the victim. The victim is transported on a board or a firm stretcher in the face-up position.

○ TREATMENT

1 Turn the victim *very* gently on his back, and immobilize the pelvis as much as possible.

2 Pass a broad cravat bandage, triangular bandage, or folded blanket about his hips, so that it extends about 2 inches above the hipbones, and about 2 inches down onto the thighs. Tie the ends firmly enough to give firm support to the pelvis, in much the same way that a corset would (Fig. 7-10).

3 Bandage the knees and the ankles firmly together, with a pad placed between the bony prominences for comfort.

4 Transport the victim to a hospital on a firm stretcher, such as a board or shutter, flat on his back (in the *face-up* position). He should be tied firmly to the stretcher, as with a victim of a broken back, so as to secure as rigid immobilization as possible.

5 Take all possible antishock measures (described in Chap. 6), as emergency surgery may be required immediately upon reaching the hospital. This injury is notorious for producing shock and intestinal and bladder complications.

8 Strains, Sprains, and Dislocations

A number of other common types of injuries are, from an emergency care standpoint, not as serious as fractures, but they also involve the body's structural system and may be exceedingly painful as well as incapacitating. Such injuries are known as strains, sprains, and dislocations and occur to the muscles, ligaments, tendons, and joints.

STRAINS

A strain is an overstretching of a muscle or group of muscles in such a way that the little individual bundles making up the muscle are torn or the tendon, by which the muscle is fastened to the bone which it moves, is stretched or ruptured.

Strains are caused by a violent, unexpected movement such as may occur when one is attempting to lift a heavy weight and slips. The result is a wrench which is violent enough to produce some degree of tearing in the muscle groups upon which the brunt of the force is thrown. This kind of accident may also occur as the result of attempting to lift a very heavy weight improperly, so that the force being exerted by the muscles themselves is great enough to produce a tear in the muscle or in its tendon.

Lower Back Strain. One of the most common and most important types of strain affects the lower muscles of the back and accounts for a great deal of lost time in industry. It is usually incurred as the result of attempting to use the back muscles alone in lifting a heavy weight, without being in the proper position to use the strong muscles of the legs and thighs to help. This type of injury can usually be avoided by keeping the back in an erect position and starting the lift with the feet firmly planted on the ground, with the knees bent. The lift is then made by straightening the legs so that the weight is distributed evenly along the strong bony structures of the vertebral column and pelvis, rather than borne by the back muscles alone.

Many other conditions, of course, may give rise to severe low back pain, which, since they present difficult problems in diagnosis, do not lie within the province of emergency care. However, as a matter of general information, such common conditions as herniated, intervertebral disk, osteoarthritis of the spine, bad posture, flat feet, constipation, spastic colon, and kidney stone should be mentioned.

Signs and Symptoms. The indications of low back strain are acute tearing pain at the time of injury which may radiate downward into leg muscles; increasing stiffness and pain on movement of the back and legs; and spasm and excruciating pain in the region of the lower back (victim may be unable to move without assistance).

Sometimes the actual occasion of injury may go unnoticed until later when a sudden spasm catches the victim unaware.

O TREATMENT

1 Rest the involved muscles in whatever position is most comfortable. Often this will be in a semireclining position, with a pillow under the knees, so as to take all possible strain off the back muscles.

2 Apply heat to the back to help relax the spasm, and give the victim an analgesic medication, such as aspirin, in adequate dosage—at least 10 grains every 4 hours. Aspirin is an antiinflammatory agent as well as an analgesic. Gentle massage also is valuable, provided it is not done directly over the affected muscles. Frequently more powerful muscle relaxants and analgesics are more helpful than aspirin in alleviating the muscle spasm and thus helping to stop a "vicious cycle." Among many, diazepam (Valium®) and meperidine (Demerol®) have proved very useful.

3 As soon as the spasm is brought enough under control to

allow the victim to be moved to a standing position or onto a table in the face-down position, apply a supportive strapping.

Usually, strapping should be applied by a physician, trainer or other qualified individual, but, when one is not available, a temporary strapping may be applied.

The basic objectives of strapping a back are to limit movement and to supply compression so as to take the strain off the affected muscles, tendons, and ligaments, thus giving them rest.

A low back strapping should not be left in place longer than 7 to 10 days on a person who is up and about, because the movement of the limbs in walking and sitting often produces chafing in the groin, especially when these areas are not protected by padding.   If the victim is compelled to stay in bed, the strapping may be left in place longer.

Procedures for Strapping the Back.   Strapping of the lower back is best accomplished with strips of adhesive tape 3 inches wide, with the victim in an upright position if possible.   The front pelvic region and the pelvic bones at the back should be protected by a broad double padding.

1   Fasten the first strip 3 inches from the middle of the body in front, and carry the strip around the back, with the lower edge slightly below the buttock crease, to a corresponding point on the opposite side.

2   Apply subsequent strips parallel to and overlapping the preceding strip by about 1½ inches.   Five such strips will usually suffice (Fig. 8-1).

Leg Muscle Strain.   Another common type of strain is known by various names, such as "tennis leg" or "golfer's leg." It consists of a tear in the gastrocnemius muscle, one of the large muscles which form the calf of the leg and actuate certain movements of the foot through the Achilles tendon, which is inserted into the calcaneus, the heel bone of the foot.   The injury is caused by excessive pull on the heel by the calf muscles when one attempts to attain a sudden burst of speed, as when running for a ball in tennis or when putting force into a drive in golf.   Arner and Lindholm dispute the widely held belief that the Achilles tendon itself is involved, but in some cases it may actually be ruptured.

The condition most commonly occurs in individuals of

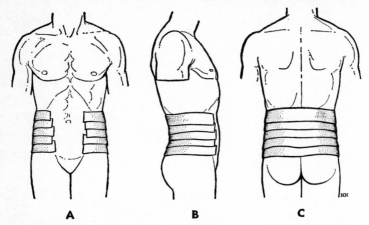

A   **B**   **C**

Fig. 8-1. Method of providing a firm adhesive tape support for injuries of lower back, particularly useful in treatment of sacroiliac strain.

middle age and, according to Froimson, is often preceded by premonitory pain in the calf of the leg a day or so before the injury actually occurs.

At the time of injury the victim may hear a slight "pop" and think he has been hit in the back of the leg by a stray ball. At first there is little pain, but when the player takes his first step the pain may be so severe that he collapses or faints. At the least, he requires assistance to walk.

On examination there is exquisite localized tenderness over the calf of the affected leg, and sometimes a defect can be felt where the muscle belly has torn. Eventually the area may become "black and blue."

Immediate treatment consists of the application of cold compresses or ice over the area of the affected muscle. After the acute local reaction has subsided in 12 to 24 hours, a strip of adhesive may be applied along the back of the leg and down on the heel, with the foot in the position that will give the greatest relaxation to the gastrocnemius muscle. This will help keep the muscle relaxed and protect it from further strain. Crutches should be used to avoid weight bearing for at least the first few days. In severer cases, disability may last several weeks.

When the patient can comfortably discard his crutches, Froimson recommends the temporary addition of an extra heel to the shoe for the involved side in order to provide a lift to the heel and further relieve strain on the gastrocnemius muscle. The extra heel my be discarded after 2 or 3 weeks. An elastic stocking also supplies additional comfort.

Vocational Injuries of Dancers and Acrobats. Because of their special training for maintaining continuous fitness and agility, professional dancers and acrobats seldom experience muscle tears. They frequently suffer joint sprains and may even sustain fractures. However, muscle or tendon tears occasionally occur, which are more disabling than ordinary bruises or sprains.

The most serious muscle tear probably occurs in the fibers of the adductor longus muscle near its tendinous attachment to the pubis (Fig. 8-2). This injury occurs in performing the so-called "split." If the injury is not too severe, and the patient is treated immediately by means of an adhesive strapping, disaster may be averted. A snug inguinal spica bandage can be applied immediately. In strapping for tear of adductor longus tendon, a circular application of 3-inch-wide adhesive tape is started high in the groin. Four turns are made around the upper portion of the injured thigh; two turns lower down are then made around both extremities to obtain maximum adduction (Fig. 8-3). By this method the opposite leg is used as a splint. In the female it may be necessary to place an indwelling catheter for a short period.

When multiple small tears are produced over a long period of time, periostitis develops at the attachment of the adductor longus tendon to the bone. Occasionally myositis ossificans supervenes.

SPRAINS

Sprains are injuries to the ligaments about a joint, or to the joint covering (capsule) itself, which produce undue stretching or actual tearing of these tissues.

Sprains may be relatively minor, or they may cause severe damage to the tissues, which requires many weeks to heal and the symptoms of which are sometimes difficult to distinguish from fracture. As a matter of fact, some sprains are so severe as to pull off a chip of bone (as in some ankle injuries), in which case the condition is spoken of as a *sprain fracture.* Most sprains are caused by a sudden twist or wrench, as when

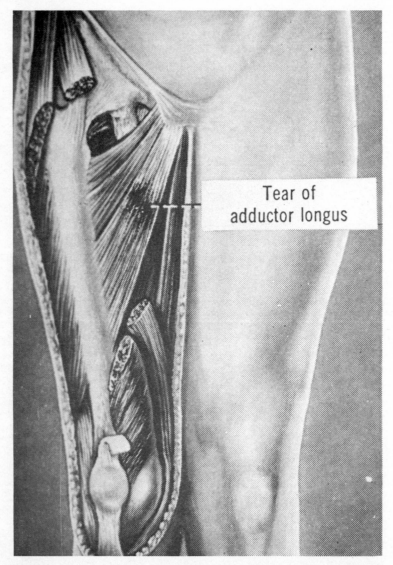

Tear of
adductor longus

Fig. 8-2. Pathologic anatomy of tears of the adductor longus muscle such as occur in professional dancers.

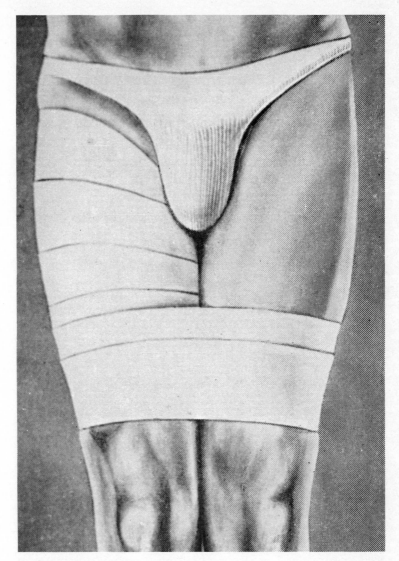

Fig. 8-3. Method of immobilization using adhesive tape in tears of the adductor longus tendon and similar injuries.

the foot is unexpectedly caught in an obstruction while walking or running, which results in the severe twisting of the joint.

A sprain may not be distinguishable from fracture, except by x-ray. However, there may be severe pain at the site of the sprain, swelling, loss of function in the affected part, black-and-blue discoloration and tenderness in the general area.

One of the most common forms of sprain is *neck sprain,* which occurs so frequently as the result of an auto accident (see page 277). Neck sprains or strains may also occur without any apparent injury in older persons with osteoarthritis of the cervical vertebrae.

O TREATMENT

The general treatment of sprains is directed in its early stages to minimizing the swelling and leakage of blood into the injured tissues.

1 Put the injured part at complete rest, and elevate it whenever possible.

2 Use cold applications, in the form of fresh water ice whenever possible, for the first 24 hours, during which time an elastic bandage may be used to give support, some degree of immobilization, and, at the same time, supply gentle pressure to help counteract swelling. Because of its elasticity, the bandage will "give" as the part continues to swell for a time, whereas a regular bandage or adhesive tape would not. Nevertheless, be sure not to apply an elastic bandage too tightly.

3 When it seems unlikely that there will be further swelling, suitable immobilization and firmer support should be applied, so that the victim can again begin to use the part with some degree of comfort and without danger of doing further damage.

As a rule, the application of adhesive tape for the purpose of immobilizing a sprained joint should not be considered a first-aid measure, but should be left to a physician or trainer. There are, however, circumstances when a doctor cannot be procured and under which a properly qualified first-aid worker would be justified in applying an adhesive-tape strapping. For that reason, simple strappings will be described for the most common sprains, namely, those of the wrist, knee, and ankle.

For a Wrist

1 Using 1-inch-wide adhesive tape, start at the base of the hand and place circular strips about the joint, overlapping each turn ½ inch. Six strips will usually suffice (Fig. 8-4A).

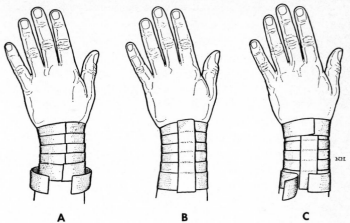

Fig. 8-4. Simple wrist strapping for sprain.

2 Place a perpendicular strip over the ends and fasten with two circular strips (Fig. 8-4*B* and C).

It is important that this strapping be applied firmly enough to give the desired support, but not so tight as to interfere with the venous circulation of the wrist and hand. Otherwise, a painful and possibly dangerous degree of congestion will be produced which will cause more harm than good and seriously interfere with rapid recovery.

For a Knee

1 Using 1-inch-wide adhesive tape, start the first strip on one side of the leg 6 inches above the joint, carry it down the leg to a point directly beneath the kneecap, cross to opposite side and end 6 inches below joint.

2 Start the second strip opposite to the start of the first and follow a similar course.

3 Start the third strip at the point where the first strip ended, carry it up the leg to a joint directly above the kneecap, cross to the other side, and end where the first strip began.

4 Start the fourth strip at the end of the second strip and carry it up the leg to the upper edge of the kneecap, cross to the opposite side, and end at the start of the second strip.

5 Subsequent strips should overlap each other by ½ inch and be continued until the joint is covered.

6 Finishing strips should be 2 inches wide and nearly encircle the leg.

Adequate support and compression of the knee joint can often be obtained by using an elastic bandage (Fig. 8-5). It also will be helpful in the temporary treatment of injury to the cartilages of the knee and will aid in the control of swelling. Anchor a 3-inch-wide elastic bandage several inches below the knee joint, carry it in a circular fashion to a point well above the joint, each turn overlapping the preceding turn by 1½ inches, and fasten it with several strips of adhesive tape. Compression bandages are of value in aiding absorption of fluid in and around joints.

For an Ankle. A sprained ankle is a very common injury; it occurs with considerable frequency on the street or about the home, usually as the result of tripping over rugs, slipping on a wet pavement or highly waxed floor, or turning one's foot on a curb or on dark cellar steps; and it is also commonly sustained by athletes.

Because of the frequency of this injury, it is desirable that anyone trained to render emergency care understand the nature of the injury itself and how it may be effectively treated if a doctor is not readily available.

There are two main types of ankle sprain: one resulting in a torn tendon when the foot is turned forcibly *outward* and the other when the foot is turned forcibly *inward* (Fig. 8-6).

Sprain fractures may occur when the injury is such as to cause a tendon, in addition to being torn itself, to tear off a fragment of the bone to which it is attached. Not uncommonly, the tip of the tibia or fibula may be torn off in this manner.

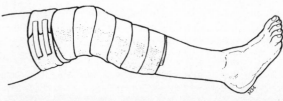

Fig. 8-5. Compression bandage for a knee, using elastic bandage 3 inches wide.

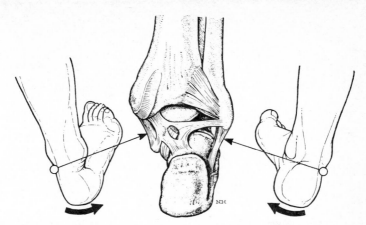

Fig. 8-6. Diagrammatic representation of the tears in the tendons on each side of the ankle joint, which may occur in various types of sprained ankle.

○ TREATMENT

Immediately after an ankle sprain occurs, the leg should be elevated, so as to put the limb at complete rest, and ice cold compresses or fresh water ice applied for 12 to 36 hours, until the acute pain and swelling have subsided.   Then firm pressure with an elastic or other type of bandage is applied to support the foot in the correct position, rest the injured structures, and provide limited use until a firm strapping can be applied and the limb restored to fairly active function.

There are times when, in an emergency, the victim's ankle must be given sufficient support so that he can use the foot enough to transport himself to a point where more suitable treatment can be obtained.   Such support can be temporarily achieved by using a cravat, or any other suitable bandage, tied firmly about the ankle in a figure eight.

The shoe need not be removed for this purpose, although it is better to loosen the laces to permit easy removal of the shoe later on, when swelling may be more severe (Fig. 8-7).

After 24 hours or so, when the swelling is down and the victim is ready to try a little weight on the foot, an ankle strapping may be applied.   While strapping is best done by a doctor, a little practice on a well ankle will enable the first-aider to learn to do a satisfactory job.   As a matter of fact,

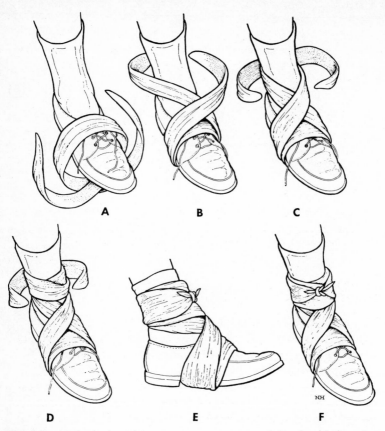

Fig. 8-7. Method of applying temporary support to injured ankle by using a figure-eight cravat over a shoe which has been loosened to allow for swelling.

many athletic trainers are experts and put on an excellent strapping in a matter of a few minutes.

It should be emphasized that only a simple sprain, with little or no displacement, should be treated immediately with adhesive strapping. However, in sprains of this type, weight bearing can often be permitted promptly.

One method of ankle strapping is as follows (Fig. 8-8):

1 Using 1-inch-wide tape, start the first strip 5 inches above the ankle joint, on the inner side of the leg, close to the Achilles tendon. Carry the tape down the leg, under the heel, up on the outer side of the leg, and fasten it slightly higher than the starting point.

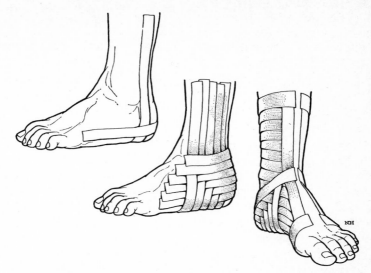

Fig. 8-8. Application of the well-known Gibney ankle strapping, one of the most widely used methods for athletic injuries.

2 Start the second strip at the base of the big toe, follow the inside edge of the foot, go around the heel, and end at the base of the small toe.

3 Then, alternately apply perpendicular and horizontal strips as follows: the third and subsequent perpendicular strips are placed parallel to and overlapping ½ inch of the previous strip. The fourth and subsequent horizontal strips are placed parallel to and overlapping ½ inch of the previous strip. The size of the ankle will determine the number of strips to be used.

4 To complete the strapping, place two perpendicular strips along the front edges of the strapping, and anchor these with three strips placed semicircularly around the foot, beneath the ankle bones, and around the calf so as to leave a free circulatory path open along the instep and the shin.

Sprain Fractures

If there is any question as to the existence of a fracture, the patient must receive medical aid as promptly as possible, as treatment may be difficult and its success depends upon getting it early. In the meantime, weight bearing must be absolutely forbidden; the part should be elevated with a light compression bandage, and cold in the form of fresh water ice applied. In 36 to 48 hours much of the acute reaction will have subsided, and a decision can then be made as to the best method of immobilization. In severe cases, ambulation may be delayed for a matter of weeks.

DISLOCATIONS

Where there is a freely movable joint, there exists the possibility of a dislocation. This may come about by either the stretching or tearing of the fibrous tissue capsule which holds the joint together, thus allowing the bones which form the joint to slip out of place. A dislocation occurring in a ball-and-socket joint means that the ball part simply slips out of the socket.

Some joints are much more prone to dislocation than others. Dislocations of the jaw, shoulder, elbow, wrist, fingers, hip, knee, ankle, and toes are common in everyday life.

A dislocation occurs as the result of a twisting force applied to a bone near a joint, from sudden spastic muscular contractions, from an extension of the forces which also produce sprains, and from falls in which the force is transmitted directly to the joint. The resultant stretching lets the bone slip out of its socket.

Symptoms

In general, the signs and symptoms of a dislocation are: rigidity and loss of function of the injured part; unnatural shape of the affected joint; lengthening or shortening of the affected limb; very severe pain about the joint; and marked swelling.

General Procedures

Until medical aid is available, immobilize the part by splinting it, by placing it in a sling, or both. Make the patient as comfortable as possible while waiting for a doctor. If medical aid is *not* available, you will have to try to set the dislocation.

Some dislocations are not easy to reduce. If, after trying *once*, you do not succeed, let the patient rest a minute and then try again. But multiple failures only serve to further injure the part and may lead to an unstable joint after reduction has eventually been effected under anesthesia.

Obviously, certain situations are so complicated that they are beyond the scope of emergency aid; in such cases, there is little choice but to get the victim to a hospital as quickly as possible, with the dislocated part suitably immobilized for transportation. However, dislocations of the jaw, fingers, and toes, and occasionally other dislocations can be handled satisfactorily by the well-trained first-aider.

Jaw. Dislocation of the lower jaw may occur during a yawn, during the extraction of a tooth, when taking too big a mouthful of food, or as the result of direct force applied to the lower jaw while the mouth is open. Usually both sides are dislocated, although sometimes only one side may have slipped out of its socket.

In this type of dislocation, the mouth stays open and, in fact, cannot be closed. The condition is very painful and may not be easy to correct.

○ TREATMENT

Reducing a dislocation of the lower jaw is accomplished in the following manner, with thumbs wrapped in heavy gauze or a large handkerchief:

1   Place the thumbs over the lower molar teeth as far back on each side of the jaw as possible (Fig. 8-9).

2   Then, with the fingers of each hand under the victim's chin, press the thumbs firmly downward.

3   As the back portion of the jaw is felt to move downward and backward, lift the chin upward.

4   As the jaw starts to return to its proper position, slip the thumbs out of the way alongside each jawbone, since the jaw snaps into place with a strong click. (If the thumbs are far enough back to be in the way, they may be painfully squeezed against the upper jaw.)

Sometimes, considerable force is required to accomplish reduction of the dislocation. Occasionally, it may not be possible without an anesthetic to relax the muscles. In such a case, setting the dislocation, of course, requires medical aid. Once the dislocation is reduced, apply a cravat bandage to hold the jaw firm and give it support until the ligaments have healed.

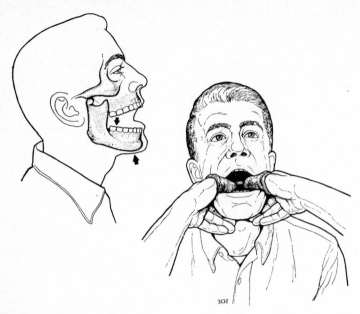

Fig. 8-9. Method of reducing a dislocation of the jaw by pressing downward and backward with padded thumbs.

Shoulder. This condition usually is the result of a fall on the shoulder, of a direct blow, or of forces transmitted to the shoulder joint because of a fall on the elbow or hand. It presents a very serious situation, since there may be associated damage to nerves and blood vessels in the region, as well as an accompanying fracture of the head of the upper arm bone.

A common mistake is to treat a fracture of the bone of the upper arm as if it were a dislocation; this error must be guarded against.

Dislocations of the shoulder constitute from 40 to 65 per cent of all dislocations. There are several types, depending upon whether the head of the arm bone slips forward or backward, but a forward dislocation is by far the most common.

○ TREATMENT

Setting of a dislocated shoulder is extremely painful and may cause further damage very easily. Therefore, if at all possible, this procedure should be left to a physician, the arm being supported with a triangular bandage until he can take care of it. However, circumstances sometimes warrant an attempt at setting under emergency conditions without medical assistance, provided the possibility of doing further damage and the necesssity for extreme gentleness are fully realized.

The simplest way to accomplish reduction of a dislocated shoulder is to have the victim seated and the operator sitting opposite him on the side of the injury. If it is feared the victim may faint, the following maneuvers may be accomplished with him lying down:

1 Bring the elbow very gently close to the victim's side and slightly toward the back (Fig. 8-10*A*).

2 Then, holding the elbow itself in this position, turn the forearm outward so that it projects more or less at right angles to the body (Fig. 8-10*B*).

3 With the forearm held in this position, slowly and gently lift the elbow upward, to form an angle of about 60 degrees (Fig. 8-10*C*).

4 Then bring the forearm quickly across the front of the body while holding the elbow in the raised position (Fig. 8-10*D*).

If setting is accomplished, the head of the arm bone (humerus) will slip back in place with a sharp click. The arm should then be supported with a triangular or cravat bandage.

Do not try again to set the shoulder if the first attempt was not successful. In any case, successful or not, get the victim to a doctor for examination as soon as feasible.

Elbow. This condition usually is caused by a fall upon the hand or by a violent twist of the forearm. There are four types, the most common being a backward displacement of the bones of the forearm at the elbow joint. The condition is easily recognized by the deformity of the joint, an inability to bend the elbow, and great pain.

Reduction of an elbow dislocation is rarely possible without an anesthetic, and it should *never* be attempted without adequate medical aid. It is far better to splint the entire arm so as to immobilize the elbow joint in the position in which it is found, and to get the victim to a hospital as quick as possible.

Wrist. Dislocations of the wrist are not common, but, when they do occur, they usually are caused by a fall on an extended hand. The resulting deformity resembles the pre-

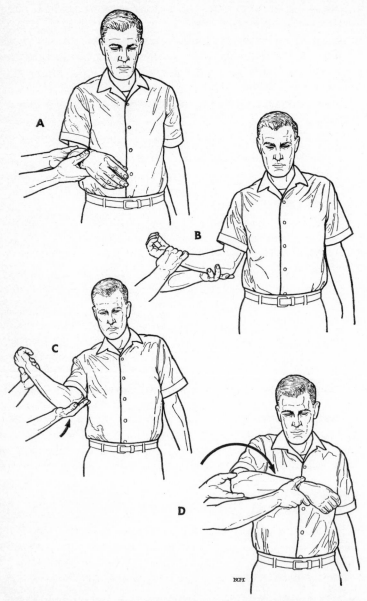

Fig. 8-10. Procedures for setting a dislocated shoulder. (A) Elbow held close to side. (B) Rotate forearm outward. (C) Raise elbow forward. (D) Rotate forearm across the front of the victim.

viously described fracture of the wrist, and it often is difficult to distinguish between them.

For this reason, and because setting may require an anesthetic, it is better to treat the condition as if it were a fracture, to splint the wrist accordingly, and to get the victim to a doctor as promptly as possible.

Finger.

1 Grasp the finger just *above* the dislocated joint, with the palm of the victim's hand turned downward.

2 Holding the finger firmly with the other hand just *below* the dislocation, exert a *strong, direct* pull on the joint. This maneuver is usually successful. If it is not, splint the finger loosely and obtain the help of a doctor (Fig. 8-11).

There is one special exception, which should be noted, known as "football finger," an injury described by Wenger. It occurs usually to the fourth finger when a player grabs an opponent's shirt as he is breaking away, and the finger is momentarily hooked in the jersey. There is a sudden sharp pain which is usually ignored until after the game. The injury is often hard to diagnose and consists of avulsion of the flexor profundus tendon, which is the one that bends the finger. Early x-ray diagnosis and immediate operation are most likely to bring about a successful result.

Thumb. Do not attempt to set a dislocation of a thumb. Because of its complicated anatomy, reduction may require anesthesia and perhaps a minor operation. Cover the thumb with a protective compress, support the hand in a sling, and seek medical aid.

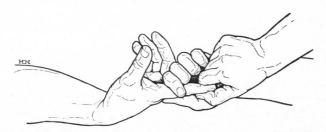

Fig. 8-11. Procedure for reducing a simple dislocation of a finger, applying pull on each side of the affected joint.

Hip. Hip dislocations are caused by falling on a foot or a knee. Great force is required to produce this kind of injury, because the ligaments about the hip joint are very strong. There are several types of hip dislocations, and setting should not be attempted except after thorough x-ray study and with the victim under anesthesia.

Emergency care consists of placing the victim on a firm board, so that he is firmly secured with his knee and foot raised on a pillow or suitable substitute, and transporting him to a hospital (Fig. 8-12).

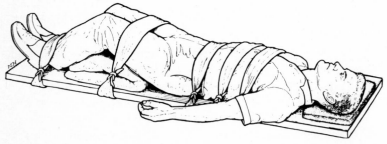

Fig. 8-12. Procedure for immobilizing a victim with a dislocation of the hip in preparation for transportation.

Knee. This type of accident can only be caused by extreme violence and is not common. Posterior dislocation is more common than anterior; the great danger in a knee dislocation is injury to and possible rupture of the popliteal artery, which runs across the joint at the bend of the knee. In these cases the circulation should always be checked at the ankle.

Signs and Symptoms. The condition is easily recognized by the obvious deformity, inability to bend the knee, and great pain.

This is a surgical reduction. The leg should be immobilized in the position in which it is found and the victim transported to the hospital as quickly as possible.

The kneecap may be rather easily dislocated, but can generally be reduced without anesthesia.

Ankle. Dislocation of an ankle without an accompanying fracture is a rarity and should be treated as if it were a fracture. Therefore, setting this type of dislocation should *not* be attempted except by a physician.

Toes. This type of injury often results from blows upon the tips of the toes.

Setting may be effected by bending the toe backward and exerting a strong pull. Sometimes this does not work because a tendon may have slipped in between the heads of the bones; in such a case an operation will be required. If the simple maneuver does not work, it is wise to make no further attempts at setting, but get the victim to a physician.

9

Burns and Other Conditions Caused by Abnormal Temperatures

Temperatures that are too high or too low may affect the body in a number of ways, either locally or generally. For instance, the application of excessive heat or cold to a localized area results in a burn or in frostbite, as the case may be. On the other hand, staying for a prolonged period in a place where the temperature is extremely high may, under certain conditions, result in several types of illness, such as heat cramps, heat exhaustion, or heat stroke.

Burch and Giles* have stressed the effects that climate— temperature, humidity, and barometric pressure—has upon man's health.

We are all aware, of course, of the tremendous increase in respiratory illnesses during the winter or during cold waves in the warmer parts of the country, but the increase in morbidity during these periods is not due solely to these conditions per se. Respiratory infections, particularly, injure and kill hundreds of thousands of people of all ages suffering from coincidental chronic illness, especially old people and those with heart disease.

What is not widely realized is that a similar increase in morbidity and mortality of patients with chronic illness also occurs during the summer. Deaths from cardiac disease soar

---

* Burch, G. E. and Giles, Thomas D.: The Burdens of a Hot and Humid Environment on the Heart. *Modern Concepts of Cardiovascular Disease*, Vol. XXXIX, No. 8, August, 1970. (By permission of the American Heart Association, Inc.)

during heat waves, when there is a sudden onset of hot and humid weather, and especially among old people. Each year many people die from excessive heat, particularly during heat waves that develop suddenly when acclimatization has not had time to develop.

True, heat exhaustion and heat strokes themselves account for many deaths, but it is the effect of heat on patients with cardiovascular and other chronic debilitating diseases that is responsible for the greatest morbidity and mortality.

One of the major reasons for this is that the cardiovascular system itself exercises a primary role in maintaining the thermal equilibrium of the body, so that when this system is diseased, it is vulnerable to injury from extreme climatic conditions. For this reason, death from coronary thrombosis or myocardial infarction, stroke, emphysema, and related conditions increases sharply during the summer months in southern cities, whereas in the more northern areas the greatest mortality occurs during the winter months.

An additional factor of special interest is emphasized by the detailed studies made by Hodgson with respect to the relationship between levels of air pollution as measured by sulfur dioxide content, particulate matter, and day-to-day temperature changes. The results showed that both particulate matter and temperature stresses are important in the death rates of those over 65 years of age, with particulate matter alone more significant in the daily mortality variations of those below that age. In both groups, the data supported a strong implication that all measurable air pollution is harmful from a medical viewpoint.

All these factors are of importance in relationship to emergency medical care, since abnormal temperatures at either end of the comfort scale can greatly increase the incidence of those types of illness subject to such environmental influences; these difficulties are further intensified by the presence of atmospheric pollution.

Under such conditions, an emergency situation may occur at almost any time and in any place—in the home, at the beach, or at work. It is, therefore, necessary to understand the factors which can lead to such medical crises and what to do to meet the immediate emergency situation until professional medical aid can be obtained.

BURNS

Probably the most common type of thermal injury is that resulting from direct application of heat in one form or another to the skin, resulting in a burn. A burn may also involve the underlying tissues, causing destruction of the cells in the involved area. The ability of the burn to heal spontaneously depends upon the *depth* to which the injury extends; for this reason, a burn is generally classified as first, second, or third degree to indicate its depth or seriousness (Fig. 9-1).

Burns are painful, but, paradoxically, deep burns may be less painful than relatively superficial ones, since the nerve endings in the deeper burns are wholly destroyed. This fact may be used to reassure the victim by pointing out that, because his burn is giving him great pain, it may not be as serious as it appears.

Close to 7,000 people are killed by fires, burns, and associated causes each year. About 2,000 children under the age of 14 die as the result of fire each year, the deaths for those under 5 numbering almost 1,000; many more survive, but with serious injuries. Explosions of space heaters where kerosene is fed by gravity to burn in an open flame for the heating of individual rooms have caused many fatal burns. Most, if not all, of these accidents might have been prevented.

It is particularly important to keep hot liquids such as coffee, tea, or water out of reach of small infants. In a typical

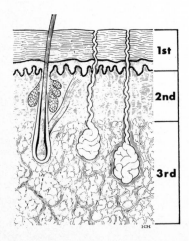

Fig. 9-1. Diagram of the layers of the skin in relation to the depth, or degree, of a burn.

case, a toddler reaches up to the table and tips over a cup of coffee or tea upon himself, inflicting a very painful and often a very deep burn, particularly if the hot liquid is held in prolonged contact with the skin by the clothing.

Those that are burned by direct contact with flame (about a third of the cases) are the most serious and sustain the deepest and most extensive burns. The type of clothing worn at the time of the accident is of importance and was the subject of a study by the American Academy of Pediatrics and the National Fire Protection Association. The object of the study was to learn the role of fabric flammability in clothing fires and included 84 cases of burn injury in which ignition of clothing itself was a causative factor in the burn.

Interestingly enough, all the fabrics involved met the requirements of presently established standards for normal flammability, and of the 124 samples studied, 94 were of cotton exclusively. Others consisted of rayon, acetate, and nylon. Wool was involved in only one case. Most people think that cotton and rayon are safe, but actually these fabrics are among the most flammable, with the synthetics varying in flammability, and wool being the least flammable.

Many persons are under the impression that the new synthetics are more flammable than the old natural materials, but, in general, the opposite is true. Rayon is not any more flammable than cotton, but all other synthetics are less flammable and some will hardly burn at all. They do, however, have a property that is most important in the question of burn injuries. When set afire, they tend to soften, some actually melting, to form a syrupy liquid or a sticky tar-like substance which sticks to the skin.

While all clothing is, of course, flammable to some degree, there are other factors involved which determine the seriousness of the injury. The design of clothing, for instance, plays a major role. Approximately 40 percent of the clothing that burned in the cases studied consisted of loose-fitting night wear —pajamas, housecoats, robes, and nightgowns, with blouses and shirts being involved in nearly one-third of the cases.

Prevention of Burns

Fire-prevention practices, particularly in the home, are of the utmost importance in reducing the incidence of burns and deaths caused by burns. Almost invariably, burn accidents occur as the result of ignorance, carelessness, neglect, or just plain bad housekeeping or bad maintenance practices.

Some Basic Concepts in the Treatment of Burns

Severe burns are among the most difficult of all medical problems to handle and require the greatest medical skill and understanding of the difficult physiological problems which arise. Modern burn treatment has been eminently successful in saving the lives of many people who only a few years ago would have died, but the proper treatment of the burned patient is a team effort requiring the greatest skill and the modern apparatus available in the better equipped hospitals. A burn victim must be given the best of modern medical care as promptly as possible.

The treatment of major burns, as it might be expected to apply in a major civilian disaster, may be divided into five phases, listed in the order in which they should be carried out:

1 Relief of pain.

2 Prevention and treatment of shock.

3 Emergency dressing of burns.

4 Employment of the most feasible antibiotic therapy available, to minimize the occurrence of infection.

5 Maintenance of body fluids.

It warrants reemphasizing that in addition to relief of pain, treatment designed to prevent and care for shock should not wait until the burn can be properly dressed, as valuable time may be lost. As has already been stated, because definitive medical care may not be available for an indefinite period, the best emergency care that can be provided under the circumstances must be given.

In the home treatment of burns, there are some very important "don'ts" to remember. Although some of the practices have become firmly entrenched in people's minds over the years, modern medical science now knows them to be wrong. These include the following:

1 Don't use tannic acid jelly in any form. Such treatment, popular years ago, is now known to be dangerous.

2 Don't use picric acid ointments—they also are dangerous.

Besides, they are not very effective and stain everything they touch.

3 Don't use butter or other fats on a burn—they are hard to get off, may introduce infection, and may irritate the burn.

4 Don't use absorbent cotton on an open burn—it will leave particles of cotton in the wound. However, absorbent cotton may be used to apply medications to a tender burn in which skin is intact.

5 Don't use boric acid soaks in treating large burns or boric acid ointment over large areas; enough boric acid could be absorbed to be dangerous.

6 Don't open blisters if there are many of them. They should be treated by a doctor, since there may be other complicating factors.

Types of Burns

First-degree Burns. A first-degree burn is a superficial injury, characterized merely by reddening of the skin, even though the reddening may be quite intense. A sunburn or a mild scald (as by steam from boiling water) is an example of this type of burn. First-degree burns, while they may be very painful (as in the case of moderate sunburn), will not cause scarring and will heal of their own accord.

O TREATMENT

The use of very cold wet compresses or fresh water ice packs for the treatment of both first- and second-degree burns has come into great favor. This form of treatment seems to lessen the pain quite remarkably and may very well lessen the degree of tissue destruction. By this means, for instance, what might be the more serious second-degree burn type (see below) may possibly be converted into simply a first-degree burn. The method is certainly worth trying whenever feasible.

Subsequently, the involved areas may be coated with an antiseptic water-miscible-type ointment which also has local anesthetic properties. This kind of ointment not only relieves the pain, but prevents the damaged skin from drying out and cracking and minimizes the possibility of infection. Any ointment used for burns should be of the type that can be easily washed off, rather than one that is greasy and difficult to remove without painful rubbing.

Second-degree Burns. A second-degree burn is characterized by deep reddening and blistering because of the extension of the injury into the deeper layers of the skin and the capillaries found there. Such damage results in the leakage of fluid (plasma and electrolytes) from the blood into the tissues, thus raising up the top layers of the skin to form blisters.

A second-degree burn, while deeper than a first-degree one, still does not injure the tissues to such a depth that they cannot heal by themselves when treated with reasonable care. This is an important point which is not always recognized. Burns that are entirely second degree cause little scarring and do not require skin grafting, although, by the very extent of the body surface which may be involved, they may make the victim very ill and present a serious problem.

A severe sunburn with blister formation is a second-degree burn; the unwary person is liable to get a combination of first- and second-degree burns on his first day at the beach if the sun is very hot and he does not take proper precautions.

○ TREATMENT

Second-degree burns, if they are deep or extensive, require competent medical care. The immediate primary objectives are to relieve pain, prevent shock, and minimize infection.

In the ordinary, relatively mild second-degree burn with blister formation, such as commonly occurs about the house, relief can be quite promptly obtained in the following way:

1 Gently clean the skin of any grease or dirt, using sterile absorbent cotton or a gauze pad and a mild antiseptic soap. Pat gently; *do not rub!*

2 If the grease is stubborn, it can be wiped off the skin with an ordinary household dry-cleaning solvent (*not* carbon tetrachloride), followed by soap and water.

3 Before applying an ointment, soak the part in a solution of bicarbonate of soda, made by adding 2 heaping tablespoonfuls to a quart of boiled tap water which has been cooled until it is quite cold.

4 After soaking the part for about 20 minutes and drying it gently with a sterile compress, a good burn ointment, as described above, should be applied.

Blistering. Opening blisters increases the possibility of infection; however, if this is done properly, there is little danger, and the burn will heal more quickly. Most blisters may be opened safely by painting the blister with a nonirritating antiseptic and making a small opening near the *base* of the blister with a needle that has been sterilized by heating to redness over a match flame or a gas flame. (Treatment of extensive blistering should be handled by a physician.) A sterile absorbent gauze pad should then be applied and bandaged firmly in place. To prevent sticking, the gauze pad may be lightly coated with an antiseptic burn ointment.

If a person has suffered extensive, as well as deep, second-degree burns, it will eventually become necessary to contend with the problems of shock, infection, and serious disturbance in the individual's metabolic equilibrium. Medical aid should be sought at once. While awaiting such aid, follow these procedures:

1 Remove clothing from around the burned areas by cutting it away if necessary; and place the victim in a reclining position with his feet raised (shock position).

2 If any cloth sticks to the burn, do not attempt to remove it, but simply cover the area with a dry sterile dressing.

3 Since swelling may be severe and may come on early, remove all rings, bracelets, and similar articles immediately—even from an *unburned part*.

4 Fluids may be given by mouth—as much as the victim can comfortably take.

5 Keep the victim comfortably warm, but not overheated. Do not cover a burn victim directly with a blanket. Blankets are usually germ-laden and scratchy. Use a clean sheet, with a blanket over it if necessary.

6 The burned areas should be covered with sterile dressings or pieces of a freshly laundered sheet, and the victim removed to a hospital as quickly as possible.

Many bad sunburns represent extensive, but still fairly superficial, second-degree burns. After having tried a prolonged soak in a tub of cold water, these usually can be cared for adequately as follows:

1 Cover the burned areas with a water-miscible burn ointment, or continue to use cold wet compresses.

2 Give fluids by mouth—as much as can be tolerated—in order

to dilute toxic substances in the blood, which even a bad sunburn can produce.

3 Aspirin, acetaminophen (Tylenol®), or a similar medication will be helpful in relieving general discomfort.

A word should be said here concerning prolonged and repeated exposure to the sun. It is great to lie on the beach when you are young and get a good tan with or without various sunscreening concoctions. Some of the better ones do screen out a large proportion of the burning rays of the sun's spectrum, but it is all relative; if you get a burn or a tan, obviously a certain proportion of the sun's rays have gotten through to your skin. This may be fine while your skin is young; but when you age and your skin ages, you begin to pay the penalty. Limited exposure is of especial importance in the case of young babies, whose skin is very delicate.

The penalty takes the form of prematurely aged skin, so-called sailor's skin, and the formation of keratoses and "sun cancers," known medically as rodent ulcers or *basal cell epitheliomas,* which may take many forms. They constitute the most common form of skin cancer found in the United States. While, as suggested by Jansen, these lesions are technically malignant, they only rarely metastasize or spread to any degree locally unless treatment is neglected.

Fortunately, there are many modalities for treating this type of cancer, including x-ray, electrodesiccation, and surgical excision. Whatever form of therapy is selected by the physician, the important point is to seek treatment as soon as a lump or a sore on the skin, which does not heal readily, is discovered.

Another important point to be emphasized with respect to overexposure to the sun is that many drugs—often prescription drugs—are photosensitizing; in other words, they can provoke skin reactions of various types when the person using them is exposed to the sun for unduly long periods, or, in some cases, only a very short exposure will cause a reaction.

The list of such compounds is far too long to be included here, but certain commonly used ones are the oral contraceptives and certain hormones, various diuretics, several psychotherapeutic drugs, the corticosteroids, sulfonamides and their diuretic or antidiabetic derivatives, and even some of the sunscreening lotions themselves. There are many others.

The best advice is—beware!—and if you are taking any medication or other preparation, ask your doctor or pharmacist if it is all right to expose yourself to the sun while taking it.

Third-degree Burns. Third-degree burns involve the entire thickness of the skin, with or without charring. Such a burn can rarely heal by itself and requires the best surgical care. Without proper care, there may be months or years of contending with infection, disability, and scarring. Third-degree burns, depending upon their extent, offer the most difficult surgical problems, and in their care every effort is made toward skin grafting of the involved areas at the earliest feasible moment. If grafting is omitted in burns of this type, the only way nature has of healing the wound is by contracture—drawing the undamaged areas together—she cannot by herself replace the part that has been destroyed except by scar formation. It is with such wounds that plastic surgery performs its greatest miracles.

Third-degree burns, if extensive, give rise to burn shock, particularly if initial preventive measures have been inadequate, as well as many medical complications. The mechanisms of burn shock have already been reviewed (see page 179).

Joshi has shown, in a clinicopathologic study of fatally burned children, that congestive heart failure was a prominent contributing factor in their deaths. In all cases the burns were infected, and there were serious fluctuating disturbances in acid-base and protein balance. All these factors reflect the enormous difficulties, from a medical point of view, in providing adequate care for the seriously burned patient—child or adult.

O TREATMENT

From the standpoint of first aid, it must be assumed that some degree of shock is present or imminent, and this must be combated by technics already described (see page 181 et seq.). Otherwise, no attempt should be made to treat the burned areas, except to remove obvious foreign matter, such as burned clothing, and to cover the burns with a clean cloth or sterile dressing.

The extent of the burns, which supplies a rough rule of thumb as to the amount of fluid required per 24-hour period, can be estimated on the basis of the burned area as a percentage of the total body surface (*vide infra*). As much of the required fluid as possible should be given by mouth, as well as whatever sedative is available.

Be sure to mark down the exact amount of any medication given to the victim and so advise the attending physician.

The victim should be transported in a reclining position if possible, with his feet raised, and arrangements should be made to keep him warm and to continue giving him fluids until the hospital is reached.

Fourth-degree Burns.   The term *fourth-degree burn* is used by some specialists to designate a burn which affects the tissues underlying the layers of the skin.   This means that the burn is so deep that muscles, tendons, nerves, blood vessels, and even bone may be involved.   The signs and symptoms and the treatment of fourth-degree burns are an extension of those mentioned in the discussion of third-degree burns.

A fourth-degree burn is caused by intense heat, as from blazing structures, chemical (including gasoline) fires, and during war, from flamethrowers.   This type of burn would be a problem in nuclear warfare.   In industry, small areas of fourth-degree burns may occur as the result of spattering with molten metal.

In the treatment of severe burn victims, it is important to be able to estimate quickly the proportion of a victim's total body area which has been burned in order to know, for instance, how much blood, plasma, and other fluids will be required to control burn shock.   A rule of thumb which has been found useful is to give, during the first 24 hours, 1 milliliter (about 1/30 of an ounce) of plasma (plasma substitute or whole blood) per kilogram (1 kilogram = 2.2 pounds) of body weight for each percent of body surface burned (Fig. 9-2).

Since plasma or whole blood would not be available in the home, comparable amounts of water, saline (1 teaspoonful salt per quart of water), or sugar water (1 tablespoonful per glass) should be given by retention enema (see page 595), in addition to whatever fluids the victim can take by mouth.

Two other important points to remember about burns in general are that, first, it is often impossible to tell for several

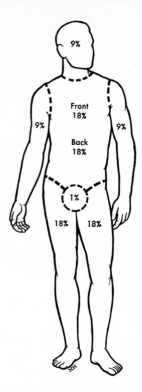

Fig. 9-2. Diagram showing approximate areas of various portions of the body, for use in calculating the extent of burns or other injuries.

days how badly a person has been burned; what appears to be simply a deep second-degree burn may turn out to be of a more serious nature (or, sometimes, less serious). This is particularly true, as emphasized by Salisbury et al., of electrical burns since, when first seen, their appearance gives little clue as to their severity. Until the nature of a burn becomes quite clear, treatment must consist largely of an effort to combat shock and to control infection.

Secondly, any person who has been burned as the result of an explosion or a blast of superheated air must be assumed to have sustained burns of the lungs. Such victims must be carefully observed, since first, they *must* be provided with an adequate airway to prevent respiratory obstruction, and, secondly, symptoms do not appear for about a week after the burn. There then develops a characteristic cough producing bloody mucus, and the victim becomes acutely ill.

The sense of well-being which, at first, the victim seems to enjoy, can be very misleading; he should be kept under observation for several days before reaching any optimistic conclusions.

Electrical and Chemical Burns

Electrical Burns. These result from arcing between a source of high electrical power and a person's body or from being struck by lightning. Electrical burns are not particularly common about the home, but they do occur with some frequency in industry.

Because electrical burns vary widely in type and extent of injuries, and it is often impossible to assess the extent of the damage for some time, they pose a difficult problem in treatment. There are major secondary effects, involving the heart and respiration, which are of more immediate urgency than the burn itself; therefore, in any case of electrical burn, obtain medical aid as soon as possible and in the meantime treat as a case of electrical shock, if so indicated (page 188).

Chemical Burns. Chemical burns of any degree may be produced by contact with strong acids or alkalies or with a corrosive chemical. Frequently, further damage may be done by the neutralizing agent which is used in an attempt to counteract the effects of the original chemical. This may occur in three ways: (1) the neutralizing agent itself may be too strong and may burn the tissues; (2) in neutralizing the original substance, the heat of chemical reaction may be so great as to burn the tissues further; (3) the reaction products formed as the result of the neutralization may themselves be damaging to the tissues.

○ TREATMENT

1 Remove, immediately, all contaminated clothing, and treat the burn by long and thorough drenching with water. Many plants and laboratories are equipped with showers for this purpose, located at strategic points so that, in potentially hazardous areas, a worker is only seconds away from the nearest shower.

2 After thorough washing, treat an *acid burn* by flooding it with a dilute solution of bicarbonate of soda (2 tablespoonfuls to 1 quart water), and an *alkali burn* with a dilute solution of vinegar (about half vinegar and half water).

Surface carbolic acid burns should be flooded with alcohol and then thoroughly washed.

After thorough irrigation and neutralization, chemical burns should be dressed with water-soluble antibiotic ointment and covered with a sterile nonadhering-type dressing.

Chemical Burns of the Eye. If the chemical gets into an eye, extensive flushing of the eye (not with just an eyecup) is essential. The easiest way to accomplish adequate flushing is to fill an enema bag with warm tap water to which 1 teaspoonful of salt has been added to each quart. Raise the bag just high enough so that a gentle stream from the end of the rubber hose flows into the eye. Don't wait to start until the salt solution is made up; start with tap water and use the salt solution when someone else has it ready. After thorough flushing for at least 15 minutes, a soothing antiseptic *ophthalmic* ointment may be instilled into the lower conjunctival sac. Even an apparently mild burn should be seen by an ophthalmologist, since chemical burns, like electrical burns, are slow to heal.

FROSTBITE

Frostbite is an injury to a part of the body due to freezing temperatures. It is similar to a burn in that it represents local injury or death of tissue.

The parts most commonly affected by frostbite are the ears, nose, hands, and feet. As the result of exposure to intensely cold air or liquids, the blood supply to the part of the body affected becomes so limited, because of constriction of the blood vessels, that not enough warmth is present in the tissues to prevent freezing. In severe cases, gangrene sets in and ultimately results in the loss of a portion or all of the affected parts.

A similar condition, prevalent during wartime among troops who have to spend long hours in wet, cold footwear, is known as *immersion foot* or "trench foot." This condition is also seen among outdoor workers and hunters, especially during very cold periods.

Some types of people are much more prone to frostbite

than others.   For instance, those who are nervous, easily excitable, and sweat profusely, and alcoholics who have fallen asleep under conditions where they may be exposed to extreme cold and damp conditions, very commonly sustain frostbite. Every severe blizzard brings cases of frostbite victims who have been trapped in their autmobiles and have had no way of keeping themselves warm until rescued; the same applies to mountain climbers who may get lost or trapped by a severe storm with little means of keeping warm.   Various winter sports enthusiasts may sustain frostbite without realizing it, or may become exposed to prolonged cold as the result of being lost or injured.   In any event, frostbite is common and may often require treatment under somewhat primitive conditions.   For that reason, it is important to know what to do and what not to do.

That some portion of the body is about to suffer from frostbite is heralded by the warning symptoms of a tingling sensation and numbness, which may then become painful with a violet red flush to the skin.   Burning and itching develops and, if the freezing process continues, eventually all sensation is lost and the skin becomes dead white.

There have been many theories regarding the treatment of frostbite, from rubbing the part with snow to gradually letting it thaw out at room temperature.   Nothing could be worse than rubbing it with snow, since frostbitten tissues are extremely susceptible to further injury, and rubbing the part with snow or anything else only serves to increase the extent of the damage.   Thawing out at room temperature is a long and painful process, and probably does little from a definitive viewpoint toward saving damaged tissue from eventual death.

We know from animal studies and from clinical observations that frostbite occurs when the temperature of the involved tissues is lowered to about 22°F.   Under ordinary room temperature conditions it takes a long time for tissues this cold to be warmed back up to body temperature.   It therefore seems logical that the involved tissues should be reheated as rapidly but as gently as is physiologically possible, and studies have indeed shown that when the involved parts are immersed in warm water which is maintained at a temeprature from 103 to 107.5°F., the optimal effect is obtained.   Water temperatures higher than this might further damage the already traumatized tissues, and temperatures any lower than this would not bring about the desired degree of warmth.

With this method of rewarming, the amount of permanently damaged tissue usually turns out to be much less than might at first have been suspected. In severer cases it takes quite a long time to determine just what tissues are permanently damaged and may require amputation, and what tissues will eventually heal by themselves.

In many cases the part may appear at first to be severely damaged and to require amputation, but later proves not to require surgery and relatively little tissue is lost.

In addition to rewarming, every effort should be made to protect the frozen area from further injury, so that it is important to remove very gently anything that may cause constriction, such as boots, socks, or gloves. If it is the feet that are involved, obviously the victim should not be allowed to walk.

Measures which help to improve the general condition and comfort of the victim include hot, stimulating fluids such as tea or coffee, coffee being especially good as it is both a stimulus and helps to dilate the blood vessels as well. In many cases, as the part begins to thaw, the pain is severe enough to require an analgesic.

After thawing is complete, rhythmically raise and lower the part to stimulate the return of circulation. Pressure on any part of the frostbitten area must be avoided; except under hospital conditions, it is probably best to keep it covered with a dry, soft sterile dressing, to help avoid infection.

The victim should not be allowed to smoke, as the effect of tobacco is to constrict the blood vessels further and impair circulation.

If the severity of the injury is great enough to require hospitalization, there are other procedures which may be followed to hasten restoration of the circulation, such as the use of drugs which will bring about marked dilatation of the blood vessels in the extremities, but the value of this type of treatment is still open to debate.

Except in very minor injury, the victim should receive medical care as promptly as possible, and in the meantime every effort should be made to keep the frozen part warm and to prevent infection and further injury.

The most important thing about frostbite is to be on the

alert for signs of it; when the first warning symptoms appear, take such steps as may be possible to protect the affected part.

HEAT CRAMPS

This is a relatively simple and easily controlled condition which develops in some individuals who are subjected to prolonged exposure to high temperature and who drink large amounts of water because of excessive sweating, hence losing a great deal of body salt. Heat cramps are common among workers in heavy industry and may also occur about the home during periods of marked physical exertion when the weather is excessively hot.

Signs and Symptoms. Indications of heat cramps are severe muscle cramps and pain (especially in the calf of a leg and in the abdomen); faintness and dizziness; exhaustion.

O TREATMENT

The treatment of heat cramps consists simply in administering adequate amounts of salt. In mild cases, salt taken in 5- to 10-grain coated tablets will allay the symptoms; more severe cases may require medical attention to promptly relieve the condition by giving salt intravenously. Salt solution (1 teaspoonful per quart of water) by mouth is quick acting but may be nauseating to some people.

Plain salt tablets also may cause nausea in some individuals; therefore, coated tablets are preferable, since the salt is then released in the upper intestine instead of in the stomach, and nausea is minimized. It also helps to prevent nausea if the tablets are taken with a full glass of cool, *not* ice-cold water. Those who perspire excessively should take salt as preventive treatment during the very hot days of summer. This will help to confer an improved sense of well-being and tend to lessen perspiration.

Since heat cramps can be prevented by maintaining an adequate intake of salt, in many industrial plants tablets are made available in dispensers placed in convenient places. Salt tablets should also be kept in the home during the summer, since salt has been found to be useful in minimizing proneness to fatigue, prevalent during very hot days, though actual cramps may not be present.

HEAT EXHAUSTION

Another condition in which high environmental temperature is a contributing cause is heat exhaustion. (A careful distinction must be made between *heat exhaustion* and *heat stroke*, since different treatments are necessary for each of these conditions.)

Signs and Symptoms. Heat exhaustion is the less serious of these two conditions. It occurs most commonly in those not used to hot weather, those who have a tendency to perspire excessively, and in women much more often than in men. In its early stages it is characterized by fatigue, lassitude, and faintness, followed by profuse clammy perspiration, whiteness of skin (*redness* in heat stroke), loss of consciousness—usually brief, cold, clammy skin, weak and thready pulse, and shallow breathing.

The whole appearance of the victim suggests an ordinary case of fainting, but one should be alert to the possibility of heat exhaustion, especially if the weather is very hot or if the individual has been working in a hot, close environment.

Although the skin may feel cold, the body temperature will be found to be either normal or only slightly above normal. This is important, since it is a point which serves to differentiate this condition from the much more serious one of heat stroke.

The development of heat exhaustion starts with the accumulation of large quantities of blood in the skin, in the body's attempt to increase its cooling efficiency under temperature conditions to which the individual is not accustomed. This accumulation causes a substantial loss of circulating blood volume and a decreased output of the heart, which results in a decrease in the blood supply to the brain. If this is severe enough, the victim will faint. Usually, the fainting is transient, since the body processes readjust themselves quickly; but sometimes, more positive restorative measures are required than for ordinary fainting.

O TREATMENT

1 Remove the victim to as cool and comfortable a place as possible, place him in a reclining position, loosen or remove as much of his clothing as possible, and assist the body to cool by using an electric fan or by placing cool moist cloths on his forehead and wrists.

2 If the victim does not respond rapidly, hold aromatic spirits of ammonia near his nose, to act as a stimulant.

3 If these measures are not immediately effective, raise his legs above his body and bandage each leg rather tightly, from the ankles toward the body, in order to force the blood from the legs back into circulation.

4 Since this condition is often associated with depletion of the body's stores of salt, give the victim a salt solution (salt dissolved in water) or salt tablets, by mouth if the victim is conscious; if he is not, by means of a retention enema.

Upon recovery, do not allow the victim to sit up for some time; keep him quiet in a cool place until he feels entirely recovered. Cool, sweetened drinks are helpful, especially sweetened iced coffee, since coffee acts as a stimulant. If necessary, a teaspoonful of aromatic spirits of ammonia in a glass of cool water may be given.

HEAT STROKE

Knochel has pointed out that this condition is more eruditely known as siriasis since it is most commonly associated with the "dog days" of July and August when the dog star, Sirius, rises each morning with the sun, bringing about the association with heat stroke.

The most important feature of heat stroke (sometimes also referred to as *sunstroke*) is the extremely high body temperature which accompanies it. It is a far more serious condition than heat exhaustion.

Heat stroke occurs much more often in males than in females and is more common in elderly people and in those addicted to alcohol. Physical exertion is a definite contributing factor; and an attack is much more likely to occur when the humidity is high than when it is low, even at the same temperature.

The underlying cause of heat stroke is intimately connected with a cessation of sweating or inability to dissipate the heat generated by heavy muscular exertion, which accounts for the excessive rise in body temperature. It is the high fever which causes permanent damage to various organs, such as the brain, kidneys, or liver, and which makes heat stroke so dangerous unless it is treated promptly and efficiently.

Signs and Symptoms.   Usually, the victim is observed after he has collapsed, and his skin will be flushed, very dry, and very hot.   If he is seen shortly after his attack, the flushed appearance will be striking and, together with the fact that the weather is extremely hot or the humidity high, will be a clue to his condition.   However, if profound *circulatory* collapse follows, his face will turn a deathly gray pallor—a sign that indicates a grave condition.

In many cases, the body temperature reaches 106°F and has been known to go as high as 112°F.   The diagnosis is based on a very high body temperature that is not readily explainable by some other obvious cause.   A body temperature over 105°F, occurring during hot weather in a collapsed or unconscious person with a red, hot, dry skin, strongly indicates treatment for heat stroke; the chances are remote that the person is suffering from some other condition.   In the case of an ordinary stroke, for instance, in which the appearance of the person may be similar to that in heat stroke, the body temperature would not be so strikingly high.

○ TREATMENT

This is a grave emergency, and medical aid should be summoned quickly.

Treatment must be begun immediately to assure a favorable outcome, for the danger lies in actual "cooking" of the tissues from the prolonged high fever; therefore, the body temperature must be lowered quickly by every means possible.

1 Place the victim in a tub of very cold water, containing cracked ice if possible.

2 When the body temperature has been lowered to about 100°F, remove the victim to a bed, wrap him in wet, cold sheets, and expose him to several electric fans to increase the rate of evaporation.

3 Check his temperature every few minutes, and if it shows a tendency to rise, place the victim in a tub of cold water again.

4 If the victim cannot be quickly plunged into cold water, try to lower his body temperature by whatever means are available, such as wet sheets (after first removing all his clothes) and forced draft (an electric fan or a hand fan).

5 Administer rectal irrigations or retention enemas of ice water, by using an ordinary enema bag found in practically every household. This will prove helpful in absorbing body heat and lowering the temperature.

Many persons who suffer from heat stroke have previously had various forms of heart disease, so that cardiac damage may be a complicating factor of the attack. For that reason, it is *not recommended* that the victim be placed in full reclining position until he is seen by a doctor, since to do so in a case of severe heart damage might prove fatal. A low, semireclining position is probably safest, but it is important to get the victim to a hospital as quickly as possible.

Recovery from heat stroke is very slow, and careful medical supervision is essential. It should be emphasized again, however, that the eventual outcome depends on the immediate early treatment—the *quick* reduction of body temperature.

10 Vehicular Accidents and the Multiple-Injury Victim

It has been said that the automobile has become the most dangerous weapon ever placed in the hands of a civilian population. In round figures, there are about 56,000 deaths and about 2 million disabling vehicular injuries a year. Since the beginning of this century, the number of people killed in auto accidents is more than double the total number of our battle deaths incurred in all wars in which the United States has ever participated.

Injury is one of the nation's greatest health problems. Each year about 10 million people sustain disabling injuries, 400,000 are permanently disabled, and 114,000 die.

An important fact was pointed out by Fitts in the Scudder Oration on Trauma: "Although deaths from accidents rank fourth—behind heart disease, cancer and stroke—the number of productive years eliminated by trauma raises it in importance. Almost half of those killed from accidents are below the age of 35, and of the total number of deaths from ages 1 to 35, accidents account for almost half. Taking people from all age groups, we find that accidents, because the average age of the accident victim is much lower than that of the other three killers, ranks third in the number of expected years eliminated—twice the number of strokes."

As mentioned in Chapter 2, the leading cause of death in the United States of persons under 39 years of age is accidents, and motor vehicle accidents account for over 40 percent of all accidental deaths. Total cost amounts to about 20 billion dollars a year.

Except in rare instances, the automobile doesn't become dangerous until it starts moving with a human being behind the wheel! Therefore, the problem is one of *human* engineering, and the question is, basically, what makes human beings have automobile accidents. A tremendous amount of research at several of our leading universities, much of it sponsored by the automobile manufacturers themselves, has gone into trying to find out. In any case, all drivers should be taught basic first-aid procedures before being given a license to drive.

We know, for instance, that, for a variety of deep-seated psychological reasons, some people are much more likely to have accidents—any kind—than others, and some individuals certainly should never be allowed behind the wheel of a car. The difficulty is that this is a situation which is almost impossible to control. The sorting out of characteristics of individuals who are more likely to have accidents than the rest of the population has already been reviewed in the discussion of accident proneness earlier in this book.

The greatest single cause of auto accidents is alcohol. The drinking driver is involved in more than 50 percent of the deaths, with ejection of the occupants from the car being the leading cause of death. There is a great deal of misunderstanding about the effect of alcohol on one's capabilities, the usual feeling being "Shucks, a few drinks won't hurt me—I can hold my liquor." Give a tyro a drink or two, and he suddenly becomes a great expert!

The truth of the matter is that the average person shows some impairment of driving skill with as little as 0.05 percent of alcohol in his blood. This level is not, however, enough to convict him of drunken driving, as most laws require a level of 0.15 percent or higher. Most of the problem lies between these two extremes—the chap who has had a few at a cocktail party is not really sober, but thinks he is perfectly capable of handling his own car even under our modern high-speed conditions. Unfortunately, statistics consistently prove how wrong he is. What we need, therefore, are better and more understanding laws that will take this particular type of situation into account; enforced use of seat belts alone would save a great many lives.

Next to alcohol, speed and reckless driving account for the greatest number of deaths—about 30 percent.

Excessive speed brings tremendous forces to bear with the sudden stopping of a vehicle at the moment of impact. As a result, the passengers and driver are thrown against the dashboard and windshield, the steering wheel, and the back of the front seat or are actually thrown out of the car—a common cause of death in such accidents. Hence, the parts of the body most frequently injured are the head and neck, the chest, with the extremities coming third.

The most important ways to avoid such injuries are the conscientious observance of speed limits and the use of safety belts—or even safety harnesses. It has been thoroughly demonstrated that, even in high-impact crashes, a safety belt is the best single protective feature that can now be provided. If properly installed and used, it will prevent more than 60 percent of the deaths and severe injuries which would otherwise have occurred. In spite of the fact that some injuries may occur, pregnant women should also wear seat belts, since the increased protection outweighs the potential hazard.

The remaining 20 percent of auto accidents are the result of a number of factors. Among them are fatigue, which in some cases may actually result in the driver falling asleep at the wheel; various medical conditions, such as a heart attack, a stroke, an epileptic seizure, or the sudden loss of consciousness from any one of several causes; and mechanical failure of the car (Fig. 10-1).

There are certain other special factors that may contribute

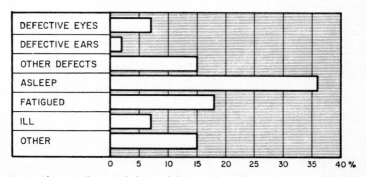

Fig. 10-1. The correlation of driver defects with traffic accidents. Especially important is the factor of driver fatigue.

to or cause an accident. One of these is carbon monoxide, which can seep into a tightly closed car, even though the car is moving. Carbon monoxide quickly causes a person to become drowsy and lose consciousness, even before he realizes that anything is wrong.

It has also been found that those who smoke from 20 to 30 cigarettes a day may show a very substantial amount of carbon monoxide in their blood, and night vision, as well as overall performance, may be impaired by excessive smoking.

In addition, there are many drugs, used for such ailments as motion sickness, allergies, colds, and drowsiness, which may have powerful side effects and *cause* drowsiness and even hallucinations, when the driver thinks he sees something that really isn't there and swerves to avoid it. This alone has caused many accidents.

Furthermore, as has already been noted, various types and degrees of medical impairment may be a precipitating factor in many accidents. Typical examples would be deficient eyesight, epileptiform states, Meniere's syndrome, and cerebral vascular deficiency in older people.

Certain states have enacted legislation which requires the reporting of epileptiform seizures (recurrent convulsive seizures, recurrent periods of unconsciousness, or loss of motor coordination due to epilepsy or related conditions) directly to the Division of Motor Vehicles. This information is considered confidential, and it is used only for determining the eligibility of such an individual to operate a motor vehicle after careful medical screening.

Narcolepsy, another potentially dangerous neurologic disease because the victim is unable to stay awake and is compelled to fall asleep, undoubtedly is responsible for many vehicular as well as other types of accidents. It is estimated by the American Medical Association that the condition is suffered by from 400,000 to 600,000 individuals, of whom between 200,000 and 300,000 are estimated to be motorists. In a study of 100 narcoleptic drivers, it was found that a substantial number had either come close to having accidents or had actually been involved in multiple accidents; only two denied that their condition represented a very real hazard to driving. Obviously, anyone with this disease should not drive under any circumstances.

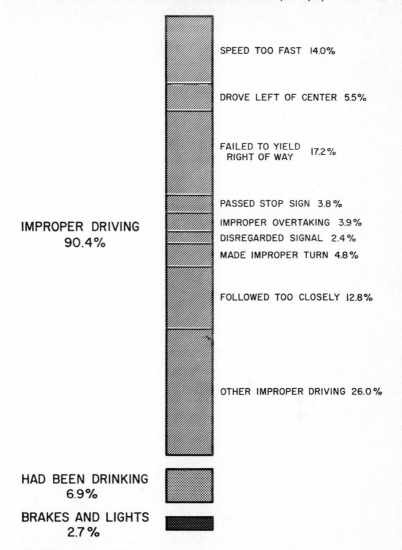

Fig. 10-2. Statistical breakdown of the many contributing causes of auto accidents.

The worst of it is that all these factors, or most of them, can be brought together in one situation, thus increasing the danger (Fig. 10-2). For example, take the all-too-common situation of bumper-to-bumper driving which may result in excessive inhalation of carbon monoxide (from running motors and poorly ventilated cars) and exasperation which often leads to chain smoking and intemperate actions; throw in emotional stress, irritability, and fatigue so common on the return trip at the end of a weekend, and the result is a keg of dynamite on wheels!

The most neglected passengers of the car are young children. Only a small percentage of parents insist upon their children riding in the back seat, and only a few provide comfortable safety seats (ideally the child should ride backwards) with suitable restraining devices, according to the age of the child.

Under present circumstances children are extremely vulnerable to injury in even a small accident and the young child reacts very differently to injury and even to intelligent first-aid measures than does an adult. According to Richardson et al., even a minimal injury in children may produce very serious effects.

It has been pointed out by the Physicians for Auto Safety that, in 1972, 1,000 children under 5 were killed in auto accidents, and more than 77,000 were injured. Shouldn't we use a little discipline and protect our children (and pets)?

In this connection, the American Academy of Pediatrics Committee on Accident Prevention, in a statement on Auto Safety for the Infant and Young Child, has issued the following safety guidelines:

1 Mother's lap is NOT safe.

2 All car doors should be locked.

3 Children must never be unrestrained in the front seat of a motor vehicle or in the cargo section of a station wagon.

4 Infants and children under age 4 years or 40 lbs. should not use standard safety belts. Lap belts alone exert too much pressure on the abdominal area of a small child and may cause injuries in a forward crash. If a safety belt must be used because nothing else is available, the risk of injury can be reduced by using a small pillow between the seat belt and the child which will reduce the likelihood of abdominal injury in a severe crash.

5 For infants and young children, special restraints have been approved by the American Academy of Pediatrics and the Committee on Auto Safety, and are available from reliable auto dealers. To be effective in preventing injury or death

in a crash, the recommended restraints must be installed according to the manufacturer's instructions. Children over 4 years of age and over 40 lbs. in weight may wear regular seat belts. . . ."

After noting the death of a little child left in a parked car during a warm summer day, as the result of excessive heat buildup within the car, Roberts and Roberts initiated an experimentally based study of temperatures inside parked cars during late summer, under various conditions, in Baltimore, Maryland. Some had their front windows open halfway. They found that temperatures rose to a point where a child (or pet) would be extremely uncomfortable or perhaps die. Temperatures in similarly parked cars in the southern United States may rise to as high as 130 to 140°.

Clearly, leaving your child or pet in a closed or semiclosed car on a hot summer day can cause injury or death. Shouldn't this mean something to all driving parents?

The answer to most of these problems is driver education plus a critical self-analysis of one's own fitness to drive, and consideration for the car's occupants.

A training course should be a requirement for everyone of driving age, from teen-agers to adults, and made a part of the regular school curriculum. Such courses, which many schools now have, should cover not only the proper technics of driving, but should stress safety features and practices as well as the dangers of drinking, speeding, and all the other factors which contribute so heavily to auto accidents.

Everyone should be aware of the danger signs that may indicate an accident-prone personality in himself.

If you want some idea of how you measure up, ask yourself the following questions which are based on factors most commonly found in individuals who have had accidents:

Is your physical condition medically safe, as determined by at least a yearly checkup by your doctor?

Do you start out with an attitude of consideration for others and a safety-conscious observance of the traffic laws—even though you might not agree with them?

Can you quickly recognize potential hazards when you see them?

Can you judge speed and distance accurately, and is your vision *really* adequate?

Is your reflex-reaction time fast enough to meet the demands of today's driving conditions?

Are you impulsive—inclined to take chances at the last split second?

Are you nervous or apprehensive?

Are you often depressed, or do you tend to worry too much?

Are you frequently overtired?

Do you pay constant attention to your car, the road, and the other drivers near you, or do you tend to daydream or think out your problems while driving?

Do you have a strong sense of responsibility toward your own passengers as well as toward the occupants of other cars?

You know, as well as anyone else, what the answers to these questions should be. If you come up with too many wrong ones, it is better to take stock of yourself and not to drive until you are satisfied that you have found the right answers. Above all, when you do drive, follow these few simple rules for your own safety and happiness as well as for that of others:

1 Be sure your car is in absolutely safe mechanical condition— steering mechanism, front wheel bearings, brakes, horn, windshield wipers, defrosters, and tires. Carry an adequate first-aid kit, flares, and a flashlight. These may save your life.

2 See that the back and front seats of your car are equipped with safety belts, and make sure that you and the children use them.

3 Don't let little children stand with their faces near the windshield. If you had to stop suddenly, they could very easily be killed.

4 Courtesy is the best policy; give the other driver a break, and observe all the traffic rules—you'll get there faster.

5 If weather conditions are hazardous, such as road icing or poor visibility, play it safe and delay your trip until conditions improve.

6 Don't drive if you are overtired, feel ill, or are taking medicines which might make you drowsy or impair your judgment.

7 Don't drive if you have been drinking, and never ride with a driver who has been drinking—even if you have to walk home!

A slight switch on the Golden Rule is probably the most important axiom of all: Drive unto others as you would have them drive unto you.

TYPES OF AUTO-ACCIDENT INJURIES

Because of the tremendous impact forces usually involved in almost any type of auto accident in which injury is sustained, it is more often the rule, rather than the exception, that there will be more than one type of injury in any given victim, and these are more often of a complex, rather than a simple, nature.

In a detailed study of 1,000 automobile accidents involving over 2,000 occupants, it was found that over 74 percent of the individuals sustained some degree of injury.   In over 72 percent of these, injury to the head occurred in some degree.   In almost 37 percent of the cases, the chest and the chest and spine were involevd.   In 29 percent of the cases, the upper extremities sustained injury and in 47 percent, the lower extremities.   In over 15 percent of the cases, there were injuries to the abdomen, pelvis, and lumbar spine, and in about 7 percent, the neck and cervical spine were involved.

Multiple injuries were extremely common and usually consisted of head injury combined with injury to another part of the body, so that the chances of having to treat an auto-crash victim for more than one injury are very high.

Essentially, injury results from the continued forward motion of the passengers, while the car itself has been brought to a very sudden stop as the result of an impact.   Because of this, any one of a number of things can happen; for instance, the individual riding next to the driver, unless he is protected by a safety belt, may well be projected through the windshield and sustain multiple lacerations and cuts of the face, neck, and arms.

What may be even more important is the fact that, in passing through the windshield, the victim may strike his chest on the dashboard and sustain a crush injury of the chest; a penetrating wound of the chest wall, thus producing a sucking wound of the chest; or a fractured skull or, at least, a concussion.

These serious conditions will be missed unless a thorough

and careful examination of the victim is carried out and all the possibilities are borne in mind, without being distracted by the flurry and excitement occasioned by the usually profuse bleeding of the more superficial and often less important cuts about the face.

The first few chapters of this book have been devoted to a description of specific types of wounds, such as lacerations, puncture wounds, tears of the aorta, fractures, and dislocations, and their probable physiologic results, such as severe hemorrhage, shock, and unconsciousness. It is extremely important to bear in mind, in handling an auto-accident victim, that practically any combination of these conditions may have occurred.

Unfortunately, as many prominent surgeons have noted, the gap between what is being done to medically retrieve the injured and what could be done is wider than for any other disease situation. As Fitts points out: "Waller found that a disproportionate number of deaths from injury are in rural areas, due to lack of good transportation and the ready availability of good hospitals. He showed that the mortality from motor vehicle accidents was higher in rural and mountain counties in California than in urban counties. The National Safety Council reports that 70 percent of the motor vehicle deaths occurred in rural areas and in communities with populations under 2500." But even many city emergency departments' procedures and equipment for handling accident victims (Phase II) leave much to be desired and are now the subject of intensive study looking toward improvement in all areas of emergency care.

In addition, stimulated by the National Highway Safety Act of 1966, many worthy organizations are concentrating on Phase I operations—the emergency care and transportation of injured from the scene of the accident to the hospital. That such a need exists is pointed up by a study of 159 auto accident deaths conducted by Frey, Huelke, and Gikas. Of these, it was considered that 28 victims probably could have been saved. This would have required specific resuscitative measures of endotracheal intubation, intravenous fluid therapy, and aspiration of tension pneumothorax. In 15 of the 28 patients, to have proved lifesaving, these measures would have had to be instituted at the scene of the accident, during transit to the hospital in 11 instances, and within the hospital in 2.

While volunteer ambulance crews perform a dedicated service to the community, there is an increasing need for a more advanced level of technical training in the using of modern rescue and resuscitation equipment, as well as the use of various supplemental items which in the past have not been standard ambulance equipment.

In recognition of these needs, the Committee on Trauma of the American College of Surgeons has recently issued an expanded list of essential items recommended as standard inventory for every effectively equipped ambulance.* The list includes the following items:

1 Portable suction apparatus with wide-bore tubing and rigid pharyngeal suction tip.

2 Hand-operated bag-mask ventilation unit with adult-, child-, and infant-size masks. Clear masks are preferable. Valves must operate in cold weather, and the unit must be capable of use with oxygen supply.

3 Oropharyngeal airways in adult, child, and infant sizes.

4 Mouth-to-mouth artificial ventilation airways for adults and children.

5 Portable oxygen equipment with adequate tubing and semi-open, valveless, transparent masks in adult, child, and infant sizes.

6 Mouth gags, either commercial or made of three tongue blades taped together and padded.

7 Sterile intravenous agents, preferably in plastic bags, with administration kits.

8 Universal dressings, approximately 10 inches by 36 inches, compactly folded and packaged in convenient size.

9 Sterile gauze pads, 4 inches by 4 inches.

10 Soft roller self-adhering type bandages, 6 inches by 5 yards.

11 Roll of aluminum foil, 18 inches by 25 feet, sterilized and wrapped.

12 Two rolls of plain adhesive tape, 3 inches wide.

13 Two sterile burn sheets.

14 Hinged half-ring lower extremity traction splint (ring 9 inches in diameter, overall length of splint 43 inches) with

* Subcommittee on Prehospital Emergency Services on behalf of the Committee on Trauma, American College of Surgeons. BULLETIN of the American College of Surgeons, May 1970.

commercial limb-support slings, padded ankle hitch, and traction strap.

15 Two or more padded boards, 4½ feet long by 3 inches wide, and two or more similarly padded boards, 3 feet long, of material comparable to four-ply wood for coaptation splinting of leg or thigh.

16 Two or more 15-inch by 3-inch padded wooden splints for fractures of the forearm. (By local option, similar splints of cardboard, plastic, wire ladder, or canvas slotted lace-on may be carried in place of the above 36-inch and 15-inch boards.)

17 Simple inflatable splints in addition to Item 16 above or as substitute for the short boards.

18 Short and long spine boards with accessories.

19 Triangular bandages.

20 Large-size safety pins.

21 Shears for bandages.

22 Sterile obstetrical kit.

23 Poison kit.

24 Blood pressure manometer, cuff, and stethoscope.

It will be noted that the present list contains seven new items—intravenous agents, blood pressure manometer, cuff and stethoscope, and obstetrical kit, a poison kit, inflatable splints, aluminum foil, and burn sheets.

Of these seven items, the intravenous agents are essential if the patient is to be treated for shock at the emergency scene and during transportation to medical facilities. Although the technic of infusion is a recommended part of the basic training program for technicians, the exact agents to be used and their uses should be determined by the local physician responsible for crew training.

The technic of blood pressure monitoring is readily acquired during the in-hospital sessions of the basic training program.

The obstetrical kit should contain as a minimum sterile gloves, scissors, umbilical cord clamps or tapes, sterile dressings, towels, and plastic bags. Satisfactory disposable units are available. Burn sheets may be used as drapes if necessary.

Consultants knowledgeable in the field of poison control recommend that syrup of ipecac and activated charcoal be the contents of the poison kit. In the conscious patient, emptying of the stomach by vomiting is considered the optimum treatment in poisoning, except when poisoning is due to corrosives or petroleum products.

Inflatable splints are satisfactory for fractures at and below the knee and at and below the elbow. The hand and foot must be included, and the splint is to be inflated only by lung pressure. Pressure in the splint must be controlled, especially in situations where it is applied in cold weather and, shortly thereafter, the patient is transferred to a heated ambulance.

Aluminum foil is useful as an occlusive and nonadherent dressing.

An effective emergency incubator may be constructed by wrapping a premature infant in foil, leaving its face free.

Ordinary bed sheets—wrapped sterilized, and packaged in plastic bags—provide excellent dressings for burns of any magnitude.

The short and long spine boards (see page 275 et seq.) are essential for safe removal of various injured patients, especially those with actual or suspected damage to the spine. Either board is also useful in providing a firm surface on the wheeled stretcher for performance of cardiopulmonary resuscitation. The straps of 2-inch belting should be at least 9 feet long and equipped with slip-through friction catches.

The "Universal" dressing unfolds to 10 inches by 18 inches or to 10 inches by 36 inches and affords adequate coverage for any wound. It may be used also as padding for splints. When two dressings are folded together lengthwise, they form an effective cervical collar which may be held in place either by safety pins or by wrapping with a soft roller bandage.

The Universal dressing is available commercially but is easily made locally by cutting bolts of standard "A.B.D." material into 36-inch lengths, folding these from each end to the center three times, and packaging each in a paper bag, the end of which is sealed by stapling. After sterilization, each packaged dressing is placed individually in a plastic bag which also contains a 6-inch soft roller bandage.

The hand-operated bag-mask ventilation unit is superior to the mechanical resuscitator or pulmotor. It is simply constructed, it performs adequately, and the operator may make immediate pressure adjustments simply by changing his hand pressure. The unit is also much less costly than the mechanical resuscitator or pulmotor.

The major advantage of the bag-mask unit is that it permits the technician to direct attention to the patient rather than to apparatus.

For effective pharyngeal suction a minimum vacuum of 12 inches of mercury (20 inches optimal) and free air flow of over 30 liters per minute at the delivery tube, with rapid draw-down time, is required.

Litters, and safety and housekeeping equipment, are not specified, since it is assumed that these basic items, as well as *installed* suction and oxygen, will be carried.

Supplemental Medical Equipment. In anticipation of more advanced training in the use of specialized equipment for greater numbers of technicians, and the occasional presence of physicians at the scene of emergencies, additional equipment may be carried in a sealed container, depending on local conditions and decisions. These items are:

Tracheal intubation kit
Pleural decompression set
Drug injection kit
Venous cut-down kit
Minor surgery kit
Tracheostomy or cricothyrotome set
Urinary catheters
Portable cardioscope and defibrillator

Unless a rescue vehicle accompanies an ambulance on every accident call, certain access and extrication equipment also should be carried. The time element in life-threatening problems is so critical that if the technicians must await the arrival of such equipment, lives that could be saved will be lost. Specifically, these items are:

One wrench, 12 inches, with adjustable open end
One screwdriver, 12 inches, with regular blade
One screwdriver, 12 inches, Phillips type
One hacksaw with 12 wire (carbide) blades
One pliers, 10-inch vise-grip

One 5-pound hammer with 15-inch handle
One fire axe butt with 24-inch handle
One 24-inch wrecking bar (bar and two preceding items can either be separate or combined as a forcible entry tool)
One crowbar, 51 inches, with pinch point
One bolt cutter with 1¼-inch jaw opening
One portable power jack and spreader tool
One shovel, 49 inches, with pointed blade
One double-action tin snip, minimum of 8 inches
Two manila ropes, each 50 feet long and ¾ inch in diameter

A power winch is optional. A front-mounted winch, with a minimum capacity of 2 tons, is recommended, particularly in areas where it would not otherwise be readily available. In addition to rated cable, the ambulance should carry a 15-foot rated chain with one grab hook and one running hook.

Handling the Multiple-Injury-Victim Situation. Three basic principles should be borne in mind in all accident situations: first, the possibility of a much more serious type of injury existing than is immediately apparent on first inspection; secondly, it may be necessary to undertake lifesaving measures before the victim (or victims) is removed from the vehicle (it is essential that the victim's ability to breathe be assured and that serious bleeding be controlled to the best degree possible before undertaking what may be prolonged steps toward removal of the victim); third, never attempt to right an overturned vehicle until the occupants have been removed. Access first must be gained to the vehicle, whatever emergency measures taken that are immediately required, and the victims carefully prepared for removal from the vehicle by means of a backboard or other suitable measures. To right the vehicle with the victims still in it may give rise to further disabling or even fatal injury.

Spinal Injuries. Two types of injuries, in particular, should be mentioned because of their frequency of occurrence and their potential seriousness. The first is injury to the spine, including the neck and back, and the second is the so-called "whiplash" injury of the neck.

Fractures of the neck and back are extremely common in

auto accidents, usually as the result of the victim being forced down under the dashboard or crumpled up against the back of the front seat because of the force of the impact.   Being thrown into such positions sharply bends the spine so that the vertebrae become dislocated or actually broken and exert a bending or shearing force on the enclosed spinal cord.

Also, as pointed out by Ommaya et al., neck injuries may cause or be accompanied by serious brain damage, including unconsciousness, hemorrhage, and contusion of the brain and cervical cord.

As previously mentioned (see page 211), notice should be taken of whether the injured person was using a seat belt.   It is true that seat belts prevent an accident victim from being thrown out of the vehicle and offer a high degree of protection against fatal injury.   A study by Steckler, Epstein and Epstein showed that: "The seat belt prevents ejection and, therefore, prevents many serious injuries.   One study of safety belt effectiveness compared injuries among 933 drivers and occupants of the right front seat who used belts and 8,784 who did not. After accounting for the influence of speeds of cars, accident type, and seats occupied, the authors concluded that users of safety belts sustained 35 percent fewer 'major-fatal' grade injuries than nonusers."

Nevertheless, by virtue of this very lifesaving restraining force which seat belts exert, they can produce both abdominal and lower spine or pelvic injury, and this possibility must be kept in mind in handling any vehicular accident victim who had his seat belt in place at the time of the accident.

O TREATMENT

In removing an injured person from an automobile, it should always be borne in mind that since some type of back injury is very liable to exist, always have adequate help when moving the victim so that the least possible strain or twisting force will be put on any part of his spinal column, including his neck.

An excellent way of accomplishing this has been emphasized by J. D. Farrington.*   He recommends the use of two sizes of spine boards, one short and one long (Fig. 10-3).   The

---

* BULLETIN of the American College of Surgeons 52(3): 121–130, May–June, 1967.

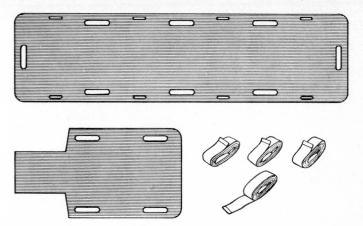

Fig. 10-3. Spine boards are of great value in safely moving the injured, particularly those with possible spinal injury. The short board is used to move sitting victims with cervical injury; the long board is used for those with back injuries, and as a means of extricating the injured from wreckage. The victim is affixed to the board by means of 8-foot-long straps.

short board is used for immobilizing the multiple-injury victim who may be in a sitting position, whether or not he only may be suspected of having sustained a spinal injury. In cases where a cervical injury seems a probable part of the patient's injuries, the board is used in conjunction with a supporting cervical collar. This is easily made up on the spot from two heavy dressings folded lengthwise wrapped snugly about the victim's neck and fastened with safety pins in the rear (Fig. 10-4). The short board is then used to carefully immobilize the victim's spine and head while he is in the upright position, so that he can be removed from the vehicle with a minimum of twisting (Fig. 10-5).

In situations where the victim is accessible, as when thrown from the car and is suspected to have a spinal injury in addition to other possible injuries, or when he must be extricated from between the seats of a vehicle, the long board is used. To do this, it is slid along the back or front of the victim, as the case may be, and he is then fastened securely by means of straps passed through the hand holds. The victim and board may then be worked out of the vehicle as a unit.

A special use for a combination of the long and short boards occurs if the victim is too large to be lifted out. He may be

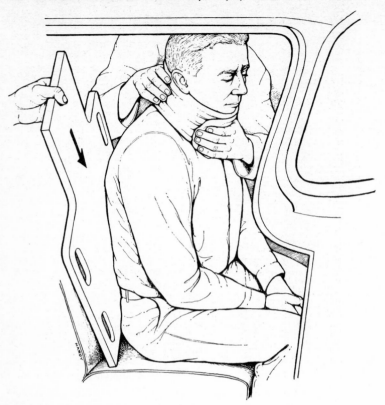

Fig. 10-4. Method of using an extemporized cervical collar and short spine board to extricate victim with possible neck injury safely from car.

removed as a unit on the long board by first securing him to the short board, turning him so that he is placed flat on the seat, thus making his leg accessible for definitive splinting. Then the long board is slid under him and the short board. The short board with the victim on it is then pulled along the long board until properly positioned and secured by straps. The victim can then be lifted out on the long board and he should remain on it until he reaches the hospital. The use of the long board also facilitates removal of many victims even though they may not have spinal injury per se.

Another technic which Farrington has shown to be useful is the use of a 6-foot sling of 1-inch rope for extricating a victim trapped under a vehicle or in such a position in a vehicle that he is otherwise inaccessible (Fig. 10-6).   In the latter case, the sling is used to carefully pull the injured person onto the long board, which has been previously pushed into position under the head and shoulders.   The victim can then be removed from the vehicle with relatively little likelihood of further damage, even though he may have a spinal injury.

Once the injured person is out of the automobile, *continue to handle him as if he had a back injury until it is known for certain that he has not.*   How the victim is handled at this time may determine whether he will be paralyzed for life or whether he may ultimately recover the function of those limbs which may be paralyzed only temporarily.

Whiplash Injuries.   The so-called "whiplash" injury is extremely common, even in relatively minor accidents when no other injury may have been sustained.   It may produce either mild effects or relatively marked neck disability, sometimes accompanied by a strong psychologic factor, which may last for several months or years.

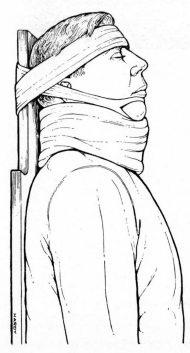

Fig. 10-5. The victim is safely immobilized by firm fixing of head (and upper part of body) to short spine board before moving.

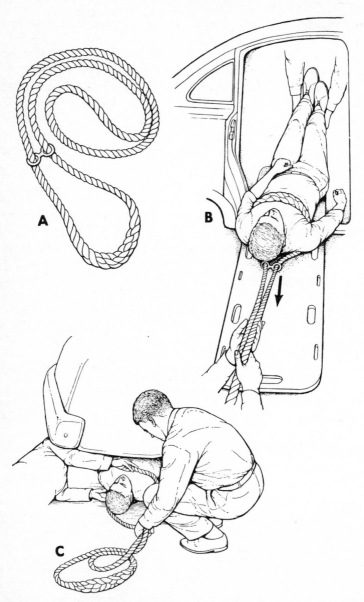

Fig. 10-6.   A 6-foot-long rope sling used in conjunction with the long spine board is very useful in extricating a victim from within a car or from underneath it.   It is also invaluable in other types of heavy rescue work.

A whiplash injury of the neck is the result of a collision, which exerts a sharp forward thrust on the passenger or the driver of the vehicle. Usually, the victim is seated in a relaxed position and the impending accident is totally unanticipated. The strong forward thrust causes his body to bend forward suddenly, with most of the force being exerted on his neck and upper part of his spine. After the body has bent forward as far as it will go, it recoils, snapping the neck and head sharply backward; this cycle may be repeated several times, in a series of such oscillations within a period of a few seconds (Fig. 10-7). The resulting injury is essentially a straining and bruising of the ligaments and muscles of the back; in many of the cases the lower spine may be involved as well.

In at least half the cases, a cerebral concussion also occurs as the result of the sudden mechanical deformity and pressure on the forward part of the brain when the head and neck are suddenly whipped backward after the first acute forward bend.

Signs and Symptoms. In such persons, there may be a momentary lapse of consciousness, lasting from just a few minutes to as long as half an hour. Though the period of unconsciousness may be quite short, the victim may remain bewildered, stunned, and dazed for some time and usually develop severe frontal headache from within a few minutes to several hours or days after the accident.

The most common symptom of whiplash injury is sharp,

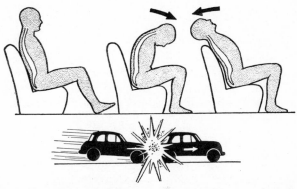

Fig. 10-7. Diagrammatic illustration of forces creating whiplash injury, showing normal position, neck being whipped forward, and head and neck rebounding backward.

intermittent pain in the back of the neck, radiating up into the skull, the lower jaw, down around the shoulders and front part of the chest, and sometimes into the upper extremities. The pain is a result of injury to the nerves in the neck.

In about a fourth of the cases, there may be a dislocation of an intervertebral disk in the neck, a complication which is indicated by sharp pain and changes in the sensation in one upper extremity, which sometimes alternates between both extremities.

A psychoneurosis may develop in victims of whiplash injury, which is extremely persistent and difficult to alleviate. Authorities who have studied the problem state that the circumstances inherent in a whiplash injury make all victims prone to the development of such a disturbing emotional reaction, and it has been found that such a condition is the most important factor in delaying complete recovery.

O TREATMENT

Quick relief of symptoms in whiplash injuries is sometimes difficult, and this is understandable in the light of the nature of the anatomical structures which have sustained injury. On the other hand, the strong emotional complex associated with continued pain, which is often present, has led trial lawyers to quip that nothing will cure a whiplash injury as rapidly as a handsome settlement!

Severe cases, including those which show evidence of emotional disturbance, of concussion, or of a fracture or dislocation of the neck, should, of course, be hospitalized. In milder cases this may not be required and the physician will permit treatment at home, with bed rest and, if indicated, a cervical collar. Often symptoms do not come on for several hours or days after the accident; this is at a time when the victim may be experiencing the greatest emotional disturbance over the incident.

Possible Preventive Measures

Because of the distressing and persistent nature of whiplash injuries, preventive measures are important. About 15 percent of auto accidents causing injury or property damage are rear-end collisions, usually when the first vehicle is stopped at an intersection; roughly 90 percent of whiplash injuries are the result of rear-end collisions.

Accidents of this type can be largely avoided by following a few simple rules which evolved as the result of detailed study by medical investigators. These are as follows:

1 Keep brakes in good condition.

2 Stay a safe stopping distance behind the car ahead.

3 Be alert for sudden changes in traffic conditions, especially for a quick stop by the car ahead.

4 Allow a driver who is following you too closely to pass, since he is quite likely to drive into the rear of your car if you don't.

5 Make use of proper hand signals to indicate stops and turns.

6 When stopping, observe the driver behind in the rearview mirror to be sure that your signal is seen, and, at the same time, you may be able to move ahead enough to avoid his crashing into you.

7 Use your safety belt. In addition, a properly adjusted head rest on the back of the seat will do much to absorb and prevent whiplash forces.

If it is obviously going to be impossible to prevent the car in back from colliding with yours, the best protection is to take your foot off the brake if the road in front is clear, and cover and support the head and neck with your arms or, if you have time, fall in the same protected position across the seat of the car.

Kneecap Injury.   Another kind of injury which is common in both the minor and major types of auto crash is fracture of the kneecap or cutting of the big tendon which holds it in place. This happens, as a rule, when the passenger is catapulted forward and strikes his knee against the lower part of the dashboard, thus exerting a severe crushing force on the kneecap, which may break into many pieces. The fragments are usually retained inside the capsule of the tendon which encloses them, and the part can eventually be repaired surgically. Sometimes the damage is so severe that it is necessary to remove the kneecap and, by plastic surgery, repair the knee joint itself.

Chest Injury.   In many auto accident cases, the chest of the driver or one or more other occupants of the vehicle strikes the steering wheel, cowl, or some other obstruction with sufficient force to create a contusing but nonpenetrating injury. This type of trauma can, of course, be extremely painful and may produce substantial internal damage to the lungs or other vital organs within the thoracic cage.

Myocardial Contusion. Zinsser and Thind have described the effects of myocardial contusion resulting from this type of injury and have observed that it may result from even relatively minor trauma, such as might be caused by being thrown against the dashboard in even a very low speed collision.

The original symptoms are more or less typical of myocardial infarction with severe precordial or retrosternal pain, with cardiac arrythmia being one of the most frequent signs as mentioned by Doty et al. There is not the acute prostration characteristic of a true coronary thrombosis, however. The pain is usually of relatively brief duration, although generalized chest aching and soreness may persist for some time.

Nevertheless, upon the original examination a heart attack is often suspected and an electrocardiogram is therefore of great importance, as well as other studies including serum glutamic oxaloacetic transaminase determinations. The typical finding in myocardial contusion is transient (though sometimes persistent) right bundle branch block, occasionally accompanied by other relatively minor changes in the general pattern.

As emphasized by Zinsser and Thind, an electrocardiogram should always be done in cases of chest trauma, if for no other reason than as a matter of record, since abnormal tracings have been described in apparently normal symptomless individuals but having a history of previous chest injury. A record made at the time of injury would help resolve the question of existing heart disease.

O TREATMENT

The treatment of simple cardiac contusion consists of bed rest and careful EKG monitoring with suitable supportive and sedative therapy. The important point is that cardiac injury must be suspected in every case of chest trauma, particularly if sustained in an automotive accident.

Crush Injuries of the Chest. Another important type of injury, which must be borne in mind and which has already been mentioned, is a crush injury of the chest. Again, this results from severe impact forces which occur when an individual strikes a barrier within a vehicle or is catapulted onto the pavement. The effect is actually to cave in part of the chest, and there may or may not be a sucking wound of the chest wall, tension pneumothorax, or flail chest (q.v.). Rupture of the esophagus is not uncommon, and, as previously emphasized, in many fatal cases the aorta has been completely ruptured or extensively lacerated (see page 164).

It is thus quite evident that in handling any auto-accident victim, one is faced with a potentially complicated situation which demands an effective, logical approach in order to determine the nature and seriousness of the accident and the course of action which will best serve the injured.

Snowmobile Injuries.   A fairly recent advent on the vehicular accident scene, with its own sequelae of injuries, is the snowmobile.   Predictions put a million vehicles in the hands of winter sport enthusiasts in 1970, and many of these will travel over rough terrain at speeds in excess of 60 miles per hour.   Most snowmobiles are designed to carry the driver plus one passenger, with attachments for a trailer to carry supplies plus children.

As these machines travel over rough territory and strike all sort of obstructions, the driver and his passenger get a terrific jolting, resulting in sudden severe flexing of the spine with vertically transmitted force, which frequently results in compression fractures of the lower thoracic and upper lumbar vertebrae.   Other injuries occur when the occupants are thrown from the vehicle or as the result of a head-on collision with a boulder, an automobile, or another snowmobile. Barbed wire fences have a way of producing extensive lacerations on sudden and unexpected impact.

The majority of injuries occurs to teen-agers and young adults, usually male, according to Mongé and Reuter. Seventy-five percent occur during the late afternoon or evening; alcohol was found to be a factor in about two-fifths of the cases.

Chism and Soule, in a study of snowmobile injuries in 103 patients, found, in addition to one fatality, many types of trauma, including fractures and dislocations, sprains, lacerations, and contusions. Practically every major bone or joint was involved, in addition to a pneumothorax injury and one case of kidney laceration. These authors point out that while snowmobiles serve many valuable utilitarian services in many parts of the world, most accidents result from excessive speed and irresponsible operation.

The Committee on the Pediatric Aspects of Physical Fitness, Recreation and Sports, of the American Academy of Pediatrics, issued the following very pertinent comments in 1974:

"The number of deaths in the snowbelt states has reached as high as 20 to 30 per month in the snow season. The National Electronic Injury Surveillance System (NEISS) reported 476 injuries from snowmobiles in the fiscal year ending June, 1973. The national injury figures approximate 18,898. Nine percent of the 476 injuries were listed in the under-14 age group. When considering the number of miles, and the number of users, the statistics are of even more significance. In Michigan (1971) there were 1,835 injured. The *under*-15-year group numbered 298.

"Head injuries top the list of fatal injuries, with drowning a close second (National Safety Council). The lower extremity leads the nonfatal injury list as the most frequently involved part of the body. Yet trauma is not the only source of injury. Frostbite is an ever-present risk in this sport with the windchill index frequently at minus 30°F or below. A nonreported injury thus far is hearing loss. Some states require a noise level not exceeding 82 dB-A, but measured at *50 feet from* the snowmobile. The 1974 snowmobiles have been tested at the *ear level of the driver* and the results disclosed a range from 92 dB-A to 111 dB-A. (Industrial noise limits for U.S. factories are: Workers may not be exposed to more than 115 dB-A for over 15 minutes per day, 110 dB-A for 30 minutes, 105 dB-A for 60 minutes.) Later models do show some improvements in padding, better handling, safer coverings, but they are also of higher horsepower (some models reach 80 miles per hour).

"Of the 28 states that require snowmobile registration, 8 also require a training program for the under-16 driver. The age limit of some states is as low as 10 years for the training programs. Twelve states have no age limit and have no minimum age to operate on public land.

"The Committee suggests a few do's and don'ts for the young snowmobiler:

DO take a good training course.

DO join a snowmobile club (they tend to be the most safety oriented).

DO test drive each machine.

DO know the laws.

DO learn the terrain and surface conditions (how thick is the ice over the area traveled, etc.).

DO learn safe driving techniques.

DO use a buddy system.

DO wear appropriate clothing (frostbite protection) and helmet and goggles.

DON'T let a child drive (it is a powerful machine, as is a car).

DON'T tailgate.

DON'T travel on railroad tracks, private property, or public roads.

DON'T wear long scarves or stocking caps.

"The snowmobile may be a lifesaving tool, or a fun vehicle, or an instrument of pain and destruction—the choice is up to the user."*

General Concepts in Handling Crash Victims

This is perhaps the most challenging situation that can face anyone rendering emergency aid, including the physician. Obviously, there can be no rules that will cover all cases, but there are certain basic guiding principles which, if properly carried out, will greatly enhance the victim's chances of survival during transportation to the hospital and his ultimate recovery.

In the first place, remember that thoroughness is much more important than haste, except to remove victims from such danger as the car catching on fire. If however, there is no immediate danger, wait for adequate help rather than trying to move any victim single-handedly, unless it is obvious that help will not be available within a resonable period of time.

* Reprinted by permission of the American Academy of Pediatrics.

It may be of interest to mention in this connection that the factor of haste has been studied by a group of clinical investigators who found that, in a series of some 2,500 consecutive ambulance runs, haste in transporting the injured was actually unnecessary in 98.2 percent of the cases. In other words, in some 2,455 patients transported by ambulance, there would have been no difference in the ultimate outcome if all traffic regulations had been obeyed. In less than 2 percent of the cases was extreme speed considered essential. It must also be taken into consideration that the danger factor of a speeding ambulance could have increased the severity of the patients' injuries, while in itself constituting a traffic hazard.

As far as handling the victim himself is concerned, definite rules have been set forth by a number of medical authorities who have specialized in the treatment of injuries and have developed certain basic principles as a guide for the less experienced. If these are followed, bearing in mind the basic principles of emergency care already set forth, the chances of an ultimately successful outcome will be greatly enhanced.

Not all of these principles can be carried out at the scene of the accident, nor can all of them be performed by someone who is not especially trained, as, for instance, are the medical corpsmen in the armed services. Whenever possible, of course, the injured should be attended by a physician before being moved; frequently a physician will stop at the scene of an accident and offer expert help, although he is not legally obligated to do so. It is a well-known fact that the first physician to see the victim, whether he works at the scene of the accident, in his office, or in an emergency room of a hospital, has the greatest opportunity to successfully resuscitate the casualty and pave the way for an optimum ultimate result.

It has been emphasized repeatedly by the Committee on Trauma of the American College of Surgeons that lives can be saved if ambulance personnel are well trained, ambulance vehicles are equipped adequately and operated safely, and all communities and operators insist upon meeting and maintaining high standards for the organization and operation of emergency ambulance services. The standards established by the Committee on Trauma include requirements for appraisal and immediate care at the site of injury or illness, followed by safe and comfortable transportation to a hospital. This should be the goal of any organization operating an emergency ambulance service.

Many of the volunteer first-aid and ambulance squads throughout the country have done an excellent job in establishing high standards for dedicated emergency aid to the injured and ill, and it seems quite probable that, as the result of the expertise which comes from study and practice, much secondary injury has been prevented and many lives saved simply through proper handling and emergency service rendered at the site of the emergency, before transportation begins.

It goes without saying that the ambulance itself must be properly equipped and sufficiently large so that emergency aid, such as resuscitation or the administration of fluids, can be continued while enroute. Many modern ambulances are adequate for this purpose, for the most part are expertly and safely operated, and are maintained with a great deal of pride by their crews.

When more than one victim is involved in an accident, the injured must be cared for according to the seriousness of their injuries and the facilities available at the moment. If a victim is so badly injured as to be obviously beyond help, one must move on to the next for whom there is some hope of saving life.

Before starting any first-aid assistance, reassure the victim that you have been trained to know what to do and will take care of him in the best manner possible.

The first problem that must be faced is to remove the victim from the wreckage, although in some instances, as has been indicated, it will be necessary to render assistance in the wreck before an attempt can be safely made to get the victim out. Proper removal of the victim from the wreckage is probably the most important single act of assistance that can be rendered in the light of his future welfare. It is at this point that an injury, however severe, that might be curable through surgery, can be turned into a permanent disability in the flash of a single second.

First things must come first, with the most vital systems of the body being given priority. Make sure that the respiratory system is unobstructed and that the injured person can breathe, for it is obvious that, even though he may be bleeding profusely, if he cannot breathe, for whatever reason, he will not survive.

Therefore, it is important (1) to gently adjust the position of the victim's head in order to make sure that he has an unobstructed airway; (2) to prevent the aspiration of vomitus or foreign matter; and (3) to compensate for blood loss.

If the person is unconscious, he should be placed on his side and his mouth kept open. Using a handkerchief, clear the mouth of all foreign bodies, such as dirt, stones, or the person's own dental plates, and make sure that his airway is unobstructed.

Look for a sucking wound of the chest. If present, it should be closed immediately with *anything* that can be used as a large bulky dressing—even a blanket or folded newspapers firmly bound against the chest wall, if nothing else is available.

In some instances, it will be necessary to initiate artificial respiration; under these circumstances mouth-to-mouth or mouth-to-airway is the best method (see pages 123 and 128).

Having assured yourself that the victim is breathing properly and has an adequate airway, search for and control the source of hemorrhage. Hemorrhage can usually be controlled by direct pressure over the bleeding area and control maintained by the application of a pressure dressing. As stated elsewhere in this book, a tourniquet should be used *as a last resort,* but in some situations it may be necessary as a lifesaving measure. If you do use one, make sure that it is properly applied; once applied, it should *not* be removed until the injured person has been taken to the hospital and facilities are available to cope with a hemorrhage and possible shock. Occasionally, because of its nature or location, bleeding cannot be adequately controlled at the accident site, and this constitutes one of the major reasons for *rapid* transportation to the hospital.

Deep lacerations of the face, scalp, head, and neck are common in auto accidents and often bleed profusely. There is little use in wasting time trying to patch up each injury— definitive surgery will take care of this at the hospital. Simply cover the multiple wounds with a properly secured heavy compression dressing and move on to the next most urgent requirement.

A point should be made here which has been emphasized by Berens; it relates to burns incurred by victims of various types of accidents, including vehicular accidents, while lying on the pavement awaiting assistance or transportation.

As Berens has shown, the pavement can get surprisingly hot (up to 172°F or more) even on relatively cool days, and black asphalt surfaces get much hotter than white concrete surfaces since they absorb more and reflect less heat. A person lying unconscious, unable to move, on such a surface can sustain severe burns on exposed areas of the body in a relatively short period of time.

These facts should be borne in mind in caring for accident victims. If the pavement surface feels hot to touch, the accident victim may well sustain a burn if allowed to lie directly on the pavement. Put some protective material *under* him and protect his hands and head, particularly, until he can be moved.

The next major consideration is to properly prepare the victim for transportation to the hospital; there are certain pitfalls to be avoided. These include improper positioning, inadequate splinting of broken limbs, inadequate control of hemorrhage, and inadequate help or inadequate facilities for moving or transporting the victim.

The most important of these is transportation of the victim in the proper position. If he is unconscious, place him on his side or, if necessary, on his abdomen, with his head turned to one side in order to avoid aspiration of the stomach contents into his lungs or blockage of the windpipe.

In cases of spinal injury, it is absolutely essential that the injured person be transported on a rigid support, such as a door or shutter, if a backboard is not available in the *face-down* position. If such a support is not available, place him face down on a blanket, but do not move him until at least six people are available to do this without twisting his body in any direction. In cases of probable injury to the cervical spine, one individual should be assigned the task of holding the victim's head, with slight traction and so that it does not turn in any direction on the axis of the spine. When a fracture of the neck is suspected, the victim should be transported in the *face-up* position.

If the injuries include burns, no attempt should be made

to treat them at the site of the accident; cover them with a clean dressing of some kind, simply to provide protection until the victim can be gotten to a hospital.   If his body is extensively burned, he should simply be covered with a clean sheet. Do not make the mistake of covering such an individual with a blanket for two reasons: (1) blankets are usually dirty, even though they look clean, and are a fertile source of bacterial contamination; (2) if you have ever had a severe sunburn, you know how very uncomfortable a blanket can be when in contact with the burned area.

If the burns are extensive and there are facilities available for administering fluids to the victim, by mouth, rectum, or intravenously, administration should be started immediately and carried on even during his transportation to the hospital.

Sometimes in severe accident cases, the question comes up as to whether or not to administer sedatives or narcotics, such as morphine, at the site of the accident.   A common mistake is to give morphine when it is not really needed or to give so much that the symptoms of possible underlying injuries are masked by the time the victim reaches the hospital, thus making it exceedingly difficult to make a complete survey of his injuries.   It is true that in some cases it is desirable to administer morphine or its equivalent before beginning transportation of the victim, but *under no circumstances* should morphine or any other narcotic be given to a victim who is unconscious or in severe shock or who has a head injury or a blocked airway.   To do so may cause the death of the victim.

In handling an accident case, another extremely important point should be borne in mind: the accident may have been caused by or have been the result of an acute sudden illness, such as a heart attack or a stroke.   While the victim may superficially appear to be in shock, it is obvious that, if the possibility of a heart attack is not considered and he is treated for shock in the conventional manner, his life would be placed in serious jeopardy, and such a mistake might well prove fatal.

On the other hand, if this possibility is considered and the victim is carefully observed before proceeding with any form of emergency care, it is unlikely that such a mistake will be made.   As has been pointed out by an outstanding authority, "The high venous pressure, bulging veins, and defective action of a disabled heart are in sharp contrast to the low venous pressure, collapsed veins, and regular cardiac rhythm of shock."

In the event there is any doubt as to whether the victim may have had a head injury or a stroke or a heart attack, he should not be put in the conventional shock position. Also, in the presence of any injury to the chest or difficulty in breathing from any cause, the shock position should be avoided, since it would cause the shifting of the weight of the abdominal contents downward against the diaphragm, thus further hampering the victim's effort to breathe.

Before beginning the transportation of the victim to the hospital, make certain that adequate measures have been taken to conserve body heat, by means of a light blanket or two, being careful to avoid overheating, and that means have been provided for giving the admitting physician at the hospital an adequate history of the accident and, if possible, of the victim himself. Sometimes it is possible for a member of the family, who may have witnessed the accident, to accompany him, and in such an instance, the pertinent personal history of the victim would be available. In any event, it is often helpful for the doctor to know just how the accident came about, as this might well provide a clue to the nature of the victim's injuries or illness.

Many ambulances are equipped with oxygen; it is often desirable, particularly in head injury or heart attack cases, to begin the administration of oxygen immediately, on the way to the hospital, since this will aid in preventing a sharp drop in blood pressure and in minimizing the likelihood of the victim going into profound shock. As a general rule, however, it is not desirable to attempt to administer other drugs until the victim can be admitted to the hospital and the exact nature of his problem determined.

When the victim reaches the hospital, he should quickly be given a thorough examination in the emergency room, in order to determine the exact extent of his injuries, to institute the proper definitive emergency treatments promptly, and to minimize the possibility of overlooking any less obvious, but possibly serious, injuries.

As a rule, no surgery will be performed until the necessary measures to combat shock and loss of blood have been taken. In addition, specific examinations, such as x-ray, will be carried out, in the emergency room if possible, so as to avoid unnecessary movement because of the ever-present possibility of doing further damage.

In some cases, the administration of oxygen, started in the ambulance, will be continued, and a catheter will be inserted into the bladder in order to determine whether any injury has occurred to the urinary tract as well as to keep track of the urinary output of the victim. If there is blood in the urine as it comes from the catheter, it is of course, strong evidence of injury to the bladder, the ureters, or the kidneys, and surgical exploration and repair may be required promptly.

The victim with multiple injuries constitutes a difficult medical and surgical problem, since any or all systems of the body may have sustained some type of injury; in addition, there may be some complicating serious underlying medical condition, such as a heart attack, diabetes, or infectious disease.

Regardless of what the ultimate situation may be, the importance of adequate preliminary care by the first person on the scene, be he a trained first-aider, a physician, or a member of a trained ambulance squad, cannot be overemphasized.

Remember that doing the wrong thing is worse than doing nothing at all. Do not act in haste, but be as objective and as effective as possible with the means at hand.

Usually it is possible, through some means or another, to summon medical aid. Many areas of our country are served by highly effective and well-trained first-aid squads utilizing the best of modern equipment. These individuals, together with the local medical facilities which back them up, contribute much toward minimizing the terrible toll of the traffic-accident holocaust. The traveling public owes a debt of gratitude to these volunteer services and should support them whenever possible.

11 Treatment of Poisoning

Many substances in everyday use, such as medicines, certain cosmetics, cleaning agents, plant and insect sprays, bleaches, and the like, when accidentally or deliberately misused, cause illness or death. Furthermore, household appliances and equipment, as well as the family's motor car, that are not checked regularly account for additional illness, and, often deaths from carbon monoxide. A general knowledge of the potentially harmful effects of these various items and an understanding of how to combat their toxic effects is important. The emergency care rendered within the first few moments after exposure to a poison may spell the difference between life and death.

Because of the widespread incidence of poisoning of all kinds and the need for exceedingly prompt and effective action in even the most unusual cases, a nationwide network of poison control centers has been set up in or near all major population areas.

The centers are especially equipped to handle all types of poison cases, and they maintain a detailed file of the ingredients of all new and potentially dangerous products, regardless of their nature. With such facilities and special knowledge, these centers offer the best chance of survival for any poisoning victim. In the event of suspected poisoning, either call a center for assistance or get the victim to a center as quickly as possible. If none is nearby, take the victim to the nearest hospital emergency room as soon as possible after rendering immediate first-aid assistance.

We suggest that you look up the phone number of the Poison Control Center in your area, and list it under "Emergency Telephone Numbers" on page 615 of this book.

PREVENTION OF POISONING

The most important factor in the prevention of accidental poisoning is reasonable care and common sense in using and storing potentially poisonous substances and in maintaining and using equipment which, in the course of either normal or defective operation, may give off poisonous fumes. This can be accomplished by following a few simple rules:

1 Do not keep medicines, cosmetics, cleaning fluids, rat poisons, and insecticides where they can be reached by children. Especially, do not carry medicines in a purse or handbag, which may be easily accessible to young children. Shulman and Reddy, in a survey of the contents of purses, including those of mothers, found an amazing variety of potentially powerful drugs, varying from aspirin and other "over-the-counter" analgesics and antihistamines, through powerful tranquilizers and oral contraceptives, to sleeping pills, diuretics, and nitroglycerine. Any of these preparations in sufficient amounts could kill a child. The fact that "OTC" sleeping pills may have side reactions simulating mental disease has also been stressed by Ullman and Groh in the *American Journal of Psychiatry.* Such pills would be particularly dangerous to young children.

2 Do not keep any medicinal or chemical preparations that are not clearly labeled.

3 Do not store drugs or household chemicals in food containers.

4 Be certain that the purpose and dosage of a medicine are clearly stated on the label and that you understand them before you or anyone else takes any.

5 Do not take a medicine in the dark; which means, never take a medicine without reading the label.

6 Never keep prescription drugs after they have served the purpose of the particular person for whom they were prescribed. Never give another person someone else's prescription without checking with your physician.

7 Except under medical supervision do not give aspirin or any other medicine containing salicylate to a very sick child with high fever and great loss of body fluids, in any but the exact *recommended* dosage for the age of the child, or more frequently or over longer periods of time than called for by the directions.

8 Do not keep known poisons in a medicine cabinet, the kitchen, or any place where food is stored, or where they can inadvertently become accessible to a child.

9 Do not use any kind of cleaning fluid near a flame (as a gas stove or a lighted cigarette) or where the ventilation is inadequate.

10 Thoroughly wash the hands and other exposed parts after using rat poison, plant spray, or insect spray.

11 Do not stay in a closed room in which an insect spray has just been used or allow food to remain exposed in such a room.

12 Do not operate a gasoline motor in an unventilated space, such as a closed garage.

13 Do not use a gas or kerosene stove in an unventilated room.

14 Have any appliance using utility gas or kerosene inspected regularly to be sure that it is working properly and is venting correctly.

Most poisonous substances are properly labeled with clear directions for their use. *Read the directions* on the container and follow them exactly.

HOW POISONS ENTER THE SYSTEM

By Mouth. The most common route by which a poison finds its way into the body is through the mouth. This is particularly true of very young children, since almost everything they touch goes into their mouths. Although adults should know better, they often do not seem to, since, by design or accident, they swallow such corrosives as acids or alkalies, as well as too many sleeping pills, various disinfectants which contain carbolic acid, and many other known or potential poisons.

By Inhalation. . Very often poisonous vapors or fumes, as from insecticides, cleaning fluids, leaky gas appliances, and even the family automobile, are inhaled.

By Absorption. Many substances can be absorbed directly through the skin in large enough quantities to be poisonous. This is true of some of the insecticides, plant sprays, and cleaning fluids, which are only a few, but more ordinary, of the substances that produce general toxic effects or severe local irritation which tends to increase the amount and rapidity of absorption.

Attention to a special danger from absorption of potentially poisonous substances through the skin of young infants has been stressed by the American Academy of Pediatrics. A variety of substances which are still being used in the laundering of clothing, diapers, and bedding, especially for hospital nurseries, may prove hazardous.

Cases have occurred in which premature and full-term newborn infants have contracted methemoglobinemia after their diapers were rinsed with the bacteriostatic agent 3-4-4' trichlorocarbanilide (TCC). Methemoglobinemia is a condition caused by various poisons resulting in a lack of oxygen which may lead to death or serious disturbance of the vital functions.

Reports in pediatric literature have indicated that aniline— a well-known cause of methemoglobinemia—has resulted from the breakdown of TCC during sterilization of infant diapers. It is possible for aniline to be absorbed through the skin of infants from diapers and other nursery clothing, although direct proof of the etiologic role of TCC is still lacking.

The Academy also points out that although most hospital (and commercial) laundry procedures have abandoned TCC in treating clothing and bed linens of newborn infants, sporadic instances of neonatal methemoglobinemia associated with exposure to this substance still occur.

Death and severe illness have also been reported when the sodium salt of pentachlorophenol (PCP) was absorbed through the skin. The PCP was present in the antimicrobial neutralizer product used in the final rinse of the laundry process for diapers, infant undershirts, and crib linens for the nursery.

The Academy further expresses concern over the newer laundering agents such as enzyme-detergent combinations and optical brighteners at least two of which are potent photosensitizers. It is pointed out that the biology of premature and full-term infants demands that even the most innocent-appearing substance in their environment be scrutinized for the possibility of adverse effects.   It is concluded that "Until data on toxicity are available for various substances which are proposed for introduction into the nursery, clinical judgment would dictate avoiding them."

It is essential, therefore, to establish the purity, safety, and effectiveness of any product used in laundering all articles coming in contact with a baby's skin.

By Injection.   Finally, poisons can inadvertently be injected into the system.   You may never be shot with a poisoned arrow, but bees, wasps, and scorpions do sting; tarantulas and black widow spiders bite, as do rattlesnakes, copperheads, and moccasins; and saltwater catfish, stingrays, and Portuguese men-of-war have various ways of getting their particular "brand" of poison into the unwary.

HOW POISONS ACT

Once in the system, poisons act in various ways.   The acids and alkalies produce actual burning and corrosion of the tissues with which they come in contact and may quite literally burn a hole in a person's stomach.

Sleeping pills and alcohol act as strong depressants of the central nervous system, while an insecticide, like chlordane, or a drug, like strychnine, produces extreme stimulation of the central nervous system.   Other compounds, such as cyanide and carbon monoxide, produce an asphyxial type of death by combining with the oxygen-carrying system of the blood and thus preventing oxygen from being carried to the tissues.   Muscarine, the toxic substance in certain poisonous mushrooms, acts on a special part of the nervous system to depress breathing and heart action and to increase the peristaltic action of the intestinal tract.

If effective first-aid assistance is rendered before medical aid becomes available, the physician can then make use of drugs that specifically counteract the effect of a particular poison and thus save the life of the victim.   It is the *emergency aid* to the victim that may determine the success of the medical treatment.

GENERAL PROCEDURES FOR TREATING POISONING VICTIMS

In many cases, the specific poison taken by a person cannot be determined immediately; under such circumstances, no time should be wasted in attempting to find a specific antidote.   If the poison is *corrosive*, usually indicated by stains and burns about the victim's mouth and lips, the poison should be neutralized as quickly as possible.

If the poison appears to be a *noncorrosive* one (no stains or burns about the victim's mouth and lips) give the victim an emetic, such as seven or eight glasses of soapy water, salt water, baking soda solution, or syrup of ipecac—½ ounce for a child over 1 year of age, plus at least a cup (8 ounces) of water—to make him vomit.   Use *syrup* of ipecac, *never* the fluid extract, which, according to Arena, is 14 times more potent and extremely toxic.   This procedure serves to dilute the poison and helps the body to get rid of it.   If no vomiting occurs after 20 minutes, this dose may be repeated *one time only.*

As a general rule, the best early treatment for any poison taken by mouth is evacuation of the stomach contents.   The two most common exceptions to this rule are the ingestion of a caustic poison or a petroleum distillate such as kerosene.

Medical thinking is swinging more and more toward the use of syrup of ipecac as an emetic, since it is thorough and generally safe, even for use in children.   It is also effective even in the presence of antiemetic drugs (which could be the accidentally ingested poison).   The proper dosage should be given all at once, since smaller repeated doses may not achieve the desired effect.   The presently recommended dose for children 1 to 5 years of age, the group in which most accidental poisonings occur, is 15 to 20 milliliters of syrup of ipecac.   This amounts to half an ounce or just a little over.   This dose should be followed by enough water to fill the stomach, in order to make the emetic action more effective and dilute the poison. If vomiting does not occur in 30 minutes, the dose of ipecac may be repeated. If emesis still does not occur, then the stomach must be emptied by a stomach tube and thoroughly washed out. It is uncommon for the first dose of ipecac to fail. As a matter of fact, so effective is ipecac as an emetic, both in children and in adults, that many authorities feel that it should be kept for emergency use in all homes, particularly those with small children. However, in certain cases the injection of apomorphine (a powerful emetic) is used, but only under medical supervision.

The victim should be removed to a hospital as soon as feasible after his stomach has been evacuated, but waiting for vomiting to occur should *not* delay transportation to a medical facility. It may be necessary to administer artificial respiration and, in some types of poisoning, to keep it up for many hours, or even days. For that purpose, of course, an automatic respirator is invaluable; artificial respiration, if required, should be continued using a respirator, if possible, during transportation to the hospital.

Be sure the stomach contents are saved for chemical analysis so that the nature of the poison may be determined. This step may not only subsequently prove to have been of life-saving importance, but it may well have great legal significance. If the remaining contents in the package of the suspected poison can be found, send it along with the victim to the hospital.

If the victim is seen by a physician and hospitalization is not deemed necessary, after the stomach has been entirely emptied and if the victim is conscious, hot tea or coffee may be given. Do not give alcohol in any form.

TYPES OF POISONS

Corrosive Acids and Alkalies

When the exact nature of the poison is known, certain specific steps are indicated. One of the frequently encountered groups of poisons likely to be swallowed comprises the corrosive acids and alkalies. Clues to many of these are the stains and burns about the mouth, mentioned earlier, or the presence of a characteristic odor. The common ones and their common uses are listed.

Corrosive Acids	**Corrosive Alkalies**
Sulfuric acid (automobile batteries)	Potash (lye; drain cleaners)
Hydrochloric acid (metal cleaners; masonry; soldering)	Caustic soda (soapmaking)
	Lime (building trades)
Nitric acid (industrial cleaning solutions)	Ammonia (household and industrial uses)
Oxalic acid (cleaning solutions)	
Carbolic acid or crude cresol (disinfectants)	

If any one of the substances listed above has been swallowed, as a general rule do *not* use an emetic or a stomach tube because of the danger of causing a perforation of the stomach or esophagus where the chemical may have caused severe tissue damage.

If a corrosive *acid* has been swallowed (except carbolic acid or other cresol disinfectant), give the victim limewater, chalk and water, small amounts of diluted milk of magnesia, or 1 teaspoonful of baking soda in a glass of water. The objective is *not* to induce vomiting, but simply to neutralize the acid. If vomiting does occur, try to keep the victim from straining.

If a corrosive *alkali* has been swallowed, give large amounts of lemon or orange juice or equal parts of vinegar and water.

After the first neutralization has been effected in the case of either acid or alkali, give the victim milk, raw eggs beaten up in milk, any food oil, flour in water, gruel, or similar substance, for further neutralization and for the formation of a protective coating on the tissues.

Lye.   As emphasized by Ray et al., alkali ingestion, particularly in the case of young children, has assumed especial importance in the light of the fact that several liquid drain openers or cleaners are on the market which offer severe hazards unless special precautions are taken. These products consist of strong solutions of liquid lye and are even more dangerous than the older crystalline-type lye preparations that were offered for the same purpose. The crystalline preparations tended to adhere to the tissue locally and therefore did not do such extensive damage to the esophagus and stomach as the liquid type. Because of the dangers involved, suggestions have been made that these products be removed from the market. In the event of ingestion of the latter type of product, in addition to immediate first aid measures, prompt hospitalization, with the prospect of early operation, may be the only lifesaving procedure.

The pain in these cases is usually severe, and the victim may go into shock. Medical aid should be obtained quickly, as some form of sedation will be required, as well as medical supportive measures.

Carbolic Acid (Phenol) Poisoning. Usually the clue to carbolic acid poisoning is the very strong characteristic odor of the breath and of the vomited matter. When carbolic acid is taken orally, it produces extensive local burning and corrosion, with whitening of the skin and severe burning pain in the mouth, throat and stomach. Phenol is absorbed from the gastrointestinal tract, skin, and lungs, and this causes a severe general reaction, the symptoms of which are usually slightly delayed. In general, there is depression of the central nervous system and marked irritation of the kidneys. Headache may be severe, and there is muscular weakness, dark bluish coloration of the face, rapid pulse, delirium or coma, or occasionally convulsions. The respiration is irregular, and death occurs as the result of respiratory failure.

The principal object of treatment is to remove the phenol from the stomach as quickly as possible before much absorption has occurred. The victim should be taken to a hospital, where a stomach tube can be passed and the stomach washed out with a substance that will slow the absorption of the phenol as well as dissolve and get rid of it. Olive oil (or other vegetable oil) is excellent for this purpose, but alcoholic solutions and mineral oil are not recommended since alcohol will hasten the absorption of the phenol, and mineral oil is not a very good solubilizing agent.

Until the patient can be gotten to the hospital, he should be given copious quantities of milk or evaporated milk, which should be repeated after each vomiting. It is, however, extremely important that the stomach be washed out by gastric lavage as quickly as possible, and this usually requires hospital facilities. After the stomach has been thoroughly evacuated, a large quantity of olive oil should be left in the stomach to retard absorption and sequester any remaining phenol.

Systemically, the patient should be treated as for shock and receive various supportive measures, including the administration of antibiotics, copious amounts of isotonic sodium chloride solution by vein in order to promote diuresis, blood transfusions, or exchange transfusions where these are indicated, oxygen and artificial respiration, and specific treatment of the esophageal burns in the hope of preventing subsequent contraction and stenosis.

Local burning of the skin by carbolic acid can be treated by thorough washing with water or 50 percent alcohol solution, and the application of glycerin or any of the vegetable oils.

It must be emphasized that any case of phenol poisoning is serious, even though the patient's condition does not seem to be poor, and he must receive medical attention as promptly as possible.

Irritant Substances

There is a large and varied group of compounds which have in common the characteristic of causing irritation of the stomach when swallowed and produce nausea, vomiting, and severe abdominal pain. Many of these irritants are found in combination with other chemicals as active ingredients in commonly used items in most households. This group includes the following:

arsenic (rat poisons; weed killers)
copper (plant sprays; rat poisons)
iodine (antiseptic)
mercury (fireworks; plant sprays; germicide)
phosphorus (fireworks; matches; rat poisons)
silver nitrate (inks; cleaning solutions)
zinc (weed killers; soldering paste; metallurgy)

Signs and Symptoms. The victim complains of a metallic taste in his mouth, the lips and tongue may appear white and shriveled; in severer cases shock is present.

○ TREATMENT

The treatment consists of washing out the stomach thoroughly, by giving the victim an emetic (ipecac), followed by whites of eggs in water or milk (except in phosphorus poisoning).

For *phosphorus* poisoning do not give mineral or olive oils or other fats because of their solubilizing action.   After the stomach has been emptied, give the victim 2 ounces of Epsom salts in an 8-ounce glass of water.

In the case of *iodine* poisoning, a mixture of starch and water should be given.

For *silver nitrate,* a strong solution of salt water should be used; this forms a compound, silver chloride, which is relatively inert and which is removed from the stomach by vomiting or gastric lavage.

POISONING BY SUBSTANCES COMMONLY FOUND ABOUT THE HOME

A wide variety of miscellaneous substances are included in this category.   If one were to take the things that might logically be found around the bathroom or in a medicine cabinet, for instance, the following possibilities should be considered.

Atropine and Belladonna.   These drugs are commonly used in many prescriptions, and if taken in an overdose—particularly by children—they produce marked symptoms.

Signs and Symptoms.   Characteristically, the skin becomes hot, dry, and flushed; the mouth and throat are so dry that swallowing or talking is difficult; and the pupils are widely dilated.   The pulse is rapid and weak; the victim may be very restless, have hallucinations, and, at times, be difficult to control; he will usually complain of double vision.

○ TREATMENT

1 If the drug has been taken by mouth, induce vomiting and give strong tea.

2 Control fever by ice packs and other procedures similar to those used for the treatment of heat stroke (see page 255).

3 If respiration is inadequate or failing, artificial respiration is indicated.

Medical aid should be procured promptly. The specific antidote is pilocarpine (obtainable from Wyeth Laboratories) in a dose of 2 to 4 milligrams, but only a doctor can give this by injection and it would not be within the province of emergency aid.

Nitroglycerine. Nitroglycerine tablets are commonly used for the control of anginal attacks. An overdose may cause most disturbing symptoms.

It should be noted that relatively mild cases of nitroglycerine poisoning, resulting from absorption through the skin, are seen among workers who handle dynamite. Some persons are much more susceptible than others.

Signs and Symptoms. Symptoms consist of a full, throbbing headache, dizziness, tenseness of the head and neck muscles, dilated pupils, irregular pulse, pain in the chest, and weakness. In severe cases, there will be nausea, vomiting, unconsciousness, and convulsions.

○ TREATMENT

In mild cases of nitroglycerine poisoning plenty of fresh air and aromatic spirits of ammonia and coffee are usualy effective. Although the headache is very hard to relieve, it will gradually wear off.

Where a sizable overdose has been taken by mouth, medical aid should be obtained quickly; in the meantime, empty and thoroughly clean the victim's stomach with a dose of ipecac or other emetic, such as repeated doses of bicarbonate of soda, followed by repeated glasses of salt water. Because these victims easily go into shock, they should be kept warm, lying down, and given stimulants to help raise the blood pressure, which is markedly lowered by the poison. In severe cases prompt medical aid should be sought.

Salicylates. Salicylate poisoning is most commonly acquired in one of several ways: by swallowing pleasantly flavored aspirin tablets, usually by a child who believes it to be candy; by swallowing oil of wintergreen rubbing compound (which smells like peppermint); or by overdoses of either aspirin or sodium salicylate, given for rheumatic fever or for some other illness.

Of late, the incidence of aspirin intoxication has reached

alarming proportions because the drug is in such common use and because of its availability in pleasantly flavored forms for children. The greatest mortality occurs in children between the ages of 1 to 4 years. Whatever the form of salicylate swallowed, the clinical symptoms are quite characteristic.

Signs and Symptoms. The onset of symptoms of a single large overdose (as from a child's eating a whole bottle of tablets) may not occur for from 12 to 24 hours. If overly large doses are given at regular intervals over a long period of time, it may require from 1 to 4 days for symptoms of poisoning to appear.

The first and most dependable sign of poisoning is rapid, deep breathing. This sign is so characteristic that, in any instance in which there is an unexplained increase in rate and depth of breathing, the possibility of *aspirin poisoning* should be borne in mind. Hyperventilation can eventually lead to dangerous or even fatal changes in the body chemistry.

Lengthening of the clotting time of the blood causes diffuse hemorrhage into the various tissues and organs of the body; bleeding from the lining of the stomach as the result of corrosive action of the salicylate may give rise to the so-called "coffee-ground" vomitus which sometimes occurs in salicylate poisoning. There may also be a rash on the skin and actual bleeding from the gums or other mucous membranes.

If salicylate poisoning occurs in a child, he will be irritable and restless and, in severe cases, may go into convulsions. He may be in a semiconscious state or in a complete stupor, although, often, he can be temporarily aroused. Older children or adults may complain of dizziness and ringing in the ears, or they may be delirious. There may be either pallor or dusky blue color of the face, and there often is a high fever and some evidence of acute abdominal pain.

The exact amount of salicylate required to produce symptoms cannot be stated, since it varies widely with the age, weight, and condition of a person. Infants are much more susceptible than older children, especially those who are ill and eating and drinking inadequately; fever, for which aspirin often is given, tends to aggravate the effect of the drug. Furthermore, the physiologic mechanisms for excreting salicylate are less effective in children than in adults.

For these reasons, it should be realized by parents, as it is by physicians, that aspirin can be a dangerous drug and the dosage should, therefore, be carefully controlled.   The average adult dose is 10 grains per dose every 4 to 6 hours for a total of not more than 60 grains in any 24-hour period.   Half this amount is used for children 6 to 12 years of age; and one-fourth (2½ grains per dose) for children 3 to 6 years of age.

For children under 3, the physician's instructions should be carefully followed, but the maximum dose would be approximately 1 grain per year of age, given every 4 to 6 hours.

It should also be pointed out that several brands of 600 milligrams (10 grain) acetylsalicylic acid tablets ("big aspirin") are considered to represent twice the poisoning hazard of the familiar 300 milligrams (5 grain) tablet and might be inadvertently taken for the smaller dose tablet.

It should be clearly emphasized that, when giving aspirin to a sick child, he must be carefully watched; this is particularly important if he is vomiting, has severe diarrhea, or has a high fever.   Under these conditions the effects of aspirin may quickly become cumulative.

○ TREATMENT

If aspirin poisoning does occur:

1   Take the child to a hospital as quickly as possible, since there are a number of highly technical procedures which must be followed to combat the successive stages of the poisoning.

2   However, if the child is found shortly after swallowing a single large amount of the salicylate (most commonly aspirin or oil of wintergreen), his stomach should be emptied immediately by giving a dose of ipecac; at the hospital the child's stomach may be further cleansed by means of gastric lavage, using magnesium oxide as a neutralizing agent.

If, however, an increased rate of breathing is noted, absorption will already have occurred and stomach washing will be of little value.   Therefore, treat the child as for shock and, *without delay*, take him to a hospital.

Acetaminophen.   This drug is now sold in Britain, the United States and elsewhere in increasing quantities.   It has advantages over aspirin in that it can be formulated into a stable suspension which is acceptable to children.   It has good analgesic and antipyretic properties but it lacks the anti-inflammatory properties of aspirin.

However, acetaminophen lacks the anticoagulant properties of aspirin, which, of course, contraindicate the use of the latter in the face of potential bleeding situations, and it does not have the tendency to produce gastritis or tinnitus which may occur when aspirin or any salicylate is given in large doses.

Poisoning from overdosage of acetaminophen can occur and its treatment has been extensively studied since the drug may constitute a potential hazard in children, if not in adults as well.

Symptoms. According to Goulding, following an overdose no symptoms may appear for two days or so. Then there is usually loss of appetite, nausea and vomiting, but the sensorium remains entirely clear. Liver damage may occur with the appearance of jaundice on the third or fourth day, as the result of which the patient becomes dangerously ill.

○ TREATMENT

The individual should, of course, be taken to a hospital as soon as signs of illness develop, but if there is unavoidable delay, the stomach should be thoroughly washed out, and then activated charcoal given to adsorb any residual that may still be present.

Hemodialysis should be initiated as soon as possible to reduce the blood level of acetaminophen. Any liver dysfunction should be treated according to its nature, and other supportive measures are, of course, essential.

The many studies of acetaminophen poisoning conducted in adults should be helpful in evaluating this type of poisoning. But while many deaths occur each year as the result of aspirin poisoning, we know of no deaths from acetaminophen poisoning except in the exceedingly rare event of a young child choking on a tablet when he should have been given a liquid suspension, which is readily available and possesses no significant hazard. Furthermore, to our knowledge, children's tablets are not yet available in candy flavors.

Iron. Iron in various forms is widely used as a tonic and for the treatment of anemia and also is given during pregnancy. Several cases of poisoning in children who have had access to capsules of medicinal iron preparations have been reported.

It is well to be aware of the danger and to be able to recognize the symptoms, since only about half the cases of those ill enough to attract attention recover. As little as a single 1 gram (15 grain) capsule is dangerous to a child, and two capsules have caused death. As dispensed, such capsules are easily available to children. Needless to say, *all* iron-containing preparations should be kept out of any possible access by children.

Signs and Symptoms. The child becomes pale, restless, and nauseated, and there may be vomiting and very severe, bloody diarrhea. Drowsiness gradually merges into coma; the pulse appears to be weak and rapid and the skin bluish; and the child appears to be in a state of profound shock. Curiously, some of the victims then appear to improve rapidly for 12 to 24 hours, but then die suddenly, with little warning, 24 to 48 hours after the iron has been taken.

○ TREATMENT

The stomach should be emptied by stomach tube—not by emetics—in children, and washed out with sodium bicarbonate solution or a 5-percent solution of sodium dihydrogen phosphate (Fleet's enema diluted half and half). The child should be taken to a hospital as quickly as possible, as other technical supportive measures will be required. In addition, a new antidote, desferioxamine, has become available to some centers and appears to be lifesaving in many instances.

Boric Acid. Pure boric acid is often used in powdered form for preparing mildly antiseptic solutions for washing out the eyes and for wet dressings. It is also available in various concentrations in ointments for use on cuts and burns. The virtues of boric acid have been vastly overrated. It is not a good antiseptic, and is a dangerous poison under certain conditions of misuse. It has no place in the household.

Pure boric acid is poisonous when taken accidentally by mouth or when applied to extensive raw surfaces of the body.

Signs and Symptoms. The symptoms of boric acid poisoning are a bright red appearance of the skin; a generalized rash, with shedding of the skin; rapid breathing and suppression of urine. The condition is difficult to diagnose with certainty and may be confused with illness having similar symptoms.

○ TREATMENT

There is no treatment within the scope of emergency aid. The victim should be hospitalized as quickly as possible.

Camphor. Camphor is not seen in the family medicine chest as much as it used to be, but it is still an occasional cause of poisoning in children, particularly if camphorated oil is given by mistake for castor oil. Camphorated oil has little demonstrable use and should be banned from the family medicine cabinet. Tincture of camphor is sometimes used for "fever blisters."

Signs and Symptoms. The general symptoms are a burning sensation in the throat and stomach, excessive thirst, nausea and vomiting, blurred vision, dizziness, headache, and convulsions. After a few hours, the victim shows all the symptoms of being drunk. The breath or urine usually smells of camphor.

○ TREATMENT

Thoroughly empty and wash out the stomach; then administer a large enough dose of Epsom salts to rid the intestines of the poison quickly. The victim should be kept warm and the convulsions controlled with suitable sedation. Prompt medical aid is essential.

Strychnine. There is still enough strychnine around the home in some form—often not as a medicine, but as rat poison —to be responsible for the death of many children each year.

Signs and Symptoms. Usually, the symptoms come on rapidly after swallowing the poison, but may be delayed for more than an hour. They are unmistakable. There is great apprehension, shuddering, and then, suddenly, a generalized spasm which grips the entire body, causing the back to arch in such a way that the victim is resting only on the back of his head and his heels. During this period the victim cannot breathe because of the spasm, so that he becomes blue in the face, his pulse is rapid, weak, and thready, and his face assumes the horrible grin known as *risus sardonicus*. Muscular contraction during the spasm is so great as to be exceedingly painful; when the spasm passes, the victim relaxes, exhausted. He remains so until, within a few minutes, another spasm occurs. These may be brought on by a sudden noise, touch, strong light, or any sudden stimulus; therefore, these victims must be handled with exceeding gentleness and with slow movements.

○ TREATMENT

Emergency aid consists of the prompt emptying of the stomach, followed by copious amounts of very strong tea. The tannic acid in the tea combines with and neutralizes the strychnine. The mixture is then removed by vomiting or lavage and the procedure repeated as necessary.

This is an acute medical emergency, for anesthesia may be *required to control the convulsions,* and other medications must be given to carry the victim through and to support him until the effects of the drug wear off—which will be a matter of several hours in those cases which survive.

Potassium Permanganate. Potassium permanganate is often kept in the medicine chest for making wet dressings or antiseptic solutions for treating poison ivy. It is a dangerous substance which, if swallowed, acts as a strong corrosive poison, with the characteristic symptoms (see pages 299 and 300); the lips, mouth, or throat may be stained a typical bluish brown.

○ TREATMENT

Treatment consists of emptying the stomach and washing it out several times to dilute the irritant and then administering eggs whipped up in milk or water to act as a protective coating for the walls of the stomach and complex with the permanganate.

Chloral Hydrate. Chloral hydrate was formerly widely used as a sleeping powder, and still is to some extent; under proper conditions it produces normal sleep. Combined with alcohol, it makes a "Mickey Finn," which rapidly produces unconsciousness, followed, upon awakening, by a terrible headache and nausea.

Signs and Symptoms. When taken by itself in an overdose, chloral hydrate renders a person suddenly helpless and, for that reason, has been used as knockout drops for vicious purposes. The symptoms come on suddenly, with burning and dryness of the throat, collapse, shallow breathing, weak pulse, and coma. The victim appears to be in shock.

O TREATMENT

Emergency aid consists of emptying the stomach, rendering artificial respiration when required, and administering strong stimulants. Medical aid should be summoned quickly, and the victim taken to a hospital. Such a case may be so serious that ultimate survival remains in doubt for some days.

Lead Poisoning

According to the American Academy of Pediatrics, in 1972 one child died every 36 hours of lead poisoning, more than 110,000 suffered from the disease, and as many as 600,000 were found to have high lead blood levels.

In a joint statement by the American Academy of Pediatrics, the American Public Health Association, and the National Environmental Health Association, it is pointed out that "a paint chip the size of a fingernail can contain as much as 100 times what we consider to be the maximum amount of lead a person ought to have enter his or her body in a single day. Eating one such paint chip each day for two to three months can result in convulsions, severe brain damage and eventually death. Many children who survive the disease are left mentally retarded, or suffering from cerebral palsy, convulsive disorders, blindness, learning defects, kidney diseases, and other handicaps. None of these need occur if the disease is caught in time and if further exposure to the lead hazard is terminated. Unfortunately, many of the children who are seen by physicians in acute lead poisoning attacks are children who have been treated previously and then have been sent home where they start eating paint chips again."

Most cases of acute lead poisoning occur as the result of suicidal or accidental ingestion of soluble lead salts or by injection combined with edectic acid for the treatment of encephalitis (Arena). Chronic lead poisoning is more common as the result of industrial exposure; occasionally it is seen in soft water areas where lead pipes are still used as part of the water system. The water reacts with the lead to form soluble lead salts which are absorbed over a long period of time and gradually accumulate to reach toxic levels in the body.

Lead poisoning continues to be an important problem in childhood. Unless the possibility of its occurrence is suspected and the child properly diagnosed and treated early, it is capable of producing death, mental crippling, or other complications in later life.

In young children, lead poisoning is caused most frequently by the eating of old wall plaster and paint containing lead on toys or the sides of cribs, as the result of a compulsive craving (pica). The condition now ranks as one of the most common causes of childhood mortality as the result of poisoning. Children 1 to 4 years of age living in older-type houses, where lead-containing paints were widely used, are most frequently the victims.

The paint does not have to be on the surface but is, in fact, usually buried under several coats of newer-type paint which in itself may be relatively innocuous. The reason for this is that before the development of modern pigments and bases, older paint consisted essentially of various lead pigment compounds suspended in linseed oil or similar base. These pigments are used less today than formerly and have been replaced by easier-to-apply and more durable paints, which are very frequently put on over the original coat. They are not proof, however, against a toddler's teeth, so that when he chews on the side of an old crib or toy, window sills, trim, or furniture, it doesn't take him long to get down to the poison-containing layer.

Likewise, old flaking paint or plaster falling from the walls or ceiling of a child's room over a long period of time is an even greater hazard, since the mouthing of such material is an almost universal habit of young children.

Curiously enough, there is an increase in the number of clinical cases of lead poisoning among children during the summer months. This seasonal variation, although not fully explained, is in part probably due to the greater chance of exposure to lead paint on the part of children playing outdoors as compared to indoors. Many houses are painted with paint consisting of white lead in linseed oil, an older-type paint which tends to powder and flake off as the result of the weathering process. Children playing on the porches of such houses, for instance, are constantly exposed to this source of lead as it is dusted off on their clothes and hands, so that one can very easily understand how it may readily be taken into their bodies and absorbed.

The American Academy of Pediatrics has urged that a federal standard of less than 0.06 percent lead in paint is needed in order to minimize this particular health hazard to future generations of children. At the present time, lead poisoning as seen in children is related to old, deteriorated housing so that a federal standard is unlikely to have a significant impact on plumbism as *now* seen. Nevertheless, as this old housing is replaced or rehabilitated, safe surface covering should be used in order to minimize hazards to the health of future children.

The discovery of lead poisoning in adults does not pose any great problem, but in children it may, largely because the possibility of the condition occurring is not suspected until the child becomes very ill.

Symptoms. The earliest signs of trouble in children are vomiting, constipation, and a peculiar ashy pallor, coupled with loss of appetite and irritability; if a child has been taking in sufficient quantities of lead over a long enough period of time, the effect of the lead on the central nervous system may be to produce very marked irritability and, in advanced cases, convulsions and loss of consciousness. These symptoms can, of course, accompany other types of disease but, lacking some other obvious explanation, they are, in themselves, sufficient to raise the suspicion, at least, in the mind of the physician of the possibility of lead poisoning.

One danger of lead poisoning in children, as well as in adults, is the toxic effect on the kidneys, so that a child is unable to excrete sufficient quantities of urine. A damaging effect on the kidneys may also show up later in life.

The *treatment* of lead poisoning is difficult, and all but the most mild cases should be hospitalized. Fortunately, there are certain drugs, such as dimercaprol, which, by combining with the lead, aid excretion by changing it into a form that can be excreted by the kidneys and the intestinal tract. But these drugs in themselves are dangerous and have to be used under the closest possible medical supervision.

It seems likely that lead poisoning in children may be even more prevalent than is even now suspected, and it is only through public education, coupled with an acute degree of "lead consciousness" on the part of physicians and public health personnel, that the problem can be reduced.

POISONS FOUND ESPECIALLY IN THE GARAGE AND STORAGE AREAS

Carbon Monoxide. This gas is given off in large quantities by automobile exhausts and may prove quickly fatal in unventilated spaces, such as garages or automobiles with closed windows, even if the vehicle is moving. This is sometimes an important contributing factor to many auto accidents. Utility or illuminating gas may contain carbon monoxide or may create it in the process of burning where there is a limited supply of fresh air; defectively vented or operated water heaters are a powerful source of this lethal gas. Obsolete gas-operated refrigerators which have become defective are also a source of carbon monoxide poisoning.

Signs and Symptoms. It is of the utmost importance that every person familiarize himself with the signs and symptoms of carbon monoxide poisoning in order to save his own life or the life of another. They are: headache, yawning, dizziness, faintness, ringing in the ears, nausea, pounding of the heart, bright cherry-red color of skin, lethargy, stupor, and coma.

Any person experiencing the early symptoms must seek fresh air as rapidly as possible, even though he may have to exercise great will power to do so, as one effect of carbon monoxide poisoning is a lethargy which makes any effort seem to be scarcely worth the bother.

Howlett and Shephard have emphasized the dangers of carbon monoxide as an occupational hazard and enumerate several sources of carbon monoxide from which the gas may accumulate in the body making an undesirable and perhaps dangerous total. These include such things as synergism with high altitude as in flyers, hypoxia, ambient air concentrations, and smoking. Although aircrew personnel are exposed to somewhat lower total concentration than taxi drivers and baggage handlers, Howlett and Shephard state that "because of synergistic stresses and severe task demands, they are at greater risk and exposure should not exceed 40 parts per million for one hour or 15 parts per million for eight hours."

O TREATMENT

To treat carbon monoxide or any gas poisoning:

1 Move the victim into fresh air and start immediate artificial respiration if breathing has ceased or is very poor.

2 Summon medical aid as quickly as possible.

Preferably, the victim should be taken to a hospital by a well-equipped first-aid squad as quickly as possible; oxygen should be administered while continuing artificial respiration, preferably with a respirator. The oxygen not only greatly aids in dissociating the carbon monoxide from the red blood cells, but it is much needed to replace the carbon monoxide.

In addition to the oxygen and artificial respiration, there are certain drugs, which can be given by qualified medical personnel, that help in getting rid of the carbon monoxide in the blood and certain other drugs that stimulate breathing. With these aids, only cases of overwhelming carbon monoxide poisoning need die.

Carbon Tetrachloride. The principal danger of carbon tetrachloride, which has been commonly used as a household cleaning fluid, lies in the *inhalation* of its vapor; this occurs when it is used in a confined, poorly ventilated space. The great advantage of carbon tetrachloride over many other cleaning fluids is that it is noninflammable; however, the toxic nature of its vapor is much greater than that of many common inflammable solvents.

Carbon tetrachloride is also used as the chemical in a common type of hand fire extinguisher which must be used with great care, because, when the carbon tetrachloride hits the flames, it is converted into an irritant gas which is sufficiently toxic to have been considered a war gas. Therefore, in using this type of extinguisher indoors, get into the open air as quickly as possible after attacking the fire.

Signs and Symptoms. The symptoms of carbon tetrachloride poisoning are headache, dizziness, and mental confusion, followed by nausea, vomiting, and abdominal cramps. The danger lies in its toxic effect on the kidneys and liver; death results from failure of these organs.

○ TREATMENT

Treatment consists of getting the individual into fresh air as quickly as possible, removing all clothing which may be saturated with the chemical, sponging his body, and giving oxygen and artificial respiration. The victim should be hospitalized, since he will require supportive therapy and observation for probable liver and kidney damage.

Two less toxic solvents are now widely used in place of carbon tetrachloride, although these, of course, are not wholly lacking in toxicity under improper conditions of use:

Methyl chloroform (1, 1, 1-trichloroethane). This is an excellent industrial degreasing solvent and is widely used by the hobbyist in either liquid or aerosol form. It is also used in the home for removing grease spots from clothing or fabrics. It should be used only under conditions where ventilation is adequate.

Symptoms. According to Stewart, who reports four cases of intoxication and reviews the literature, this solvent, when inhaled in excessive amounts, causes dizziness and lassitude which may progress to respiraory depression, hypotension, and vasomotor collapse.

If methyl chloroform is taken by mouth, nausea, vomiting, and diarrhea result within an hour. Ingestion of this compound is not known to have caused death in humans and has a far lower potential for producing kidney and liver damage than does carbon tetrachloride.

○ TREATMENT

There is no specific treatment. The victim should be removed from the contaminated atmosphere and artificial respiration should be given if necessary. If the solvent has been swallowed, induce vomiting and repeat until return fluid is clear. Observation in a hospital is desirable, especially if intoxication is severe, since suppression of urine (oliguria) may develop as the result of the low blood pressure and require special treatment.

Trichloroethylene (trichlorethene). This is another widely used solvent in industry, for degreasing, dry cleaning, and many other purposes. It is much safer than carbon tetrachloride, but it should, of course, be used with adequate ventilation. Medicinally, it has been used as an analgesic and anesthetic for short operations and in obstetrics. Like trichloroethane and carbon tetrachloride, it is nonflammable.

Symptoms. Moderate exposure to the vapors produces symptoms similar to those of alcoholic intoxication. Excessive exposure produces narcosis and anesthesia. Tachypnea and cardiac arrythmias may occur, and death, if it occurs, probably is the result of ventricular fibrillation. Liver and kidney damage as the result of industrial exposures or those likely to be encountered in the home has not been observed.

○ TREATMENT

The same as for methyl chloroform.

Benzene (benzol, C_6H_6). According to Goldstein, this is the most dangerous solvent used in industry, largely because of its extremely toxic effect upon the bone marrow. It is used as a starting material for the manufacture of a great many products, including plastic paints, pesticides and drugs; as a solvent; and as a component of gasoline. It should not be confused with the far less toxic *benzine* also referred to as petroleum benzine or naphtha. *Benzine* consists of a mixture of hydrocarbons of the methane series and has about the same degree of toxicity as the common place mineral spirits (ligroin) and kerosene (q.v.).

Symptoms. Acute poisoning as the result of exposure to high concentrations of *benzene* may produce death very quickly, preceded by coma and convulsions, as the result of anesthetic action. Lower concentrations produce exhilaration and excitement (referred to industrially as a "benzol jag"). This stage is followed by severe headache, loss of balance control, incoherent speech, nausea and vomiting.

Chronic poisoning develops insidiously after months or even years of low-grade exposure. The symptoms are largely related to changes in the hemapoietic system, and the condition may offer a diagnostic and therapeutic challenge.

○ TREATMENT

If benzene has been ingested, olive oil, other vegetable oils, butter or cream, or even ice cream, should be given to retard absorption. Gastric lavage and vomiting should be avoided because of the danger of aspiration, since respiratory toxicity is much greater than oral toxicity.

There is no specific treatment for poisoning by inhalation other than quick removal to a pure atmosphere and artificial respiration if required. Oxygen and other supportive treatments are used as indicated.

Kerosene and Other Petroleum Distillates. Kerosene poisoning is common in certain rural and city areas where kerosene is used for heating and lighting purposes and as a solvent for insecticides. Because "pop" bottles and coffee cans containing kerosene are carelessly left about, young children can easily get hold of it and drink substantial quantities.

Children between the ages of 16 to 20 months are the most common victims. Practically all cases would be preventable if kerosene were not left lying about where very young children could get hold of it; anywhere from a tablespoonful to several ounces may cause death.

Signs and Symptoms. The child may choke, cough, gasp, appear to be strangling, or vomit immediately upon drinking the kerosene, although often he is found lying depressed or stuporous beside the container from which he drank. In about half the victims there may be abdominal pain, and almost all will show some degree of fever.

○ TREATMENT

Authorities differ on the emergency care of victims of kerosene poisoning. Some have urged the immediate emptying of the stomach by an emetic or stomach tube. Others, because of the danger of increased irritation of the lungs by sucking in the vapor or actual liquid from the stomach contents, say that emptying of the stomach should be done only under special circumstances. However, most authorities advise against inducing vomiting unless a very large amount of kerosene or other distillate has been ingested.

Take the child to the nearest hospital as quickly as possible, where the proper treatment will be undertaken on the basis of the best medical judgment. If the child does vomit spontaneously, an effort should be made to prevent his sucking the vomited matter into the lungs, by keeping his head lower than the rest of his body. A very high proportion of victims of kerosene poisoning develop pneumonia, either as the result of breathing in the fumes, actual aspiration, or absorption of toxic portions of the kerosene from the gastrointestinal tract.

Ant and Roach Preparations. Poisoning by preparations meant to kill ants and roaches can be produced by absorption through the skin, but accidental swallowing by children is the more common way.

○ TREATMENT

Since the exact nature of the poison may not be known immediately, thoroughly empty the stomach, using syrup of ipecac or some other emetic, and then flush through repeated vomitings with copious amounts of salt water, or activated charcoal, followed by diluted egg whites or milk. The case should be treated at the nearest Poison Control Center or hospital so that specific treatment can be given for whatever active ingredient is identified in the ingested preparation.

Rat Poisons (Rodenticides). Rat (rodent) poisons include many poisonous substances. A widely used and very toxic substance, known as alpha-naphthylthiourea (warfarin®) kills the animals by internal hemorrhage when swallowed or when absorbed through the pads of their feet; in proportionately larger doses it can kill human beings in the same way. (In therapeutic doses, the same compound is used to lessen the clotting tendency of the blood in certain types of cardiovascular disease.) Many rats, however, have become more or less immune to this compound and *phosphorus* is now widely used in rat poisons. It produces what is known as the "smoking stool syndrome."

The clue to yellow phosphorus ingestion lies in the history of the victim ingesting a substance containing yellow elemental phosphorus, skin burns, a garlic-like odor in the breath, vomitus or feces, or the actual "smoking of the vomitus or feces."

Signs and Symptoms. Following accidental ingestion or overdosage, the victim goes into profound shock, with subnormal temperature, congestion of the chest, convulsions, and coma. This is an acute medical emergency.

○ TREATMENT

Empty the stomach if the poison has been taken by mouth. Give artificial respiration and oxygen if possible. Get the victim to a hospital immediately.

If phosphorus poisoning is suspected, both the victim and the attendants themselves should be protected from further contamination (stools and vomitus). Simon and Pickering recommend copious gastric lavage with potassium permanganate in a water dilution of 1:5000. After lavage, mineral oil—*never a vegetable oil*—should be left in the stomach to delay further absorption. This should be done, followed by a tablespoon of bicarbonate of soda in a quart of warm water, simply as an immediate first-aid measure until medical aid is obtained. Later on, in the hospital, long-term supportive measures will be required to combat shock and treat liver and kidney damage. There is usually considerable pain during the immediate postpoisoning period, during which cardiac vascular collapse may be followed by death. If not, a relatively asymptomatic period lasting several weeks may occur, followed by general systemic involvement which may or may not produce death, depending upon the size of the dose ingested.

Insecticides. Insect killers act as poisons when inhaled or absorbed through the skin, or through ingestion. Poisoning usually results from misuse of the preparation and failure to follow directions. Certain very toxic insecticides have been used as murder weapons by surreptitiously placing them in the victim's food. All too often a poisonous substance is left in a beverage bottle or other food container, where it is accessible to small children who inadvertently drink it.

As an example of the dangers of leaving toxic pesticides in containers available to little children, DePalma, Kwalick, and Zukerberg have reported an instance in which two young children, brother and sister, drank from an unlabeled jar a mixture of parathion, chlordane, and dimpylate (Diazinon®). One died despite emergency resuscitation measures and intensive therapy, apparently having ingested the larger amount. The other survived.

The authors point out that in this particular case intoxication from the chlorinated hydrocarbon (chlordane) as well as intoxication from the organophosphates in the mixture had to be treated. Phenobarbital was used effectively along with calcium gluconate, which has been found to be useful in the control of chlorinated hydrocarbon-induced convulsions to treat the convulsions in this instance, which probably were the result of the chlordane as well as the two organophosphates in the mixture.

It is also emphasized that the specific treatment of severe parathion and dimpylate poisoning (both cholinesterase inhibitors) includes atropine sulphate in substantial doses given intravenously after any necessary resuscitative efforts have been followed and cyanosis is eliminated.

The ingredients most commonly used in the older types of household insecticides are DDT, chlordane, and the pyrethrins, in an oil base.   When in a powder base, the danger of absorption through the skin will be slight.

Signs and Symptoms.   The symptoms of DDT *poisoning* are apprehension, a feeling of tightness of the jaws and throat muscles, sore throat, nausea and vomiting, headache, and general weakness.   Few cases are fatal; usually the victim recovers fully after a few days.

Absorption of a *pyrethrin* produces hyperexcitability, incoordination, paralysis of the general muscles, as well as respiratory paralysis.   A fatal outcome is rare in humans.

Chlordane acts by absorption through the skin or lungs and produces convulsions followed by coma and marked respiratory depression.   Symptoms start within an hour after exposure, so that the cause of poisoning is usually fairly obvious.

○ TREATMENT

If the *DDT* has been swallowed, it should be removed from the stomach by induced vomiting and thorough washing out, *avoiding oils*.

Emergency treatment for a *pyrethrin* can only be supportive, and the victim should be taken to a hospital at once.

The victim of *chlordane* poisoning should be hospitalized as quickly as possible, as detailed specific treatment will be required to pull him through.

Garden Sprays.   In addition to substances already discussed, these sprays may contain nicotine, which, in fairly large amounts, may prove dangerous by inhalation or by accidental swallowing.

Signs and Symptoms.   The symptoms are muscular weakness, irritation of the throat, nausea, vomiting, convulsions, dizziness, and ultimate collapse.   The victim appears to be in shock, the pupils are dilated, and the extremities are cold and clammy.   Death may result from respiratory paralysis.

○ TREATMENT

If the poison has been taken by mouth, empty the stomach and wash out with very strong tea.   The victim should be taken to a hospital as quickly as possible, since prolonged artificial respiration and other supportive measures may be required.

Organophosphate Insecticides. There are a host of other newer garden sprays and insecticides, the toxicity of some of which is much greater than the common home-use types which have been reviewed. As pointed out by Milby, the organophosphates constitute the group of insecticides most commonly involved in serious poisoning, particularly in view of the growing restrictions on the use of DDT and related compounds.

A list of the most commonly used preparations is given in Table 11-1.

Some organophosphates, of course, are relatively safe as well as effective. Figures 1 and 2 list the various agricultural sprays as well as ones commonly used by the home gardener, in terms of their oral toxicity (Fig. 11-1) and their toxicity when in contact with the skin (Fig. 11-2).

Symptoms. The organophosphates as a group show similar pharmacologic characteristics, though in varying degrees; hence, members of the group produce similar clinical symptoms and require similar treatment.

All organophosphate insecticides may readily be absorbed through the intact skin or may be inhaled, especially if a protective mask is not worn. A history of exposure obviously puts one on the alert.

Initially, the symptoms of intoxication consist of severe headache, blurred vision, nausea and vomiting, diarrhea, profuse sweating and weakness, and abdominal pain.

There may also be shortness of breath, excessive salivation and lacrimation, irregular heartbeat, twitching of the muscles (fasiculation), and convulsions. In severe cases, shock may occur, leading to coma and death.

○ TREATMENT

Victims of organophosphate poisoning have an enormous tolerance for atropine, the antidote of choice, so that one should not hesitate to use large doses in the attempt to reverse the effects of the organophosphate intoxication. Two to four milligrams of atropine should immediately be given intravenously (this is about ten times the usually accepted therapeutic dose used in other conditions). The atropine may be repeated at up to 5-minute intervals or until the drug becomes effective, along with the use of another drug, pralidoxime chloride (Protopam®), 1 gram (25-40 milligrams/kilogram) given intra-

TABLE 11-1
SOME ORGANOPHOSPHATE PESTICIDES*

Most Dangerous†	Dangerous
TEPP (Bladan; Kilmite 40; Tetron; Vapotone)	phosphamidon (Dimecron)
phorate (Thimet)	carbophenothion (Trithion; Dagadip; Garrathion)
disulfoton, thiodemeton; dithiosystox (Di-Syston)	coumaphos (Co-Ral; Asuntol; Muscatox; Resitox)
paraoxon (E-600; Mintacol)	dichlorvos, DDVP (Vapona)
thionazin, BSI (Nemafos; Cynem)	diazinon, ISO, BSI (Basudin; Diazide; Gardentox; etc.)
parathion (E-605; Alkron; Alleron; Etilon; Thiophos; etc.)	ethion (Nialate; NIA 1240)
demeton (Systox)	delnav, dioxathion (Delnav)
mevinphos, ISO, BSI (Phosgene; Phosdrine)	**Less Dangerous**
EPN	methyl demeton (Meta-Systox)
schradan (OMPA; Pestox III; Sytam)	dimethoate (Cygon; Daphene; Trimetion; etc.)
metacide	naled (Dibrom)
methyl parathion (Dalf; Metron; Nitrox 80; etc.)	Phostex
azinphos-methyl (Guthion; Carfene; Guthathion M)	dicapthon (Di-Captan)
monocrotophos (Azodrin; Nureacron; etc.)	DEF; DeGreen; Ortho Phosphate Defoliant, etc.
dicrotophos (Bidrin; Carbicron; Ektafos; etc.)	trichlorfon, ISO (Dipterex; Tugon; etc.)
	Least Dangerous
	Chlorthion
	Ruelene
	malathion (Cython; Karbofos; Malamar; etc.)
	ronnel (Korlan; Trolene; Viozene; etc.)

* Reproduced, with permission, from Milby, Thomas H.: Prevention and Management of Organophosphate Poisoning. *J.A.M.A. 216*(13): 2131 (June 28) 1971.
† Estimate of hazard is based on acute dermal and oral toxicity in animals.

venously in 50 to 250 cubic centimeters saline. For children the dose may be 25 to 50 milligrams/kilogram of body weight. According to Milby, the combination of the two antidotes, atropine and pralidoxime, is more effective than either one alone. Supportive measures are, of course, essential. Mechanical

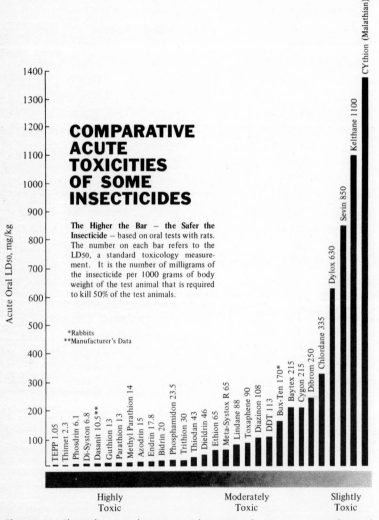

Fig. 11-1. Chart showing the acute oral toxicity of various commonly used insecticides. (Reproduced with permission of the American Cyanamid Company, Princeton, New Jersey.)

artificial respiration over a considerable period may be required, since respiratory failure is the usual cause of death. Convulsions must be controlled by the use of thiopental sodium or other anticonvulsive agent and, if the poison has been ingested, the stomach should be washed out and a saline

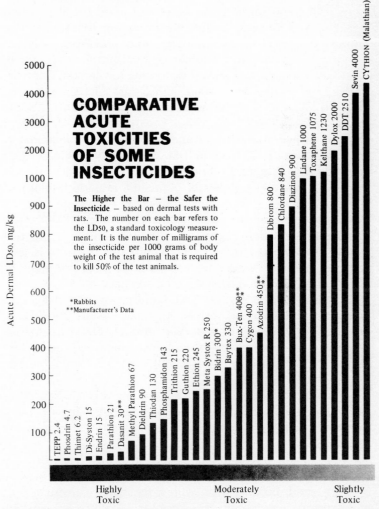

COMPARATIVE ACUTE TOXICITIES OF SOME INSECTICIDES

The Higher the Bar — the Safer the Insecticide — based on dermal tests with rats. The number on each bar refers to the LD50, a standard toxicology measurement. It is the number of milligrams of the insecticide per 1000 grams of body weight of the test animal that is required to kill 50% of the test animals.

*Rabbits
**Manufacturer's Data

Acute Dermal LD50, mg/kg

5000
4000
3000
2000
1000
900
800
700
600
500
400
300
200
100

TEPP 2.4
Phosdrin 4.7
Thimet 6.2
Di-Syston 15
Endrin 15
Parathion 21
Dasanit 30**
Methyl Parathion 67
Dieldrin 90
Thiodan 130
Phosphamidon 143
Trithion 215
Guthion 220
Ethion 245
Meta Systox R 250
Bidrin 300*
Baytex 330
Bux-Ten 400**
Cygon 400
Azodrin 450**
Dibrom 800
Chlordane 840
Diazinon 900
Lindane 1000
Toxaphene 1075
Kelthane 1230
Dylox 2000
DDT 2510
Sevin 4000
CYTHION (Malathian)

Highly
Toxic

Moderately
Toxic

Slightly
Toxic

Fig. 11-2. Chart showing the local toxicity, due to absorption through the skin, of various insecticides. (Reproduced with permission of the American Cyanamid Company, Princeton, New Jersey.)

cathartic administered. Physical contamination (clothing, skin, hair) should be corrected immediately through the copious use of water and soap or detergent. Rigorous attention to all these details is essential to prevent death in the severer cases.

Cyanide. A number of preparations used about the garden for killing moles, rodents, worms, and ants contain cyanide in some form, as do silver and other metal polishes. It is also widely used in the electroplating industry and in various metallurgical and photographic processes. Hydrocyanic acid is a common commercial fumigant for ships, warehouses, and similar structures. According to Gleason, Gosselin, Hodge, and Smith, the average lethal dose of HCN taken by mouth is believed to lie between 60 and 90 milligrams (1 to 1½ grains); this corresponds to about 1 teaspoonful of a 2 percent solution of hydrocyanic acid and to about 200 milligrams of potassium cyanide (Gettler and St. George, 1934; Gettler and Baine, 1938). Prompt treatment, however, has saved a person who swallowed 6,000 grams of potassium cyanide (Miller and Toops, 1951) and 3 to 5 grams are said to have been survived without specific therapy (Liebowitz and Schwartz, 1948). The lethality of most derivatives is proportional to the content of readily available cyanide. In nonfatal cases recovery is generally complete. Rarely neuropsychiatric sequelae may be observed, as in carbon monoxide poisoning.

Cyanide is one of the most rapid-acting and dangerous poisons known, being extremely toxic when swallowed, breathed in as vapor, or absorbed through the skin or small wounds. Many cases of cyanide poisoning, of course, are accidental, but this chemical has long been a common method of committing suicide.

Signs and Symptoms. With any but the very smallest doses the victim quickly collapses; there may be but a single convulsion, followed quickly by death as the result of respiratory paralysis.

With small, but still fatal, exposures, however, life may continue for several hours. The symptoms commonly include a bitter, acrid, burning taste with a feeling of constriction or numbness of the throat, accompanied by dizziness, anxiety, and confusion. An almost pathognomic sign is the odor of bitter almonds on the breath. Often the mouth may be covered with blood-tinged foam. At first, respirations are very rapid but then become slow and irregular.

There is at first a rise in blood pressure with a slow pulse rate. Shortly, however, the pulse becomes rapid, weak, and irregular, along with palpitations and feelings of severe chest constriction.

Unconsciousness is followed by epileptic-like convulsions and then paralysis. The skin may become a brick-red color, the pupils are dilated with protrusion of the eyeballs, and sweating may be profuse.

O TREATMENT

Treatment is based on the theory of converting a certain portion of the circulatory hemoglobin to methemoglobin in order to protect the body against the action of the cyanide ion until it itself can be detoxified metabolically. When exposure has been heavy, it is rare that treatment can be rendered quickly enough to enable the victim to survive, but the most urgent effort should be made to get him to a hospital.

If ampules of amyl nitrite (such as are carried by many people for the relief of anginal attacks) are available, inhalation from these may be tried as a means of quickly producing some degree of methemoglobinemia. Gleason et al., based on a wide experience, outline the following steps for treatment:

1 If the patient is apneic, start artificial respiration immediately. Keep the airway clear.

2 Administer by inhalation amyl nitrite (amyl nitrite perles) for 15 to 30 seconds of every minute, while a sodium nitrite solution is being prepared.

3 Discontinue amyl nitrite and immediately inject intravenously 10 milliliters of a 3 percent solution of sodium nitrite over a period of 2 to 4 minutes. If necessary, inject a nonsterile solution. Do not remove the needle.

4 Through the same needle infuse intravenously 50 milliliters of a 25 percent aqueous solution of sodium thiosulfate. The injection should take about 10 minutes. Other concentrations (5 to 50 percent) are permissible if the total dose is held at approximately 12 grams.

5 Administration of oxygen therapy may be of value in speeding detoxification reactions.

6 If symptoms recur, the injections of nitrite and thiosulfate may be repeated at half the above doses.

7 Gastric lavage should be postponed at least until after the foregoing steps have been taken. Probably the best lavage fluid is a dilute solution of potassium permanganate (1:5,000).

8 Oxygen therapy along with whole blood transfusion may become necessary if nitrite-induced methemoglobinemia becomes too severe.

Because the onset of cyanide poisoning is so extremely rapid, it is essential that the necessary supplies be immediately available in ambulances and in emergency rooms, and that personnel should be thoroughly trained in their use. Patty recommends a basic kit composed of the following items:

2 boxes (2 dozen) of ampules each containing 0.3 milliliters of amyl nitrite

2 ampules of sterile sodium nitrite solution (10 milliliters of a 3 percent solution in each)

2 ampules of sterile sodium thiosulfate solution (50 milliliters of a 25 percent solution in each)

1 10-milliliter and 1 50-milliliter sterile glass syringe with sterile intravenous needles

1 ampule file

1 tourniquet

12 gauze pads

1 small bottle of 70 percent alcohol

1 stomach tube

2 1-pint (473 milliliter) bottles of 1 percent sodium thiosulfate solution

Methyl Alcohol (Methanol; Wood Alcohol). Methyl alcohol is used around the home as a window cleaner and for burning in spirit lamps; in industry it is used as a solvent. Unfortunately, it is also used as an adulterant in cheap bootleg whiskey and wines, and often is purloined as a substitute for ethyl alcohol. Poisoning can occur from drinking it or from accidentally inhaling toxic concentrations of its vapor.

Methyl alcohol is an extremely poisonous substance; the ingestion of a fraction of an ounce has been known to cause death. Dose for dose, it is far less intoxicating than ethyl alcohol, but, even though it is promptly absorbed from the gastrointestinal tract, its effects are often delayed for as much as 12 to 24 hours. In instances of adulteration of whiskey by methyl alcohol, a large number of cases of poisoning, as well as many deaths, have been reported from a single batch. Methyl alcohol has a specific degenerating effect on the optic nerve, which may result in permanent blindness even if only a very small quantity of the poison has been consumed. Methanol is metabolized in the body to form formaldehyde and formic acid, most of which is excreted in the urine but some of which is oxidized to carbon dioxide and water. These by-products of metabolic degradation are thought to be the essential elements which produce the toxicity and lead to the extreme acidosis characteristic of this type of poisoning. Enormous amounts of alkali, usually given in the form of sodium bicarbonate, are required to combat it. Recent evidence suggests that ethyl alcohol enters into direct competition with methyl alcohol for certain enzyme systems within the body and hence greatly slows the absorption and deleterious effects of the methyl alcohol. For that reason, ethyl alcohol has found a definite place in the treatment of wood alcohol poisoning.

Symptoms. The most characteristic symptoms of wood alcohol poisoning, aside from the general symptoms of intoxication—some of which may be due to simultaneous imbibing of ethyl alcohol—are great thirst, visual disturbances, very severe abdominal pain, and occasionally convulsions.

O TREATMENT

While it may be desirable to wash out the stomach as a routine matter as soon as the victim's condition is discovered, this probably has little effect in most cases because of the rapid absorption of the methyl alcohol. The most important facet of treatment is to correct the severe acidosis by the administration of 4 percent bicarbonate of soda in 5 percent dextrose, given intravenously. Because of the very slow metabolism of the methanol within the body, it is necessary to maintain alkalinization of the victim over a long period of time until finally the methyl alcohol is metabolized and excreted.

Because of the evidence which suggests that ethanol counteracts the toxicity of the methyl alcohol, the former is given either by mouth or intravenously as required. One of the most striking characteristics of wood alcohol poisoning is the enormous thirst of the victim, which even a huge quantity of fluid fails to satisfy. Because of the severe inflammatory reaction in the optic nerves, the eyes should be shielded from light and oxygen administered for respiratory embarrassment when required. These cases die of respiratory failure and uncontrollable acidosis, but mortality is unpredictable in relation to amount of methanol ingested and the outcome often remains in doubt for many days.

POISONOUS GASES

The most important gases from the standpoint of emergency treatment are carbon monoxide and utility gas; the treatment of poisoning from these has already been described on page 300). However, there are other gases that should be mentioned, since, under certain even domestic conditions, they can prove dangerous to the point of being lethal. These are carbon dioxide, methane, hydrogen sulfide, and sulfur dioxide.

Carbon Dioxide. This gas, commonly thought of as innocuous, is routinely used as a respiratory stimulant during anesthesia and to help maintain acid base equilibrium in certain complicated types of medical cases; it is normally present in the atmosphere in a concentration of about 0.04 percent.

But concentrations of from 0.1 to 0.5 percent may produce malaise and headache; concentrations of 8 to 9 percent are in the suffocation level; higher levels may produce death.

Carbon dioxide (CO_2) is heavier than air (specific gravity 1.52) and therefore tends to gravitate to low areas and accumulate in such places as cellars, manholes, wells, silos, caves, and mines where concentrations may reach asphyxial levels. Death occurs when such areas are entered without adequate safeguards such as the use of an ordinary oxygen mask.

A potential source of danger from carbon dioxide about the home or farm arises from the large amount of "dry ice" (which is solidified carbon dioxide) used in keeping ice cream and other perishables, and has given rise to what is known as the "ice house syndrome." As pointed out by Mr. Paul Witt, of the Bureau of Mines, this may occur, for instance, when someone stores ice cream over night in "dry ice" in a small, tightly closed ice house, of which there are still many in our rural areas. The next morning someone enters the ice house and the papers subsequently report that he "died of apoplexy." The carbon dioxide level in the confined space had reached a lethal level by sublimation of the solid carbon dioxide to gaseous carbon dioxide—the mechanism by which "dry ice" refrigerates.

A similar type of case has also been reported of a young mother preparing for a birthday party for a child, who brought Dry ice-packed ice cream home and hid it in a small pantry. The mother evidently stuck her head into or near the mouth of the sack some time later. She was found unconscious by her husband, who came home to lunch apparently only a few minutes after the accident. Artificial respiration and emergency oxygen brought about a complete remission in the nick of time!

Many comparable incidents could be recounted although, fortunately, deaths from carbon dioxide are relatively uncommon.

Symptoms. Carbon dioxide produces asphyxia by replacing life-supporting oxygen in the atmosphere—a process which is hastened by the fact that the gas acts on the respiratory center to accelerate the breathing rate. Early symptoms are dizziness, ringing in the ears (tinnitus), a feeling as if the head were going to explode, diaphoresis (sweating), muscular weakness and fatigue, and a feeling of great sleepiness or lassitude. There follows a rise in blood pressure and pulse rate, then general collapse, coma, and death.

O TREATMENT

If the victim is rescued in time, the specific treatment is artificial respiration with the administration of oxygen. Resuscitation should be continued for a prolonged period even though unconsciousness persists, since recovery may eventually be achieved.

Methane. Methane (CH_4), commonly known as marsh gas, is formed in nature by decaying organic matter in marshes and mines where it is known as "fire damp." It is also present in sewer gas and gas formed by the fermentation of sewage and other organic matter in land fills, mixed with substantial amounts of hydrogen and carbon dioxide.

Commercially, methane is present in a concentration of

from 94 percent to 98 percent in natural gas. It is colorless and odorless and diffuses readily in air; a mixture of one part in ten parts of air by volume is highly explosive, but air containing 14 percent or more methane burns without exploding. The gas itself has little inherent toxicity but simply acts as an asphyxiant by replacing essential oxygen in an atmosphere so that in very high concentrations it produces narcosis followed by death from asphyxiation.

○ TREATMENT

Artificial respiration with simultaneous administration of oxygen.

Hydrogen Sulfide. Hydrogen sulfide (H_2S) is an exceedingly poisonous, colorless gas that smells like rotten eggs. It is slightly heavier than air, inflammable, and explosive when mixed with equal parts of oxygen.

According to the American Conference of Governmental Industrial Hygienists (1970), the gas has a threshold limit of 10 parts per million, is 100 percent lethal in 2 minutes at 1,000 parts per million (0.1 percent), and in as little as 100 parts per million abolishes the sense of smell, so that the victim may inhale heavy concentrations of the gas with little warning.

As an example, mentioned by Witt, in the lime gas fields of Arkansas, Louisiana, and Texas the wells produce a gas which may run as high as 65 percent hydrogen sulfide. Workers have been known to state that they no longer smelled the gas and in a few minutes were dead from its effects.

In nature, the gas is produced by the decomposition of organic matter containing sulfur compounds and is liable to be present in high concentrations in such places as cesspools, tannery vats, fat-rendering plants, the holds of fishing vessels, and, in fact, any semiclosed space where organic decomposition occurs. Many deaths have been reported from men going into sour crude tanks to make repairs and from falling into tanks as a result of metal corrosion from the action of the hydrogen sulfide. People have been known to lose the muscular control necessary to climb out of a tank in less than a minute even when they say that they do not smell the gas. In one reported incident, several men were killed very quickly by this highly toxic gas while attempting to clean the hold and bilges of a fishing trawler.

Symptoms. Externally, hydrogen sulfide is a local irritant, so that it inflames the conjunctivae and irritates the upper respiratory tract. If inhaled in small quantities, it is simply converted in the bloodstream into harmless sulfates and excreted in the urine. If toxic concentrations are inhaled, the gas paralyzes the central nervous system and death occurs very quickly as the result of rapid paralysis of the respiratory center in the brain.

Lower concentrations produce preliminary dizziness, nausea, abdominal pain, cardiac irregularity, anoxic convulsions, and coma. Unless rescue is prompt, death ensues.

○ TREATMENT

Artificial resuscitation and the administration of oxygen in an effort to counteract formation of sulfmethemoglobin in the bloodstream. Cases of hydrogen sulfide poisoning should be hospitalized and carefully observed for the development of pneumonitis as the result of the irritant effect of the gas on the lungs.

Gleason and Gosselin suggest that severe poisonings be treated with amyl nitrite and sodium nitrite as for cyanide poisoning. This therapy has had no clinical trials in sulfide poisoning but is effective in animals. Also, it is suggested that atropine sulfate (0.0006 gram intramuscularly) may contribute some symptomatic relief. Conjunctivitis may be relieved by the instillation of one drop of olive oil in each eye and sometimes by three to four drops of epinephrine solution (1:1,000) at frequent intervals (e.g., 5 minutes). Occasionally local anesthetics and hot or cold compresses are necessary to control the pain. Antibiotics should be administered at the first hint of pulmonary infection.

Sulfur dioxide (SO₂), a refrigerant sometimes found in older mechanical refrigerators, is so extremely acrid that it produces very severe irritation of the eyes and respiratory passages and therefore could cause serious poisoning only if the victim could not escape exposure. Toxic concentrations of sulfur dioxide cause the victim to choke to death because of uncontrollable spasm of the vocal cords.

Sulfur dioxide is, of course, an important factor in air pollution; its presence in subtoxic levels produces sneezing, coughing, and other manifestations of respiratory tract irritation. There now seems to be little question that in populations chronically exposed to polluting levels of sulfur dioxide in the atmosphere, the incidence of respiratory illness, particularly among older age groups, is increased.

More modern refrigerants, though not inherently toxic, can kill by suffocation. For instance, fluorocarbon 12 is a volatile liquid widely used as a refrigerant and aerosol propellant. Since it leaves no toxic residue on evaporation, it recently has been used as a "glass chiller" to produce frosted cocktail glasses. The death of a young girl who inhaled fluorocarbon 12 vapor from a balloon points up the danger that can occur if this usually innocuous compound is mishandled.

Fluorocarbon 12 is a mild intoxicant, but it can kill by suffocation if inhaled in the absence of oxygen, or by cold damage to the larynx if aspirated in liquid form. The potential dangers of inhaling this or any other substance for intoxicative effects cannot be overstated.

Vinyl Chloride and Polyvinyl Chloride. These two compounds are briefly discussed here, since both give off noxious gases under certain conditions and can be extremely hazardous.

Vinyl chloride is manufactured as a basic chemical used for many purposes in industry. Block and others have found a high rate of angiosarcoma of the liver in those engaged in vinyl chloride production; on the basis of animal studies, Tabershaw and Gaffey found cancers in the lungs, kidneys, skin, and other sites.

Falk et al. found that the premonitory symptoms, in a study of some 3,000 cases of vinyl chloride workers, were variable but that usually the first to cause the victim to seek medical attention were acute abdominal pain, weight loss, and abnormal findings in routine blood tests. Other findings have been reported which suggest that vinyl chloride poisoning is indeed a systemic disease.

Block also feels that a high rate of liver angiosarcoma occurs in workers who have either been exposed to low levels of the vapors over a period of many years, or possibly to a high level many years before the appearance of the tumor.

The greatest hazard occurs when workers enter the vats in which the chemical is made, and clean them by chipping residual material off the sides of the tank.

Prevention through the use of new cleaning technics and better respirators is needed. Treatment consists of surgical resection of the tumor, or other suitable treatment.

Polyvinyl chloride, a polymer of vinyl chloride, is used in many plastics, and it is present in many common articles such as furniture; either as covering or stuffing, or as actual structural elements; floor and wall coverings; textiles; and many other products.

As pointed out by Dyer and Esch, many plastics produce large volumes of irritant gases when they burn, making fire fighting both difficult and dangerous. When polyvinyl chloride burns, it is known to produce some 75 products of degradation, including chlorine, phosgene, and hydrochloric acid, all of which are highly toxic and strong irritants. In addition, burning plastics produce highly toxic smoke.

Sorenson, who cites a number of detailed statistics, takes serious exception to some of the statements offered by Dyer and Esch; he, nevertheless, concludes that efforts must be made to make both natural and synthetic materials safer to use.

Extreme pulmonary irritation; coupled with shock and unconsciousness, may follow exposure to the smoke of burning plastic. If actual contact is made, burning plastic also tends to stick to the skin, such as all too often has occurred with a burning plastic fiber nightgown.

Preventive measures consist of the use of self-contained breathing apparatus when fighting fires and the wearing of proper heavy-duty fire fighting apparel. Fires involving any plastics—and many of them do—are extremely dangerous.

POISONOUS BITES AND STINGS

Bees, Wasps, and Hornets. The insects which are the greatest source of danger in this regard are technically known as arthropods of the Hymenoptera group, and include the honeybee, bumblebee, wasp, black hornet, and the yellow jacket. According to the *Journal of the American Medical Association,* the venom of these stinging insects causes more deaths in the United States each year than are caused by the bites of rattlesnakes.

This is usually an example of the reaction of the body, known as anaphylaxis, to overwhelming sensitization, the whole process being set off by the injected venom. Death results in these cases from respiratory obstruction caused by swelling of the vocal cords or to severe constriction and congestion of the bronchial tubes, and anaphylactic shock.

Symptoms. In the nonsensitive individual a beesting produces nothing more than a painful swelling with redness, aching and itching. But if several stings are received at one time, enough venom can be absorbed to make the victim quite ill and perhaps cause him to develop severe hives or a generalized swelling (angioneurotic edema) of all the tissues.

If a victim has been stung many times by a bee, or happens to have been stung by bees on several different occasions over a period of time, or is severely allergic to beestings, he can be made desperately ill and may require emergency treatment to save his life. This occurrence is by no means so rare as might be expected, and if it is seen that the victim of even a single sting is becoming short of breath or shows other signs of acute distress, he should be rushed to the nearest doctor or hospital.

Wasps, black hornets, and yellow jackets, when they sting a person, retain their stingers and can sting repeatedly, thus being capable of inflicting multiple injections of venom into the same person. On the other hand, when the honeybee sinks its barbed stinger into the skin, it is unable to withdraw it. As the bee attempts to escape, it simply disembowels itself, leaving behind the stinger, with the abdominal contents and the venom sac attached. Worse yet, the muscles controlling the venom sac, although separated from the bee, continue to contract for as long as 20 minutes after the bee itself has flown off, thus driving the stinger deeper and deeper into the skin and all the while injecting additional venom from the sac. Drop for drop, the venom of the bee is just as potent as that of the rattlesnake.

O TREATMENT

Unless the victim is in distress because of a generalized reaction, remove the stinger immediately by scraping it out gently with a sharp object, such as a knife blade, the side of tweezers, or the fingernail.

Don't try to grasp the sac or stinger with fingernails or forceps, since this simply forces the remaining venom into the skin. By careful teasing with a sideways motion, the stinger and the sac can usually be extracted without squeezing additional poison into the tissues.

When the stinger and sac have been extracted, local treatment of the area by the application of strong Epsom salts soaks may provide symtomatic relief and help to reduce the swelling. The local application of an ointment containing triancinolone, hydrocortisone, or other anti-inflammatory corticosteroid also provides relief. The local itching and such other general symptoms as mild urticaria or hives that may occur can be relieved with an antihistamine such as is usually used for the treatment of hay fever and other allergic conditions. Cases of this type are not serious, and the annoyance and discomfort disappear after a few hours or days.

If the victim is known to be sensitive to bee venom because of previous stings, anaphylactic shock usually develops quickly and can be easily recognized by the fact that the victim experiences severe difficulty with breathing, becomes restless, may develop a mottled, livid blueness of the skin, begins to cough, complains of headache, and may become unconscious.

In some cases the victim may have no difficulty in breathing, but his general appearance is similar to that of profound shock, and there may be severe nausea, vomiting, and diarrhea. These are warning signs of extreme sensitivity, and the victim must be taken to a physician or hospital emergency room with all possible speed. By way of warning, it should be emphasized that if an individual known to be sensitive is stung, he *should be taken to medical aid immediately without waiting for symptoms to develop.*

If medical aid is not immediately available, a drug that may prove to be lifesaving is epinephrine injected subcutaneously. An individual who has a known acute sensitivity to beesting or has reacted badly to previous stings should never be without this drug close at hand. He, or a member of his family, should be advised by his personal family physician on how to use it to carry him through until he can get to a doctor.

There is also a drug (isoproterenol) which is absorbed very

quickly when placed under the tongue and acts similarly to epinephrine; there is also a special form of epinephrine which can be used as an inhaler and produces a very prompt effect. These are both very powerful drugs and should be used under emergency circumstances only, in accordance with a physician's previous instructions. Also, though slower acting, the antihistamines are valuable in controlling the symptoms over an extended period of time and in making the person more comfortable, but in severe cases a corticosteroid must also be used by emergency medical personnel.

In addition, when anaphylactic shock threatens as the result of an insect sting on an extremity, a constricting band should be placed between the sting and the base of the extremity to minimize the absorption of the poison into the general system.

Laryngeal obstruction due to swelling of the vocal cords usually responds rapidly to the administration of epinephrine, but on the rare occasions when it does not, a surgical incision into the trachea (tracheotomy), or a "medical tracheotomy" as previously described (page 111), may be required as a life-saving measure.

It is true, of course, that anaphylaxis can best be treated by a physician in the hospital, where oxygen, cortisone-like (corticosteroid) drugs which can be given intravenously, and other facilities are available. But under conditions where medical aid is not available and could not be expected to be quickly available, adequate foresight, having the necessary supplies on hand, and correct training may save a life that otherwise might be lost.

That a beesting may be fatal to many people has been recognized by physicians who have specialized in the study of this disorder. They have recommended a specially developed emergency kit (containing the essential materials already mentioned, together with instructions for using them) for those sensitive to beesting to tide them over until they can get to a doctor. It should be kept readily available whether the individual is at home, on a vacation or business trip, or simply engaged in routine daily activities. With one kit, manufactured by Center Laboratories, Port Washington, New York 11050, the victim can start his own treatment while on the way to the hospital. While not adequate for severe cases or prolonged treatment, it is sufficient to get a victim started until he can reach a doctor, and it should always be carried by those known to be highly sensitive.

Prevention

From a preventive standpoint, by using a very careful procedure, it is possible to desensitize some sufferers so that a sting will not be as dangerous as it might be otherwise. Also, there are certain definite recommendations to help avoid beestings.

For instance, bees are more likely to sting on bright, warm days, especially if interfered with while gathering honey. They are particularly likely to sting after a heavy rain, because they are unable to gather the nectar from flowers, which was washed away.

In addition, it is well known that all such stinging insects are attracted to brightly colored or dark, rough clothing, but, strangely enough, are not attracted to white clothing with a hard, smooth finish. Highly scented hair dressings, perfumes, and other cosmetics are also attractive to these insects; therefore, people who are sensitive to stings would do well to avoid using them.

Particular precaution should be taken with respect to young children who, if they have any allergic tendencies at all, may prove exceptionally vulnerable to beestings.

Never, under any circumstances, treat a beesting lightly, particularly if the individual has been stung on previous occasions. Promptly treat the sting locally and then watch the victim very carefully for the development for any further symptoms. If he appears to be experiencing the least generalized distress, get him to a doctor immediately.

Black Widow Spiders (Latrodectus mactans). Bites by these spiders are generally quite serious, but are not, as many people suppose, necessarily fatal. The black widow spider is about ¾ inch across and is easily identified by the hour-glass-shaped red spot on its belly (Fig. 11-3). It is found in many areas of the United States, usually around old wooden buildings and in dark places.

Signs and Symptoms. The symptoms caused by a black widow spider bite are severe abdominal pain due to muscle spasm (without nausea or vomiting), a partial state of collapse,

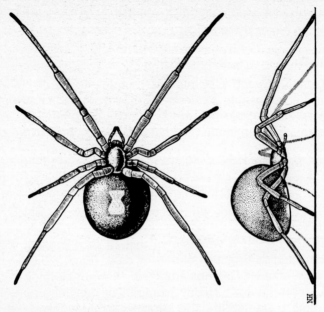

Fig. 11-3. The red hourglass marking on the underside of the round abdomen of the female black widow spider is characteristic.

dilated pupils, generalized swelling of the face and extremities, and, at times, convulsions.

○ TREATMENT

The recommended procedure has been to make a crisscross incision over the bite and suck out the poison (as for snake bites). If done very soon after the bite occurs, a constricting band may be applied just above the bite, tight, *but not so tight as to constrict the arterial blood supply*. It is questionable, however, how much good these procedures really do. The amount of venom injected by the spider is small and rapidly diffuses into the tissues. It is probably better to cleanse the bite area thoroughly and wash with hydrogen peroxide, alcohol, or other antiseptic, as these spiders are very dirty and the wound may easily become infected. The bite site is not as likely to necrose as in the case of tarantula or brown recluse spider bites. From the standpoint of emergency care, not much more can be done except to get the victim quickly to the nearest hospital.

An antivenin is available and should be given as soon as possible, in order to limit the development of further toxic symptoms. The intravenous injection of calcium lactate or calcium gluconate is helpful in relaxing the severe muscle spasm.

Brown Recluse Spiders (Loxosceles reclusa). The brown recluse spider, a member of the *Scytodidae* family, is at least as poisonous as the black widow spider. Berger feels, however, that many less serious bites which cause no major symptoms go unreported. Although many spiders are poisonous, the bites of the black widow and the brown recluse are to be feared the most within the continental United States.

Brownish in color and with a somewhat flattened body which averages ½ to ⅝ of an inch in size, both sexes of the brown recluse spider bear a dark-brown somewhat hourglass-shaped or, as generally described, violin- or "fiddle"-shaped marking on the under side of the cephalothorax; characteristically, the legs are disproportionately long in relation to the size of the body (Fig. 11-4).

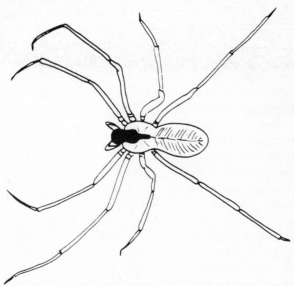

Fig. 11-4. Brown recluse spider, showing typical marking on cephalothorax. (Reproduced, with permission, from Hershey, F. B. and C. E. Aulenbacher: Surgical Treatment of Brown Spider Bites, *Ann. Surg. 170:*300–308 (August, 1969.)

Bites from this spider, though perhaps less frequent than those of the black widow spider, possibly because it is not so readily encountered, are undoubtedly becoming more common.

The species is prevalent in the southern states from Texas to Florida and ranges into Georgia, Indiana, Illinois, Missouri, and Kansas. It can be controlled by spraying or dusting with lindane or chlordane, or a combination of the two, in places likely to harbor these insects.

L. reclusa weaves a large, irregular web, and for the most part lives under stones, the bark of trees, underneath woodpiles and cement building blocks, and in other dark hiding places such as caves. It may also be found indoors in such areas as cellars and closets, and bites have occurred while donning infrequently used clothing. Bites of sleepers by spiders trapped in the sheets or blankets have also been reported with fair frequency.

Because these spiders readily find their way into clothing and trunks or other storage units, they may be inadvertently transported anywhere in the country—or the world for that matter. They live a long time and can survive a wide range of temperatures, so that for practical purposes their geographical distribution is not limited.

Symptoms. When the brown recluse spider bites, it injects a poison which, like that of the black widow spider, is a neurotoxin, but is also both hemolytic and necrotizing; it is said to be nine times more powerful than that of rattlesnake venom and produces a severe local reaction, which in many cases results in extensive tissue necrosis as well as systemic symptoms. Children react more severely than adults, and the most deaths occur in the younger age groups.

According to Fardon et al. and Hershey and Aulenbacher, who have studied the treatment of recluse spider bites extensively, there may be a mild stinging sensation at the time of the bite, or the bite may initially go unnoticed. In 6 to 8 hours, however, major symptoms begin to develop, preceded in some cases by moderate itching. At first, the bitten area becomes inflamed, quite tender, and a blister appears in its center.

In the severer cases, 12 to 24 hours later, constitutional symptoms develop with high fever, chills, grippe-like sensations, and often nausea and vomiting. In some cases a measles-like rash breaks out over the entire body about 36 hours later. After approximately 2 days, the skin around the bite begins to turn white (due to impaired blood supply); necrosis then sets in and may not reach its full extent for up to a week. At this time local pain is so severe that even narcotics may prove ineffective.

O TREATMENT

Altough bites from this spider are relatively infrequent, they are, nevertheless, dangerous. Lacking a specific antivenin, treatment must be directed along general lines. Local treatment is similar to that for black widow spider bites. The severe pain and apprehension require the use of analgesics and sedative drugs, although in severe cases these may be relatively ineffective. Shock may occur and require specific antishock therapy. Medical attention should be sought promptly.

Many physicians employ large doses of corticosteroids, antihistamines, and antibiotics in an attempt to counteract the severe reaction to the spider's poison, although experimental studies suggest that these may have only a minimal effect. They should, nevertheless, be tried. It has also been suggested that phentolamine (Regitine®) may be helpful in minimizing necrosis, since this preparation has proved useful for preventing or counteracting sloughs caused by the intravenous administration of norepinephrine.

Medication, however, often fails to prevent extensive local necrosis and gangrene. It is now accepted, therefore, that prompt deep excision of the necrotic area, with subsequent plastic restoration, is the treatment of choice in severe cases and almost immediately relieves the intractable local pain.

Tarantulas (Lycosa raptoria). Tarantula bites are generally similar in their effects to those of the black widow spider, the greatest danger arising when young children are bitten.

O TREATMENT

The treatment can only consist of measures to relieve whatever symptoms appear, as no specific antivenin is available. The wound of a tarantula bite is very liable to undergo necrosis and therefore requires careful attention over a considerable period of time. Tarantulas of this country seldom cause death, but those of the South American variety can be highly venomous.

Scorpions.   Scorpion stings, although quite properly greatly feared, are usually not very serious, except for the stings of breeds in certain parts of the United States, the tropics, northern Africa, Brazil, and certain other parts of the world.   There are a great number of varieties of scorpions, and the sting of many can be deadly.

The wound is inflicted by a stinger that is carried at the end of a fairly long tail.   While the victim may be made painfully ill, stings from the scorpions of our South and Southwest are not necessarily fatal, but the stings from African and Asiatic scorpions may be.   Children are much more susceptible to the toxin than adults.

Signs and Symptoms.   The venom of scorpions has a very strong affinity for the tissues of the sympathetic nervous system, a fact which explains the nature and severity of most of the symptoms.   There is a burning sensation at the site of the bite, followed by pain that spreads to the entire limb.   General symptoms appear within about an hour and include headache, dizziness, nausea, vomiting, and increased saliva formation. In severe cases, the victim goes into shock, then becomes greatly excited, and finally lapses into coma.

Gueron and Yaron have reported clear-cut cardiovascular effects, including changes in the electrocardiogram simulating early myocardial infarction.   In these cases, there was usually marked hypertension upon admission to the hospital, but in some cases the blood pressure was so low as to approach shock levels.

○ TREATMENT

Place the victim under the care of a physician or hospital as quickly as possible.   Antivenin against the more poisonous varieties is now available in areas of the world where scorpions are prevalent.   Considering the usual time lapse between the sting and the availability of treatment and the slow diffusion of the antivenin into the nerve tissue, large doses (20 to 30 milliliters, or cubic centimeters) are required to be effective. When administered early, however, the antivenin dramatically lowers mortality.

Masco has reported prompt symptomatic relief from the use of chlorpromazine, which is most effective when given intravenously or intramuscularly. In a small group chlorpromazine appeared to be more effective than the barbiturates of cases in providing relief from symptoms.

Bites by Mites

Chiggers. Several varieties of tiny insects of the *Eutrombicula* species of mites, generally called "chiggers" in the North and "red bugs" in the South, are found practically everywhere in the United States.

Bites by these insects cause intense itching and small, reddish welts on the skin. These symptoms may be your only warning that you have been in an infested area, because chiggers are so small that most persons cannot see them without a magnifying glass.

Adult chiggers pass the winter in protected places and become active in the spring. A few days after the females become active, they lay eggs which hatch into the first generation of the year.

The larval form of the young chigger is the troublemaker; it is a parasite—feeding on both man and animals. The larva transforms to a nymph, and the nymph to an adult. Neither the nymph nor the adult is a parasite.

Chiggers raised experimentally complete the life cycle— from egg to egg—in about 50 days.

In southern Florida and southern Texas, chiggers may be present throughout the year. In other states, the chigger season begins in May, June, or July, and lasts until September or the first frost.

In the larval stage chiggers are orange yellow or light red, with hairy bodies; they are less than 1/150 inch in diameter. A larva has three pairs of legs. Its mouth parts include two pairs of grasping palps, which are provided with forked claws.

The nymphs and adults have four pairs of legs. The bodies are hairy, about 1/20 inch long, and usually a brilliant red.

The young chiggers attach themselves to the skin of people, animals (including reptiles), poultry and other birds, and, before settling down to feed, scurry around for a choice location. The preferred areas on humans are those parts of the body where clothing fits tightly over the skin, or where the flesh is thin, tender, or wrinkled.

Like ticks, they attach themselves by inserting their mouth parts into the skin—frequently in hair follicles or pores—and inject a fluid which dissolves the tissues. The chiggers then suck up the liquefied material. When they attach themselves to animals, they become engorged in about 4 days. Then they drop off and change to nymphs. Nymphs and the adults feed on insect eggs, small insects, and organisms found on or near woody decaying material.

Chiggers are not known to transmit any disease in this country. In some parts of the world, particularly in parts of the Far East, they transmit scrub typhus, a serious disease similar to spotted fever.

Chiggers are most often found in low, damp places where vegetation is rank—for example, berry patches, orchards, woodlands, and margins of lakes or streams. But some species are adapted to living in drier places where vegetation is low, and heavy infestations may be found in lawns, golf courses, and parks.

It is not possible, simply by looking at a place, to tell whether it is infested. One trick for finding out is to stand a piece of black cardboard edgewise on the ground. If chiggers are around, they will congregate along the top edge in a short time. Chiggers may be numerous in a place one year and scarce or absent another year; and they occur in some places only for short periods.

Symptoms. The fluid which chiggers inject into the skin is highly irritating and causes reddish welts. It also causes swelling, itching, and (in some persons) fever. Chigger bites have a more severe effect on some persons, who are very sensitive, than on others.

A chigger attached in a pore or a hair follicle may be so enveloped in swollen skin that it appears to be burrowing into the skin. This fact sometimes leads to the mistaken belief that chiggers embed themselves in the skin or that welts contain chiggers.

The symptoms develop within 24 hours after the attack, sooner in those who are very sensitive. Itching is intense and, if nothing is done to relieve it, may continue a week or longer. Scratching a bite may break the skin and result in infection.

Chiggers attacking in large numbers can cause systemic illness and, in some areas, may do serious harm to domestic poultry flocks.

○ TREATMENT

Attack is almost certain if infested areas are entered without repellent protection. You may not know that you have been attacked until welts appear on the body and itching begins.

Take a very hot bath as soon as possible. Apply a thick lather, then rinse it off. Do this several times. The bath kills most, or all, of the attached chiggers, and any others that may not yet be attached.

Next, apply a dab of antiseptic to each of the welts. This will kill any chiggers not killed by the bath, and aids in preventing infection. Concentrated isopropyl alcohol (rubbing alcohol, but 90 percent isopropanol) is effective in relieving itching, as well as killing the red bugs. Ordinary rubbing alcohol, obtainable almost anywhere, usually is a dilute solution of isopropanol and may be used when pure isopropanol is not available.

Destroying the chiggers reduces the itching but does not stop it, since the fluid injected by the chiggers causes the itching. No practicable way to remove the injected fluid has been found, and no treatment is known that will give permanent relief from the itching.

Temporary relief may be obtained by using a good local anesthetic cream such as dibucaine hydrochloride (Nupercaine®) or lidocaine (Xylocaine®), and these can be reapplied as needed. Corticosteroid creams, such as triancinalone (Aristocort® or Kenalog®), are also helpful in reducing the intense inflammatory response in the skin and thus aid in relieving itching. Severe constitutional symptoms in very sensitive people require treatment by a physician.

Prophylaxis. The only protection against chigger (red bug) attack is the copious use of effective repellents applied to exposed skin areas and to the clothing as well—especially around collars, waistbands, pant cuffs, and socks.

Many repellent preparations are sold under various trade names. Read the labels carefully and search out those which contain diethyltoluamide, dimethyl phthalate, dimethyl carbate, or ethyl hexanediol, or combinations of these ingredients.

Some preparations are available in convenient aerosol form but, whatever type is used, be sure to follow label directions exactly.

Scabies. This disease results from invasion of the skin by a tiny accarine mite known as the itch mite, or *Sarcoptes scabei*.

Symptoms. Almost intolerable itching, which is often worse at night, occurs in areas where the female burrows under the superficial layers of skin to lay her eggs, where they hatch. Her burrowing raises tiny linear elevations on the skin, with a small blister at the point of entrance. The ridges of skin which form the roofs of the burrows may be up to half an inch long, usually less. The burrows contain the eggs laid by the female mite and her feces. She dies after depositing from 20 to 25 eggs. The young hatch and form new burrows as they move toward the surface of the skin; they attain adulthood in about 2 weeks, at which time mating occurs. The males then die; the females start making new burrows to lay their eggs.

Since the entire process takes place in the skin, infestation can continue indefinitely unless interrupted by treatment. Infestation occurs only by direct contact with a scabious human—rarely with a family pet. Pets have their own types of mites which usually don't infest humans; however, pets, as well as other members of the family, become infested by direct contact with the already infested human victim.

Most commonly involved body areas are the spaces between fingers and toes, the forearms and wrists, the armpits, the navel, and the genitals and buttocks. The itching may not begin for 2 weeks or more after infestation; this may be followed in 4 to 6 weeks by a rash, which is probably the result of sensitization.

Scratching often leads to secondary inflammation with a deep skin infection, so that in untreated cases the lesions may become very extensive and resemble impetigo or eczema. The diagnosis is made by demonstrating under the low-power microscope the presence of the infesting mite. Superficially, the disease may simulate many other dermatologic conditions.

○ TREATMENT

This should be under the direction of a dermatologist, and is aimed at the relief of the severe itching and killing of the mites through the use of scabicidal agents such as sulfur, benzyl benzoate emulsion, or gamma benzene hexachloride cream sold under the name Kwell®.

The usual routine is to scrub thoroughly in a very hot bath, using an antiseptic soap, and then apply the scabicide over the entire body. The process is repeated in 24 hours, and then again 4 and 8 days later.

Everyone in the family must also undergo the same routine, and all clothing should be thoroughly laundered in very hot (140°F.+) water to kill any surviving mites. Throughout the period of treatment, only thoroughly laundered clothing which has been stored at least 4 days should be worn.

Since infestation occurs under crowded conditions and as the result of poor personal hygiene, prevention is directed toward personal cleanliness, generally improved hygiene, and the avoidance of physical contact with individuals, or their clothing, who might be harboring the mites. Scabies appears to be on the increase due to a number of factors involving population movement and poor housing among others.

Insects Poisonous by Contact

There are many insects which, in various stages, are poisonous simply by coming in contact with them.

Caterpillars. There are a number of species of caterpillars throughout the world whose fine, bristly hairs are like so many hypodermic needles, each one loaded with an irritating poison. When this is injected into the skin as a result of even the gentlest contact, a rather violent inflammatory reaction or dermatitis results, and in some cases a true allegic reaction may ensue.

In addition, some of the delicate hairs very easily come loose from the caterpillar and can then be blown about by the wind. This creates a real menace, since the tiny hairs can easily be lodged in the eyes, producing a severe conjunctivitis, or get into the upper respiratory tract where they can cause irritation, inflammation and pain, or a distinct allergy.

The worst and most common offender in the United States, particularly in southern areas, is the puss caterpillar. Sometimes these caterpillars appear in enormous numbers. Circumstances have been reported in which they were so numerous that schools had to be closed, with a severe dermatitis appearing in the affected areas in truly epidemic proportions.

Symptoms occur shortly after contact with the caterpillar, beginning with intense burning pain which is followed by severe itching. Red blotches quickly appear, which soon develop into a red wheal-like rash. When there are only a few, the lesions remain separate, but in severe exposure they all run together, creating large inflamed patches which itch almost unbearably. The rash may last anywhere from a few hours to several days, depending upon the degree of exposure and the sensitivity of the individual.

The poison which these caterpillars inject is extremely powerful, so that when the exposure has been heavy, distressing systemic effects develop. Major symptoms include nausea, vomiting, high fever, and numbness and swelling of the particular area or part attacked. In severe cases, particularly if the stings have been around the neck or head, actual temporary paralysis is possible.

Moths. In a similar way, the hairs of the brown tail moth can produce a severe skin reaction, but in these cases there are rarely any systemic symptoms. The rash is typically made up of little vesicles or blisters, and is known colloquially as "brown tail rash."

Both of these scourges can be controlled to some extent by using suitable sprays to eliminate the caterpillars from the trees and shrubbery which they inhabit and to wash very carefully all clothing and bedding where the hairs might have been shed or blown.

Miscellaneous Insects. There are several kinds of bugs that can cause blisters even though they hardly touch you. For instance, there are about 200 species of insects, many of which are widely distributed throughout the United States, known as blister beetles. These are particularly common throughout the southeast and western United States; the most common one (a member of the genus Epicauta) is ½ to 1 inch in length with a soft body and long legs, so that he is able to hop about with great agility.

These beetles contain a high concentration of an irritant substance, known as cantharidin, in all their body tissues. If one of these villainous creatures happens to walk across the skin of an unsuspecting victim, and he is not molested, probably nothing will happen. On the other hand, even the slightest pressure on the insect's body, such as merely brushing him away, causes a clear amber fluid to exude from many parts of the insect's body onto one's skin.   Tingling of the area develops in about 10 minutes, followed in 8 to 12 hours by blister formation.   If the beetle is actually crushed on the skin, a giant-size blister will form and there will be considerable surrounding irritation.

Often the victim is not even aware that he has been attacked until a series of blisters seems to appear spontaneously, much to everybody's surprise.

The blisters almost always occur on exposed parts of the body and are usually contracted at night, since the beetles are night-flying and are strongly attracted to light.   However, agricultural workers are very frequently attacked during the day, since the beetles favor common agricultural crops such as soy beans, clover, and potatoes.

Best prevention rests on good insect control in the area and keeping one's body unexposed.

Snakebite.   There are four major kinds of poisonous snakes in the United States: rattlesnakes (many varieties), moccasins, copperheads, and coral snakes.   The first three belong to the *pit vipers,* so called because of a small deep pit between nostril and eye on each side of the head.   (No *nonpoisonous* snake in this country that is large enough to bite has this characteristic.)   These species are distributed widely, but are found in far greater numbers in some localities than in others (Fig. 11-5).

The bite of the pit vipers leaves a distinctive type of mark, which is distinguishable from the bite of nonpoisonous snakes. This fact is important and means that a person bitten by a nonpoisonous variety of snake need not be subjected to the measures necessary in the case of a bite by a poisonous snake.

The bite of the pit vipers comes as a lightning-like strike, a small amount of the venom being injected from two fangs in the forward portion of the upper jaw; this leaves two distinctive puncture wounds at the points of entry.   In addition, there are two additional sets of teeth marks, made respectively by two rows of teeth extending backward from the two fangs in the upper jaw, and two corresponding rows in the lower jaw (Fig. 11-6A).   The bite of a nonpoisonous variety differs in that there are six rows of teeth marks—four rows made from the

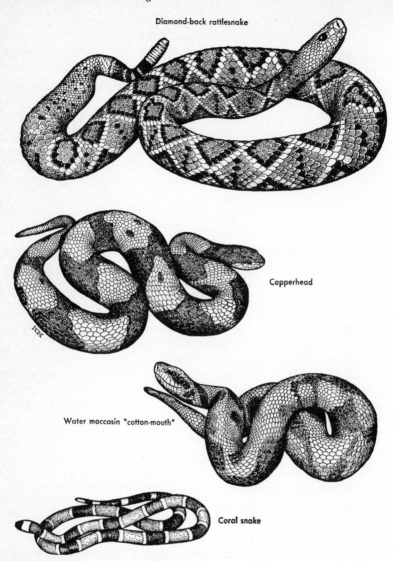

Diamond-back rattlesnake

Copperhead

Water moccasin "cotton-mouth"

Coral snake

Fig. 11-5.   Poisonous snakes found in the United States.

teeth of the upper jaw, and two from the teeth of the lower
jaw.   If the latter configuration is seen, it is certain that the
bite has *not* been inflicted by a poisonous variety, and only
minor attention to the wound need be given (Fig. 11-6*B*).

The small *coral snake*, which is marked with bands of red

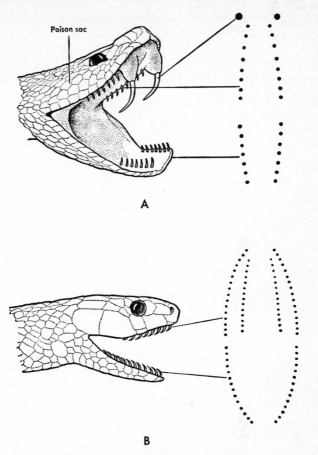

Poison sac

A

B

Fig. 11-6. Comparison of the characteristic distribution of fang and tooth marks from the bite of a poisonous snake of the pit viper family (A) and one of a nonpoisonous variety (B). (Modified from C. H. Pope and R. M. Perkins, *A.M.A. Arch. Surg. 49*:331, 1944.)

and black and with narrower bands of yellow, bites in an entirely different manner.   Coral snakes, which are *very* dangerous, attack human beings relatively rarely, but when they do, they bite and hang on, sinking their fangs with a chewing motion.   Its venom is exceedingly toxic and is similar to that of the cobra, since it acts as a nerve poison, while that of the pit vipers acts mainly as a blood and tissue poison.

Most snakebites occur on the legs; therefore, in areas where poisonous snakes are known to exist, the danger can be greatly minimized by wearing suitable boots.   In recent years, the incidence of snakebite in this country has been on the increase, however, because of the increase of all types of outdoor recreational activities.

Thus, the treatment of snakbite is of increasing importance, and has aroused much interest in the development of newer methods.   No treatment devised so far is completely successful; in some instances, death still occurs; at best some permanent disability may result, particularly in bites of the hand.

The venoms of different snakes produces their poisonous effects in different ways.   For instance, the cobra of India, the adder of Africa, and the coral snakes of this country inject powerful venoms which have a strong effect on nerve tissue but produce relatively little local tissue reaction.   On the other hand, rattlesnakes inject venoms which contain powerful enzymes and cause extensive local tissue destruction by actually digesting the tissues into which they are injected.   In addition, rattlesnake venom contains a hemorrhagic factor which has a destructive effect on the blood vessels themselves.

Signs and Symptoms.   Following a bite by any one of the *pit vipers,* there is immediate severe pain accompanied by swelling and dark-purplish discoloration of the skin.   The two puncture marks of the fangs are usually easily found but, occasionally, there is only one mark, as in the case of a bite on a finger or toe, where there is no room for both fangs to sink in.

The general symptoms consist of growing weakness, shortness of breath, increasing lassitude leading to unconsciousness, dimness of vision, rapid pulse, and nausea and vomiting.

The symptoms of *coral snake bite* are similar, with the addition of great drowsiness; the victim sinks into unconsciousness as if he were going to sleep.   Although the bite does not necessarily produce severe local pain or swelling, there may be considerable bruising, since the coral snake hangs on and chews, thus lacerating and bruising the tissues in the area of the bite.   The general symptoms set in very rapidly.

O TREATMENT

Although the victim of snakebite should be taken to a hospital as quickly as possible, certain emergency treatment cannot wait, since waiting may permit the poison to spread.   The long accepted method of treatment includes the following steps:

1 Immobilize the extremity and put a constricting band *just above* the bite and *just tight* enough to stop the flow of blood in the veins. Do *not* tighten the band enough to shut off the arterial blood supply—remember you are *not* applying a tourniquet. If you have a first-aid kit with you, use the triangular bandage for a constricting band; if not, use any article of clothing, such as a belt, necktie, stocking, or shirt.

2 When the constricting band is in place, make cross incisions a good ¼ inch deep over the fang marks, using a knife or razor blade that has been flamed, and proceed to suck out the venom, mixed with blood and lymph, which will flow from the wound (Fig. 11-7).

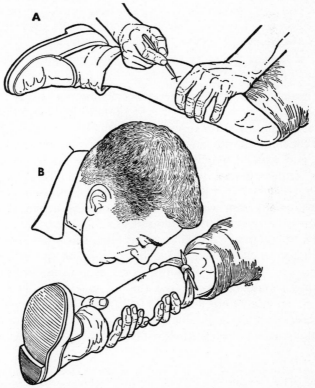

Fig. 11-7. After making deep cross-cut incisions in the bitten area, the poison is sucked directly from the wound by mouth if no suction device from a snakebite kit is available. The evacuated material is immediately expectorated.

3 If you are fortunate enough to have a snakebit kit (as you should have if you are in snake country) use the suction cup it contains for this purpose. If you have none, use your mouth—you will not get poisoned, except in the unlikely event that you have large open sores in your mouth.

4 As the swelling grows and spreads, continue to make similar cross incisions over the swollen area; perhaps as many as 30 or 40 may be required. Usually there will be no marked bleeding, only a flow of clear yellowish fluid and a little blood.

5 If you do happen to cut a small blood vessel, it is not a matter for concern; stop the bleeding with a little pressure and proceed with your task.

6 Keep the affected limb a little lower than the rest of the body, and loosen the constricting band if swelling tends to tighten it too much. Keep the body and the affected limb at complete rest in order to help slow absorption.

7 If swelling should get beyond the band, put another one just above it and remove the first.

Presumably, all this has happened in the country at some distance from medical aid. It is important, however, that as soon as possible you try to get to a hospital, where more adequate facilities for treatment and antivenin will be available.

If you were foresighted enough to have *polyvalent crotalidae antivenin* with you, inject up to about 50 milliliters (cubic centimeters) in the tissue around and above the bite. This will greatly improve the victim's chances of recovery.*

The victim should exert himself as little as possible. Do *not* give stimulants of any kind at this time, since they increase the circulation of the blood and hence the absorption of the venom. If the victim goes into shock, all possible antishock measures should be taken, but do *not* give alcohol in any form—even though it is alleged to be a "snakebite remedy."

Other Methods. On the basis of our knowledge of the toxicology of snake venoms, new methods are being evaluated

---

* Warning: Polyvalent crotalidae antivenin is prepared in horse serum, to which many people are very sensitive, especially if they have had an injection of horse serum at some prior time. If the victim of the snakebite is likely to be sensitive, an injection of a large amount of antivenin would more than likely produce severe anaphylactic shock. It would therefore be better to wait to give him antivenin until he can be gotten to a medical facility where he can be rapidly desensitized and the serum administered more safely.

for the treatment of snakebite which, on the basis of further experience, may prove significant in limiting both the mortality and the permanent disability. One which has attracted attention is so-called "cryotherapy," which simply means refrigeration of the part involved as quickly as possible after the bite has been inflicted. The theory is that this method will control the local enzymatic destruction of the tissues involved by limiting the activity of the injected enzymes, since enzymes do not act below certain critical temperatures. Freezing also has the additional effect of slowing down the circulation to the bitten part and thus slowing down the diffusion of the poison throughout the rest of the system.

Theoretically, cryotherapy should be more effective against rattlesnake venom than that from the cobra or coral snakes, but there is at least one report in the medical literature referring to a case of cobra bite which was successfully treated by this method. If for no other reason, refrigeration of the bitten part should be effective in slowing down the absorption of the venom and thus give more time for the antivenin, administered around the site of the bite and also intravenously or intramuscularly, to act.

Proponents of the method believe that all cases of snakebite, regardless of the type of snake involved, should be treated by cryotherapy as quickly as possible, but opponents of the method have pointed out that it may lead to unnecessary amputation and does not, in fact, minimize the effect of the venom in the long run.

In addition to the refrigeration treatment, the standard more conventional methods, including the administration of a specific antivenin and antibiotics, are, of course, used.

By the cryotherapy method when a bitten extremity is immersed in fresh water ice, the temperature of the tissues is dropped to about 59°F. This temperature is low enough to inactivate the enzymes of the venom but not cold enough actually to freeze the tissues. (Dangerous freezing of the tissues might result if salt water ice, which is much colder, were used.)

In other words, all the local physiologic processes are slowed, and at the same time tissue destruction, which would have occurred as the result of the action of the venom, is lessened. As a result, swelling of the part, which ordinarily would be severe, is said to be minimized, and the pain, once refrigeration has occurred, is greatly relieved.

Another advantage is said to be that when cryotherapy is employed early, or soon after the bite, there is no need to use a constricting band *except temporarily.* This is a particularly important consideration since every precaution must be carried out to make certain that adequate circulation is maintained in the affected extremity, and for that reason the refrigerated extremity must be continuously observed in order to be sure that it is not becoming too cold and that there is no damage resulting either to the circulation or to the skin itself. In addition, it is extremely important to keep the rest of the patient warm, which easily can be accomplished by the use of an electric blanket or other means.

If cryotherapy is to be employed as the method of choice under the circumstances which exist, the bitten area should be packed in plain-water ice as quickly as possible, a constricting band being applied between the bite and the rest of the body and left in place only until refrigeration of the part has been thoroughly established, and in no case for longer than 1 hour. While this is being done, the victim can be taken to a hospital. Specific antivenin can then be administered and incisions made into the bitten area, to help drain off the venom which has not already been absorbed.

Tetanus toxoid and suitable antibiotics are also administered, but strong analgesics are usually not required and, as a matter of fact, are avoided since it has been shown that they may increase the lethal effects of the venom.

When hospital facilities are readily accessible, it is better that these procedures be carried out in the hospital than attempted in the field by a layman.

One of several problems connected with cryotherapy is to know when the patient is really over his snakebite and the treatment can be discontinued. If refrigeration is discontinued too soon, all the usual symptoms flare up, the venom again becomes active and disseminates through the body, and the patient is in jeopardy. Present practice generally is to keep the patient in the hospital for at least 6 days under refrigeration. This allows sufficient time for the body, helped by the use of antivenin, to build up its natural defenses and to render the venom itself harmless.

The method undoubtedly requires further study since, although it may have advantages, it also has its hazards and limitations, and as yet it cannot be accepted without reservation. Its proponents and advocates are equally vociferous, and only time will give the final answer.

At the present time, however, as Sparger concludes, the cryotherapy method can be dangerous and has apparently resulted in a number of amputations which might not otherwise have occurred. Aside from temporary dry local cooling (with an ice bag) at the site of the bite to relieve pain, cryotherapy is *not* now recommended. For general use, the time-honored method of incision and suction, with the administration of antivenin, is considered the method of choice.

In spite of the modern improvements in the treatment of snakebite, there is still a need for wider availability of more potent specific antivenins which can be administered safely in larger doses than at present. An important aspect of the problem is that snake antivenins are prepared from the serum of horses, to which many individuals are highly sensitive, and the careless administration of antivenin without proper testing can result in reactions which may be even more dangerous than the snakebite itself.

The possibility of developing antivenins of human origin, utilizing the blood from volunteer donors who have been previously bitten and who have received booster shots of small doses of snake venom to stimulate the production of powerful antibodies in their blood, may well prove to be the answer to this important and vexing problem.

Stings of Marine Animals

A number of marine animals of various species may inflict very painful wounds but, except under rare circumstances, these are not fatal.

Stingrays (Whip Rays). There are many varieties of whip rays, some more poisonous than others, but all have in common a long whiplike tail that may inflict a very painful lash, and serious poisoning may result from the stinger, which is located near the *base* of the tail and usually breaks off in the wound. These fish rarely deliberately attack a human being unless molested, but the sting is inflicted when a stingray is inadvertently stepped on, for instance when a person is walking barefoot through warm, sunny shallows or along the undertow at the break of the beach, where this species is fond of basking in the sun (Fig. 11-8). The weight of a swimmer stepping on the ray gives the necessary leverage to elevate and cause penetration of the barb. Shuffling, rather than walking, scares the rays away and usually avoids trouble. These fish must be differentiated from the common skate, which is not to be feared, since the appendages down near the base of the tail are merely the reproductive organs and are in no way harmful.

Signs and Symptoms. The stingray produces a lacerated puncture type wound and a very painful swelling of the leg, which becomes black and blue and may result in blood poisoning. Most of the wounds occur below the knee, but in relatively rare instances may be inflicted elsewhere on the body. Because of the jagged retrorse (backward-bending) barbs on the stinging spines, deep ragged lacerations, which bleed profusely, are often inflicted rather than a simple puncture. Part of the spine may break off in the wound and require removal. Swelling of the tissues around the wound may be severe. The symptoms produced are caused both by the

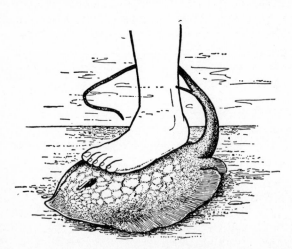

Fig. 11-8. The sting of a whip ray is inflicted when it is inadvertently stepped on. When wading where the presence of these fish may be anticipated, injury may be avoided by shuffling through the sand rather than lifting the feet, as in walking. The vibrations thus set up warn the ray off.

venom injected and the mechanical nature of the injury itself. Generalized symptoms of prostration and blood poisoning may develop and require special medical care.

○ TREATMENT

The more rapidly treatment is effected, the better will be the results, and it should be initiated by the victim himself without waiting for assistance. The basic steps are as follows:

1 Irrigate the wound immediately and profusely with the salt water at hand. This helps to wash out the poison and to prevent its spread by constricting the blood vessels.

2 Apply a constricting band as for snakebite, above the wound, as soon as possible.

3 Remove any remains of the stinger still visible in the wound, and suck out the wound, making a small incision if necessary to do so, to remove as much of the venom as possible.

4 Then immerse the leg in water as *hot* as can be borne without injury for 30 to 60 minutes. This helps to further destroy the toxin. Sometimes a minor surgical operation, which should be done as soon as possible, is required to remove all of the barb and avoid further distress.

The wound should then be further cleansed and sutured by a physician, who can also administer such additional therapy, including antibiotics and sedatives, as may be indicated by the circumstances. No specific antivenin is available. Fortunately, the outcome usually is not as serious as the bite of a poisonous snake, but in severe stings generalized symptoms resembling shock may be present.

Saltwater Catfish. These fish carry a venomous stinger at the base of the large dorsal fin, which is capable of inflicting a potentially serious wound similar in its effects to that made by the stingray. Usually the wound is incurred on the hand when an inexperienced person attempts to remove one of these fish from a fishing hook. (There is a way of doing this quite safely, but if you are an amateur you had better get an old-timer to show you how, and practice first on a dead fish.) The barb of the stinger is cartilaginous and is strong enough to penetrate shoe leather—with painful results. This has happened when the fish has been kicked to remove it from a dock.

Scorpion fish, toad fish, and star-gazers also carry venomous spines and inflict even more serious wounds; fatalities have occurred.

○ TREATMENT

Stings from the above-mentioned fish should be treated as outlined for the treatment of a stingray wound (see above). This may seem a little extreme, but experience has proved that it saves trouble and a great deal of pain and disability in the long run.

Jelly Fish.   Jelly fish, particularly the Portuguese men-of-war (*Physalia physalis*), can inflict painful stings with their long tentacles, which may make the victim feel quite ill.   In southern waters, they seem to be even more potent.   These stings are usually incurred on the legs.   An even more dangerous jelly fish is the sea wasp (*Chiropsalmus quadrigatus*), found in the seas around northern Australia, the Philippines, and in the Indian Ocean.   A closely related but somewhat less dangerous species also occurs in the waters mentioned, as well as in the Atlantic Ocean from Brazil to North Carolina.

○ TREATMENT

Treatment consists of first flushing the stung areas with seawater and then soaking the affected part with dilute ammonia water, followed by hot Epsom salt soaks, which will give relief from pain.   The leg should be kept slightly elevated.   If the glands in the groin swell and become painful, an ice bag should be applied for about 20 minutes of each hour.

It has been suggested that the toxin may be deactivated by applying an organic solvent such as mineral spirits, kerosene, or gasoline, provided any of these is immediately available. Such treatment, however, is not effective unless applied promptly, before the toxin enters the bloodstream.   Of particular note is that Adolph's meat tenderizer, sprinkled lightly over the afflicted areas, often provides effective relief.

In some severe cases, circulatory absorption may lead to very severe pain, shock, respiratory failure, and cardiac arrest, depending upon the organism and the amount of venom absorbed.   Treatment must be directed toward preventing and combating these contingencies.   The victim should be taken to a hospital as quickly as possible.   Morphine or other anal-

gestic, such as meperidine hydrochloride (Demerol®) or propoxyphene hydrochloride (Darvon®), may be required to control pain, as well as heroic supportive measures to combat
shock and anaphylaxis and tide him through a very critical
period.

Swimmer's Itch

Swimmer's itch is a widespread, sometimes painful annoyance caused by tiny, worm-like creatures known as cercariae,
which represent an intermediate free-swimming stage in the
life cycle of a huge group of small trematode worms known as
schistosomes.   A few species employ man as the definitive host
and, in so doing, produce a serious systemic disease known as
schistosomiasis.   This condition is common in Egypt, the Far
East, tropical Africa, Central America, and in certain portions
of the United States.

The vast majority of schistosomes cannot utilize man as a
definitive host.   Some, however, such as those which give rise
to swimmer's itch, can cause moderate distress in humans,
since their cercariae can penetrate the skin a short distance and
cause irritation and itching.

It has been noted that these tiny worms are definitely attracted by light and are present in greatest concentration near
the surface in warm, sunny shallows frequented by snails, the
obligatory intermediate host.   Hence, children playing near
shore or fishermen wading in the shallows are most likely to be
attacked, while those who swim in deeper water are less subject to exposure.

The cercariae can penetrate the skin while the exposed
parts are still in the water, but penetration seems for the most
part to take place as the skin dries by evaporation after leaving
the water.   For this reason, immediate drying with a towel
minimizes or eradicates the opportunity for the cercariae to
penetrate the skin and cause trouble.

Almost immediately following penetration, there is an intense itching or prickling sensation which may last for an hour
or more while the cercariae are boring into the skin.   Soon
afterward, a fiery red dimple-like eruption develops and the
whole area may become reddened and swollen.   In very sensitive individuals, almost a hive-like eruption ensues.

After a little time, this first eruption may diminish, but from

10 to 15 hours later it again appears and the itching becomes extremely intense. Small water blisters form, which later on become filled with pus. After about a week, the worst of the eruption subsides but often leaves in its place small pigmented spots which persist for some time. In sensitive individuals, or where the exposure has been extremely heavy, the amount of inflammation and irritation may be severe and the individual may actually be quite ill.

While the first attack may be quite mild, repeated attacks may cause a severe reaction and even general bodily urticaria, simply as the result of allergy to the invading cercariae.

Prevention

As a defensive measure, in addition to immediate drying of the skin, the use of protective coats of oil or grease may be helpful but, unless the preparation used is heavily applied and is tenacious, it does little good. Suitable clothing is almost certain protection and can easily be utilized by fishermen but is hardly practical for anyone wanting to do serious swimming.

In most localities the cercariae tend to emerge from the snails in greatest numbers in the morning, so that during the early part of the day there is liable to be a much higher concentration in the water than later on. Also, it is unfortunately true that during the hottest weather and reaching a peak in July, just when people most want to swim, more cercariae are present in the water than during cooler weather.

The chances of avoiding an annoying attack of swimmer's itch are better if you swim during the latter part of the day in deep water and dry yourself thoroughly as soon as emerging.

A similar condition may occur in salt water and is known as sea bather's eruption. But, unlike swimmer's itch, this condition is more likely to occur in body areas covered by the bathing suit than in the exposed parts. The lesions themselves closely resemble insect bites, and the itching is severe. The condition is almost entirely limited to the Atlantic and Gulf coasts of Florida and seems to occur only between March and September.

○ TREATMENT

The treatment of both swimmer's itch and sea bathers' eruption is purely symptomatic, and anything that will relieve the itching is the best thing to use.   In severe cases, doctors can prescribe cortisone-like drugs and antihistamines by mouth and these are of considerable value in relieving the severe itching. Ointments containing one of the more powerful corticosteroids, such as triamcinolone, are of great help in relieving the inflammatory reaction and itching.

POISONING BY CONTACT WITH VENOMOUS PLANTS

A number of plants cause a marked reaction on contact with the human skin and may produce severe general symptoms if eaten.   The most common of these are *poison ivy, poison sumac,* and *poison oak* (Fig. 11-9).

Signs and Symptoms.   The symptoms produced in sus-

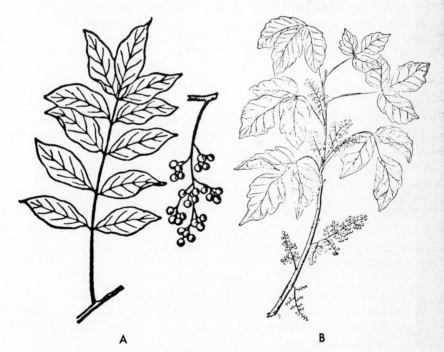

A   **B**

Fig. 11-9.   Poison sumac (A) and poison ivy (B) cause extreme irritation of the skin in sensitive individuals by direct contact with the leaves, stems, or smoke of burning plants. The appearance of poison oak, which is more common in the western sections of the United States than in the East, is superficially indistinguishable from that of poison ivy.

ceptible individuals by the irritant oils of these plants are similar for all three plants.   There is a diffuse reddening of the skin, with blister formation that itches intensely and is easily spread to other portion of the body by fingers or clothing.

In severe cases in which large areas are affected, the victim may be quite ill, with generalized swelling of the tissues and other signs of allergic reaction.

○ TREATMENT

It is poor practice to use oily ointments or alcoholic solutions of various substances to treat the condition; these only serve to spread the irritation, since the irritant is soluble in both fats and alcohol.

Although there is no specific treatment, the antihistamines help in relieving the itching; various corticosteroids, such as cortisone, hydrocortisone, or triamcinolone, taken by mouth, have been found to give considerable relief in more serious cases.   In addition, ointments containing an antihistamine or corticosteroid provide relief and suppress the inflammatory skin reaction.   *These drugs must be used under a doctor's direction,* and severe cases should have proper medical attention in any event.

Attempts at immunization against poisoning by these plants have met with slight success.   Various preparations are marketed, to be taken either by mouth or by injection, with the intent to build up an immunity against poison ivy and related plants; while these may be of some value in diminishing sensitivity in certain cases, there is no clear evidence of their producing real immunity.

Other plants that may produce similar reactions in sensitive individuals include the *buttercup, crowfoot, primrose, rue,* and *arnica* (Fig. 11-10).

In addition, there are a number of common plants which may be highly poisonous and are often used for foundation planting and for decoration about the home, or may grow wild in the woods and fields about a house.   Since some of them have attractive-looking berries, they are not infrequently eaten by children or by unwary adults.   Many other plants may contain poisonous compounds known as alkaloids which, although very toxic, in proper dosage have useful medicinal properties.

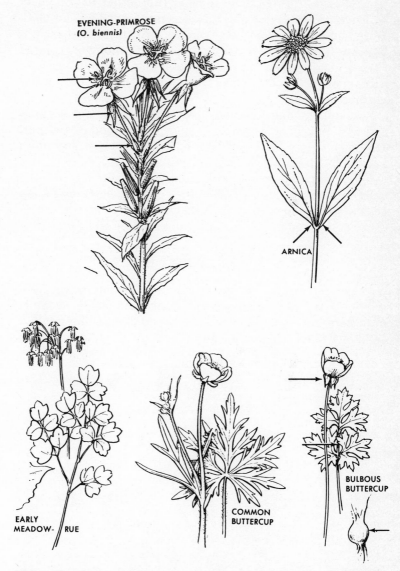

Fig. 11-10. Common field plants that may cause poisoning if eaten by children or unwary adults. (From Peterson and McKenny, "A Field Guide to Wildflowers," Houghton Mifflin.)

Poison parsley (Fig. 11-11) is a dangerous masquerader, for its leaves may be mistaken for ordinary parsley, its roots for parsnips, and the seeds for anise. The berries of the privet hedge or of ivy may be poisonous, as may be the bark of black locust trees or of elderberry bushes. As a practical matter, however, children are much more likely to eat brightly colored berries than to chew on bark, unless, as is common, they are sucking on a stick which may happen to be from some poisonous tree or shrub.

Other common poisonous plants include the *death camas* and false *hellebore*, poppies, western monkshood, rosary pea, blue nightshade, black nightshade, black henbane, and thorn apple (Fig. 11-12).

The symptoms of poisoning from these plants vary with the nature of the poisonous alkaloid they contain, but the signs are usually so acute and so obvious that it is evident that poisoning has occurred and proper medical steps must be taken promptly.

POISONING BY TOXIC FOODS

A number of relatively rare types of poisoning occur from foods which under ordinary circumstances are edible, in whole or in part, but which have been rendered toxic as the result of certain natural circumstances. Such illnesses include, for

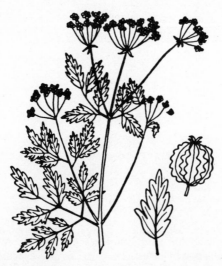

Fig. 11-11. Poison parsley.

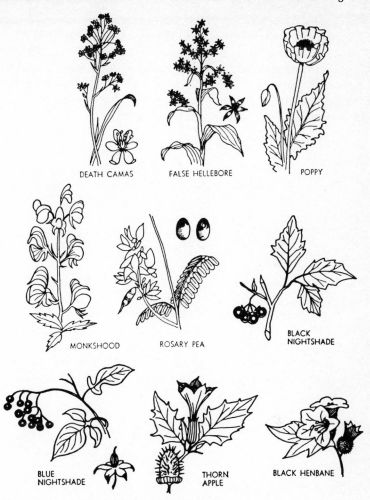

Fig. 11-12. Common plants that may be found in the fields or around the home and which may cause poisoning if eaten.

example, oxalic acid poisoning from eating quantities of the leaves of the rhubarb plant; ergot poisoning from eating bread made from rye grain contaminated with the plant disease known as *smut;* milk poisoning from drinking the milk of cattle that have fed on the poisonous weed *white snake root;* and potato poisoning from eating sprouted potatoes, which, under some circumstances, contain a toxic substance known as *solanine.*   These conditions are of little importance from the standpoint of emergency care, but acute illness caused by ingesting nonedible varieties of mushroom is fairly common.

It should be mentioned also that certain fish, while perfectly edible in one area, may be poisonous in another. Local regulations and customs should be followed as protection against this possibly dangerous condition, known technically as *ichthyotoxism* (see page 372 and following).

Mushroom Poisoning.   Large quantities of mushrooms are consumed in this country annually, and it is only natural that occasionally a poisonous variety will be picked by amateur naturalists who find them growing in woodland glades.   There is no sure trick, such as turning a silver spoon black or the way the skin peels off, by which poisonous varieties can be identified.   It is safest to obtain mushrooms from commercial sources, which are carefully safeguarded.

There are several poisonous varieties of mushroom-like fungi, but those that most often cause illness are the two species: *Amanita phalloides* and *Amanita muscaria*.

The *Amanita phalloides* contains a toxin that liquefies tissue cells all over the body, especially the red blood cells, and causes death in more than half the cases.   This fungus is found by the roadside in woody areas during the late summer and early fall.   It is from 4 to 6 inches tall and its cap is about 4 inches in diameter (Fig. 11-13).

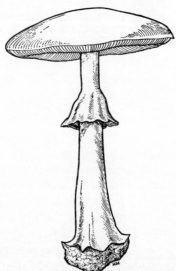

Fig. 11-13. The poisonous mushroom Amanita phalloides. It is considerably larger than the edible Agaricus campestris, as well as having other distinguishing characteristics.

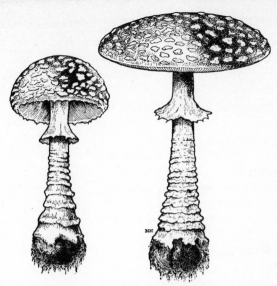

Fig. 11-14. Amanita muscaria is also poisonous but is easily distinguished from the edible variety by its larger size and general appearance.

Signs and Symptoms. Symptoms begin several hours after eating this species of mushroom and are characterized by acute abdominal pain, diarrhea, and vomiting. The attacks come in bouts with intervening periods of remission. After about 24 hours or longer, the victim may go into shock, have convulsions, and become comatose. According to Lampe, the only specific treatment known is acute hemodialysis. Death may occur after several days and may be due to serious damage to the liver and kidneys.

The *Amanita muscaria* contains the toxic drug *muscarine* which has a strong action on certain parts of the nervous system. This plant is dangerous, but it causes death less frequently than the *Amanita phalloides*. It grows by itself in sandy soil, often among scrub pine, and is fairly large (Fig. 11-14).

Signs and Symptoms. Symptoms come on in a few hours; they are characterized by violent vomiting, diarrhea, a flow of tears, excessive secretion of saliva, and profuse sweating. The victim may find it difficult to breathe, the pulse is slow, and there may be hallucinations. The pupils of the eyes are contracted. If the outcome is fatal, it is because of respiratory paralysis, which occurs in about 2 days.

○ TREATMENT

Mushroom poisoning constitutes a severe medical emergency. Until medical help can be obtained, first-aid steps include absolute bed rest, emptying the stomach by use of an emetic— if the victim is not already vomiting—and treating for shock if the signs show that this condition is imminent.

If poisoning is due to *Amanita muscaria* and if no doctor is available, place an atropine tablet (1/150 grain) under the victim's tongue every 1 to 2 hours (oftener if necessary) until symptoms abate.

If poisoning is due to *Amanita phalloides,* and mental confusion or hallucinations are present, control the victim by restraint, if necessary, until an ambulance arrives.

Shellfish Poisoning

A fairly common type of acute gastroenteritis is caused by eating shellfish that have been heavily contaminated with bacteria, have been improperly refrigerated, or stored too long before eating and have undergone some degree of putrefaction.

On the other hand acute illness from eating crabs, shrimps, lobsters, clams, mussels, or oysters may be simply the result of an allergy to the particular species. To a person not allergic to them, the same food will be quite harmless.

Signs and Symptoms. The symptoms are those of a violent intestinal upset, a generalized, blotchy reddish-blue rash with severe itching, generalized swelling, asthma, and sometimes convulsions.

○ TREATMENT

Treatment is largely beyond the scope of emergency care; therefore, get a doctor *immediately,* as the victim may be in profound collapse. In the meantime,

1   Give him a dose of Epsom salts to hasten removal of the poison from the lower intestine and to help neutralize the toxin. Since vomiting and diarrhea are already purging the poison from the intestinal tract, it is usually unnecessary to use an emetic; if required use ipecac (see pages 298 and 299).

2   Since some of the symptoms are probably allergic in nature, antihistamine drugs may help to control the itching.

3   Watch the victim carefully for swelling of his larynx, in which

case the administration of epinephrine or a tracheotomy will be required. Medical attention is *urgent*.

Gonyaulax Poisoning. A different type of poisoning is contracted by eating shellfish that ordinarily would cause no difficulty, but which at certain times of the year feed on poisonous plankton and hence have themselves become violently toxic. Contamination of shellfish, particularly bay clams, mussels, and certain species of oysters, occurs intermittently and is not limited to a specific season.

This so-called "paralytic" type of shellfish poisoning is much more serious than either that due to a simple bacterial contamination or to allergy. It is caused specifically by the poison secreted by plankton, known as dinoflagellates, which is absorbed by the particular shellfish. The condition is also known as clam or mussel poisoning.

Symptoms. The first symptom to be noted is a tingling or burning sensation around the face, lips, and the tongue, with eventually the entire body becoming involved. There follows a sense of numbness and various muscles of the body become either difficult to move or practically paralyzed. In addition, there is intense thirst, a feeling of weakness and dizziness, often pain in the joints, and excessive salivation. Contrary to the other forms of shellfish poisoning, nausea, vomiting, and abdominal pain are not characteristic features.

Unfortunately, there is no specific treatment and the paralysis becomes increasingly severe until eventually the patient dies. However, as soon as the condition is suspected, the stomach and entire gastrointestinal tract should be thoroughly cleansed by provoking vomiting by whatever means is available, followed by Epsom salts as a purgative. Copious amounts of sodium bicarbonate solution should then be given by mouth, since the toxin is destroyed in an alkaline medium. Artificial respiration may be required, and it is extremely urgent to get the patient to adequate medical facilities, in the hope that further energetic supportive measures may avoid a fatal outcome.

The toxicity of *Gonyaulax catenella,* a causative agent of this type of poisoning, cannot be overemphasized, and there is no simple way of determining which shellfish are contaminated and which are not. Usually an area where this type of contamination is known to occur is closed for fishing by the authorities and, if this be the case, discretion is certainly the better part of valor.   If there is any doubt at all about the safety of a particular shellfish anywhere, don't under any circumstances eat it.

Fish Poisoning

A similar type of problem arises in connection with fishes, some of which may be naturally poisonous; others which are considered to be excellent food fish in some areas may be highly toxic in others, again because of feeding on poisonous plankton.   This is particularly true of fish who are normal inhabitants of reef areas.   It is best to follow local custom and advice in eating fish from questionable areas.

Scombroid Poisoning.   One common type of fish poisoning involves the well-known food fishes such as mackerel, tuna, and other members of the mackerel family.   The difficulty here arises from inadequate preservation of the fish themselves, which do not have very good keeping qualities to begin with. It is thought that bacteria rapidly change a chemical compound, known as histidine, which is normally present in their tissues, into a toxic histamine analog, which produces a severe allergic response when ingested.

Scombroid poisoning can be avoided by eating only absolutely fresh mackerel or tuna, or making certain that the fish in question has either been kept under refrigeration or has been properly canned.   Fish, ungutted and uniced, lying around a boat in the sun, for even a short time, can be very dangerous.   If there is not a proper facility for refrigeration on board, release the fish as you catch them, keeping only those caught shortly before the return to shore.

If a bad fish is eaten, it will not be long before the victim is well aware of his predicament, since the symptoms develop within a few minutes.   They consist of dizziness, intense headach, dryness of the mouth, palpitation, often difficulty in swallowing, and signs of acute prostrating gastrointestinal upset, and it will not be long before huge red hives, which itch intensely, appear all over the body.   Usually these symptoms abate within 24 hours, but they can be greatly relieved after the gastrointestinal tract has been purged of the poison by the administration of any of the antihistamine drugs and a suitable corticosteroid.

Ciguatera Poisoning. Another type of fish poisoning is known as ciguatera poisoning; it can involve more than 300 different kinds of species, many of which are perfectly edible under other circumstances. The problem is particularly bad in tropical seas, around the West Indies, and in some regions poses a serious economic difficulty. It may occur without warning in a previously unaffected area. Apparently the fish that become toxic have fed on poisonous plankton and their flesh contains the toxins of the ingested organisms.

Symptoms. The symptoms of this condition are not unlike those of gonyaulax poisoning and may come on quickly, or not for a period of a day or so. There is great prostration, weakness, and generalized severe aching muscle pains. Many times there are frightening visual disturbances and a feeling of suffocation, often accompanied by definite laryngeal spasm or edema.

There is no specific treatment. The gastrointestinal tract should be thoroughly cleansed, as described for other types of fish poisoning. A victim of ciguatera poisoning is dangerously ill and urgently requires the best available medical facilities.

Unfortunately, there is no easy way of distinguishing those food fish which are safe to eat and those which have become poisonous. Perhaps the safest thing to do is to depend on local knowledge. *Ciguatera toxin is not destroyed by cooking,* although it is soluble in water and, in suspicious areas, boiling thin strips of the fish for at least 45 minutes, preferably more, and discarding the cooking water, is said to render potentially contaminated flesh less toxic. The fact remains, however, that it is far better not to eat the suspected flesh than to take a chance.

12 Recognition and Treatment of Drug Abuse

Aldous Huxley once wrote: "Most men and women lead lives at the worst so painful, at best so monotonous, poor and limited, that the urge to escape, the longing to transcend themselves, if only for a few minutes, is and always has been one of the principal appetites of the soul." It is true, as T. S. Eliot so succinctly stated, "Human kind cannot bear very much reality." Hence we have seen in the last few years the horrifying increase in use of drugs by all levels of society and all ages, in a desperate effort to secure escape from reality and a few brief moments of "paradise."

Youthful drug abuse is one of our most important and frightening public health problems. It is no longer confined to lower-class delinquents but, according to authorities at the Awareness Training Center in Tucson, Arizona, has spread like wildfire among young persons from ages 10 through 25. Those who have studied the problem often find that half the young people in high school and from 10 to 35 percent of those in junior high and grammar school have experimented with dangerous drugs, often beginning their initiation into drug abuse with marijuana and glue sniffing, soon graduating to the use of LSD, the pep pills and barbiturates; and ultimately often ending up with heroin.

Not only that, but an even worse problem is now developing. Alcohol consumption among teenagers (and now even grammar school students) is increasing at a time when use of "hard drugs" such as amphetamines and hallucinogens is decreasing. This problem is demoralizing and difficult to deal with.

So vast are the number and types of drugs available that it is impossible to give a single definition for all forms of drug addiction or habituation. Features common to these conditions or, rather, common to drug abuse in general, are dependence upon the drug, which may be either physical or psychic, or both, plus an effect which for varying periods of time permits the individual to detach himself from reality or achieve an altered state of mind which he thinks will be more pleasing to himself. That such is not always the case has to be learned by the drug abuser through bitter experience.

A variety of terms have been used for describing the relationship of the individual to his drug abuse. These include *drug taking,* which may or may not be harmful; *drug abuse,* which may be mentally, physically, or socially harmful; and *drug addiction,* in which mental, physical, and social functioning are impaired beyond the individual's ability to control his situation because the drug has fully and completely taken over the user's will to resist; he must not only have the drug at regular intervals but in ever increasing amounts to achieve the desired psychic effect.

While the terms drug abuse and drug addiction are in common use, they may, however, be inaccurate as well as confusing. The World Health Organization has pointed out that a better understanding can be obtained by the use of the term *drug dependence* of this or that specific type, according to the agent or class of agents being abused.

According to this approach, drug dependence is defined as a state of psychic or physical dependence, or both, on a drug following administration of the drug on a periodic or continuous basis. The manifestion of the state thus evoked will vary with the agent involved; for example, drug dependence of the morphine (heroin) type, the barbiturate type, or the amphetamine type, each of which produces characteristic effects.

While drug dependence is a general term, when suitably modified by the designation of the class of abused drug it is not only an aid to classification but is helpful in diagnosis as well as treatment since, *within a given group, the overall man-*

agement of the case is essentially the same for all drugs falling within that particular category, regardless of the specific drug abused. Consequently, the recognition and management of the drug abuser will be discussed from that point of view.

DRUG DEPENDENCE OF THE MARIJUANA TYPE

Marijuana, known to man for over 5,000 years, is a drug found in the flowering tops and leaves of the Indian hemp plant *Cannabis sativa.* Before 1937, it was widely used medically, including the treatment of warts, migraine, and dysmenorrhea. Currently it is under intensive investigation in all types of terminal cancer as a means of relieving suffering. It is also under active investigation as a possibly useful drug by local instillation in the treatment of glaucoma, according to Cohen.

The pharmacologic activity of the plant results from one of its main ingredients known chemically as tetrahydrocannabinol, or THC. The plant grows in mild climates all over the world, especially in Mexico, Africa, India, and the Middle East. It is also widely distributed geographically in the United States, where the drug is known by many slang terms such as "pot," "tea," "grass," "weed," "Mary Jane," and many others.

For use as a drug, the leaves and flowers of the plant are dried and crushed or chopped into small pieces. This green product is usually rolled and smoked in short cigarettes or in pipes, or it can be taken orally. The cigarettes are commonly known as "reefers," "joints," and "sticks."

The smoke from marijuana has a strong, harsh, somewhat acrid smell, very similar to that of burning rope or dried grass. Its rather sweetish odor is easily detectible and persists for some time.

The effects of marijuana smoking vary widely, largely as the result of great variation in the content of the active principle, the area and conditions under which the plant was grown, and the mood and susceptibility of the user. One of the most devastating things about the abuse of marijuana is that not only may its potency vary so greatly, depending upon what part of the plant was used in its manufacture, but it is often sold on the street adulterated or contaminated with extremely potent and dangerous drugs such as mescaline, methamphetamine, LSD, *phencyclidine* (a powerful veterinary anesthetic), or many other drugs, including an anticholinergic such as belladonna. This fact alone may account for much of the confusion which has arisen concerning marijuana use, and pharmacologic research conducted with the pure drug may have little bearing upon the results observed in actual practice.

Even more powerful than marijuana is a preparation known as hashish, the brown resin collected from the tops and leaves of high-grade marijuana plants. Hashish is many times more potent than marijuana prepared from any of the other parts of the plant. Widely employed throughout Asia, its use in the United States seems to be increasing, and again the problem of adulteration is a major factor. Many bad "trips" result from the use of the more potent drug in place of the less powerful domestic product.

In addition, it has been found, working with synthetic tetrahydrocannabinol, that high dosages of the drug brought on severe reactions in every person tested. The National Institute of Mental Health study also showed that psychotic reactions sometimes occur, for unknown reasons, in some individuals who take smaller amounts.

The use of marijuana as an intoxicating or hallucinogenic drug was introduced into the United States about 1920, and in 1937 its general use was outlawed by the Federal Marijuana Act. Arrests on marijuana charges have more than doubled since 1960. In spite of stringent laws, estimates of people in the United States who have used the drug at least once in their lives or are, in fact, habitual users vary from 4 to 20 million.

However, there is considerable feeling among informed groups that legislation with respect to marijuana may be undesirably strict, and the American Academy of Pediatrics has urged that the penalty for possessing and being in the presence of marijuana should be changed from a felony to a misdemeanor. In so doing, the American Academy of Pediatrics emphasizes that since marijuana is not considered a narcotic but, rather, a hallucinogen and does not produce addiction as such, "it is inappropriate to continue to have this drug subject to the narcotic laws, i.e., the Harrison Narcotic Act."

The penalties for possession and being in the presence of marijuana are severe in terms of their immediate and long-term effects on the individual, the statement points out, and the

Academy's opinion is largely based on the nature of the drug and the cultural circumstances associated with its use. This may be particularly true, since undoubtedly many young people view the identification of marijuana as a narcotic, with all the attendant severe punitive connotations, as another example of hypocrisy and lack of justice in America today.

Nevertheless, the Academy emphasizes that marijuana, as a potentially harmful drug, should not be legalized in any amount at this time, feeling that legalization, if ever, should be deferred until a maximum degree of research and study on the matter can be accomplished.

Perhaps the greatest danger of marijuana lies in the fact that in so many cases it simply provides a stepping stone to the use of more dangerous drugs. A high percentage of heroin addicts report that they started with marijuana, although it is probably true that most marijuana smokers do not go on to more dangerous abuses.

Symptoms

When good quality marijuana is smoked, a deep inhalation will produce an effect within a few minutes which may continue for an hour or more and can be maintained over long periods by continued inhalation. The effects thus attained are much more rapid than when the drug is taken by mouth.

Following inhalation of marijuana smoke, the hallucinogen quickly enters the bloodstream and reaches the brain by a route the exact nature of which is not known. At any rate, it produces subjective effects, including unreasonable hilarity, disorientation as to time, euphoria, and impairment of judgment and memory—often accompanied by irritability and confusion. In some individuals there appears to be an increase in perception, so that they feel they have a greater insight into art and music; various forms of antisocial behavior and sleep disturbances are common. Often the user of marijuana becomes so engrossed in his habit that all will to accomplish anything constructive is lost.

Physically, the individual frequently shows evidence of over-reactivity of the central nervous system, manifested by tremulousness, incoordination, and general unsteadiness. Typically, one frequently sees a characteristic injection of the scleral blood vessels, or conjunctivitis (the tell-tale "red eye"), and of the mouth and throat. This is not due to the irritant qualities of the smoke; it occurs also when marijuana is ingested. Chronic bronchitis and asthma are common.

Contrary to what many people believe, marijuana has no specific aphrodisiac qualities, any such effect being due merely to the loss of inhibitions. While marijuana is often used by those who are inherently mentally unstable, there is at present no good evidence that the drug may produce a major psychosis or lasting mental changes. However, a type of acute phychosis has been reported by Talbott and Teague among soldiers in Vietnam, associated with the use of various powerful cannabis derivatives. Symptoms cleared under conservative and supportive treatment without evidence of permanent damage. It is clear, however, that marijuana as used in the Orient is much more dangerous than the relatively benign product distributed in this country.

While the argument still rages concerning the possible adverse genetic effects of chronic marijuana smoking (there may well be, although the picture is still confused), several other important considerations are evident: Driver reaction time may be seriously affected and large doses may lead to a variety of adverse physical effects. The question of potential adverse effects upon the lungs has yet to be determined. There is also experimental evidence to suggest a causal relationship with various types of birth defects. Heavy use of marijuana (particularly Oriental cannabis) may lead to serious psychotic defects.

While young people will try almost anything for "kicks" in an effort to discover and achieve various psychic effects, the problem is by no means limited to youthful abusers, but has become an important factor among industrial workers and other adult socioeconomic groups. However, with the rise of alcoholism among school children, there seems to be some drop in the abuse of "hard drugs."

○ TREATMENT

There is no specific treatment for reactions arising from drug abuse of the marijuana type. For the most part, the symptoms will subside rather quickly, providing the patient is given support and reassurance.

Symptoms arising from powerful adulterants which may be present in the marijuana must be treated on the basis of the presenting findings. A "bad trip" caused by other adulterating hallucinogens such as LSD or mescaline usually will wear off without antidotal therapy other than possibly a mild sedative or tranquilizer. As a general rule, it is advisable to avoid giving "therapeutic" drugs except on the basis of some clear-cut and specific indication, placing the greater reliance on psychologic support and understanding.

In the series of acute psychotic reactions reported by Talbott and Teague, it was felt that the use of phenothiazine tranquilizers and various sedative drugs did little more than individual and group psychotherapy, and the use of drugs in this type of reaction was therefore largely abandoned.

It also should be remembered that the reaction being exhibited by the patient may not be due inherently to marijuana, but to one of the many adulterants commonly present in illicitly distributed preparations. The use of drugs in the treatment of a so-called marijuana "high" should be carried out with great care lest a more severe type of reaction be precipitated.

In general, physical protection of the individual, rest, and reassurance are the major factors in the handling of all but the most severe marijuana type of reaction.

DRUG DEPENDENCE OF THE HALLUCINOGEN (LSD) TYPE

LSD, one of the most widely publicized and in some respects perhaps the most sinister of the mind-distorting drugs, is a powerful man-made chemical known as lysergic acid diethylamide, or LSD for short. It was developed in 1938 from one of the alkaloids, ergot, found in a common fungus that grows on rye and is easily synthesized in any chemical laboratory. It is exceedingly powerful, a single ounce being enough to provide 300,000 average doses.

The group of drugs known as hallucinogens, of which LSD is the most prominent member, contains a large number of other psychedelic or mind-affecting drugs. These include psilocybin ("magic mushroom"), an indole found in the mushroom *Psilocybe mexicana;* mescaline, the most active alkaloid present in the buttons of a small cactus ("mescal" or "peyote," technically known as *Lophophora williamsii*), as well as in the seeds of some morning glory varieties ("ololiuqui," *Rivea corymbosa* L. Hall f.; *Ipomoea violacea* L.); dimethyltryptamine (DMT); phencyclidine (PCP); and dimethoxy-4-methylamphetamine (STP, which stands for serenity, tranquility and peace). These are in addition to a host of similar acting but less well-known agents.

The mushroom, cactus buttons, and morning glory seeds have been used for centuries by various Indian tribes in connection with religious ceremonies or have been employed in the treatment of illness, usually as part of some religious ritual.

The psychedelic drugs in general have a particular appeal for psychologically and socially maladjusted persons who take the drug for thrills, to alter a mood, to "enhance" perception and psychological insight, or to achieve some occult religious experience. Drugs in this category are usually taken by mouth, their use being periodic over short periods of time rather than continuously. The period during which the individual is under the influence of the drug is known as a "trip." It may vary from ½ hour to 36 hours or more.

Symptoms

The general pharmacologic effect of drugs in the hallucinogen group is to induce a high state of excitation of the central nervous system. This is reflected by marked changes in mood, often accompanied by anxiety, distortion in sensory perception, i.e., seeing sound and hearing color, visual hallucination, delusions, depersonalization of a feeling of disembodiment or dissociation of the spirit from one's own body, dilatation of the pupils, and an increase in body temperature and blood pressure.

The first effects are likely to be sudden changes in the physical senses. Walls may appear to move, colors seem stronger and more brilliant. Users are likely to "see" unusual patterns unfolding before them. Flat objects seem to stand out in three dimensions. Taste, smell, hearing, and touch seem more acute. One sensory impression may be translated or merged into another; for example, music may appear as a color, and colors may seem to have a taste.

One of the most confusing yet common reactions among users is the feeling of two strong and opposite emotions at the same time—they can feel both happy and sad at once, or depressed and elated, or relaxed and tense.   Arms and legs may feel both heavy and light.

Effects can be different at different times in the same individual.   Researchers have found, even in carefully controlled studies, that responses to the drug cannot be predicted.   For this reason, users refer to "good trips" or "bad trips" to describe their experience.

In some cases the effect of the drug is so acute as to severely frighten the user; he is thrown into a life or death panic and may commit physical acts which will bring about serious injury to himself or others, or even death.   Such an individual is said to be having a "bad trip," and he must be protected both from himself and from his environment until the psychic-amplifying effects of the drug have worn off.

Sometimes the effect of LSD or other hallucinogen on a susceptible individual will be such that he loses all sense of proportion and judgment and believes that he has unusual abilities which, of course, do not exist.   For instance, deaths have occurred in people under the influence of LSD who thought they could fly and have accordingly jumped out a window.   In another situation, a person under the influence of a drug may think he has unusual strength and will stand in the street in an attempt to push a truck or automobile aside, thus promptly getting himself run over.   In other words, the principal danger to life and limb from the hallucinogenic drugs is from the psychic effect they have on the individual rather than the actual toxicity of the drug itself.

A severe "panic" reaction or markedly irrational behavior is the manifestation of hallucinogenic drug abuse most commonly requiring emergency care.

○ TREATMENT

The treatment of an acute reaction to a hallucinogenic drug is largely expectant.   As has been indicated, individuals using the hallucinogens tend to be highly suggestible; hence, while protecting the victim of a bad drug reaction from himself as well as his environment, additional control should be attempted by "talking the patient down."   He should be taken to some quiet place, free of observable police presence if possible, and a calm, friendly rapport established.   It is important to try to find out when and what drug was taken.   Often such information can be elicited by questioning along the lines of "How long ago did you drop it?" This approach will tend to reassure the victim by making him realize that his present condition is the effect of something he has actually taken, the reaction to which will gradually wear off, and that the person taking care of him understands his predicament. He should be continually assured along these lines, in addition to repeated attempts to orient him as to time and place. With repeated assurances that his condition is due to a drug, that the effects are wearing off, and that he is soon going to be all right, he will gradually come down off his "high"; in this way, his confidence and self-control will be reestablished.

It is possible to end a "bad trip" quickly with certain drugs such as chlorpromazine (Thorazine®), diazepam (Valium®), or chlordiazepoxide hydrochloride (Librium®). As a general rule, it is safer to avoid the use of drugs whenever feasible because of their possible adverse interaction with some unknown contaminant of whatever hallucinogen the patient has ingested. For example, deaths have been reported when chlorpromazine has been given to end a "bad trip" caused by LSD when the LSD has been adultered with atropine, belladonna, or some other anticholinergic drug. If it is felt that the situation is sufficiently urgent to require the use of a drug to terminate the reaction more quickly, diazepam probably is preferable to chlorpromazine because of the lesser likelihood of a severe hypotensive effect and less chance of a severe adverse drug reaction in the event of adulteration. It should be realized that chlorpromazine may potentiate the effects of certain hallucinogens, especially STP—which often contains belladonna-like adulterants.

If chlorpromazine is used, it should be given in doses commensurate with the weight of the patient, not in relation to the severity of the symptoms. The dose for an average size person would be 50 milligrams intramuscularly or 100 milligrams by mouth. Providing no drop in blood pressure or other adverse effects appear, this dose can be repeated every 45 minutes to 1 hour until symptoms subside. If the blood pressure drops significantly when the patient stands, the chlorpromazine should be discontinued and the patient returned to the reclining position. It is rarely necessary to give a vasopressor agent such as levarterenol to counteract this type of complication.

A severe anticholinergic crisis may be counteracted by administration of 2 to 4 milligrams of *physostigmine sulphate* either intramuscularly or by mouth. This is a short-acting drug and may need to be repeated in an hour or so, but it should be used with caution and with careful observation of the patient as a safeguard against overtreatment.

Even without drugs, a victim often can be "talked down" in 15 to 20 minutes to the point where he will be calm enough to wait for the effect of the drug to pass. Friends or other drug users who are not "on a high" can be helpful in the "talking down" process and may be permitted to take over, provided no actual medical emergency exists.

This process is safer than an attempt to abruptly terminate a "bad trip" through the use of counteracting drugs, because of the great likelihood that one may not be dealing with a pure LSD reaction, for instance, since it is quite possible that the original drug was not pure but contained adulterants which could produce a severe or even fatal interaction.

DRUG DEPENDENCE OF THE COCAINE TYPE

Cocaine is the oldest of the central nervous system stimulant drugs and has been abused in one form or another for centuries. When used in sufficiently large quantities, it is capable of inducing a high degree of euphoric excitement and hallucinatory experiences.

Although cocaine produces probably the highest degree of psychic dependence of all commonly abused drugs, it causes neither the development of tolerance nor of physical dependence. It is, however, the strong psychic dependence which leads to such a profound and dangerous type of drug abuse.

According to the World Health Organization, abuse of cocaine takes several forms. The most common is the century-old custom of coca leaf chewing, which is practiced habitually by certain Indian tribes of the Andes. The leaf, mixed with lime juice, apparently in an effort to release the active principle, is used almost continuously to reduce sensations of cold, fatigue, and hunger. With this form of abuse, release of the alkaloid and its absorption generally are too slow, or quantitatively too small, to induce mental changes that would lead to abnormal behavior.

Cocaine was used many years ago in medicine as a vaso-constrictor and as a local anesthetic, but with the availability of superior and far less dangerous preparations both its availability and its use for legitimate purposes have sharply declined.

Despite its vasoconstrictive properties, cocaine is readily absorbed through the mucous membranes, and, even when used for legitimate medical purposes, a high degree of euphoric stimulation was often observed. However, in recent times, with the phrenetic search of socially maladjusted individuals for new and more exciting forms of drug abuse, a most dangerous usage has evolved—the intravenous injection of cocaine at frequent intervals; the effect is short lasting but, for a brief period of time, the user is said to enjoy the most satisfying ecstasy.

Symptoms

Unfortunately, cocaine abuse appeals particularly to persons with psychopathic tendencies, which are often brought to light by this devastating use of the drug. With the feeling of great muscular and mental strength which ensues, the individual is led to overestimate his capabilities; this fact, associated with various delusions and auditory, visual, and tactile hallucinations, combine to create an extremely dangerous situation.

The chronic cocaine abuser is characteristically nervous, tremulous, apprehensive, and easily startled. The pupils are often dilated, and the heart rate may be rapid, accompanied by an elevated blood pressure. In addition, the abuser of cocaine often suffers profound physical disturbances, including nausea, loss of appetite, sleeplessness, loss of weight, and convulsions.

In a sense, in any single individual, the overabuse of cocaine is more or less self-limiting, since the user reaches such a state of excitement that he literally cannot stand it and he seeks some form of sedation. Unfortunately, he often seeks the sedation which he requires in the form of morphine, often injecting the morphine along with the cocaine, a combination known as "speed ball."

○ TREATMENT

Cocaine undergoes very rapid destruction in the body, so that huge amounts can be consumed within a 24-hour period when relatively small doses are used at any given interval. But in spite of this, cocaine does not produce true tolerance. In addition, there is no evidence that physical dependence on cocaine develops, and as a result there are no characteristic withdrawal symptoms when the use of the drug is abruptly stopped.

There is no specific treatment, but if the patient is extremely nervous or hallucinating, he should be given up to 500 milligrams of a quick-acting barbiturate such as sodium pentobarbital intravenously to produce the required sedation, or one of the phenathiazine tranquilizers (such as chlorpromazine). In extreme cases, morphine in doses of 20 to 30 milligrams is an effective antidote but obviously must be used cautiously with the patient under close observation, since any depressant drug may dangerously enhance the respiratory depression caused by cocaine poisoning.

The great dangers of cocaine addiction are the unleashing of strong psychopathic tendencies in the user and the enormous psychic dependence which develops from use of the drug.

DRUG DEPENDENCE OF THE AMPHETAMINE TYPE

Amphetamines, first produced in the early 1920s for medical use, are powerful central nervous system stimulants and, for that reason, have a great ability to combat fatigue and sleepiness. In the past, they have also been widely used as appetite depressants but, because of their numerous side effects and the fact that tolerance readily develops, they have largely been abandoned for this purpose in favor of other agents.

The best known amphetamines are amphetamine sulfate (Benzedrine®); dextroamphetamine sulfate (Dexedrine®); and methamphetamine hydrochloride (Methedrine® and Desoxyn®). Some of these amphetamines are also sold in combination with certain barbiturates; for instance, the combination of methamphetamine hydrochloride and sodium pentobarbital is sold under the brand name of Desbutal®. A combination of dextro-amphetamine sulfate and the barbiturate amobarbital is marketed under the brand name of Dexamyl®, the theory being that the barbiturate will have a quieting action on the stimulant action of the amphetamine, which occurs more or less as a side effect of the drug.

There are two other well-known preparations which have essentially the same type of action as the amphetamines: one is phenmetrazine hydrochloride, marketed as an appetite depressant under the trade name of Preludin®, and methylphenidate hydrochloride which is marketed as a mood elevator under the name of Ritalin®.

All these drugs are legally available only on prescription. About 20 percent of all medical prescriptions for mood-affecting drugs are stimulants. The amount produced by the drug industry each year is enough to provide each American with 25 doses. The Food and Drug Administration reports that about half the supply (if not more) enters illegal channels for nonprescribed use; several varieties of stimulant drugs are produced in black market laboratories and are easily obtained from illegal sources.

The black market drugs are often mislabeled and are frequently adulterated with some other agent to increase the "kick." It is these adulterants that are so often responsible for bizarre and frequently dangerous reactions and pose a serious hazard to the medical treatment of these cases during the withdrawal period.

Amphetamines are abused and misused by people of all ages from all walks of life, but today young people are becoming the greatest abusers. Drivers and students also take drugs of this type when attempting long trips without rest or cramming for examinations, and athletes have been known to use them in order to supposedly attain extra strength and stamina. Reputable sporting associations have banned this type of use both in human athletics and in horse and dog racing.

Some people add insult to injury by using amphetamine-type drugs as stimulants and then "letting themselves down" with depressive drugs such as the barbiturates. The amphetamines are used to a marked extent by people who abuse alcohol and/or barbiturates. In such instances there is a dependence developed on more than one drug.

A particularly dangerous practice is the use of the drug methamphetamine intravenously—a technic known as "speeding." Intravenous administration produces bizarre mental effects often associated with sexual function—sometimes to the point of orgasm. This type of abuse has been increasing sharply in recent years throughout the world, and at the present time methamphetamine is the most widely abused of the central nervous system stimulants that can be injected intravenously ("main-lining").

The effect is an intense "high" of relatively short duration but, as the effects begin to wear off, the injection is repeated, so that so-called "speed runs" may be continued for long periods of time. Because tolerance to amphetamines develops rapidly, the dose must be constantly increased to obtain the ultimate effect, or "total body orgasm" as it has been termed.

A further unfortunate feature of the amphetamines is their extraordinary capacity to induce tolerance which, because it increases slowly, eventually permits the use of amounts of drug several hundred times greater than the recommended therapeutic dose. Although such huge doses may not prove fatal, they produce profound behavioral changes that are psychotic in nature and include hallucinations, delusions, and other marked mental aberrations. Such effects are greatly intensified by intravenous administration.

An additional complication of the intravenous injection of methamphetamine has been reported by Citron et al., who noted extensive necrotizing angiitis in young drug absuers who had used a variety of narcotics, hallucinogens, central nervous system stimulants and depressants. The common denominator seemed to be methamphetamine, alone or in combination with LSD. Complications included renal failure, hypertension, pancreatitis, and edema of the lungs. Postmortem findings in four cases revealed the characteristic generalized vascular changes, especially in the kidney, liver, pancreas, and intestine.

Although the amphetamines do not induce true physical dependence, withdrawal from the use of the drug is far from symptomless. If a stimulant drug has been used for a long period of time to mask chronic fatigue and the need for sleep, it stands to reason that when this drug is stopped, these symptoms will reappear in intensified form. It is for that reason that once the amphetamine drugs are stopped, there follows a period of depression, which is both psychic and physical, and which often the victim seeks to relieve by reinitiating the use of the drug. It should be pointed out that while no really true physical dependence develops, there is a likelihood of a strong psychological dependence, so that the continued use of the drug is practiced and becomes a habit for mental or emotional reasons, with the person getting used to and turning to the drug for its effects whenever he feels the need.

The urge, however, is not as strong as that encountered with morphine, heroin, the barbiturates, alcohol, and other drugs that create true physical dependence. Withdrawal from the amphetamines, therefore, is not life-threatening and usually requires only psychological treatment without the aid of specific counteracting agents.

One dangerous feature of the amphetamines is that they can drive a person to do things beyond his physical endurance but leave him totally exhausted. Heavy doses may cause a temporary toxic psychosis, usually accompanied by auditory and visual hallucinations, which may be severe enough to require hospitalization. Abrupt withdrawal of the drug at this time can result in deep and sometimes suicidal depression.

Symptoms

When amphetamines or related compounds are used legitimately under prescription by a physician, moderate doses can check fatigue and produce feelings of alertness, self-confidence and well being, although, when the drug is stopped, there is a letdown feeling or depression hangover. Larger doses of the drugs, or too frequent doses, cause the jitters, irritability, unclear speech, and tension. People on very large doses of the amphetamines appear withdrawn, with their emotions dulled, and seem unable to organize their thinking.

Aside from their psychic stimulating effect, amphetamines increase blood pressure, with an increase in heart rate, and may cause an increase in respiration and palpitation or arrythmia of the heart. The pupils become dilated, the mouth may be dry, and often there is sweating (especially of the palms of the hands), headache, diarrhea, and paleness, particularly if the individual tolerance level for the drug is exceeded.

The respiration may be shallow and rapid, and there may

be a sharp rise in body temperature. In cases in which an overdose has been taken, the victim may be very confused, have paranoid ideas of persecution, and be extremely irritable and aggressive, especially after using methamphetamine ("speed") intravenously.

Those who use amphetamines continuously and in large doses are usually irritable and unstable, and, like other heavy drug users, show social, intellectual, and emotional breakdown. A large dose of an amphetamine given intravenously to an individual whose tolerance is low may result in death.

Another point to be emphasized, quite aside from the pharmacologic dangers of using these drugs intravenously, is the high rate of serum hepatitis that develops as the result of using unclean or unsterile needles and syringes by more than one individual (as in main-lining within a group), and the formation of multiple indolent abscesses at the site of injection.

○ TREATMENT

The medical treatment of amphetamine intoxication is largely supportive in nature, under as quiet circumstances as possible, with the victim being offered understanding, psychologic support, and encouragement.

As a basis for treatment, Espelin and Done have provided an assessment of the degree of amphetamine poisoning as set forth in the following table:

Symptoms	Severity
Restlessness, irritability, insomnia	1+
Tremor, hyperreflexia	
Sweating, mydriasis, flushing	
Hyperactivity, confusion	2+
Hypertension, tachypnea, tachycardia, extrasystoles	
Fever (mild)	
Sweating, etc.	
Delirium, mania, self-injury	3+
Marked hypertension, tachycardia, arrhythmias	
Hyperpyrexia	
Above, plus:	4+
Convulsions and coma	
Circulatory collapse and death	

On the basis of their experience, chlorpromazine is used in all cases of 2+ severity or greater. In patients who have used an amphetamine alone, 1 milligram per kilogram is given intramuscularly. However, as emphasized by Cohen, the amphetamines as purchased on the street are often "cut" with various anti-cholinergic drugs (atropine scopolamine and related belladonna alkaloids) to increase the "high." If such a possibility exists, the phenathiazine should not be used. If it is suspected that an amphetamine-sedative combination has been ingested, 0.5 milligram chlorpromazine per kilogram body weight is given intramuscularly and repeated in 30 minutes if necessary to control excitement. If necessary to control hypertension, an alpha-adrenergic blocking agent such as Dibenzyline® may also be given. In very severe cases, hemodialysis or peritoneal dialysis should also be used as a lifesaving measure.

Once the individual is over the acute phase of withdrawal, he should be offered psychiatric guidance since many of these individuals are mentally unstable to begin with or they would not have resorted to the abuse of such a powerful group of drugs.

DRUG DEPENDENCE OF THE BARBITURATE TYPE

The barbiturate drugs have the opposite effect on the central nervous system to that of the amphetamines. Whereas the amphetamines stimulate, the barbiturates, like alcohol, depress.

The consumption of barbiturates in this country has reached astounding proportions; it has been estimated that of all prescriptions written by physicians for mind-affecting drugs, one in four is for a barbiturate. There are a great many such drugs on the market for legitimate medical purposes and in general they are divided into two categories—the short-acting drugs with quick onset of action and those drugs having a more prolonged effect with a slower onset of action.

The most widely used, and incidentally abused, drugs in the short-acting group are pentobarbital (Nembutal®) and secobarbital (Seconal®). In the longer-acting group, the most common drugs are: phenobarbital, which has long been available and was formerly marketed under the trade name

Luminal®; sodium amobarbital (Amytal®); and sodium butabarbital (Butisol®).

The first barbiturate was synthesized as long ago as 1846 from barbituric acid, and the use of this type of drug has been expanding tremendously ever since.

The barbiturates have many legitimate uses in medicine; when taken in normal medically supervised doses, they exert a depressive action upon the central nervous system, skeletal muscles, and heart muscle.   Unfortunately, many tons more of barbiturates are consumed in this country each year than are required for legitimate medical purposes.

Users may react more strongly at one time than another, and barbiturates distort how people see things and slow down their reactions and responses.   For this reason, they are an important cause of automobile accidents and may well be a factor in other types of accidents, especially industrial accidents.

Since barbiturates are so easily obtained both legally and illegally, they provide one of the most common forms of suicide.   The victim simply takes an overdose and sleeps his life away if not discovered in time.

The barbiturates are not only physically addicting but the dose must be continually increased to obtain the desired effect as the body develops tolerance.   There are many features in common between barbiturate addiction and narcotic dependency; many experts feel that barbiturate addiction may be even more difficult to cure than narcotic addiction since there is no specific counteracting drug available to ease the withdrawal symptoms as in the case of narcotic addiction.

In the case of the barbiturates, if the drug is terminated abruptly, the withdrawal symptoms may be violent, with cramps, nausea, delirium, and convulsions, and in some cases even sudden death.

Symptoms of Barbiturate Abuse

The barbiturates slow both the heart and respiratory rates and tend to lower the blood pressure.   In higher doses the effects resemble alcoholic intoxication, with mental confusion, slurred speech, staggering gait, and disorientation.   The ability to think, to concentrate, and to work is impaired, and emotional control is weakened.   Chronic users may become irritable, easily angered, and want to fight or assault someone. Finally, they may fall into a deep sleep.

Acute Barbiturate Intoxication

The principal indications of this type of poisoning are drowsiness, mental confusion, hallucinations, slurred speech, very shallow breathing, and weak pulse. The pupils of the eyes are *not* contracted as in opium poisoning.

In toxic cases, the pupils are normal (in contrast to the pinpoint pupils of narcotic overdose), but both the blood pressure and respiration are markedly depressed; there is a partial loss of deep tendon reflexes; characteristically there is staggering and loss of balance accompanied by confusion and drunkenly slurred speech. In severe overdosage the patient may be in deep shock and coma, a situation which may easily lead to death.

Shubin and Weil stress that the degree of shock in the comatose patient may be severe and complicated by potentially lethal cardiac arrythmias caused by inadequate ventilation as the result of the severe respiratory depression.

Hence, mechanical respiration with constant monitoring of the respiratory exchange is essential if a fatal outcome is to be avoided. On the other hand, it has been shown that pneumonia is the major cause of death in acute barbiturate intoxication and that the incidence of pneumonia correlates strikingly with the number of those undergoing endotracheal intubation.

The fast-acting barbiturates, such as pentobarbital and secobarbital, produce coma quickly, but the effects wear off relatively rapidly. The reverse is true of the longer-acting drugs such as phenobarbital and barbital compounds. About 1,500 deaths due to barbiturate intoxication occur each year.

For purposes of assessing the degree of intoxication and determining the intensity of treatment required, barbiturate poisoning has been divided into five classes as follows:

Class	Symptoms
0	Asleep but can be aroused and answer questions
I	Comatose but reacts to painful stimuli
II	Comatose; does not react to painful stimuli but basic reflexes present

III Comatose; no reflexes; not dangerously depressed respiration and circulation

IV Comatose; no reflexes; depressed respiration and circulation.

O TREATMENT

1 If the drug has been ingested within 4 hours, give the victim an emetic (syrup of ipecac if available) or induce vomiting by whatever means possible; wash out the stomach repeatedly by giving the victim large amounts of warm water to drink. As much of the barbiturate as possible must be removed. After 4 hours, lavage retrieves little drug and may be dangerous in semicomatose individuals.

2 Patients in Class 0 require little additional treatment except continued stimulation, such as forced walking, until intoxication wears off. All other classes should be removed to a hospital as soon as possible.

3 Administer artificial respiration by respirator (not endotracheal intubation), if possible using oxygen, in all but Class 0 cases during transport.

Through the use of mechanical respirators, which may have to be used for many days or even weeks, and intensive supportive therapy, including transfusion and the maintenance of fluid and electrolyte balance with the administration of at least 3,000 cubic centimeters of fluid a day, fewer cases are proving fatal. Though not entirely without the possibility of inducing further complications, "forced diuresis," using mannitol or other diuretic agent, is effective in removing four to six times as much barbiturate from the system as unassisted renal excretion. A. L. Linton et al., have shown that the type of diuretic used is of not such importance as maintenance of the electrolyte and fluid replacement.

O TREATMENT OF ADDICTION

The treatment of barbiturate addiction must be based on gradual withdrawal over a period of several weeks, preferably in a hospital. Many months are required for the body to return to its normal state and for the individual to completely recover from his barbiturate addiction. As a matter of fact, experts of the World Health Organization consider that the abstinence syndrome is the most characteristic and distinguishing feature of drug dependence of the barbiturate type. It begins to appear within the first 24 hours of cessation of drug taking, reaches a peak in intensity in 2 or 3 days, and subsides very slowly.

Two of the most dangerous features of the withdrawal syndrome are a precipitous drop in blood pressure on standing and convulsions of the "grand mal" type, in other words, convulsions which simulate those of a severe epileptic seizure. Delirium may also occur, which is similar to the delirium tremens which may accompany alcohol withdrawal.

As a rule, convulsions and delirium do not occur at the same time in the case of barbiturate withdrawal. Generally the patient may have one or two convulsions during the first 48 hours of withdrawal and then become actually psychotic during the second or third night. These psychotic episodes may be extremely serious and include paranoid reactions, reactions resembling schizophrenia with delusions and hallucinations, withdrawal into a semistuporous state, and even disorganized panic.

It should be emphasized, however, that the daily dose must be increased markedly above the usual therapeutic level before these severe symptoms will occur on withdrawal. Although the individual may develop a certain amount of psychic dependence on ordinary therapeutic doses, these usually can be reduced and ultimately withdrawn completely without any serious difficulty occurring.

O TREATMENT OF BARBITURATE WITHDRAWAL SYNDROME

Treatment should be undertaken in a hospital, preferably supervised by an anesthesiologist or other experienced clinician. In mildly or moderately addicted individuals, gradual reduction of the amount of barbiturate consumed may be all that is required.

In more severe cases, the addict is put on a known test dose of a barbiturate, usually pentobarbital, and observed 90 minutes later. The objective of administering the pentobarbital is not only to control the withdrawal symptoms but also to establish a mild intoxication which is manifested by a slow jerking movement of the eyeballs (nystagmus) on lateral gaze, slight disturbances of speech, and swaying but not actually falling in the Romberg (finger to nose) test.

If this end point is attained on the first test, 200 milligrams of pentobarbital is then given orally every 6 hours, with the patient being examined 90 minutes after each dose, since the pentobarbital itself has cumulative effects.   If the individual is still tremulous, agitated and twitching 90 minutes after the first dose, it was insufficient and additional drug must be given until the desired effect is achieved.

After the stabilization dose has been established, the patient is maintained on that dose for a day or two, after which the dose is slowly reduced in decrements of 100 milligrams or less daily until the patient ultimately is off barbiturates.   If the procedure is hastened too rapidly, untoward symptoms, such as a precipitous fall in blood pressure or high fever, will occur and the process must be begun over again.

Since death may result from too abrupt withdrawal, it is obvious that the withdrawal procedure must be undertaken in properly controlled clinical surroundings under the supervision of qualified personnel.

Once the patient is off the drug, social and phychological rehabilitation and stabilization are essential to minimize the chances of recurrence.

Synergism of Barbiturates and Alcohol

Special mention should be made of the dangers related to the concomitant use of alcohol and barbiturates.   Both drugs are strong depressants of central nervous system functions, and each potentiates the action of the other.   Hence a normal dose of 1 to 3 grains, depending upon the barbiturate used, which in the vast majority of cases would do nothing more than produce a desired degree of sleep, can produce a lethal effect in susceptible individuals *if alcohol is taken before or about the same time as the barbiturate*.   Even though the amount of alcohol consumed may not have been enough in itself to produce intoxication, alcohol, as has been said, is also a strong central nervous system depressant, and the combined effects of the barbiturate and alcohol become dangerously additive.

Many individuals overuse barbiturates as an escape mechanism from the problems of life which harass them, and these same individuals are also prone to use of alcohol.   The barbiturates are also used to combat the jittery aftereffects of drinking and to calm alcohol-produced restlessness and sleeplessness. Hence, it is commonly possible for these two extremely powerful drugs to be combined at the same time in the same individual—with very dangerous possibilities both for themselves and others.

It is also important to note that there is a definite and common syndrome of drug *dependence* of the *barbiturate-alcohol* type. This is characterized by the following criteria as summarized by the World Health Organization:

(a) Psychic dependence of varying degree that may lead to periodic rather than continuous abuse, especially with alcohol.

(b) The definite development of a physical dependence that generally can be detected only after the consumption of amounts considerably above the usual therapeutic or socially acceptable levels. Upon the reduction of intake below a critical level, a characteristic self-limited abstinence syndrome ensues, the symptoms of which, in the case of barbiturates, can be suppressed not only by a barbiturate-like agent but also, at least partially, by alcohol. The reverse situation exists in the case of alcohol.

(c) The development of tolerance which is irregular and incomplete, so that there is considerable persistence of behavioral disturbance dependent upon the pharmacodynamic effects of the drugs. There is a mutual, but incomplete, cross tolerance of some degree between alcohol and the barbiturates.

The problem of detoxifying the barbiturate-alcohol addict is a difficult one since the abrupt withdrawal of barbiturate can be fatal under certain circumstances. Treatment must be carried out in the hospital under carefully controlled clinical conditions.

Another consideration is that alcohol adversely potentiates the action of many commonly used drugs, often causing an ordinarily safe drug to have dangerous effects. For instance, the use of psychotherapeutic agents is widespread in this country; the number of individuals using various tranquilizers every day of their lives is on a scale comparable to or exceeding the use of barbiturates. Since these drugs exert strong effects on the brain, they can work in conjunction with alcohol so that the effect of each is greatly increased. It is quite possible for an individual who would normally be able to tolerate one or two drinks without showing any obvious effects to become drunk on the same amount of alcohol if he is on even the recommended dose of a tranquilizer.

The situation is made even more dangerous by the fact that many people believe that if one pill is good, two pills are twice as good and don't follow either their doctor's directions or the label on the bottle. They take more than is good or safe for them and thus get into real trouble.

Further difficulty is caused in the case of the tranquilizers by the fact that there is not only a mutual potentiation between the tranquilizer and alcohol, but the several commonly used tranquilizers *produce a marked lowering in the rate of excretion of the alcohol* from the blood, thus serving to prolong its toxic effects.

DRUG DEPENDENCE OF THE ALCOHOL TYPE

Acute alcoholic intoxication is, unfortunately, commonplace, and only rarely is it arrived at by accident, unless a lack of judgment on the part of the consumer of alcohol can be considered accidental. Frequently, a situation arises in which an intoxicated person requires emergency care. One large metropolitan hospital admits over 10,000 acute alcoholics a year.

Wortis has stated that: "Among the fatal acute poisons in this country, carbon monoxide ranks first and ethyl alcohol second. Deaths from acute alchoholism include many accident and traffic casualties, but about one-third are believed to be due to the direct toxicologic effect of alcohol."

Alcohol produces true drug dependence, both psychic and physical, and the development of tolerance is well known, although it is not as complete as in the case of morphine-like drugs. In this context alcohol is an addictive drug, but one which is socially countenanced in most societies and cultures.

Psychic dependence develops in all degrees and, as is the case with other dependence-producing drugs, is the result of the interrelationship between the pharmacodynamic effects of the drug—the major sites of action being the gastrointestinal tract and the central nervous system—and the personality complexes of the user.

Tolerance to alcohol develops along two lines. First, during continuous drinking there is an increase in the amount of alcohol required to maintain a given blood level; in addition, both psychological and physiological adaptation occurs so that in performance tests the chronic alcoholic is able to achieve a better rating and shows less impairment at a given alcohol blood concentration than a nonalcoholic individual.

Physical dependence occurs and results in a destructive withdrawal syndrome when alcohol is withheld or reduced below a critical level.

Epilepsy or delirium tremens may occur when alcohol is suddenly withdrawn from a chronic alcoholic. Alcoholic epilepsy, characterized by typical grand mal seizures (q.v.) but a normal electroencephalogram except during the actual seizure, may set in 6 to 48 hours after withdrawal. In about 30 percent of the cases this is followed by delirium tremens manifested by tremors, sweating, nausea, tachycardia, hyperreflexia, postural hypotension, and, in severe grades, convulsions and delirium. The last-mentioned condition is characterized by confusion, disorientation, delusions, and vivid visual hallucinations. The intensity of the alcohol abstinence syndrome probably varies with the duration and amount of alcohol intake. The mortality rate, when the alcohol abstinence syndrome is severe, averages at least 8 percent.

Miles has devised a scale relating the blood alcohol concentration to clinical intoxication in nonaddicted persons which may be summarized as follows:

TABLE 12-1

Blood level	Symptoms
30 mg/100 ml	= mild euphoria
50 mg/100 ml	= mild incoordination
100 mg/100 ml	= obvious ataxia
300 mg/100 ml	= stupor
400 mg/100 ml	= deep anesthesia, could prove fatal

It should be pointed out that while these figures are valid provided the blood alcohol concentration increases at a steady pace over a 2-hour period, they are not valid for the chronic alcoholic because of the marked tolerance which the chronic drinker develops so that he can drink more and show less effect than the uninitiated. Blood alcohol concentrations between 500 and 800 milligrams per milliter are fatal.

Mark Keller, editor of the *Quartely Journal of Studies on Alcohol,* in a personal communication, has pointed out that there is sound satistical evidence of the degree of involvement of alcohol in all types of accidents (in addition to auto accidents), including nonfatal ones and in the majority of accident fatalities.

In a study of driving and drinking, by Borkenstein, it was shown that the chances of being involved in a traffic accident go up steeply as the blood alcohol level rises above 0.05 percent. But the median blood alcohol concentrations of persons involved in automobile accidents in two areas (one in California, one in Ohio) studied by Hyman were 0.23 and 0.28 percent! These data at least raise the suspicion that any of these alcohol-accident involved people may be chronic alcoholics. A second accident involvement certainly enhances such a probability. Linnoila and Hakkinen have also shown that should the alcoholic driver also happen to be taking either codeine or diazepam (Valium®), driving ability is further impaired, particularly since diazepam increases the effects of alcohol.

Table 12-2 restates the effects of alcohol in terms of common-type drinks consumed, assuming an "average" 150-pound nonalcoholic person. The figures require adjustment on the basis of weight, the rapidity with which drinks are consumed, and hence the rate at which alcohol is accumulated in the system, and the amount of alcohol to which the individual is accustomed.

In a sense, the psychotoxic effects of alcohol are the result of the correlation between several factors—the sensitivity of the individual's central nervous system to alcohol, the amount and rate at which the alcohol is ingested, and the rate at which the alcohol is metabolized. Parker and others have also shown a strong relationship between alcohol and heart disease, producing a definite clinical entity known as alcoholic cardiomyopathy. Alcohol is absolutely contraindicated in such persons and probably should be withheld in cases of coronary thrombosis.

Alcohol is rapidly absorbed unaltered from the gastrointestinal tract—about 80 percent from the intestines and the rest from the stomach—and slowly excreted. Fatty food, milk, and water increase absorption rates. The average individual can metabolize about ⅓ ounce per hour.

The major portion of alcohol consumed is oxidized—

broken down into other chemicals, mostly acetaldehyde, acetic acid, carbon dioxide, and water—by the liver and to a lesser extent by other tissues. Two percent or less is lost through the kidneys, lungs, and skin. Alcohol can be detected in the blood 5 minutes after ingestion, and the maximum concentration is reached in from ½ to 2 hours. The energy of oxidation amounts to 7 calories per gram per hour; alcohol is used isodynamically by the body in the same manner as fats, sugar, and proteins.

Signs and Symptoms. The symptoms of intoxication are too well known to require enumeration, but one or two points should be emphasized. First, in dealing with an intoxicated person, it should not be forgotten that some other illness, such as diabetes, may also be present.

Besides being a local irritant when taken into the stomach in any sizable quantities, alcohol acts as a strong depressant on the central nervous system—not as a stimulant, as many people think. Because its effects are largely anesthetic in nature, an intoxicated person's inhibitions are removed early, and this is followed by gradual impairment of judgment.

The reflexes are slowed, and the more alcohol that is consumed, the greater is the impairment of coordination. It is for these reasons that driving ability becomes so profoundly affected; the victim's judgment and coordination—two absolute essentials to the proper operation of an automobile—are so disrupted that the individual is not capable of making the decisions required of him. It has been shown that a driver with a blood concentration of 155 milligrams per milliliter is 55 times more likely to have an accident than a nondrinking driver. As little as 40 milligrams per milliliter impairs driving ability in even an expert driver. And the worst of it is that the more intoxicated the person, the better he thinks he can drive.

As the rate of absorption of alcohol into the system gradually equals and then exceeds the rate at which the body can metabolize it, a toxic condition is reached which the victim can no longer physiologically withstand. At this point all the hilarity, joviality, euphoria, slurring speech, and other manifestations of drunken behavior subside. The depression of the central nervous system has now become so great that the stage of excitement has passed. The flushed countenance disappears, the victim turns white, breaks out into a cold sweat,

TABLE 12-2
SOME EFFECTS OF ALCOHOLIC BEVERAGES*

Amount of beverage	Concentration of alcohol attained in the blood	Effects	Time required for all alcohol to leave the body
1 highball (1½ oz whisky) or 1 cocktail (1½ oz whisky) or 3½ oz fortified wine or 5½ oz ordinary wine or 2 bottles (24 oz) beer	0.03%	Slight changes in feeling	2 hr
2 highballs or 2 cocktails or 7 oz fortified wine or 11 oz ordinary wine or 4 bottles beer	0.06%	Feeling of warmth—mental relaxation —slight decrease of fine skills—less concern with minor irritations and restraints	4 hr
		Increasing effects with variation among individuals and in the same individual	
3 highballs or 3 cocktails or 10½ oz fortified wine or 16½ oz (1 pt) ordinary wine or 6 bottles beer	0.09%	Buoyancy—exaggerated emotion and behavior—talkative, noisy or morose	6 hr

		at different times		
4 highballs or 4 cocktails or 14 oz fortified wine or 22 oz ordinary wine or 8 bottles (3 qts) beer	0.12%		Impairment of fine coördination—clumsiness—slight to moderate unsteadiness in standing or walking	8 hr
5 highballs or 5 cocktails or 17½ oz fortified wine or 27½ oz ordinary wine or ½ pt whisky	0.15%		Intoxication—unmistakable abnormality of gross bodily functions and mental faculties	10 hr

* Reproduced with permission from Greenberg, Leon A.: What the Body Does with Alcohol. Popular Pamphlets on Alcohol Problems, No. 4. Rutgers University, Center of Alcohol Studies, New Brunswick, N.J.

probably vomits, shows many signs of shock, and lapses into unconsciousness—he has "passed out."

In the average case, the victim will "sleep it off" after several hours; however, if the alcohol in the blood has reached toxic levels, a fatal outcome is possible, and immediate hospitalization is required.

○ TREATMENT

1 Induce vomiting, even if the victim has already vomited, in order to empty his stomach, and wash it out further with a solution of salt water (about 1 teaspoonful of salt to a quart) to get rid of any remaining alcohol and to soothe the inflamed lining of the stomach.

2 Follow with a large dose of epsom salts or other saline cathartic to purge the intestines.

3 Treat the victim as for shock (see Chap. 6), and keep him warm and out of drafts, as pneumonia readily develops in chronic alcoholics.

If the intoxication is severe, the victim will require intravenous fluids, especially saline and glucose solution, to restore the body's fluid balance and to help protect the liver against the toxic effects of the alcohol. It has also been suggested that fructose, rather than glucose, should be administered, since it seems that this sugar can speed up the metabolism of alcohol to some degree.

In the meantime, as a first-aid measure, stimulants may be tried in order to revive the victim and to get his cooperation. To do this, break an ampul of spirits of ammonia and hold it beneath his nose. As soon as he can swallow, give him a teaspoonful of aromatic ammonia in a glass of water; this stimulant has a surprisingly sobering effect in some cases. Hot black coffee with sugar should be given in quantity when consciousness returns.

No sedatives of any kind should be given, except under competent medical advice. The most satisfactory and safest drug for controlling maniacal degrees of intoxication is paraldehyde. It can be given by mouth (⅓ ounce in fruit juice or cold water) or as a retention enema (½ to 1 ounce in vegetable oil).

If the patient is in coma, no sedation should be given, but diuresis by the intravenous administration of mannitol should be evoked. In those cases in which the blood alcohol level is so high as to threaten life, hemodialysis has proved to be a life-saving measure.

As soon as the victim has recovered sufficiently, he should be given hot food, preferably hot cereal with plenty of sugar. This will help to soothe the inflamed lining of his stomach and intestinal tract (acute alcoholic gastroenteritis) and give him the energy he so badly needs.

A person under the influence of alcohol must be observed carefully and, if necessary, cared for. If he is conscious, he will undoubtedly resist your efforts to assist him. Great tact is essential in dealing with these cases. Under no circumstances let an intoxicated person convince you that he is "perfectly alright."

It should also be pointed out that in handling any case of alcoholic intoxication, consideration must be given to the fact that a great many drugs cause unusual or bizarre reactions when combined with alcohol, many of them increasing the effects of the alcohol or slowing its excretion from the body. Hence, one may not be treating a simple case of intoxication, but may be dealing with a combination of alcohol and, for example, any of several of the tranquilizers, oral antidiabetic agents, or other drugs.

One of the most pathetic problems of our times is the occurrence of delirium tremens in school children as the result of increasing alcoholism among those of almost all ages. Many of these are the children of alcoholic parents or the proverbial "social drinkers." So common is alcoholism among school children that Sherwin and Mead make the point that delirium tremens should at least be suspected in any school child exhibiting abnormal behavior patterns. The symptoms may even appear in little babies recently delivered of alcoholic mothers.

Somewhat along the same line, as shown by Hanson et al., is the so-called Fetal Alcoholic Syndrome, in which the child of the drinking mother may show a wide variety of birth defects, some of which may be difficult or impossible to correct, or may even require major surgery. In addition, following birth, the baby may suffer alcoholic withdrawal symptoms.

The Alcoholic Withdrawal Syndrome

As has already been indicated, there may follow the serious problem of the abstinence withdrawal syndrome, consisting of tremulousness, hallucinations, epileptic seizures, and delirium, the most grave of all being delirium tremens. This condition often occurs in the long-term excessive drinker who may have been admitted to a hospital as the result of an accident, or for an operation, or who develops some unrelated intercurrent infection or other illness (for which he perhaps may not have yet been hospitalized).

After 3 or 4 days without alcohol, delirium sets in and may last from a few days to several weeks. In about 80 percent of the cases, the duration with proper treatment is no more than 72 hours.

This and related withdrawal syndromes require hospitalization for adequate control and treatment. The symptoms can be relieved by the restoration of alcohol, but because of its relatively short duration of action, other equivalents are preferred. These include paraldehyde and various tranquilizers, especially chlorpromazine and chlordiazepoxide hydrochloride (Librium®) or diazepam (Valium®), probably the safest.

Supportive therapy includes the parenteral administration of fluids, the restoration of the acid base equilibrium, and the correction of respiratory alkalosis. There is some evidence that a deficiency of magnesium may be of significance in these cases and, if present, should be corrected; but there is also strong evidence that the respiratory alkalosis and hypoxia may be the major factor in the causation of the principal symptoms.

In addition to specific measures, a high caloric, high vitamin diet is of great importance in restoring the alcoholic's well-being.

DRUG DEPENDENCE OF THE MORPHINE TYPE

This type of dependency, commonly referred to as narcotic addiction, derives from the abuse of a group of drugs which are strong analgesics or pain killers, and all of which are strong central nervous system depressants.

Most of these drugs are related to morphine both in chemical structure and derivation. They include opium, morphine itself, hydromorphine (Dilaudid®), paregoric (camphorated tincture of opium), and, perhaps most important and dangerous of all, diacetyl morphine, the notorious heroin.

There are a number of other related drugs in this group, including meperidine (Demerol®) and codeine; these are not very likely to be abused since they have low addiction potentials, even though they are technically classed as narcotics.

The most dangerous and widely abused drug is heroin, which possibly exerts a more destructive influence on the user and on our society than any other drug. As in the case of all narcotics, a strong psychic dependence develops very early following its use and may even occur after only a single dose. There also develops a strong physical dependence which rapidly increases in intensity and is directly dose-related. This means that the drug user must keep taking larger and larger doses in order to maintain a relative degree of psychologic and physiologic equilibrium. If for one reason or another he cannot obtain his drug, the effect on the body is nothing short of disastrous and the withdrawal symptoms are overwhelming. It is this rapid development of tolerance which is one of the most striking features of heroin addiction and morphine-type dependence in general.

The problem is particularly acute in Vietnam and similar areas where pure heroin is readily available at extremely low cost ($3 a vial). The same amount and grade in this country would cost about $200 or more. Because of its high potency, the drug is responsible for a spiraling death rate as the result of overdosage. It is not unlikely that in time we may be confronted with the same type of problem in this country, economic and social factors permitting.

Heroin is usually taken by mixing into a solution and injecting into a vein. The drug quickly depresses certain areas of the brain and reduces hunger, thirst, and the sex drive. Because addicts usually have little appetite, malnutrition may be a severe secondary problem in this group of drug abusers.

Symptoms

The first emotional reaction to heroin is a reduction of tension, easing of fears, and relief from worry, resulting in a "high" which may be followed by a period of inactivity bordering on stupor.

It is not difficult to recognize the chronic narcotic users. The pinpoint pupils, which the addict often tries to conceal by means of dark tinted sunglasses, and the typical scars or pigmentation over readily accessible veins are characteristic. Sometimes the individual will have his arms tattooed in an attempt to conceal the puncture marks made by the needles which he uses to inject the drug.

Cases of nonfatal overdosage are seen with considerable regularity in the hospital emergency room. The condition should be suspected in any comatose or semicomatose individual showing evidence of severe central nervous system depression, respiratory depression, lowered blood pressure, and pinpoint pupils. There may be signs of acute pulmonary congestion leading to pulmonary edema, although the respiratory rate will paradoxically be slowed because of the severe depressant effect of the overdosage of the narcotic.

The telltale puncture marks or actual ulceration from infected needle sites are a dead giveaway to the patient's condition (Fig. 12-1).

In addition to indolent local infection resulting from the use of filthy needles, it has been stated by the U.S. Public Health Service that drug addicts, as the result of using unsterilized needles, share a major responsibility for the worst outbreak of hepatitis in our nation's history.

A further pathetic difficulty arises when a baby is born of an addicted mother. Following birth the baby must suffer terrible withdrawal pangs, although modern treatment may ease the symptoms somewhat.

O TREATMENT OF ACUTE NARCOTIC INTOXICATION

From an emergency medical point of view, the two major problems which arise in connection with narcotic addiction are the effects of acute intoxication and the development of withdrawal symptoms.

If the overdose has been great enough, the victim will be in shock and require specific antishock methods. Severe respiratory depression also must be treated promptly by either manual or mechanical means such as by the use of a respirator, and by the use of a narcotic antagonist such as nalorphine (Nalline®) in a dose of 2 to 10 milligrams, or levallorphan tartrate (Lorfan®) in a dose of 1 milligram. Both of these drugs are given intravenously.

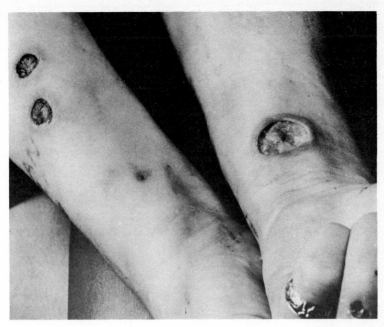

Fig. 12-1. Localized ulcerations on the forearm of a heroin addict due to mixed infection as result of using unsterilized and unclean needles to inject the drug. (Reproduced, with permission, from Birdwood, George: A Pill for the Maladies of Society? *Wld. Med. J. 17*(2): 26–31, 1970.)

The response is usually dramatic, with an increase in the respiratory rate and dilatation of the pupils. Both of these drugs must be used carefully for two reasons: (1) too large a dose may precipitate an acute abstinence syndrome, and (2) narcotic antagonists are metabolized rapidly in the body and the dose may have to be repeated at relatively short intervals to maintain the respiratory rate until the opiate itself has been metabolized.

Withdrawal Symptoms

The typical withdrawal syndrome sets in approximately 18 hours from the last dose of narcotic. The intensity of the symptoms will vary according to the degree of addiction. The main characteristic is that it involves all major areas of nervous activity, including marked changes in the behavior pattern of the individual, and excitation of all components of the autonomic nervous system as well as those of the central and somatic systems.

The symptoms themselves include all degrees of anxiety, restlessness, generalized body aches and pains, acute insomnia, yawning, running of the eyes and nose, excessive sweating, dilated pupils, gooseflesh, hot flushes, vomiting and diarrhea, fever, markedly increased respiratory rate accompanied by a rise in blood pressure, severe abdominal and muscular cramps, dehydration (excessive loss of fluid), severe loss of appetite, and a concomitant loss in body weight.

O TREATMENT OF WITHDRAWAL SYNDROME

The specific treatment of the withdrawal syndrome is methadone hydrochloride, along with suitable sedatives and tranquilizers when these are indicated.   Diazepam (Valium®) has been found to be quite effective and may do almost as well as methadone in controlling withdrawal symptoms.   Propoxyphene napsylate (Darvon-N®) has been found useful.   A number of other specific agents are currently under extensive clinical investigation, in the hope of extending the dose interval and lessening the "cheating" by some addicts who take heroin as well as the methadone or other detoxifying drug.

Methadone is a narcotic-type drug which has powerful analgesic effects comparable to those of morphine.   Its usefulness in the treatment of heroin addiction results from the fact that it blocks the euphoric effects of heroin and the craving for the drug without producing the extremely deleterious effects characteristic of heroin addiction.   Methadone is itself addicting, but somewhat less so than either heroin or morphine, and its use must be carefully supervised.   However, since it does not exert the ill effects of heroin and related drugs, it can be effectively used in helping to restore an addict to a normal life and eventually, it is hoped, free him of his addiction.   In addition, unlike the other narcotics, methadone exerts a long-lasting effect when given by mouth and does not have the drawback of having to be injected.   It probably offers the best hope for the successful treatment of heroin addiction presently available.

Generally speaking, the usual dose of methadone is 10 to 20 milligrams given orally for a total of 40 to 60 milligrams the first day.   Each day thereafter the dose is reduced by 5 or 10 milligrams, so that after a week or 10 days the patient should be relatively symptom-free without the administration of the drug to which he had become addicted, but treatment may have to be continued over a much longer period.

The use of methadone itself is not without hazard, and it is often overprescribed in the detoxification of opiate addicts. Medication should be limited to the use of oral dosage forms. While dosage must be patient-related, the dangers of methadone overdosage cannot be too strongly stressed, and urine monitoring is required to indicate possible concomitant use of other drugs which can lead to dangerous cumulation.

Methadone is still classed as an experimental drug when it is used in the *maintenance* of narcotic addicts. It may be used legally for this purpose *only* by investigators who have an effective Investigational New Drug Application granted by the Federal Food and Drug Administration. However, it has recently been announced that the Food and Drug Administration plans to sanction increased use of methadone as a substitute for heroin, although arguments still rage as to its true fundamental value in bringing about permanent detoxification. To this end, maintenance treatment of patients 18 years and older with oral dosage forms of methadone will be available at some 450 drug addiction centers throughout the United States. The drug will be available only in approved centers and hospital pharmacies. The restrictions do not preclude the use of methadone for severe pain or for the detoxification of addicts in hospitals.

In order to avoid iatrogenic addiction, it is imperative, before selecting a patient for treatment, to determine unequivocally that he is indeed a helpless addict. For the youngster who merely experiments with drugs or may be only acutely intoxicated, other forms of treatment should be utilized.

All addicts do not respond adequately to methadone maintenance. The rate of failure is lowest among those addicts who show sincere motivation to free themselves from their addiction, and those who believe that methadone represents a real solution to their problems.

Unfortunately, many narcotic-dependent individuals are also addicted to barbiturates, the withdrawal symptoms of which may be even more difficult and critical to treat than those of narcotic addiction, as has already been discussed. In such a case, of course, the barbiturate addiction must be treated as well as the narcotic addiction along lines already suggested.

A relative newcomer to the drug abuse field is oxymorphone-hydrochloride (Numorphan®). This is a synthetic opiate produced by Endo Laboratories, Inc., Garden City, New York. Illicit traffic in this narcotic is on the increase.

An increasing number of opiate addicts have sought prescriptions for this drug from physicians, and Numorphan® tablets have already found their way into the black market under the nickname of "blues," presumably because of the blue color of the tablets. "Blues" are traded for approximately $2 per tablet.

Addicts state that the "high" obtained by injecting Numorphan® is "as good or better" than the euphoria produced by heroin. While intended legitimately for parenteral use, rectal suppositories and oral tablets are also manufactured, and the latter are apparently easiest to obtain. At any rate, the most common form of abuse is with the oral tablet, which is dissolved in water, brought to a short boil, and then injected intravenously.

The drug is about ten times more potent on a milligram-for-milligram basis than morphine. It is addictive and leads to the development of tolerance with prolonged usage. As with morphine and related compounds, *nalorphine* is an effective antidote in the event of overdosage.

Medical authorities feel that the narcotic addict is essentially a sick person who is in desperate need of help to keep him from reverting to his drug abuse after his acute symptoms of physical addiction and withdrawal illness have been relieved.

It is for that reason that the most difficult part of treatment comes after the individual is out of the hospital, since drug taking may have become a way of life for him, including the friends he has and the kind of job he can get. His personality has been abused and distorted; a fresh start in life for such an individual is far more difficult than for one recovering from an ordinary illness.

The narcotic addiction problem affects everyone in every walk of life, whether he is an addict or not, and has a tremendous social impact on our society.

A summary of essential data concerning the most commonly abused drugs appears in Table 12-3.

TABLE 12-3

SUMMARY OF COMMONLY ABUSED DRUGS

Abused Drug	Slang Name†	Drug Description	How Used	Principal Effects	Signs and Symptoms of Acute Intoxication	Withdrawal Syndrome	Principal Treatment
Marijuana (Cannabis): Hashish Tetrahydro-cannabinol	Joints; sticks; reefers; weed; grass; pot; muggles; mooters; Indian hay; locoweed; mu; giggle-smoke; griffo; mohasky; Mary Jane	Marijuana is the dried flowering or fruiting top of the plant Cannabis Sativa L, commonly called Indian hemp. Looks like fine, green tobacco. Active principle is tetra-hydrocannabinol. Hashish is a powerful preparation of cannabis	Smoked in pipes or cigarettes, or taken as a tea. Hashish is infrequently made into candy, sniffed in powder form, mixed with honey or butter	A feeling of great perceptiveness and pleasure, even with small doses. Erratic behavior, loss of memory, distortion of time and spatial perceptions, and hilarity without apparent cause. Marked unpredictability of effect	Pupils normal; conjunctivae red; tachycardia and postural hypotension. Sensorium often clear; distortion of perception and body image. Hallucinations rare	No specific syndrome	No specific treatment. Avoid drug therapy if possible, because of adverse reactions with possible adulterant. Chlorpromazine may be used cautiously in severe cases, but better to let effect of marijuana wear off alone with only psychic support
Hallucinogens: Lysergic acid diethyl-amide Psilocybin Mescaline	LSD; acid; "25"; Mushrooms; mescal button; mescal beans; cactus; button; bad seed; Mesc	LSD-25 is a lysergic acid derivative. Mescaline is extracted from peyote cactus. Psilocybin is synthesized	In tablet, capsule, ampul (hypodermic) form or in saturated sugar cubes	All produce hallucinations, exhilaration, or depression, and can lead to serious mental changes, psychotic manifestations	Pupils dilated, reactive to light; blood pressure elevated; tendon reflexes hyperactive; sweating; goose-	No specific syndrome	Largely supportive with reassurance and protection until effects wear off. A "bad trip" can be ended

TABLE 12-3 (continued)

Abused Drug	Slang Name[†]	Drug Description	How Used	Principal Effects	Signs and Symptoms of Acute Intoxication	Withdrawal Syndrome	Principal Treatment
Dimethoxy-4-methyl-amphetamine Dimethyl-tryptamine	STP DMT	from Mexican mushrooms. STP and DMT are synthetic		festations, suicidal or homicidal tendencies	flesh. Anxiety; sensorium often clear; distortion of body image and of sensory perception; kaleidoscopic visual hallucinations; delusions		quickly by the cautious use of chlorpromazine or diazepam. Latter may be safer because of the danger of anticholinergic adulterants. Physostigmine counteracts anticholinergic crisis
Cocaine	The leaf; snow; speedball (when mixed with heroin)	Extracted from the leaves of the coca bush. White, odorless, fluffy powder; looks like crystalline snow	A surface-active anesthetic taken orally by abusers or, most commonly, intravenously alone, combined or alternating with heroin. Coca leaves are also chewed with	Oral use said to relieve hunger and fatigue, and produce some exhilaration. Intravenous use produces marked psychotic effects, hallucinations with paranoid tendencies. Repetitive	Dilated pupils, hyperactive, exhilarated paranoia. Convulsions and death may occur from overdose. Very strong psychic but no physical dependence and no tolerance (tachyphylaxis)	None	No specific treatment. Sodium pentobarbital is used if patient is severely hallucinating, to produce necessary sedation. In extreme cases, morphine may be required

				doses lead to maniacal excitation, muscular twitching, convulsive movements		
			lime, producing the effects of the contained cocaine			
Amphetamine	Bennies; copilots; footballs; hearts; pep pills	Amphetamines are stimulants, prescribed chiefly to reduce appetite and to relieve minor depression. Often used to promote wakefulness and/or increase energy	Orally as a tablet or capsule. Abusers may resort to intravenous injection	Normal doses produce wakefulness, increased alertness, and a feeling of increased initiative. Intravenous doses produce cocaine-like psychotic effects. Amphetamines can cause hypertension, abnormal heart rhythms and even heart attacks. Excess or prolonged usage can cause hallucinations, loss of weight, wakefulness, jumpiness and dangerous aggressiveness.	Pupils dilated, reactive to light; blood pressure elevated; cardiac arrhythmia; reflexes hyperactive; dry mouth; sweating; shallow respiration; high fever; circulatory collapse. Sensorium usually clear in milder cases; in severe cases, confusion, paranoid ideation, stereotyped activity, irritability, and aggressive behavior especially after "speed" injections	Classical physical dependence does not occur; "withdrawal" symptoms, such as somnolence, muscle aches, ravenous hunger, depression and apathy, do	Largely supportive until effects of drug wear off. Chlorpromazine is given cautiously for the more severe cases. If necessary, Dibenzyline® is used to combat a hypertensive crisis. In critical cases, dialysis is a lifesaving measure

TABLE 12-3 (continued)

Abused Drug	Slang Name†	Drug Description	How Used	Principal Effects	Signs and Symptoms of Acute Intoxication	Withdrawal Syndrome	Principal Treatment
				Tolerance and psychic dependence develop readily; no physical dependence. No characteristic withdrawal syndrome			
Methamphetamine	Speed; crystal; "meth"; splash	Stimulant, closely related to amphetamine and ephedrine	Orally, as tablets or in an elixir, or intravenously ("speeding")	Effects resemble amphetamine but are more marked, with extreme exhilaration, and toxicity greater. Produces an intense "high" of short duration when used intravenously. Repetitive dosage produces dangerous effects	Extreme restlessness and irritability; violence and paranoid reaction possible	Similar to amphetamine, but with excessive psychotoxic effects, sometimes with fatal outcome	Same as for amphetamine, but therapeutic demands may be even more critical

| Central nervous system depressants: Barbiturates: Pento-barbital Seco-barbital Amobar-bital Amo-seco-barbital mixture

Various tran-quilizers | Yellow jackets Red devils Blue heavens

Rainbows | Barbiturates are sedatives, prescribed to induce sleep or, in smaller doses, to provide a calming effect. Legally restricted to prescription use. Dependence producing both psychic and physical, with variable tolerance. Signs of physical dependence appear with doses well above therapeutic level | Orally as a tablet or capsule. Sometimes intravenously by drug abusers | Small amounts make the user relaxed, sociable, good-humored. Heavy doses make him sluggish, gloomy, sometimes quarrelsome. His speech is thick and he staggers. Sedation and incoordination progressive with dose, and at least additive with alcohol and/or other sedatives and tranquilizers. Such mixtures may be extremely dangerous and even lethal | Pupils normal; blood pressure and respiration depressed; nystagmus on lateral gaze; tendon reflexes depressed; shock; slurred speech. The appearance of drunkenness with no odor of alcohol characterizes heavy dose. Confusion may cause unintentional repetitious administration to a toxic level. Potentiation with alcohol particularly hazardous. Sedation with variable ataxia. Coma and death from respiratory failure | Tremulousness; insomnia; high fever; clonic blink reflex; convulsive seizures; cardiovascular collapse. Agitation; delirium; psychosis. Barbiturates are addictive, causing physical as well as psychic dependency. Characteristic withdrawal syndrome differs from opiate syndrome | Addiction: Gradual withdrawal over several weeks Acute withdrawal symptoms: Restoration of maintenance dose followed by carefully controlled withdrawal Acute poisoning: Gastric lavage only if drug has been taken orally within 4 hours. Maintain airway; prolonged artificial respiration; antishock procedures. Plasma expanders or whole blood. All supportive procedures |

TABLE 12-3 (continued)

Abused Drug	Slang Name†	Drug Description	How Used	Principal Effects	Signs and Symptoms of Acute Intoxication	Withdrawal Syndrome	Principal Treatment
Narcotics: Heroin Morphine Codeine Opium Hydromorphone (Dilaudid®) Many others	Snow; stuff; H; junk; M; dreamer; many others Schoolboy Lords	Heroin is diacetylmorphine, an alkaloid derived from morphine; it does not occur in opium. A white, off-white, or brown crystalline powder, it has long been the drug of choice among opiate addicts. Its possession is illegal. Morphine is the principal active component of opium. Morphine sulphate: white crystalline powder, light porous cubes or small white tablets.	May be taken by any route, usually by intravenous injection	Heroin is like morphine in all respects except faster, more powerful and shorter acting. Powerful central nervous system depressant and analgesic	Pupils pinpoint, fixed; blood pressure and respiration depressed; coma; shock; pulmonary edema, with slow, shallow respiratory movement. Sensorium depressed, although some patients may be alert and appear normal	Pupils dilated, reactive to light; pulse rate, blood pressure, temperature, and respiratory rate elevated; muscular aches and twitches; nausea; vomiting; diarrhea; dehydration; chills; rhinorrhea; lacrimation; gooseflesh; yawning; extreme restlessness followed by sleep	Acute intoxication: Counteract respiratory depression with Nalline® or Lorfan® intravenously. Antishock treatment required Withdrawal symptoms: Methadone is specific. Diazepam also effective in providing sedation and partial relief of most symptoms

Codeine is a
component of
opium and a
derivative of
morphine, in
most respects
a tenth or less
as effective as
morphine,
dose-wise

* This table was prepared, with additions, from material contained in *The Medical Letter*, Vol. 12, No. 16, Aug. 7, 1970, and in "A Guide
to Some Drugs Which Are Subject to Abuse," published by the American Social Health Association, September, 1970.

† Generally speaking, so many vernacular slang terms are used that only the most common are given here.

MISCELLANEOUS DRUG DEPENDENCE

A drug which in recent years has found favor along the street is *methaqualone,* the abuse of which has been reviewed extensively by Inaba et al. The drug was introduced many years ago by the William H. Rorer Company under the name of Quaalude® as a prescription drug. It is now known by a variety of slang terms such as "love drug," "heroin for lovers," "luding out," and many others. The Food and Drug Administration has recently placed it in Schedule II, which makes prescriptions for it nonrefillable.

It is questionable whether the many promotional claims made for it as a nonaddicting barbiturate can be justified; in all probability, it does produce addiction or drug dependence, with subsequent withdrawal symptoms, as has been reported by several authors. Its alleged aphrodisiac properties appear to be largely a figment of the imagination.

Since many addicts also use other drugs such as heroin, acute detoxification must be handled carefully. The most useful drugs for this purpose seem to be phenobarbital, diazepam (Valium®), and aloxone hydrochloride.

Ketamine is another drug that is finding favor along the street, although on a somewhat more limited basis. It is an intravenous anesthetic used in *human* surgery and produces hallucinations during the recovery period which are indeed psychedelic in nature. Unfortunately, the author can vouch for this since it was administered to him during a surgical procedure, and the results were most unpleasant!

On the street, the drug is usually taken by mouth. Shaffer states that for treatment a barbiturate or diazepam may be administered cautiously as necessary during the emergency period when there may be strong hallucinating, but otherwise cough and gag reflexes and the usual vital signs are not depressed.

Phenycylidine is a *veterinary* anesthetic and tranquilizer marketed under the trade name Sernylan®. It appears to be readily available to drug abusers and its misuse appears to be increasing. In general, as pointed out by both Tong et al. and Lidin et al., it produces symptoms, not unlike those of epilepsy, accompanied by pinpoint pupils, acute psychosis, drowsiness, hypertension, marked agitation, and a variety of signs suggesting central nervous system involvement. The onset of symptoms begins about 2 to 4 hours postingestion, sometimes as early as 30 minutes.

Treatment consists of supportive measures, together with the judicious use of phenytoin (Dilantin®), phenobarbital, or diazepam by injection.

Another drug which may be dangerous, but is not widely abused in the usual sense, is propoxyphene hydrochloride (Darvon®). Sturner and Garriott reviewed the literature and reported 41 cases, including deaths, over a 2-year period.

Indiscriminate use of this drug is obviously dangerous—the author has seen a severe reaction following the prescribed ingestion of one capsule; the drug should never be used following the ingestion of alcohol.

Treatment is supportive; many cases can be "talked down" until the effects of the Darvon® wear off, and medication should not be used unless specifically indicated. As indicated by Fraser, the prescribed antidotes are nalaxone hydrochloride, or levallorphan tartrate (Lorfan®).

Tricyclic Drugs. This dangerous class of drugs, containing a large group of antidepressant drugs which has been extensively reviewed by Arena and by Burks et al., has great importance in treating children as well as adults. It includes such well-known names as Aventyl® (nortriptyline), Elavil® (amitriptyline), Norpramin® (desipramine), Pertofrane® (desipramine), Tofanil® (imipramine), Vivactil® (protriptyline), and others which are not yet well-known.

These drugs may produce cardiac arrhythmias, heart block and other marked disturbances which show up on an electrocardiogram. In addition, there are other signs simulating acute atropine poisoning; these include excessive thirst, vomiting, drowsiness, dizziness, bowel and bladder dysfunction, and other generalized symptoms including weird movements of the extremities, convulsions and disturbances of blood pressure. The most serious period occurs during the first 12 hours postpoisoning. In cases of overwhelming poisoning, death may occur very rapidly, before any treatment can be effective.

O TREATMENT

Supportive treatment is essential, with special attention to the control of cardiac arrythymias. Arena, and Burks et al., agree that physostigmine is the specific antidote of choice. The preparation used by Burks et al. is marketed, under the name Antilirium®, by O'Neal, Jones & Feldman, Inc., 1304 Asby Road, St. Louis, Missouri 63132, and is a mixture of physostigmine salicylate, sodium bisulfite and benzyl alcohol.

It is reported that all signs, including coma, are temporarily reversed within a few moments following intravenous injection of physostigmine, but the dose must be repeated as frequently as necessary until symptoms abate. When the case appears to be life-threatening, the drug is repeated at short intervals in order to maintain life.

13 Emergencies of Infancy and Childhood

Many emergencies arise during the early years of life. Some of them are accidental and are largely preventable; others arise from natural causes and are only partly preventable. For some emergencies, there are certain definite first-aid measures which not only may keep a child alive until medical aid can be obtained, but, sometimes, may even avoid the necessity for medical aid.

In some emergencies medical aid might not be immediately available for any one of various reasons, as, for instance, a storm, a disaster, or the more urgent conditions of other patients; therefore, it is most important to know how to provide proper care for a stricken child, for in few other areas of emergency care can doing the wrong thing work more harm.

Assessing the Situation

Any situation involving a hazardous emergency in childhood is, admittedly, the more difficult because of the understandable emotional concern for the child's welfare. Yet, an objective and realistic attitude will not only do much to reassure the child and help him to minimize the seriousness of his illness, but will accomplish much more for the child's actual welfare. Therefore, it is important that the parents or relatives view the situation objectively and, with as little emotionalism as possible, do whatever may be immediately indicated, call a pediatrician, or get the child to a hospital promptly.

When the doctor is called, give him the facts as clearly and concisely as possible. Many emergencies are not as bad as they seem, and if your doctor has the facts, he may be able to tell you, over the telephone, what to do before he can see the patient. He will also be in a better position to know what special equipment or drugs might be needed and will be better able to judge correctly the urgency of the emergency and act accordingly.

Recognizing Illness

It is of extreme importance to both teachers and parents to be able to recognize, in advance, signs of illness in a child, in order to prevent a critical condition or even death. While many illnesses appear to strike with suddenness, there are often preliminary warnings which may be apparent for several hours or days before the main signs and symptoms of the disease appear.

How many children have been permitted to remain at school when they are already half sick or coming down with an acute intestinal upset, measles, or some other contagious disease! There is danger here not only to the sick child, but to his schoolmates; yet to the careful observer, clear-cut warning signs are almost always present and should be heeded when first observed, not when the child has been taken suddenly and acutely ill that night or the next day. Nowhere does the ancient admonition "He that has eyes to see, let him see" more aptly apply.

One of the earliest and most important signs that should always arouse suspicion is the change from a normally bright and happy child to one who looks peaked and seems to be a little dull, apathetic, listless, and, perhaps, irritable.

Perhaps his eyes are bloodshot and the lids slightly swollen; perhaps he has a running nose. Although these signs may indicate nothing more than an ordinary cold, the bloodshot eyes should suggest the possibility of measles—a possibility which would be even greater if his body temperature were much above normal and if measles were prevalent in the area.

Often, children will vomit suddenly and without warning; this can be the first apparent sign of an impending acute illness, which may be anything from an acute septic sore throat to meningitis, but vomiting is too often dismissed simply as an "upset stomach."

Fever is one of the most important signs of impending acute illness. Fever is universally recognized as an indication of disease and in most cases the relationship between an existing disease and the fever it causes is obvious. A child with measles runs a fever, or a person with pneumonia runs a fever, and the relationship is clear-cut and obvious.

In many instances, however, the relationship of the existence of disease to the presence of fever is not obvious, and it often takes medical detective work to discover the underlying causes of the fever.

Children, for instance, will sometimes run a fairly high fever for 3 or 4 days at a time without any obvious symptoms, and without any serious restriction on their activities. Very often no obvious cause can be found for such a rise in temperature and, while a detailed diagnostic search might turn up the cause for the increased temperature, the condition may correct itself before anything definite can be found and the justified alarm of the parents at the child's high temperature often has proved groundless. Sometimes the fever subsides, the child breaks out with the typical rash of roseola and solves the whole problem for everybody. However, the outcome may not always be so gratifying, so that any fever of significant duration should, of course, be investigated.

Some newborns may run a high transitory fever, particularly breast-fed infants. This is not indicative of any particular disease condition; since it is very readily corrected by the administration of suitable amounts of fluid, it is often referred to as dehydration fever.

In spite of these simple examples, however, there are many situations in which fever may be present over long periods of time and be caused by some serious underlying disease which for one reason or another has proved difficult to discover. Often the child or adult may run a low-grade fever without realizing it, other than possibly feeling dragged out and easily fatigued.

There are many hundreds of causes of fever; discovering the cause of a fever is not always an easy process, but it is always an important one. No one runs a fever "normally," and if a rise in body temperature persists for more than a few days or recurs at periodic intervals, a relentless search must be undertaken to discover its origin, as protection against the possibility of the existence of some serious disease.

Abdominal pain is another of the most important medical symptoms, since certain types of pain may signal that something is seriously wrong with any of the organs lying within the abdominal cavity. Often the type and distribution of the pain, along with other associated symptoms, will give a clue as to where the difficulty lies.

It is quite possible to have rather severe generalized abdominal pain as the result of various disorders which, while they may be serious, are not necessarily life-threatening nor require surgical treatment. Such conditions would commonly include acute allergy to food, various types of food poisoning, and even such relatively mild infections as the so-called "intestinal flu."

Abdominal pain is generally categorized as upper or lower in location, and dull, sharp, or crampy in nature. It is also important to know whether the pain is localized or whether it radiates to some other portion of the body through adjoining nerves. In children these facts are sometimes difficult to ascertain.

In a child suffering with appendicitis the pain starts in the pit of the stomach, gradually shifting to the lower right side, with accompanying acute tenderness and rigidity of muscles in the lower right of the abdomen (see page 554). Also, he may have complained previously of tiredness, and loss of appetite, and had some degree of nausea, vomiting, and slight diarrhea or constipation.

In very young children, acute abdominal pain raises the question of another intestinal condition known as intussusception (see page 464). In this condition, the symptoms consist of a very severe cramp-like abdominal pain which is much greater than that ever accompanying the ordinary gastrointestinal upset. There is usually prostration and vomiting, followed by loose bowel movements which at first contain mucus and then pure blood.

Diseases of the urinary system, which strictly speaking is not in the abdominal cavity, can cause most excruciating abdominal pain; so can infections of the lungs, such as pneumonia.

While some types of abdominal pain are characteristic of

the underlying disorder, the diagnosis of abdominal pain may be extremely involved, subtle, and complex, particularly in children. Although abdominal pain may or may not be serious, it should never be neglected as a symptom.

Other warning signs include persistent sneezing, a dry, hacking cough, chills (or a constant complaint of chilliness), a flushed face (indicating fever), hoarseness or a sore throat, generalized muscular aches, an earache, dizziness, and headache.

If the youngster shows only one or two of these symptoms, nothing very serious may be wrong, but, if several are present, it is better to do some checking up. Put the child to bed, for a while at least, take his temperature, and take a good look at his general appearance. For instance, are any rashes beginning to show or is he having any trouble breathing? Also, if he has vomited, does he have pain anywhere? Epidemic vomiting (caused by a virus), for instance, is not usually accompanied by real pain; appendicitis usually is. When in doubt, call a physician and let him be the judge of whether anything is seriously wrong.

Chronic illness may have a more serious and permanently damaging effect on a child than many of the run-of-the-mill acute illnesses, since a chronic condition may long go unnoticed while the child gradually falls behind at school, becoming the butt of ridicule and social neglect. A chronic illness works physical changes which, by the time they are noticed, may be irreparable.

For instance, persistent sores at the corners of his mouth may very well be the result of a severe vitamin B deficiency which can seriously impair the child's health and general efficiency if his diet has been substandard or otherwise inadequate. In the well nourished child, such sores (cheilosis) may more likely be due to allergy, or a yeast or fungus infection.

Many children are "mouth breathers." The commonest cause of this condition is enlarged adenoids, which when they are infected, as they often are, make the child irritable, listless, subject to night terrors, and physically and mentally inadequate. Enlarged infected adenoids are also the commonest cause of infected ears and partial or complete deafness in children. The child may also suffer attacks of dizziness for the same reason. The cause of mouth breathing should always be carefully investigated.

Often, one or more lumps, or swellings, in the neck may be visible. These are most often due to swelling of deep-lying structures known as *lymph glands,* indicating chronic infection in the throat, of the scalp, or sometimes an even more serious condition. There are many other signs too numerous to mention. It is well known, for example, that a child with cross-eyes is suffering under a tremendous handicap; a deaf child, equally or more so. If a child is not doing well at school or has behavior problems, is he partially deaf or suffering from eye trouble? Find out. Is he overweight or underweight? Is his posture bad? These physical conditions don't just happen; there are always reasons for them. It is the obligation of every parent and of every teacher—and of everyone else responsible for the care of children—to observe them constantly and, when something out of the ordinary is noted, to seek sound medical advice. By so doing, you may not only save a life, but you will certainly help to make it a healthier and happier one for the child.

School Emergencies

There are, of course, some emergencies for which there are few, if any, measures that can be taken by an untrained person, but for which prompt medical aid is essential. These are mentioned here only to emphasize the importance of being able to recognize that an emergency exists and, hence, obtain proper treatment for the child. Such emergencies frequently arise during school hours, so that a teacher must be alert to recognize an acutely ill child, or one, on the other hand, who is simply malingering.

Needless to say, the teacher must be backed up by an effectively organized system for handling such emergencies whenever and wherever they arise, either on the school premises or on the way to or from school if the school system is responsible for the child's transportation.

Such a system must also provide some sort of simple data retrieval mechanism that will provide immediately available information with respect to each child's health situation, including any special health abnormalities which a child may have, such as diabetes, epileptic tendencies, severe allergies, abnormal heart condition, or another physical disability. The teacher or some other individual to whom the responsibility is specifically assigned should be able to notify immediately someone whom the child's family has designated, often the family doctor, in the event that the child does meet with a sudden acute illness or has an accident. Other background information is, of course, essential and includes such routine items as the home address, home phone number, the business address, business phone number, if any, along with previously agreed-upon specific instructions as to what the parents desire to be done in the event of an emergency.

In addition, the emergency setup should provide some means of lessening the burden placed on the teacher by specifying, and providing for their automatic notification, one or more individuals on the school staff who have had basic first-aid training to assist in the handling of whatever emergency comes up. Often such an individual would be the school nurse, but in large establishments it has been found effective to have specially trained first-aid squads throughout the school who are immediately available and will be able to assist in handling the early phases of the emergency. A precise procedure should be set up which can be routinely followed like clock work. Through the use of such a system, the child's best health interests are protected, and much lost motion and excitement are avoided. It is further recommended that regular drills be held with various simulated emergencies, much as fire drills or civil defense drills are held periodically, so that when the real thing comes aong, there won't be any slip-ups.

Many emergencies of childhood are the result of some kind of injury. In this country, about 12,000 children die accidentally each year; 40,000 to 50,000 are permanently injured; and about 1,000,000 come under medical care as the result of some sort of accident. Most of these accidents are not the fault of the children, but are preventable by the parents, through proper education and discipline of their children and simple measures designed to keep the young child from hurting himself.

Many accidents, although similar to those which may occur in adult life, are, in some of their aspects, peculiar to childhood; therefore, their emergency care is the concern of every parent, teacher, or any other person who may have the responsibility for the safety and welfare of young children.

HEAD INJURIES

One of the most common emergencies of childhood is severe head injury, usually as a result of falling. Because of the thinner bony structure of the skull, there is greater likelihood of brain damage, and children with head injuries go into shock very easily. Any damage sustained may be aggravated by improper handling; for this reason, it is absolutely essential that the first-aider, in handling a case of injury in childhood, *do nothing* until he is sure what is the right thing to do.

No head injury in a child, however trivial it may seem, should be neglected. In any case of doubt, adequate x-ray studies should be made. A period of close medical observation is mandatory in order to determine the extent of possible damage to the brain and to be sure that serious symptoms do *not* develop 24 or more hours after injury.

Simple Concussion. A simple concussion does not involve any permanent organic damage to the brain, and the child recovers completely after a period of unconsciousness or semi-consciousness (see page 52).

Congestion of the Brain. A more severe type of injury is congestion of the brain, with actual swelling of the injured brain tissues, which causes definite symptoms, including drowsiness or unconsciousness, nausea and vomiting, severe headache, and shock.

Brain Contusion. Brain contusion represents an actual bruise of the brain and may be serious, since the child may not only go into profound shock, but may suffer consequential aftereffects.

Any of the more serious degrees of brain damage may or may not be accompanied by a fracture of the skull, but this condition should always be suspected and looked for. Certain types of skull fractures urgently require surgery.

From the standpoint of emergency care, any head injury in a child must be taken seriously, although he may only have received—and by the law of averages, probably only *has* received—an ordinary "bump on the head." In such a case, however, he probably will not be unconscious. If the child is a little groggy or is actually unconscious, he may or may not have a serious injury, but he should be treated as if he had.

Under no circumstances should the child be allowed to get up and walk around, nor should any attempt be made to restore consciousness by any such means as slapping him. It does not seem that it should be necessary to say this, but it has actually been tried—with disastrous consequences.

○ TREATMENT

1 Keep the child lying flat and as warm and comfortable as possible, using methods already described.

2 If the child is not fully conscious, do not attempt to give him any fluids by mouth or any form of sedation—even aspirin.

3 Obtain the services of a doctor *immediately,* and do not move the child until the doctor has seen him.

4 If this is not possible and the child must be taken to a hospital, transport him on a stretcher, lying flat on his back, with as little movement or handling as possible.

If the child is to be treated at home, it is of great importance that he be kept quietly in bed, *without* a pillow under his head, and that he be *watched closely* for signs of abnormal drowsiness which may presage the onset of coma, or loss of bloody fluid from the ears, nose, or mouth. These are grave signs and make hospitalization imperative.

MEDICAL EMERGENCIES

There are a number of medical conditions of a more or less emergency nature which occur in childhood, in addition to those which may occur in later life, and which are discussed in Chapter 15, "Common Medical Emergencies."

While it is impossible to cover all acute conditions that might occur under an emergency situation, the most common ones of especial importance in childhood are discussed here.

Foreign Bodies

Children very commonly inhale foreign objects into their respiratory tracts or swallow things that get stuck in their throats, and commonly, they put foreign objects into various other body openings where they do not belong. Even certain foods, given them by well-intentioned adults who should know better, may act as foreign bodies, since the child is unable to chew them properly or is not yet old enough to have acquired adequate eating technics. Probably the worst offenders in this respect are raw carrots, celery, bacon, and either nuts alone or foods containing nuts. Other assorted articles which may cause a serious emergency include bones, coins, various kinds of hardware, jacks, safety pins, and swallowed teeth.

Burrington, and Rogers and Igini, very properly emphasize the dangers of pull tabs on aluminum beverage cans, which the child may easily drop into the can (indeed some are taught to do so) and then swallow them. Any child with unexplained respiratory difficulties or unexplained chest pains should be suspected of having this problem. Recently, an even more dangerous type of opening has been put on the market by one of the leading beverage manufacturers. In this case the opener is so designed that the top automatically drops into the can or, in several we have tried, remains partially affixed as on a hinge; in either case it is there, just waiting to be swallowed or inhaled.

The subject, together with suggested details of treatment is discussed on pages 113–114. The important thing, unless efforts to dislodge a foreign body causing respiratory obstruction are immediately effective, is to get the child into the emergency room of the nearest hospital as fast as possible.

Convulsions

The occurrence of convulsions is merely a symptom of some underlying trouble and is not a disease in itself (see also pages 55 and 514). They may be caused by a great many unrelated conditions, particularly in young children. For example, a convulsion in a child may be indicative of a serious disorder or may merely herald the onset of an acute infectious disease; it may be of short or long duration or may recur in rapid succession; and a strong-willed child may bring on a convulsion by holding his breath deliberately until he turns blue in the face and lapses into unconsciousness. In so doing, he may set up a cycle which will perpetuate itself for some time. Any convulsion should be viewed as potentially serious until the discovery of the cause proves otherwise.

Often, the mother is alone with the child when a convulsion occurs and cannot leave him immediately, even to summon medical aid; therefore, she should know how to handle the immediate situation until such time as further help can be sought.

One of the more common causes of convulsions in children is epilepsy (see page 514). Often, attacks of this nature have been handled by the mother, another member of the family, or a teacher on previous occasions and hence the attacks cause no undue alarm. A typical epileptic seizure requires no particular treatment or hospitalization, following recovery, except rest. The child should be spared embarrassment and his classmates made to understand the nature of his disease, so as to avoid ridicule and harassment.

It is the convulsion that occurs for the first time and without warning that is frightening.

○ TREATMENT

   1   Regardless of the cause of convulsion, place the child immediately on something soft and safe, such as a wide bed or rug, where he cannot hurt himself if he thrashes about.

   2   Loosen all his clothing so as to minimize the likelihood of his being choked or of bones being broken by the twisting of garments about an extremity, such as an arm.

   3   If he is on a bed, stand guard over him so that he will not throw himself to the floor.

   4   If the child vomits, prevent his choking by keeping him on his side rather than on his back—*never* on his face, since he might smother.

Most convulsive attacks do not last long, but when they do, special medical measures are required to terminate them. In most cases other than epilepsy, particularly those that are the beginning of an acute illness, sponging with cool water, cold compresses on the head, or ice bags applied to the back of the neck and head may be very helpful.

If these measures do not terminate the attack fairly promptly, get medical help, since, if the attack is allowed to continue for a prolonged period of time, actual damage to the brain itself may result.

The physician will in all probability give the child a sedative by injection if the attack does not lessen within a short period of time. In the event of disaster conditions in which a doctor cannot be procured for some time, aspirin or acetaminophen tablets may be crushed in a little water and given by bulb syringe as a retention enema. The dosage is two times that recommended to be taken by mouth for a child of any given age (see page 306).

Do *not* put the child in the bathtub. For a long time this seems to have been the popular notion of how to treat convulsions in children, but it is a dangerous procedure, for the child may hurt himself severely on the sides of the tub or may easily get out of control and drown. Furthermore, no objective can be attained in this manner which sponging with cool water will not give.

In convulsions preceding or caused by a very high fever, a factor which is responsible for many cases, it is desirable to reduce the child's body temperature as rapidly as possible. This is best done by wrapping him in a cool moist sheet, blown upon by an electric fan. The rapid evaporation of water from the sheet takes the heat away from the child's body. Cool sponges, ice packs, and cool enemas are also helpful in reducing the temperature.

Breath Holding

Spells of breath holding in children may sometimes lead to fainting or convulsive-like twitching as the result of the relatively mild degree of cerebral anoxia which the child is temporarily able to achieve. The frightened parents (even a physician not experienced in dealing with children) may think the child may be having a sudden attack of epilepsy. Such, however, is improbable, and, except in very severe cases, the differentiation is easily made.

Breath-holding spells are comparable to temper tantrums and usually occur as the result of the child's frustration, parental friction, insecurity, fright, or as the result of punishment. Attacks of breath holding usually occur only in young children, most often between the ages of 6 months and 4 years.

The usual sequence of events is that the child becomes mildly hysterical, hyperventilates, and then stops breathing. If he holds his breath long enough, he will become somewhat cyanotic and may faint and show opisthotonus (spasmodic arching of the back) or convulsive twitching. As a rule, these attacks are benign and of short duration. Any attempt to deal with the child during the attack would prove fruitless, and punishment would only make matters worse.   Attacks of this type seem to have a high familial incidence.

The attacks may occur once or twice a day, or only on relatively rare occasions, the frequency presumably being related to the degree of the child's security and the prevailing level of family tranquility and harmony.

Livingston, in distinguishing severe breath-holding spells from epilepsy, points out that in breath holding the precipitating factor is always present and preceded by crying, that cyanosis occurs before loss of consciousness, and that typical opisthotonus nearly always occurs.   The electroencephalogram is usually normal.

In epilepsy there is usually no apparent precipitating factor (except perhaps watching television), there is no crying preceding the attack, cyanosis rarely sets in before the height of a long seizure, and opisthotonus rarely occurs.   In most cases, the electroencephalogram is indicative of epilepsy.

It should be emphasized that there are, of course, cases the symptomatology of which is not clear-cut, so that detailed measures in the hospital sometimes must be taken to make an accurate diagnosis.

O TREATMENT

Generally, children tend to "outgrow" these attacks, but Gellis is impressed with "the number of children with this condition who, as they grow older, abandoned the breath holding portion of the syndrome but exhibited simple attacks of syncope when subjected to pain, fright or anger."

Essentially, the treatment is based on achieving a secure emotional adjustment of the child to his environment and to the parents, making every possible effort to understand the child's responses to his total environment.   It is important to avoid those frustrations which give rise to anger reactions which in essence are the underlying cause of breath-holding episodes.   Basically, what the child is attempting to attain is security, emotional love, and recognition as an individual.

Infections

Common Cold.   The specific cause of this condition, which is a type of upper respiratory infection, has never been determined, but it is now thought to be initially caused by viruses, with secondary bacterial infection of the nose and throat. Everyone, at one time or another, has a cold. However, colds are much more serious in babies and young children than in adults because of the possible complications which may result from them.

As everyone knows, the common cold is highly contagious. Susceptibility is heightened by fatigue, improper diet, undue exposure to drafts, and rapid changes in environmental temperature.

Signs and Symptoms. Aside from a running nose, sniffles, general malaise, dry cough, sneezing, sore throat, and mild fever, the child may be constipated and lose his appetite. This latter is probably because of the temporary loss of much of his sense of smell and taste, so that there remains little incentive to eat.

The symptoms are similar to those that herald the onset of a dozen or more diseases of childhood. However, nothing much more happens in the case of a cold, although, as has been repeatedly emphasized, in any upper respiratory infection one must be on constant guard against involvement of the ears, and there is always the possibility of the disease getting down into the chest and affecting the lungs or bronchi. In the case of an ordinary cold, however, and with the proper precautions, this is not very likely.

○ TREATMENT

Keep the child in bed as long as he has a fever. Give him aspirin, in proper dosage to control the fever and to provide a little relief from general discomfort, and a nutritious diet with plenty of fluids—especially fruit juices.

If the cough is annoying or severe, the doctor will probably prescribe a cough medicine. Nose drops should be used judiciously to provide relief from nasal congestion and to keep the eustachian tubes open, thus minimizing the likelihood of middle-ear infection.

It is extremely necessary to teach children, who are old enough to learn, the importance of blowing their noses *gently,* with their *mouths open,* so as not to force the infection up into their ears. Also, they should learn not to stifle a sneeze for the same reason (but precaution, of course, should be taken not to sneeze in other people's faces).   If the child complains of earache, consult a physician promptly.

To date, no specific treatment for the common cold has been discovered, despite the recurrent newspaper stories and advertising claims of proprietary medicines.   The sulfonamides and antibiotics are rarely indicated unless the possibility of some more serious infection exists.   A common cold generally runs its course in a week or so.

Tonsillitis.   Many young children contract this illness after their first year, and the onset is often both severe and abrupt.

Signs and Symptoms.   The child's temperature may rise as high as 104°F, and he may vomit or show signs of acute gastrointestinal upset.   He complains (mostly by signs because it hurts him to talk) of headache, chilliness, stiff neck, aching joints, and an acutely sore throat, and he has great difficulty in swallowing.

One look at his throat makes the diagnosis clear.   The tonsils are enlarged and inflamed and they may be covered with a membrane of pus or with spots of a dirty-yellow color in the crypt-like spaces.   The disease is similar to, and often associated with, acute pharyngitis.

It is important to bear in mind that, whenever acute tonsillitis occurs, it may be simply the storm warning for some other disease, such as diphtheria.   The potential complications of acute tonsillitis are the same as those for acute pharyngitis (see page 445).

O TREATMENT

In severe cases, specific antibiotics or sulfonamides should be used under a physician's direction.   If, in an unusual instance, no doctor can be reached, take the following measures:

1   Place hot or cold compresses around the child's throat, to give some relief.
2   If the child is old enough, encourage him to gargle with warm saline (1 teaspoonful of salt to a quart of warm water).
3   Keep the child in bed, in a warm, slightly humid room.   _

The doctor also may order some candy-flavored antibiotic throat lozenges, but one should guard against the overuse of chewing-gum aspirin, since excessive use may cause the formation of water blisters in the mouth and the aspirin probably has little, if any, *local* effect.

Earache. Earache is such a common affliction that few of us go through life without experiencing this malady at some time or another—particularly during childhood. The ear, being a complicated and essentially vulnerable organ, may get a number of things the matter with it, all of which can cause earache of one kind or another.

Wax in the ear, if it becomes hard and caked, can cause trouble, and even such an odd occurrence as something getting into the ear from the outside may often be unsuspected and produce earache. (See pages 89 and 90.)

Otitis externa. This simply means infection of the tissues of the external ear canal and is another cause of earache. This condition is not limited to children and may occur at any age; it is commonly contracted from swimming in contaminated waters and in many instances is due to a fungus infection. In the tropics, where fungus infections are rampant, most external ear infection is due to bacteria and usually clears up under proper local treatment with the newer antibiotics.

Symptoms. The infection may be extremely painful, and is accompanied by redness and swelling of the tissues of the canal—and a feeling of annoying fullness in the affected ear. Sometimes the hearing itself is impaired due to the blockage of the canal by the swelling and inflammation.

Often what is taken for a fungus or bacterial infection of the canal is not really infection at all but is a type of eczema arising from various causes. There also is a special type of shingles which manifests itself in the canal rather than elsewhere on the body and is extremely bothersome.

Otitis media. This is of more serious nature; it is infection of the deeper or middle portions of the ear behind the ear drum. This condition is common in childhood and is present to some degree in almost every acute upper respiratory infection. The reason for this is that in young children the eustachian tube, leading from the ear into the throat, is relatively short and straight and hence easily allows infection to ascend from the nose and throat into the middle ear (Fig. 13-1).

Symptoms. It is important to recognize the symptoms of

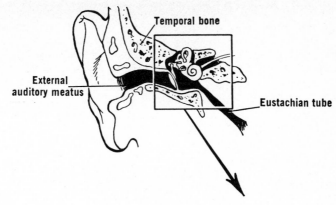

Fig. 13-1. Cutaway view showing how the eustachian tube connects the middle ear with the nasopharynx.

middle-ear infection, particularly in very young children, since aside from the extreme pain, if the infection is not relieved promptly, it may lead to rupture of the eardrum itself. Before the days of the antibiotics, uncontrolled middle-ear infection was the major cause of mastoiditis, which was then very common. Fortunately, it is now rare as the direct result of the effectiveness of the modern sulfa drugs and antibiotics.

The characteristic symptoms of otitis media usually come on a day or two after the onset of a common cold. The child becomes restless, frequently turning his head from side to side as if he could not get comfortable, obviously growing sicker while his body temperature may jump to as high as 105°F. In fact, in a child who has a very high fever but who otherwise seems only moderately sick, acute earache is one of the first things to think about. If the child is old enough to talk, he will complain of severe pain in the infected ear and will be deaf on that side. If he cannot talk, he will be crying because of the pain, which usually is worse at night or may come on suddenly in the middle of the night, and he may be brushing and pulling at the affected ear as if he were trying to get rid of it.

○ TREATMENT

Obviously, such a situation calls for prompt medical attention. Fortunately, the antibiotics are so effective that if the condition is caught early enough, it will clear up promptly without the necessity of opening the eardrum to provide drainage for the infection.

However, if there is delay in starting treatment beyond a certain point, the eardrum will become very reddened, swollen and bulging from the pressure of the pus behind it, and at this stage must be opened to prevent the infection from spreading even deeper to the delicate structures within the internal ear.

If the condition goes unsuspected or neglected, the drum may rupture by itself but the infection, instead of clearing up, becomes chronic and drainage persists. In these cases it is often difficult to effect a complete cure and to restore healing.

Middle-ear infection is certainly nothing to temporize with, and the sooner a doctor is called in, the better.

From a long-range standpoint, the important thing about all conditions which may affect the ear is the effect that they may have on the hearing itself. Too often this aspect is neglected and the child or adult without realizing it may have seriously impaired hearing as the result of some previous disease.

Inflammation of the Eyes. Inflamed eyes can be due to many causes varying from the mere irritating effect of dust in the air during the hot, dry months; sunburn of the eyes themselves; or strain and headache from increased glare to actual foreign bodies in the eyes, such as cinders or specks of dirt; allergic reactions; or infection.

Pink Eye. The common tendency is to call any inflammation or redness of the surface of the eye, or conjunctiva, pink eye. Actually, most cases of inflamed eyes are not true pink eye, or acute catarrhal conjunctivitis, as it is technically known; but when this condition does occur, it can be highly contagious.

This type of infection is particularly prevalent during childhood and may be caused by several common types of germs. When caused by the so-called "Kochs-Weeks bacillus," it may be highly contagious and occur in severe outbreaks, especially in institutions, before its nature is fully recognized and proper therapeutic measures taken. Since it is readily spread to other children having close contact with the patient, special precautions must be taken to prevent its spread. The disease may occur at any age and is most common during the fall and spring months.

The child with pink eye usually first complains that there is "sand in his eyes"; he will rub his eyes a great deal since the itching may be intense.   He may also complain that the light hurts his eyes and that they "burn."

The symptoms are usually worse toward evening, and they vary in severity with the degree of inflammation.   The condition occasionally may be limited to one eye, but usually *both* *eyes* are involved, either immediately or after 2 or 3 days.

The eye itself will be quite inflamed and will have a peculiar, brilliant "pink" color.   The eyes may be swollen and there will be a yellowish discharge which tends to dry and crust on the lids.   This is not seen when the inflammation is due simply to wind, eyestrain, or from too highly chlorinated swimming pools—or swimming in the ocean where the water has a high degree of salinity.

Since the cause of true pink eye is bacterial or, in some cases of viral origin, the specific treatment is with some suitable anti-infective agent which must, of couse, be administered under the direction of a physician.

In the meantime, however, cold compresses along with rinsing the eyes with an isotonic collyrium are very helpful in relieving the pain and reducing the inflammation.   The child or adult should be kept as quiet as possible and isolated from close contact with others until the condition has been brought under control.

Vernal Catarrh.   Another type of inflammation of the eyes which is commonly confused with (or called) pink eye is so-called "vernal catarrh."   This condition is not infectious but is due to allergy.   Its greatest incidence is in the summer and early fall, during the height of the pollen and hay fever seasons, and it may actually be a part of the symptoms of so-called "hay fever."

The cause is a sensitivity to pollens, dust, various dyes, or the dander of animals, but in some cases the true underlying factor is difficult to discover and the condition is often very hard to clear up.   It may recur at the same time year after year until a suitable treatment is found or the patient outgrows his sensitivity.

The symptoms simply consist of inflammation of the eyes, characterized by a bloodshot appearance, itching eyelids, and a watery discharge.   The condition is not uncommon in children and is sometimes seen in adults.

The basic treatment consists of an attempt to discover and eradicate the offending agent and the use of suitable anti-allergic drugs, both systemically and topically applied to the eyes in the form of ophthalmic ointments. Often the treatment for this condition must be shared jointly by an eye doctor and an allergist.

Sty. Another eye condition which is very common, particularly in children and young adults, is the well-known sty, or hordeolum. The sty itself is usually caused by an acute localized staphylococcal infection of one of the tiny glands or hair follicles along the margin of the eyelids. Sties are frequently associated with chronic staphylococcal infection of the margins of the eyelids (blepharitis), chronic ill health, and anemia. An older notion that sties are caused by uncorrected errors of refraction is probably not valid.

A sty appears as a red inflamed conicle swelling, which is quite painful, on the edge of either the upper or lower lid, often near the nose. The lids themselves may be quite swollen and inflamed. As the inflammation progresses, the center of the swelling turns yellow because of pus collecting just below the surface. It may eventually break and discharge a drop or two of thick yellow pus, unless opened earlier by the physician.

Wet compresses as warm as the child can comfortably stand, applied for 20 minutes every 3 to 4 hours coupled with an antibiotic ophthalmic ointment, give a great deal of comfort and help to bring the sty to a head. If the infection is at all feverish, or is recurrent, the youngster should be seen by an ophthalmologist so that the proper medication can be prescribed and the child checked to see if he needs glasses.

Quinsy (Peritonsillar Abscess). This type of sore throat is an acute infection and inflammation of the tissues immediately surrounding a tonsil; it is more frequent in young adults than in children. It usually occurs following a bout of acute tonsillitis or pharyngitis and seems to happen just when the person appears to be getting better.

Signs and Symptoms. Fever suddenly flares up; the throat becomes acutely sore again, especially on one side, only much worse than before; and there is marked prostration. There is also great difficulty in opening the mouth, swallowing, and speaking; the neck is sore, tender, and stiff; and the lymph glands are enlarged and can easily be felt, if not seen, on the affected side on the exterior of the neck. Often, sharp, knife-like pain shoots toward the ear on the affected side and causes acute suffering. This condition should always be suspected when a secondary rise in fever and a very sore throat follow a siege of tonsillitis. Do not make the mistake of attributing the reappearance of symptoms to a slight persistence of the previous tonsillitis or pharyngitis.

O TREATMENT
Regrdless of the patient's age, quinsy is a serious condition, and a doctor should be called promptly. Unless an antibiotic is used promptly, the inflammation may localize into an abscess which must eventually be opened. Early and effective therapy, however, often prevents formation of the actual abscess and the condition subsides without complication.

Pharyngitis. In this acute inflammation of all the throat membranes, they become fiery red and covered with a film of pus and mucous discharge. Although in older children the tonsils are also involved, in young infants, in addition to the throat membranes, the soft palate and uvula may also be affected. In either age group, the disease may make its appearance as a separate entity or in connection with some other severe respiratory infection or with any of the acute contagious diseases of childhood.

It is usually an infection caused by staphyloccoci or hemolytic streptococci, but it may also be due to a viral infection. The first type, a bacterial infection, is usually much more acute, but is often more easily cleared up by sulfonamides or antibiotics than is the so-called "virus" type.

Signs and Symptoms. In young infants, the cry is hoarse and short, as if it hurts the child to cry—which it does. Swallowing is very painful, and young children, especially, will appear very ill. Older children will complain of pain behind the angle of their jaws.

An abrupt attack of vomiting usually ushers in this disease, along with irritability, general weakness, and discomfort. The body temperature may rise to 104°F, and the lymph glands along the sides of the neck may be enlarged and tender.

Acute pharyngitis does not ordinarily last for more than 2 or 3 days, but there is always the danger of complications. Laryngitis, for example, often accompanies the disease, and acute inflammation of the middle ear (see pages 440 and 441) should be closely watched for. Streptococcal pharyngitis may also lead to an acute form of kidney disease or to inflammation of the glands of the abdominal cavity. This causes pain which is sometimes very difficut to distinguish from acute appendicitis.

The potential complications of acute pharyngitis in young children may be much more serious than the disease itself; therefore, it should never be dismissed lightly.

○ TREATMENT

For the viral form there is no specific therapy, but some relief can be obtained by applying either cold compresses (or ice) or hot-water bags to the neck and by using aspirin or a similar drug to relieve discomfort. The child should be encouraged to drink as much fluid as possible and given a diet of soft, easily swallowed food.

If he is old enough, he should be encouraged to gargle, using saline solution (1 teaspoonful table salt to a quart of warm water).

For the bacterial type of infection, these measures may be supplemented by penicillin, which in certain forms can be given by mouth very effectively in accordance with a physician's directions.

Abscess of Back of Throat (Retropharyngeal Abscess). This occurs in infants and young children, but is now encountered less often because of early treatment of tonsillitis or pharyngitis with the sulfonamides or antibiotics. In its acute form, it is an infectious inflammation of the lymph nodes underlying the mucous membrane of the throat. It almost always follows some other acutely inflammatory disorder in this region—often acute pharyngitis; it may, on rare occasions, appear after scarlet fever or measles.

Signs and Symptoms. The onset is very sudden, the child being obviously very ill without any apparent explanation. The fever is alarming at 104 to 105°F, accompanied by severe prostration. The posture of the child is characteristic (Fig. 13-2). His head is drawn far back to one side; his mouth is kept open to relieve pressure on the inflamed pharynx; and his breathing is harsh and noisy. It obviously hurts him to swallow, and as the disease progresses, it becomes harder and harder for him

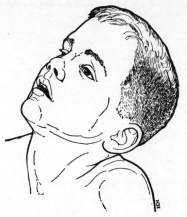

Fig. 13-2. Typical posture of a child with retropharyngeal abscess.

to breathe.   The cry has a peculiar nasal quality and sounds muffled, almost strangled.

It takes about 5 days to a week or longer before a visible abscess forms.   When it does, a bulge on one side of the throat will be seen, which may be large enough to crowd the uvula to one side.   A bulge may also be seen or felt on the outside of the neck, just below the angle of the jaw, in front of the big neck muscle (Fig. 13-3).

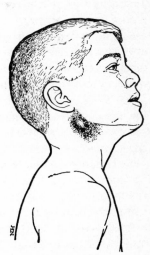

Fig. 13-3. Characteristic external appearance of swelling caused by retropharyngeal abscess.

○ TREATMENT

An abscess of the back of the throat is a serious condition and calls for close medical supervision and vigorous antibiotic therapy, using one of the penicillins. This is a serious situation and demands *immediate* medical attention. As soon as the abscess becomes soft it must be opened—in the hospital or, if necessary, under emergency conditions in the home—by a physician. Careful nursing is of critical importance because of the tender age of the child, and the weakening effect of the underlying disease that led to the attack.

Croup (Acute Spasmodic Laryngitis). This condition is an infection of the larynx that has an effect roughly similar to that of a bowling ball knocking over one pin which, in turn, knocks over another. That is, the infection seems to set off an undue amount of spasm in the larynx and that, in turn, has an excessive spasmodic effect on the vocal cords. Once the croupy "barking," strangling-type of cough, accompanied frequently by a harsh gasping for breath, is heard by a parent, it is seldom forgotten. And the frightening feeling at being sharply awakened—for the attacks usually come late at night or in what up to that point was sometimes called the "quiet hours" of early morning—by these distress signals from the crib is neither a happy nor an uncommon experience for most parents.

Signs and Symptoms. Usually, these show up following a cold or similar infection. During the day, except for perhaps some hoarseness, the child appears fairly well, but, after he goes to bed, he develops a hard, metallic-sounding cough which at first may be so slight as to be unnoticed. About midnight, however, the trouble starts. The cough becomes very hard, with a striking barking sound. And because of the laryngeal spasm, he may have great difficulty in drawing his breath. His attempts to do so resulting in a loud, shrill, strident sound.

In severe cases, the child is in great distress, but he rarely has more than a degree or so of fever, his pulse is rapid, but (quite naturally in this particular instance) the breathing is slow and labored. The lack of adequate air exchange often accounts for a bluish tinge about his lips and the beds of his fingernails.

The attack gradually subsides after a few hours, and, exhausted, the youngster falls asleep. These attacks often occur on three consecutive nights, the third attack being milder than the first two. In susceptible children (frequently those inclined to be nervous) attacks may occur every few weeks during the winter or early spring, but they are rare during warm weather.

○ TREATMENT

The doctor may prescribe standby procedures to be used when there are signs of an impending attack. Often the attacks may be prevented by this medical measure taken at home early in the evening: You can usually give the child some relief by keeping him in a very warm atmosphere of high humidity. The use of a steam vaporizer (either an electric one or a teakettle on an electric plate) or a steaming kettle under an improvised tent of sheets or blankets over the child's bed may be recommended. (For directions, see page 603).

The acute attack itself should be treated by a doctor, since it is sometimes necessary to induce vomiting with an emetic dose of ipecac, followed by a sedative, to bring relief. But no matter how frightening or distressing these attacks seem, it is reassuring to remember that they rarely result in a serious outcome. Many attacks can be relieved simply by holding the child upright over one's shoulder, wrapped in a blanket to keep warm, for 20 to 30 minutes.

Pneumonia. Of the many kinds of pneumonia, we need only consider here three main types. Two of them are caused by bacteria and are known as *lobar pneumonia,* which involves specific lobes of a lung, and *bronchopneumonia,* which is more diffuse and involves the smaller bronchi and bronchioles (the finely divided endings of the bronchial tubes within the lung itself that bring air to the tiny air cells, the *alveoli*), as well as patches of the lung tissue itself. The third type is called *viral pneumonia* which, as its name implies, is caused by a virus, usually of the influenza type. In older children, a similar disease is known as *primary atypical pneumonia,* which may be complicated by a superimposed streptococcal infection.

Signs and Symptoms. These vary with the type of infection and the age of the child. In lobar pneumonia, the onset is often abrupt, with severe chills, convulsions, vomiting, or diarrhea, accompanied by a fever which suddenly shoots up to a temperature of 104°F or higher. The child appears acutely ill; his pulse and respiration are very rapid. At first there is a hard, dry, painful cough which later on, in older children, produces a rust-colored sputum; in young children no sputum is visible because it is swallowed. In severe cases the lips or skin may have a bluish tinge.

The child may complain of a severe pain in his chest over the involved lobe of the lungs. In the diffuse form (bronchopneumonia), pain is less localized because the infection is more spread out. In the absence of specific antibiotic therapy, the disease lasts for 8 days or more; the fever may subside abruptly by *crisis,* or begin to subside gradually—in which case it is by *lysis.* With the new, highly effective antibiotic drugs, the course of the disease is often shortened.

The symptoms of viral pneumonia, however, are less well defined. This type of disease often follows an upper respiratory infection; the onset is gradual and can be noted by the child becoming worse instead of better at the time when he should be beginning to pick up. But the condition may also occur spontaneously. There may be a very hard, dry cough and difficulty in breathing; the child is obviously acutely ill. Yet, strangely enough, the body temperature shows little relationship to the real severity of the disease. It may be only a little over 100°F in very ill children, and as much as 105°F in those who really are not so ill.

O TREATMENT

The important difference, from the standpoint of treatment between the bacterial and viral pneumonias is that the first yields rather readily to sulfonamide or antibiotic therapy, while the latter does not; and viral pneumonia can, therefore, be treated largely on a symptomatic basis. In fact, there is some evidence which suggests that antibiotics actually work harm in viral pneumonia, unless there is a concomitant secondary infection, by suppressing nonpathogenic bacteria which tend to hold the virus in check, without affecting the virus itself. For that reason, while specifically indicated in the bacterial pneumonias, antibiotics are used with great caution in viral pneumonia.

In any case, the child can be made more comfortable by keeping him in a semisitting position, in a warm, moderately humid room and by giving him a cough medicine and a light nourishing diet.

In very severe cases the child must be placed in an oxygen tent, either at home or in the hospital. Proper medical and nursing care are of the greatest importance in the treatment of any type of pneumonia case.

Pus in the Urine (Pyuria). Urine containing pus is really more a symptom than a disease. It is the result of infection in the bladder or kidneys and is more common in girls than in boys, especially those under 2 years of age.

When the infection is in the substance of the kidney itself, the condition is called *pyelonephritis;* when it is in the pelvis of the kidney, it is known as *pyelitis;* and when it is in the bladder, it is *cystitis.* Sometimes a localized collection of pus forms in the kidney, and then it is known as an *abscess,* or a *carbuncle, of the kidney*—a serious condition requiring surgery. If for any reason the flow of urine is obstructed, the condition becomes more difficult to clear up until the obstruction is relieved.

Signs and Symptoms. The most definite symptom of this condition is pus and blood cells found in the urine by microscopic examination, which, by the way, is one of the most important tests that can be done in any case of childhood illness. Fever is the most common sign, coming in recurrent attacks after reaching 104°F or more. There may be severe shaking chills along with the fever and, in acute cases, profuse sweating. In less severe or chronic cases, simply the failure of the child who is chronically listless, nervous, and irritable to do well and gain weight properly may be the only observable danger signals. In all cases of this kind that cannot be explained by some other cause, infection of the urinary tract must always be suspected.

○ TREATMENT

The treatment of urinary tract infections is difficult and depends largely on the correction of any obstruction in the urinary tract and the use of a correct antibiotic or sulfonamide, as prescribed by the doctor, to combat the particular infecting organism. Of extreme importance are bed rest and proper dietary and fluid intake. All possible measures should be taken to prevent the condition from becoming chronic, since then it becomes even more difficult to cure. In infections of the urinary tract certain sulfonamides may be more effective than antibiotics and should be administered along with copious amounts of fluid, in accordance with the age of the child and the directions of your physician.

Epidemic Vomiting. In this condition, which is probably due to a virus, the child, who seems to be perfectly healthy, is seized with an attack of vomiting. It may come so suddenly that a "catastrophe" occurs before he can get to the bathroom. This frequently happens in the schoolroom, since the illness is epidemic in nature and may involve many children at the same time. The incubation period probably is about 2 to 3 days.

Signs and Symptoms. There are no apparent warning symptoms. After the initial attack of vomiting, the child often experiences a rather severe headache, lassitude, and a general feeling not unlike that of a mild attack of grippe. There may be several vomiting sessions; the child may run a slight fever; he may feel faint or dizzy; and—to add insult to injury—he may suffer from a more or less violent diarrhea.

The child's throat may be quite red and his tongue coated, and with some rather prominent red markings. Although the youngster doesn't usually complain of a sore throat, he may talk about a fullness or tenderness around the "pit of his stomach." One is always reminded of the possibility of appendicitis (see page 000), but the history of epidemic vomiting infrequently suggests inflammation of the appendix, plus the fact that many children are "down with the same thing." In case of doubt, however, a physician should be consulted immediately.

○ TREATMENT

There's no specific treatment for epidemic vomiting. Since the child probably will not want to eat, it is best to withhold food. He may also complain of a bad taste in his mouth and have a bad breath. A mouth wash is often very welcome. The attacks usually do not last for more than 24 hours. When the child (or adult) shows a desire for food, hot tea, beef bouillon, or grape jelly (for its sugar content) on toast are often well tolerated.

Infectious Hepatitis. This is an acute, infectious, inflammatory disease of the liver which may occur in similar forms in both children and adults, although it is usually much less severe in children. It results from infection with either of two types of viruses, transmitted by different means, but which produce similar symptoms.

One, known as *SH virus,* is present in the blood of many individuals without producing symptoms of disease, but, when passed to another person by means of whole blood or plasma transfusions, produces an acute inflammatory disease of the liver. This condition, known as *homologous serum jaundice,* has an extremely long incubation period—from 60 to 135 days —a factor which baffled understanding of the condition for a long time when so much blood and plasma were being used during World War II. Since this is mainly a hospital problem, we need not discuss this type of hepatitis further.

The other main type of hepatitis and, for our purpose, the more important, is caused by *IH virus (infectious hepatitis virus).* It is transmitted by carriers who harbor the organism in their gastrointestinal tracts and can therefore contaminate food, water, and milk. The incubation period of this type of hepatitis is relatively short, averaging between 2 to 4 weeks.

Hepatitis may occur in epidemic outbreaks in camps, schools, and institutions for children, and, although they may occur at any time during the year, the greatest incidence seems to be in the fall and early winter. Newkirk et al. also offer some evidence that hepatitis *B* virus infection may be transmitted by certain species of *Hymenoptera,* including bedbugs.

The onset of the disease is quite variable and, though it is usually fairly acute, may resemble the onset of a number of other acute infectious diseases.

Signs and Symptoms. These include, generally, a loss of appetite, followed by chilly sensations, grippe-like symptoms, pain in the eyes, nausea, vomiting, and occasionally, diarrhea. Very often these signs and symptoms are related to the presence of an upper respiratory infection. After a few days the symptoms subside, only to recur 1 to 2 days later in a much more intensified form. At this time, the gastrointestinal manifestations, together with extreme weakness and fatigability, are the major symptoms. The breath is extremely foul-smelling, as is the odor of the stools, and the child may complain of generalized abdominal pain.

After a few days or so, the observant mother may notice a deepening yellow color to her child's urine, and in another

2 to 3 days, the skin will take on the deep orange yellow of jaundice. As the jaundice increases, the child may or may not complain of an itching of the skin. The stools become light clay-colored, and the liver may become markedly enlarged and very tender. It is important to emphasize here that jaundice is not an essential symptom of the disease, and quite often children do not exhibit it, although it does occur in the majority of cases.

With the onset of jaundice, the fever, which has been running around 102°F, subsides, although other symptoms, such as poor appetite, nausea, and a tendency to constipation, continue, though not as severely as before.

During the next 2 to 3 weeks, with the gradual disappearance of jaundice and other symptoms, the child begins to feel quite well again, although his tolerance for physical exertion is very limited and will continue to remain so for a long time to come. While recovery is taking place, there may be a continuance of mild gastrointestinal symptoms, and the child may remain weak and irritable until fully recovered.

The disease is particularly liable to relapse, in which case the recurrence may be much worse than the original attack. In rare instances, infectious hepatitis may pursue a very rapid course and prove fatal. In any event, its seriousness must not be discounted because of the possibilities of complications in later life, such as cirrhosis of the liver.

○ TREATMENT

Treatment consists of prolonged bed rest, followed by a most sheltered convalescence, as there is no specific treatment for the disease itself at the present time. Gamma globulin in substantial doses is useful in some cases to modify the intensity of the already-established disease, if used early. The diet should supply a high caloric intake and should have a high-protein, high-carbohydrate, moderate-fat composition.

The best available hospital care is essential, as the child is extremely ill, and the treatment involves a number of highly technical laboratory procedures.

Prophylaxis. Prevention, as in any gastrointestinal infection, depends upon avoidance of fecal contamination of foodstuffs by food handlers, who may be carriers of the disease, or by flies and other insects and of water supplies contaminated by sewerage. This latter source has been responsible for several reported outbreaks in summer camps.

When there is reason to suspect that exposure to contaminated food or water has occurred, the same type of gamma globulin that is used for modification or prevention of measles and for providing temporary immunity to polio also gives temporary protection against an attack of hepatitis.

Nonspecific Diarrhea. Diarrhea may be caused by many factors, from simple indigestion to more severe conditions caused by actual bacterial or viral infection of the intestinal tract's lining. Such infections produce a more or less uniform set of symptoms, characteristic of a specific disease such as bacterial or amebic dysentery.

Signs and Symptoms. In nonspecific diarrhea there are profuse and frequent watery bowel movements immediately after meals or many times a day. The onset may be gradual, with symptoms becoming worse as the illness increases, or it may be abrupt, with high fever and all the signs of acute illness. The child's stool may be sour-smelling and contain particles of undigested food, or, in the case of bacterial infection, it may contain mucus, pus, and blood. The child may show varying degrees of prostration, loss of weight, fever, and listlessness. In severe diarrhea, dangerous dehydration may occur because of the great loss of fluid and vital body chemicals.

O TREATMENT

Treatment depends on eliminating the cause and maintaining the necessary balance of body fluids and essential body chemicals. In mild cases where there is no infection or other complication, a light diet is usually all that is necessary. Unless there is an identifiable specific infectious agent causing the diarrhea, antibiotics or sulfanilamides generally are not used. However, there are several preparations on the market, under a variety of trade names, containing kaolin and pectin and various antispasmodic agents, especially diphenoxylate with atropine sulfate (Lomotil®), which are useful in more quickly relieving the distress and discomfort of this condition.

Rat-bite Fever. This acute infectious disease is usually caused by the bite of a rat or other rodent.

One form of the disease manifests itself suddenly after an

incubation period of from 7 to 22 days or longer following the bite. The second form, exhibiting essentially the same symptoms, has a much shorter incubation period, and the general reaction is much less severe.

Signs and Symptoms. These are swelling, pain, and dark-red or purplish discoloration at the site of the bite which, during the incubation period, appears to have healed. There is usually a rapid temperature rise, severe headache, loss of appetite, nausea, and grippe-like symptoms. Simultaneously, the original wound develops into an angry-looking sore and becomes covered by a black crust often surrounded by little water blisters. This local reaction is accompanied by swelling and tenderness of the lymph glands and by a temperature which may rise to 105°F, frequently preceded by a chill.

In 5 to 6 days the fever usually subsides, and for 3 to 9 days it remains normal and then again shoots up. During the periods of relapse, the reaction at the site of the bite subsides, but flares up again with each subsequent recurrence of the fever.

A purplish skin eruption, which is characteristic, often appears during the first or subsequent flare-ups. This varies in appearance and distribution, but is most commonly found on the arms, legs, or trunk. When there is no fever it fades, only to reappear in the same or in new locations during the flare-ups. At some stage severe muscle and joint pains occur, and there may be a central nervous system involvement, shown by dizziness, ringing in the ears, delirium, or coma.

○ TREATMENT

The administration of antibiotics, especially the new semi-synthetic penicillins, usually promptly ends the chronic course of the disease, which otherwise might last weeks or months. Fatalities have been reported from the more severe types of this condition, but none is known to occur as a result of the milder form.

Cat-scratch Fever (nonbacterial lymphadenitis). This fairly common systemic illness has only recently come to be recognized in this country as a specific disease. Its exact cause is unknown, but it is believed to be due to a virus transmitted by the scratch or bite of a domestic kitten or cat, which itself shows no evidence of disease. It has also been observed after dog bites or scratches and after having been stuck with thorns or porcupine quills.   The incubation period is about 3 to 10 days.   It is most common in the fall and winter.

Signs and Symptoms.   Principally, the indications are mild prostration, grippe-like aches and pains, mild fever, and enlargement and tenderness of the lymph nodes in the general area of the wound.   About this time, redness and swelling develop at the site of the original scratch or bite, which had seemed to be healing or to be fully healed.   In very severe cases the child may show evidence of brain inflammation or actually go into a coma, but fortunately this is rare.

The disease runs a relatively mild course for from 1 to 3 months, usually clears up uneventfully, and is not considered particularly dangerous.

○ TREATMENT

Bed rest during the height of the disease is the principal treatment.   Antimicrobial drugs are ineffective.   The local wound should be treated as indicated by the doctor.   The patient need not be isolated, but careful disposal of discharges and dressings may be important in avoiding further transmission of the disease.

Common Allergic Conditions

Asthma.   This condition is caused by spasm and constriction of the bronchi, together with swelling and congestion of the lining mucous membrane, and an increased amount of bronchial secretion, all of which combine to interfere with the normal passage of air to and from the lungs.   The mechanics of respiration work in such a manner that, during an asthmatic attack, it is easier to pull air in than it is to force it out, so that not all the amount of air taken in can be expelled with each breath, and some remains trapped in the lungs.   Thus, enough fresh, oxygen-carrying air cannot get into the lungs, as they are already partially filled with the stale, trapped air.   This lack of oxygenation causes a bluish color in the child suffering a severe attack, and the constriction of the bronchi gives rise to the characteristic wheezing which is most marked as the child attempts to force air out.

Asthma may be caused by sensitizing substances, either in the air or in food, or as the result of substances injected into the body, such as certain toxins or serums, or by sensitivity to the poisonous products of chronic infection. A severe form, known as status asthmaticus, which is refractory to the usual treatment, poses a life-threatening problem and requires prompt hospitalization.

Signs and Symptoms. There are the general signs of a "head cold," especially in children during a preattack period. Characteristically, there is great difficulty in breathing; wheezing is distinctly audible; and in many cases, there is a hard, tight cough. Often, too, there is marked nasal congestion.

Breathing may become so blocked that the child turns blue, and the youngster is in great distress, especially at night, when the attacks tend to become much worse. In an effort to breathe, the child sits bolt upright and often subconsciously presses downward with his hands in order to help his respiratory muscles. He also tries very hard to cough up the congesting mucus in his chest, but usually cannot breathe in enough air to do this successfully. His heart will be seen to be "pounding" and at a very rapid rate; often, the large veins in the neck are extremely swollen and stand out like cords.

The sight of a child suffering an acute asthmatic attack is most distressing and, to parents inexperienced with this form of illness, very frightening, as, indeed, it is to the child himself. This is another instance where calmness and loving sympathy will do much for the youngster until the attack gradually wears off, breathing becomes easier, and all the symptoms abate. Once the child is able to raise the mucus which is blocking his breathing, his condition improves rapidly.

Meanwhile, the parents may take comfort in that fact that, despite the somewhat terrifying aspect of the child at this time, fatalities as a direct result of an acute attack are rare. However, repeated attacks can lead to poor general health, emaciation, and conditions within the lung which, in themselves, may be very serious.

○ TREATMENT

The treatment of asthma, from the standpoint of the underlying allergic condition, as well as the acute attack, requires the most careful medical attention in order to provide relief as promptly as possible, to find the underlying cause, and to prevent the condition from becoming chronic.

Drugs (such as ephedrine and similar compounds, and

aminophylline) which dilate the bronchial tubes are used to help the acute attack, but these must be given in accordance with specific instructions, since they are powerful and hence potentially dangerous if used incorrectly or over too long a period. By and large, the antihistamine drugs are not as effective in treating asthma as in hay fever. Asthma constitutes a difficult medical problem and every effort must be made to clear up the condition as promptly as possible, because once there are permanent changes in the lungs, the child is open to chronic invalidism in later life. On the other hand, a substantial number of infants and children appear to outgrow the condition, probably as the result of a gradual desensitization.

Prophylaxis. Because the prevention of asthmatic attacks is of such paramount importance, once the sensitizing agent is known, every effort must be made to remove it from the child's environment or, if necessary or possible, to move the child to another area. Sometimes the sensitizing agent is very simple to identify, as, for instance, the feathers or kapok in the pillow on which the child sleeps. In such a case, the child's condition can easily be corrected by purchasing a nonallergenic pillow and by keeping feathers of all kinds or kapok completely out of his environment. Other sensitizing agents, particularly those thought to be of bacterial origin, are much more difficult to isolate and require patience, kindly understanding, and just plain hard detective work.

Hives. This is another type of allergic condition, manifested by welt-like eruptions on the skin, which result primarily from a dilatation of the capillaries, thus producing a loss of fluid into the skin tissues. Almost any allergy can cause hives, but the most common are allergic reactions to food (especially to fish, strawberries, chocolate, eggs, and milk) and those to sunlight, heat and cold, insect bites, and many kinds of drugs.

Signs and Symptoms. The indications of hives are swelling, redness of the characteristic salmon-pink color, and severe itching. The typical picture of hives is so well known that further description is unnecessary.

○ TREATMENT

Relief from the intense itching may be obtained from cool applications or baths of bicarbonate of soda or Epsom salts or from the oral administration of some antihistaminic drug. In very severe cases (*giant hives*), it may be necessary to administer injections of epinephrine, in repeated small doses supplemented by one of the corticosteroid drugs prescribed by a physician, in order to terminate an attack.

The standard type of skin test is usually of little help in determining the cause of hives, and the search depends on careful consideration of the history and the elimination, one by one, of suspected substances. Ultimate cure rests either on the elimination or avoidance of the offending substance or, if possible, on desensitization to it.

Angioneurotic Edema. This condition may have an allergic or neurologic basis, or both. It is manifested by widespread dilatation of the walls of the small blood vessels of a *whole* segment of the body, rather than by the somewhat *localized* changes that produce hives.

Signs and Symptoms. In this disturbance, because of an acute allergic reaction, or for some unexplained reason various parts, such as the hand, eyelids, ears, lips, tongue, or vocal cords, swell up to many times their normal size. Depending on the part affected, the result of the swelling may be almost ludicrously disfiguring (temporarily), but it may actually endanger life. If, for instance, the vocal cords are involved, the child may die of respiratory obstruction unless the swelling can be controlled by an antihistamine drug, by the administration of epinephrine, or, if these fail, by a tracheotomy. An adequate dose of epinephrine is almost always effective. As has been noted, not uncommonly in childhood, a simple beesting will provoke a most serious reaction, and many children have died in such cases through lack of prompt medical or surgical treatment.

○ TREATMENT

It is most important to realize that, when a child shows evidence of angioneurotic edema and has any difficulty whatsoever in breathing, a potentially dangerous situation exists. Medical aid must be sought immediately, even though at the beginning the condition may not seem to be serious. In other words, beestings and other allergic phenomena *can* be dangerous. If there is any doubt at all about the seriousness of a child's condition, get him to a doctor at once. If medical aid is not available, as under disaster conditions, an antihistamine should be given by mouth in maximum recommended doses. If relief is not immediately evident, epinephrine should be given by injection in repeated small doses (0.1–0.2 milliliter) until the condition subsides; however, the antihistamine drug should be continued.

Anaphylaxis (Anaphylactic Shock)

This subject is discussed in detail on page 185.

Miscellaneous Conditions

Colic. Man's gastrointestinal tract is subject to many troubles from the cradle to the grave. The one most commonly to hit him first is colic, which, while it sounds like a specific disease, is not. It is hardly ever seen in hospital nurseries; instead, it usually waits until the baby has been brought home to plague already anxious parents.

The term *colic,* as generally used, refers to spasmodic cramp-like abdominal pain which is the result of intestinal spasm. Colic usually starts suddenly and within a short time after feeding. The anguished cry of the baby, expressing both pain and surprise, is distinguished from that of hunger, which is far more gradual and ceases with a satisfied gurgle when the child is fed.

In severe cases the abdomen is distended, the baby draws his legs up, cries more or less continuously, and acts as if he were in considerable pain. There is no fever and, aside from the signs of stomach ache, the baby doesn't show any other symptoms of illness.

Usually the attack stops with the baby belching up air or stomach contents, after which he falls into an exhausted sleep until he wakes up hungry and starts the cycle all over again. Sometimes it takes a long time to get these babies to sleep and relax.

Many explanations have been given as to the cause of colic, most of them erroneous or secondary to the real reason. It is easy to say that the baby swallows air during feeding, is overfed, that the feeding formula is not correct, or that the infant has a specific allergy, for instance to milk. Any or all of these things may be true in varying degree, but the true underlying cause of most cases of colic is that man's gastrointestinal tract is an acutely sensitive barometer of his emotions, and the newborn babe is no exception.

Most babies reflect their subconscious reactions to the parents' tensions, frictions, and apprehension, by colic. Another interesting thing is that colic occurs for the most part in the first born and is infrequent in the second or subsequent children.

Hence, from a psychologic point of view, colic is not a disease but is a problem situation in which both parents and child are adjusting to a new environment. The difficulty arises mostly from a lack of preparation for the responsibilities of parenthood, brought about by the various myths of modern society which lead the prospective parents into anticipating the arrival of a quiet, sweet little infant who sleeps most of the time and poses no problems—physical, emotional or otherwise.

Quite the contrary is often the case, and there is a daily assault on the parental nervous system by a dynamic little animal who cries, struggles, gets soiled and wet, hiccups, and, when he is really going strong, can turn everything around him topsy turvy. This situation, of course, places heavy new demands on the parents and requires considerable personal self-sacrifice, for which many parents are not prepared emotionally.

On top of all this, the parents are not experienced in the ways of infants, are inept and apprehensive in carrying out the many little tasks required for the care of the infant, and all this is made painfully evident to the youngster—usually during the periods when he is most unhappy, particularly as a result of the fact that every time the baby cries, they think something terrible has happened.

It is perfectly normal for a baby to cry, since it is his only means of communication by which he can make his wants and reactions known. Young babies are extremely sensitive to their environment and react by crying to loud noises; uncomfortable, tight, or too warm clothing; soiled diapers; and hunger.

In addition, babies demand and thrive on a great deal of love, fondling, and human contact, and they have an overwhelming need for security which is best exemplified by the pleasure of being held, fondled, and played with. Any ambitious and thinking infant will cry lustily to get these things.

Hence, while it is true that there may be underlying organic causes of colic in infants, the origins of colic are for the most part emotional and, in many cases, once the parents understand the situation, correctable.

○ TREATMENT

In most cases of colic, therefore, prevention is more effective than treatment; "burping" the baby after each feeding, of course, is important, along with gentle, loving, but assured handling. The possible effect of an allergy, such as to milk, is corrected by adjusting the diet or by eliminating the offending substance. Undue concern and obvious nervousness on the parents' part will aggravate the condition, for tense, apprehensive feelings are easily communicated to a baby. Obviously, this type of relationship should be avoided. This is one situation in which the famous admonition—keep calm—so often applied to first aid, really has some meaning!

Acute Gastric Indigestion. Similar to the colic of infancy is the condition called *acute gastric indigestion* which occurs in older children. It is extremely common and results from overeating, improper eating (too many green apples!), overfatigue, nervous exhaustion, and apprehension, which tend to upset the proper functioning of the natural digestive chemicals.

Signs and Symptoms. The child may or may not complain of fullness in the pit of the stomach and a feeling of nausea. Often, he "turns green about the gills" and suddenly vomits— usually copiously and several times within a short period. The vomiting appears to relieve the distress, and recovery is often amazingly prompt.

○ TREATMENT

No particular treatment is necessary, except for a light diet until the child clamors for more food. Tea with a little lemon often helps to settle his stomach. The most important problem, of course, is to be sure that the condition is not a forewarning of an acute infectious disease or appendicitis. Take the child's temperature, try to find out what he might have eaten to make him sick (often the vomited matter provides irrefutable and otherwise unobtainable evidence), and watch him until you are sure that nothing more serious is developing.

ACUTE SURGICAL EMERGENCIES

There are a number of acute surgical conditions that are common during childhood. While there is no specific emergency care other than to obtain the services of a doctor quickly, it is important to be able to recognize the presence and nature of the emergency in order to deal with it promptly.

Pylorospasm and Pyloric Stenosis. Both of these conditions result from the closing of the outlet of the stomach so that little or none of the child's food can pass on. If it is due simply to a spasm of the muscle (pylorus), which acts like a valve at the discharge end of the stomach, it is known as *pylorospasm*. If the muscle is congenitally closed off, the condition is known as *pyloric stenosis* and requires an operation, which is usually quite simple and safe. Pylorospasm is often an allergic condition and can be treated medically.

Signs and Symptoms. The symptoms of both the conditions are failure of the baby to gain weight and to do well generally, thin, dry, loose skin, and projectile vomiting soon after taking the formula. This condition is much more common in boys than in girls and afflicts infants who would usually be of the lusty, robust type.

Intussusception. Another condition in young infants occurs when a part of the intestine slips into the portion immediately below it, much as one turns in the foot of a sock to facilitate putting it on. This condition, which is seen almost entirely in children under 5 years of age, is known as *intussusception,* and constitutes an acute surgical emergency.

Signs and Symptoms. The symptoms, which may not be unlike those of appendicitis, consist of very severe cramp-like abdominal pain which is much greater than that ever accompanying the ordinary gastrointestinal upset. There is severe prostration and vomiting, followed by loose bowel movements, which at first contain mucus and then pure blood. Characteristically, the lump in the abdomen where the intestine has become infolded can be felt by the hand.

With such symptoms present, the child must receive surgical attention *immediately,* as the success of the treatment depends entirely upon the promptness with which the intussusception can be corrected either by conservative measures or surgically.

Appendicitis.   This subject is discussed in detail on page 554.

14 Acute Infectious Diseases

Those infectious illnesses which are transmitted by direct contact with the patient or with specific infectious material form a special category commonly referred to as contagious diseases, and are of special significance with respect to children's illnesses. They are very commonly transmitted by droplet infection. The droplets, which are spread largely by sneezing, coughing, and talking, are loaded with infectious germs which are breathed in by the uninfected person. Contagion may also be spread by toys, towels, eating utensils, or similar articles.

As a means of minimizing the spread of contagion, the child should be taught to follow these five simple rules:

1 Keep away from anyone who is sneezing or coughing. Never sneeze or cough in another person's face. Try to cover your mouth with a handkerchief or your hand, or turn your face away when coughing or sneezing.

2 Always use only your own personal belongings, such as toothbrush, hairbrush, towels, and handkerchiefs. Never play with the toys of a child who has a cold.

3 Always wash your hands thoroughly after using the toilet and before eating.

4 Do not drink water in a public place unless from a sanitary drinking fountain or from a fresh, disposable paper cup. Do not drink milk or sodas unless from a freshly opened bottle or from a fresh paper cup, except under special circumstances.

5 Avoid crowded places as much as possible in times of any epidemic.

The contagious diseases which most frequently occur during childhood include chickenpox (varicella), measles (rubeola), German measles (rubella), scarlet fever, diphtheria, meningitis, mumps, whooping cough (pertussis), and polimyelitis. The first four, together with smallpox, are characterized by typical eruptions on the mucous membranes (*enanthem*) and on the skin (*exanthem*) and by shedding of the skin when the disease is over (*desquamation*). The diseases with these characteristics are known, therefore, as the *exanthemata*.

By artificially conferring protection on the child through active immunization (injections of specially weakened disease germs or their toxins), modern biologic science has made it possible to prevent a number of the more serious contagious diseases. Immunization, in effect, provides all the protective benefits of experiencing the illness without actually having to go through its natural, prolonged, and often dangerous course. In other words, an individual can be protected against many diseases without ever having had them or even experiencing any discomfort, except, in some instances, for feeling mildly ill for a few hours or a few days (see immunization schedules in the Appendix).

STAGES OF CONTAGIOUS DISEASES

Most acute contagious diseases run a somewhat similar clinical course which may be divided into the following five well-defined stages:

1 The *incubation period,* which is the interval between actual infection and the appearance of the first symptoms

2 The *prodromal stage,* which lasts from the onset of the first symptoms to the height of the fever or, in the case of eruptive diseases, until the development of the typical eruption

3 The *fastigium,* which is the interval between the end of the prodromal stage and the fading of the eruptions

4 The *defervescence,* which lasts until the temperature returns to normal

5 The *convalescence,* which lasts until normal health has been regained

Diseases with a Rash

Smallpox (Variola). Although smallpox now is almost completely eradicated, in the United States, it is clinically a very serious disease which may be confused with a severe case of chickenpox. It is desirable to at least be familiar with the clinical features of smallpox, even though the majority of physicians have probably never seen a case.

Signs and Symptoms. The incubation period is from 7 to 17 days. It is communicable 2 to 3 days prior to the appearance of symptoms and until all scabs and crusts have disappeared. The onset is sudden, violent, and accompanied by chills, vomiting, or convulsions, and the temperature jumps rapidly to 104°F or more, with a simultaneous increase in pulse rate and respiration.

Frontal headache and low back pain are severe, a combination which, together with the marked general prostration, is strongly suggestive of smallpox.

Small, dark-red blemishes appear and later become elevated. On the fifth or sixth day, fluid appears in the earlier lesions and an irregular red area surrounds each blister. At this stage, the lesions have the shape, size, and feel of a split pea in the skin and are characteristically dimpled. By the ninth day the fluid turns to pus, and the lesions become larger.

Lesions may also occur on the mucous membranes of the inside of the mouth, pharynx, conjunctiva (the lining of the inner surface of the eyelids), or genitalia. On about the twelfth day the lesions begin to subside, and itching may become intense. Eventually, the scabs are cast off, leaving characteristic scars, or pits, which often cause disfigurement on the face.

○ TREATMENT

This disease is extremely serious and requires the closest medical supervision at all times, preferably in a contagious disease hospital. Of greatest importance in preventing spread of the infection is isolation of the patient and disinfection of all excreta, including the discharge from the lesions. The severe generalized symptoms require various medical measures for their control.

In spite of the fact that there is no specific treatment for smallpox, *consistently* good nursing care is very important.

Prophylaxis. Natural immunity to smallpox, except for a slight, transient, congenital immunity in newborn infants of vaccinated mothers and those who have already had the disease, is nonexistent; everyone is susceptible. Acquired active immunity can only be obtained through an attack of the disease or by vaccination.

Vaccination with cowpox virus—which is simply smallpox virus in a modified form and causes a similar disease in cattle—has been universally recognized as an efficient protection against smallpox, although its use is not without hazard. In the major part of the United States as well as many parts of the world, where vaccination has been compulsory, smallpox has become an uncommon disease. As a matter of fact, the Advisory Committee on Immunization Practices of the U.S. Public Health Service has expressed the belief that the risk of smallpox in the United States is so small that the practice of routine smallpox vaccination is no longer indicated in this country except for immunization of personnel involved in health services and of travelers to and from continents where smallpox has not been eradicated. The committee also emphasizes the following contraindications to smallpox vaccination under any circumstances: (1) eczema and other forms of chronic dermatitis in the person to be vaccinated or in a household contact; (2) pregnancy; (3) altered immune states from disease or therapy.

The American Academy of Pediatrics also agrees that the risk of smallpox in the United States is now insufficient to justify continuing the routine primary vaccination of infants and children. This position is particularly justified in view of the fact that smallpox vaccine occasionally results in severe reactions, some of which may be fatal.

It should also be mentioned that a means of passive immunization is now available in the form of vaccinia immune globulin (human)—VIG, which will prevent or modify smallpox if given intramuscularly within 24 hours after known exposure. VIG is also used in the treatment of accidental vaccinia of the eye, severe eczema following vaccination, or severe generalized vaccinia.

There is some evidence that the use of VIG for established vaccinal keratitis may result in scarring, and that the topical application of a drug known as idoxuridine (IDU) used alone may be a preferable form of treatment. The Hyland Laboratories, Los Angeles, California, were approved by the Division of Biologics Standards to market VIG in 1969.

Chickenpox (Varicella). Chickenpox is an extremely contagious disease, the general symptoms of which are mild. Characteristically, an eruption, consisting of crops of blisters and pimples, appears which clears up in a few days, leaving scabs, but usually no scars.

Infection probably occurs through the nose and mouth and is transmitted by direct contact with a person ill of chickenpox or shingles, through a third person, or by infected personal articles. It is caused by the varicella-zoster(V-Z) virus, which also is the cause of herpes zoster (shingles).

Most cases occur in young children, and neither race, climate, season, nor sex appears to have an influence on the incidence of this disease. Because it is so highly contagious, the spread of chickenpox is often difficult to control.

Signs and Symptoms. The usual incubation period is about 2 weeks, although it is possible for the onset to occur as early as the tenth or as late as the twentieth day. It is communicable from about a day before the appearance of the rash and for about a week after vesiculation occurs.

In young children, the early symptoms are frequently unnoticed, but in older children and in adults, the appearance of the rash is preceded by loss of appetite, headache, grippe-like symptoms, and a temperature of 101 to 102°F or higher.

The onset of the rash is sudden. Following the appearance of one or two small spots or blisters, there may be a rapid development of a huge number of others appearing in groups. The eruption appears first on the body and scalp, but may also occur in the mouth or on the surface of other mucous membranes. A characteristic feature of the rash is that lesions of all sizes and stages of development may be found at the same time on any area of the body.

The blisters begin as small rose-colored spots, which develop into pimples about the size of a pinhead. Then a tiny blister containing clear fluid forms in the top of the pimple. Itching is intense. The blisters may or may not be surrounded by an area of redness, and scar formation does not occur unless a secondary infection has been caused by scratching.

Ordinarily, the typical chickenpox rash does not run together, but scratching will greatly increase the number of pocks in a given area.

The disease runs its course in about 2 weeks. By the end of 9 days most of the pocks have formed scabs, which in another 4 days have loosened and are easily rubbed off.

Chickenpox patients are infectious from at least 24 hours prior to the appearance of the eruption until 7 days thereafter; but the patient is potentially contagious for several more days unless he has taken a thorough shampoo and bath.

O TREATMENT

Treatment is primarily aimed at relieving the itching and preventing the leisions from becoming infected. Itching can be alleviated by applying bicarbonate of soda (5 percent solution) or calamine lotion to the lesions, and by administering antihistamine drugs (available on a physician's prescription). Give suitable doses of aspirin when necessary.

To prevent infection after crusts have formed, use an antibiotic ointment prescribed by the pediatrician. Occasionally it is also necessary to give antibiotics by mouth to control severe secondary infection. In mild cases, however, calamine lotion or a similar preparation is all that is required. Keep the child scrupulously clean, and prevent him from scatching, thus reducing the chances of secondary infection and scarring.

Unless the case is very severe, the child may be allowed up and about, but he should be kept isolated for about 1 week from the time of onset or until all lesions have crusted. As soon as a case of chickenpox or any other contagious disease is suspected, the doctor should be notified.

It must be further emphasized that chickenpox in adults can be a very serious disease with potentially dangerous sequelae including varicella pneumonia and or encephalitis. For that reason the disease in adults very definitely requires hospitalization.

Measles (Rubeola). Measles is one of the most contagious diseases and was extremely prevalent, especially in children, until an effective vaccine became available. As a result, its incidence has decreased sharply. It is characterized by inflammation of the eyes (conjunctivitis), sensitivity to light, running eyes and nose, fever, typical sores in the mouth, and a rash.

Although measles is usually transmitted by direct contact with the patient or by droplet infection from secretions of the nose and throat, it also may be carried and transmitted by an uninfected third person, such as a doctor or nurse attending the patient, and by the urine of an infected person.

The highest incidence occurs during March, April, and May, and it seems to run in cycles, with some years showing a higher incidence than others.

Signs and Symptoms. The average incubation period is from 10 to 12 days, although a limit of from 7 to 14 days is commonly given. If a modifying dose of human immune serum globulin has been given, this may be extended to 3 weeks or more. The disease is communicable from 5 days before the appearance of the rash and through the first few days of rash.

The onset of the disease is gradual, with lethargy, headache, irritability, and fever becoming increasingly severe just prior to the appearance of the rash. The symptoms suggest a severe cold, with sneezing and a harsh, dry cough. The eyes typically become puffy, swollen, and reddened, and a generalized inflammation of the eyes and sensitivity to light develop early and may be extreme. Inflammation of the eyes, characterized by a bloodshot appearance and a tendency to tear, is often the very first indication of the development of measles and may be noted before any of the other symptoms appear. These symptoms last until the temperature has returned to normal.

On about the second day of fever, scattered reddish-brown spots develop on the back of the mouth or throat, and by the fourth or fifth day, congestion becomes marked and the lining of the mouth and throat is a brownish-red color.

On the second or third day, spots appear on the mucous membrane of the mouth, which resemble grains of white sand sprinkled on a red background. These are known as *Koplik spots.* They are best observed in strong daylight and may be missed entirely in artificial light. They disappear as the rash becomes fully developed.

The typical rash of measles appears 3 to 4 days after the onset of fever and about 36 hours after the appearance of Koplik spots. The temperature reaches its maximum of 104 to 105°F at the time the rash appears and then drops rapidly to normal as soon as the eruption has fully developed.

The rash, which is reddish brown, appears first behind the ears or on the forehead and cheeks. On the second day, it spreads downward to involve the trunk and on the third day, covers the arms and legs. Fading of the rash progresses in the order of its appearance. Itching and burning are common and frequently are intense. Pressure causes the rash to fade except in very severe cases.

When the rash has become general and the fever drops, the patient feels much better, although the glands in the neck may swell slightly.

The rash lasts, on the average, for 5 days. With its disappearance, the skin flakes off for 2 or 3 days. Whereas in scarlet fever the hands and feet are usually involved, in measles this occurs seldom. The cough and a brownish discoloration of the skin may persist from 1 to 2 weeks, but, in children especially, a normal state of well-being is rapidly regained, barring a complication.

The patient is contagious from at least 3 days before to 5 days following the appearance of the rash.

The complications of measles are due to a secondary infection, which may affect the respiratory tract, brain, or kidneys and may be very serious; therefore, it is wise to observe the patient and to watch for any subsequent symptoms, even though he seems fully recovered.

○ TREATMENT

Good nursing care is essential in treating a patient with measles. The patient should be kept in bed, and, because of his sensitivity to light, the room should be darkened; however, good ventilation should be provided. To loosen the cough and congestion of the chest and throat, keep the room as humid as possible; steam inhalations are usually beneficial and welcomed by the patient. Calamine lotion is often used to relieve the itching. Bicarbonate of soda baths may also help. If necessary, a cough medicine and aspirin may be used to alleviate coughing and fever.

The child should be encouraged to eat, and he should be served adequate bland meals at regular intervals. As much fluid should be given as the patient will tolerate. Medical supervision is important to guard against possible complications.

Prophylaxis. Years of research have resulted in the development of three types of vaccine, one consisting of inactivated (killed) measles virus vaccine, the other two both live vaccines utilizing two strains of virus—one the so-called "Edmonston" strain and one the "Schwartz" strain.

While at first all three vaccines seemed to prove both safe and effective, in the course of extended experience it was found that unusual local and systemic reactions occurred when children who had received inactivated vaccine later encountered natural measles or received live attenuated measles vaccine. It has therefore been recommended by the American Academy of Pediatrics that prophylaxis with inactivated measles vaccine be discontinued, and that only live attenuated vaccine be used. Recent findings have shown that immunization may best be deferred until about 15 months of age. During measles outbreaks, or whenever a high incidence of measles may be anticipated, live attenuated vaccine should be given any time after the age of 6 months. In any case a second inoculation is recommended at 15 months of age or later.

Although the live attenuated vaccine may be administered safely with or without the simultaneous administration of measles immune globulin, most physicians will wish to use the two combined because of the lessened frequency of clinical reactions. It is currently recommended that live attenuated vaccine be given to children at the age of 1 year or older, since children under this age still have protective substances in their blood, which they received from their mothers, but which are gradually lost as they get older. The vaccine would be neutralized by these protective substances and would not give the permanent protection that it would if it were given after 1 year of age.

Pregnancy is the most important contraindication to the use of live measles virus vaccine. Neither should the vaccine be used in the presence of severe febrile illness, untreated active tuberculosis, or in cases of malignancy.

However, measles can be prevented in children who have some concomitant illness, have been exposed to the disease, or who are receiving some form of therapy which contraindicates the use of life vaccine, by an injection of immune serum globulin (ISG). This should be given to all children under 2 to 3 years of age—to chronically ill children, and to healthy ones whose brothers or sisters are ill with other diseases, such as tuberculosis, whooping cough, and, especially, rheumatic fever.

The ISG is given intramuscularly as soon as possible after the child has been exposed to measles, and it is followed in 8 weeks or more by a dose of live vaccine.

In older children and adults who have not had measles, injections of immune serum globulin can be given to prevent or modify the course of the disease in the event of exposure. This procedure permits the person to have a mild infection which will confer upon him active immunity and protection against subsequent attacks of the disease. It is important that the gamma globulin be given within 6 days of exposure, since after this time, even much larger doses seem to have little effect.

German Measles (Rubella). German measles is a contagious disease, characteriezd by mild general symptoms, swollen glands, and a transient, rose-colored eruption which may resemble that of both true measles, roseola infantum, and several other rash-producing diseases. It affects young adults as well as children. It is caused by rubella virus which is found in the secretions of the nasopharynx, and the blood, urine and feces of infected persons. Transmission occurs by droplet or by direct contact with the infected persons, or by fresh contamination of articles by their secretions.

Signs and Symptoms. The incubation period is from 14 to 21 days but most cases develop late in the second week after exposure. The disease is communicable from 7 days before to 5 days after the appearance of the rash.

Sore throat and headache are usually mild and may be overlooked. The patient rarely feels sick enough to go to bed. The rash, which appears first on the face, but shortly spreads over the entire body, may be the first noticeable symptom. It is composed of tiny rose-pink spots, in contrast to the brownish-red color of measles. The rash, which easily fades on pressure, lasts only 2 to 3 days, although it may disappear in an even shorter time.

Typical of the disease is the enlargement of the glands in the neck, particularly those at the base of the skull, and, occasionally, others, such as those behind the ear, are involved. The swelling and tenderness last from 2 days to 1 week, but usually disappear shortly after the rash.

The principal danger of German measles lies in the possibility of mothers contracting it during the early months of their pregnancy, with the resulting deformity of the child in from 10 to 20 percent of the cases. The greatest danger occurs during the first trimester of pregnancy. For this reason it is a desirable occurrence when girls develop an active protective immunity by contracting the disease before reaching the child-bearing age.

Parents should keep a careful permanent record of when each daughter contracted the disease, for reference later on during her married life. It is equally important to know that up to the time of her marriage she had *not* yet had clinical German measles.

The question of whether to use ISG as a prophylactic agent in exposed expectant mothers, or those likely to become pregnant, has been a matter of controversy for many years.

Present recommendations are that prophylactic measures should be considered for women only in the first trimester of pregnancy. The available evidence with respect to the use of immune serum globulin (human)—ISG—indicates that it may modify or suppress the clinical manifestations without actually preventing the presence of the infecting virus in the blood-stream. For this and other reasons, routine use of ISG for the prophylaxis of rubella in early pregnancy remains open to question.

From the standpoint of active immunization, live rubella virus vaccine is recommended for boys and girls between the ages of 1 year and puberty. Vaccine should not be administered to infants less than 1 year old because of possible inter-ference from persisting maternal rubella antibody.

Children in kindergarten and the early grades of elementary school deserve initial priority of vaccination because they are commonly the major source of virus dissemination in the com-munity. A history of rubella illness is usually not reliable enough to exclude children from immunization.

Vaccination of adolescent or adult males is of much lower priority because so few are susceptible. However, the vaccine may be useful in preventing or controlling outbreaks of rubella in circumscribed population groups.

Pregnant women should not be given live rubella virus vaccine. It is not known to what extent infection of the fetus with attenuated virus might take place following vaccination, or whether damage to the fetus could result. Therefore, routine immunization of adolescent girls and adult women should not be undertaken because of the danger of inadvertently administering vaccine before pregnancy becomes evident.

Women of childbearing age may be considered for vaccination only when the possibility of pregnancy in the following 2 months is essentially nil; each case must be considered individually. This cautious approach to vaccinating postpubertal females is indicated for two reasons: (1) because of the theoretical risk of vaccination in pregnancy, and (2) because significant congenital anomalies occur regularly in approximately 3 percent of all births, and their fortuitous appearance after vaccine had been given during pregnancy could lead to serious misinterpretation.

It has been noted that live rubella vaccine grown in canine kidney tissue cultures may give rise to moderately severe joint pains and some cases have required hospitalization. Most reactions of this type occur 4 to 6 weeks after immunization, and for the most part the symptoms disappear spontaneously. This problem has not been noted with rubella vaccines made in other types of tissue culture, but caution must be taken to make sure that the child may not be sensitive to the particular tissue in which the virus was grown, as indicated on the label of the vial.

O TREATMENT

Little specific care is required, except for keeping the child in bed until the temperature is normal. Special care should be taken against contagion which might infect a pregnant woman, especially during the first trimester. If such a situation is possible, isolate the child for at least 5 days following the appearance of the rash. Occasionally an adult may be made quite ill by German measles, but the treatment, including bed rest, must be symptomatic.

Scarlet Fever (Scarlatina). Scarlet fever is but one of a large group of diseases caused by hemolytic streptococci; the group includes streptococcicosis, streptococcal pharyngitis, and erysipelas. Scarlet fever is an acute, highly contagious disease characterized by a sudden, severe sore throat, vomiting, high fever, and a typical skin rash.

Transmission is largely by direct contact with a person who

is ill with scarlet fever or a human carrier, but it is also possible for the disease to be transmitted by contact with personal belongings, such as bedclothes, books, towels, eating utensils, toys, and the like, of those who have the disease, and by pets, such as cats and dogs, as well. Also, there have been many occurrences of milk-borne epidemics.

Scarlet fever is most frequent from 2 to 10 years of age and is about twice as common in winter as in summer, the peak usually being reached in March.

Not all persons are susceptible to the disease, and most adults are immune. A doctor can determine whether or not a person is immune to scarlet fever by means of the Dick test, which is based on the local reaction to a small amount of scarlatina toxin injected into the skin. There are no practical, specific preventive measures. The disease is communicable as long as the patient is ill.

Signs and Symptoms. The incubation period of scarlet fever may be from 1 to 7 days, but from 2 to 5 days is the rule.

The onset is sudden, with high fever, sore throat, and vomiting; convulsions frequently occur in very young children. The fever rises abruptly and may reach a maximum temperature of 104 to 105°F on the first day, but in mild cases may not go above 101 to 102°F. The throat is usually painfully sore, the mucous membrane of the back of the throat becoming a bright red, with closely massed dark-red spots or scattered ulcers.

Vomiting frequently occurs abruptly, without warning, and is often the first evidence of illness. Severe headache and prostration are marked, the pulse rate is rapid, and swollen glands are common.

The rash of scarlet fever, which makes its appearance within 12 to 36 hours, consists of a generalized redness, which gives the skin the appearance of red gooseflesh. The rash is first seen in the folds of the joints, the groin, buttocks, and small of the back. Itching is slight or absent. Whiteness, in a ring about the mouth, is present in most cases and is a clue to the disease. The rash reaches its height in 1 to 2 days and fades out within a week.

The appearance of the tongue is characteristic. At first it is heavily coated, swollen, and roughened. The coating then disappears, and the tongue becomes bright red, and by the fourth or fifth day, it has the typical strawberry-like appearance (which is a definite diagnostic sign of scarlet fever) that has given rise to the term *strawberry tongue*.

○ TREATMENT

Scarlet fever is a serious disease, and its treatment must be closely supervised by a doctor. During the acute state, complete bed rest is absolutely essential. Strict precautions should be taken against the spread of contagion.

Aspirin or acetaminophen may be used to control fever and discomfort. Most cases run a short and mild course because of the high degree of effectiveness of various penicillin preparations in this disease. The sulfonamides, which were effective, are no longer used very much because they do not reduce the occurrence of rheumatic fever as a sequela. If the temperature is above 104°F for more than 2 or 3 hours, sponge baths should be given and other fever-reducing measures taken as directed by the doctor.

Skin care and cleanliness are important. If necessary, a bland cream may be used to relieve the scaling and itching which follow the rash.

Fortunately, most cases of scarlet fever are today readily controlled with penicillin given either parenterally or orally, and complications do not occur as frequently as in the past. Nevertheless, medical supervision is important to guard against possible complications that may affect the kidneys, the middle ear, or the heart.

In addition, patients who have a history of rheumatic fever, chorea, or who have rheumatic heart disease should be given continuous prophylaxis using either penicillin G or sulfadiazine according to designated schedules. Prophylaxis should be administered, continuously, throughout the year, well into adult life.

Roseola Infantum. One of the most common causes of skin eruption and high fever in infants is roseola infantum. This condition probably occurs almost universally between the ages of 4 months and 3 years of age, but in many cases the symptoms aren't severe enough to be noticed.

Roseola infantum usually sets in with abrupt fever, although the mother may have noticed lassitude and irritability shortly beforehand. The first striking thing, however, is that the child has a fever, which may run up to as high as 105°F. Surprisingly, in spite of the high fever, the youngster does not act as if he were severely ill and usually is quite active and alert.

The fever continues for 3 to 5 days, reaching its height in the afternoon, and is relatively low in the morning. There are no specific symptoms other than those resembling a slight cold and some irritability. Vomiting may occur, particularly if the child is overfed, but this does not seem to be a specific characteristic of the condition. Usually the fever terminates abruptly, although in some cases it may come down slowly during the recovery period.

About a third of the affected youngsters have an inflamed throat, and in some of the cases tiny pin-point pink elevated spots can be seen on the soft palate and uvula. About a fourth of these children get mildly infected ears, although the degree of inflammation rarely is such as to cause much discomfort.

The most characteristic thing about roseola infantum is that the rash comes on after the fever breaks. It is most pronounced on the neck and over the trunk, but it may appear on the face and the extremities to some degree. It may not show up until as late as 48 hours after the fever subsides, although in most cases it comes out just about the time the fever breaks.

The rash consists of characteristic rose-pink spots which do not itch. The eruption may last anywhere from 2 or 3 hours to a couple of days, when it gradually fades out, leaving no scar and no pigmentation.

The cause of the disease is not known with certainty, but studies conducted both in monkeys and in human beings strongly suggest that it is due to a specific virus which has not yet been isolated.

The incubation period is probably between 10 and 21 days following exposure, but in some cases it may be much longer than this. The source of infection is probably healthy individuals who harbor the agent. Some authorities believe that the causative virus is universal in distribution and that adults may remain carriers for life, thus creating a huge reservoir of infection. As a result, it is almost impossible for susceptible infants to escape becoming infected during the period when their protective immunity is low.

O TREATMENT

There is no specific treatment, since no antibiotic or other therapeutic agent currently existing seems to have any beneficial effect.   The main procedure is to keep the child as comfortable as possible and control the fever in order to minimize the chances of convulsions.   For this the physician will usually prescribe a suitable antipyretic and cooling sponge baths when required.   Certain mild barbiturate drugs in small doses also seem to be helpful in calming the child and allaying convulsions.

Rocky Mountain Spotted Fever.   Rocky Mountain spotted fever is a tick-borne disease characterized by an acute onset with chills and fever, a macular or maculopapular eruption, headache, restlessness, and muscle pains.   Though second infections have been reported, recovery from spotted fever is generally believed to confer lifelong immunity.   The infectious agent is *Rickettsia rickettsii*.   According to Peters, there has been an alarming increase in the prevalence of the disease, an increment of over 50 percent having been observed in 1969 alone.

At first considered a disease of the western United States, from which it obtained its name, cases of Rocky Mountain spotted fever may occur in almost any state.   Although it has been frequently claimed that the disease in the West has a higher mortality than along the eastern seaboard, an analysis of morbidity and mortality statistics with reference to age distribution does not support such a conclusion.   In both sections of the country, strains of rickettsiae of equally low and high virulence have been isolated.

At least two common strains of ticks are carriers: *Dermacentor andersoni* in the West and the dog tick, *Dermacentor variabilis,* in the East.   Laboratory experiments indicate that there are other potential vectors, especially ticks that feed on wild rabbits.   The greatest incidence of the disease is during the spring and summer months after the ticks have emerged from the ground and have entered into the adult stage.

Rocky Mountain spotted fever is innocuous for the tick and hereditary transmission occurs.   Ticks obligatorily feed on mice and other small rodents as well as dogs and large mammals, but they have been known to go without a blood feeding for as long as 4 years. Animals bitten by infected ticks develop a symptomless infection and may act as temporary reservoirs of the disease for uninfected ticks which may feed on them. Hence the disease may exist indefinitely in nature, with man only an accidental victim.

Symptoms. The average incubation period of Rocky Mountain spotted fever in man is from 4 to 8 days in severe infections and from 3 to 14 days in milder cases. Because there is a marked variation in the virulence of the infection as well as a difference in individual human resistance to the disease, three characteristic clinical types are described. These have been divided categorically into mild, severe, and fulminating types.

In none of these is there a typical lesion at the site of the bite, and regional lymphadenopathy is not a characteristic feature.

In the mild form of the disease, the symptoms range from mild intensity to a moderate degree of prostration. In this type the temperature does not exceed 102.5°F, and the pulse rate remains under 90 beats per minute. There is usually a prodromal period, lasting 2 or 3 days, of malaise, irritability, and chilly sensations. The disease itself is ushered in by a chill and slowly rising temperature, which reaches its peak about the fifth day. Headache and pains in the bones and joints may be severe. The patient is restless and may have a slightly dusky color.

The exanthem appears on the fourth to sixth day, accompanied by amelioration of the constitutional symptoms but no drop in temperature. The skin lesions are bright red, scattered, and maculopapular in type, and during the early stages disappear on pressure. As the disease progresses, the lesions darken in color, become diffuse, and will not disappear on pressure. The rash *appears first on the wrists and ankles,* but as new crops of lesions appear, the abdomen and back are also involved. At the height of the exanthem there is an actual extravasation of blood into the tissues, so that when the lesions eventually disappear, pigmentation remains in these areas for some time.

In untreated cases, the temperature remains elevated for

about 3 weeks, then gradually falls by lysis over a period of 3 to 8 days. While the constitutional symptoms can be distressing, the patient is occasionally not sick enough to take to his bed or to consult a physician. It is probable, therefore, that many of these infections remain unreported.

In the severer cases, the onset is sudden with a hard chill and prostration, marked malaise, sweating, severe lumbar back pain, frontal and occipital headache, conjunctivitis, photophobia, nausea, nosebleeds, mental confusion, and muscular incoordination. The temperature rise is abrupt, reaching 104°F in 3 days, which is usually not exceeded except in fatal cases.

The eruption appears on the second or third day characteristically on wrists and ankles first. The palms of the hands, the soles of the feet, and not infrequently the mucous membranes are also involved. The macules are bright red, but soon darken, and do not disappear on pressure. Through a process of coalescence irregular hemorrhagic blotches are formed, which may remain as pigmented areas for several months.

The disease pursues an exceptionally stormy course, and convalescence is slow. The acute symptoms last approximately 3 weeks, at the end of which time the temperature slowly falls.

Cases of the fulminating type are even more severe, involvement of the nervous system being especially marked, and there is marked toxemia. Incontinence, convulsions, opisthotonos, and tremors are common enough to be characteristic.

The exanthem appears early and pursues a rapid course to form a confluent hemorrhagic eruption which progresses to actual necrosis and sloughing. The most commonly affected parts are the external genitalia, the buttocks, the dependent portions of the body, and the soft palate. The course of the disease is exceedingly rapid. The patient relapses into coma, and the temperature may rise to lethal levels despite intensive countermeasures.

The diagnosis of Rocky Mountain spotted fever is confirmed by specific laboratory tests on the patient's serum.

Cases of Rocky Mountain spotted fever are not infectious and therefore need not be isolated, nor is quarantine of contacts required. A vaccine for active immunization is available, but its use is now recommended only for workers exposed to high occupational risk and those with particularly heavy tick exposure.

Complications. The most common complications of Rocky Mountain spotted fever are pneumonia, phlebitis, hiccough, and hemorrhage from the nose, kidneys, and intestines. Concurrent conditions as the result of the tick bite which must not be overlooked as possibilities are bacterial septicemia, tularemia, and tick paralysis. The last is an especially important consideration if the bite has occurred on the back of the neck, which is a common location for the ticks to lodge.

Prophylactic Measures. Persons whose occupations or recreational activities necessitate exposure to tick bites should wear high boots and heavy socks and examine themselves several times daily for the presence of ticks, particularly around the collar line. The ticks should be pulled gently from the skin or clothing and never crushed. Infections have occurred among dog owners who, in removing *Dermacentor* ticks, have crushed them between their fingers. It is estimated that a tick must feed about an hour before transmitting the infection to man.

Active immunization with vaccine probably should be reserved for those whose occupations or recreational activities require a high degree of risk to tick infestation. The vaccine is commercially available; although it does not prevent the disease, according to Peters and others, its course is more benign in the vaccinated than in the unvaccinated individual.

○ TREATMENT

Specific treatment consists of the use of chloramphenicol or one of the tetracyclines. These drugs are especially effective if given early in the course of the disease. In seriously ill patients, adjunctive corticosteroid therapy may be required.

Infectious Mononucleosis. This disease is somewhat more common in boys than in girls and seems to affect principally older children and young adults. As yet the cause is unknown, but certain studies suggest that the etiologic agent is a herpes type virus (Epstein-Barr–"EB" virus), although recent evidence suggests that other serologically related viruses may be the cause in some cases. The disease is probably transmitted from infected persons by droplets from the nose or throat, by saliva, or by direct intimate contact.

The exact incubation period is not known but probably varies between 2 and 6 weeks. The period of communicability may only be during the phase of acute illness. The disease may occur sporadically or in moderate epidemics, but it does not seem to be highly contagious. The principal characteristic is a large increase in the type of white blood cells known as *monocytes.*

Signs and Symptoms. Usually the onset is gradual (but sometimes may be sudden), with a temperature up to 103°F, grippe-like symptoms, and an acutely sore throat. Often, headache is present in varying degrees, sometimes appearing as the first and most prominent symptom. In the more severe cases, practically all the lymphoid tissues are involved to some degree, and there is a very marked enlargement of the glands of the neck, the groin, and the armpits. Sometimes the spleen may become so enlarged as to rupture. The liver may be affected in about 80 percent of the cases, but this is of neither the type nor the severity seen in infectious (viral) hepatitis.

About 4 days after the onset, a red pimple-like rash or lesions resembling hives may appear on the chest, back, hands, and feet. This, however, never becomes as intense as it does in some of the common contagious diseases and fades in 5 days or so. Not uncommon are rather severe nosebleeds, and at times there may be blood in the urine.

This condition is extremely difficult to diagnose with absolute certainty, since its symptoms vary so widely and may simulate so many other conditions, but the findings by a microscopic examination of the blood can be strongly suggestive when considered with the symptoms and certain serologic tests on the blood. Recently, a sensitive reagent has been introduced which greatly facilitates positive identification of this condition.

○ TREATMENT

Treatment for infectious mononucleosis is nonspecific and consists generally of prolonged bed rest, which is essential. Although all of the new antibiotics have been tried, thus far experienced observers question their real value in this disease, unless there is a complicating secondary bacterial infection. Fortunately, the outlook for the patient's recovery from this disease is generally good, except for the possibility of rupture of the spleen, although convalescence may last as long as several weeks or months.

Diseases without a Rash

The following common contagious diseases of childhood do not have a typical rash, although some form of skin eruption may appear at some time during their course.

Mumps (Parotitis). Mumps is a highly contagious disease, caused by a myxovirus related to the influenza para-influenza group, and characterized by swelling of the parotid salivary glands and, in older children and adults, by involvement of the testicles, ovaries, or pancreas. Most cases occur between the ages of 5 to 15 years, but rarely after the age of 40. Immunity is acquired through an attack of the disease, although second attacks have been reported.

Communicability is probable 7 days before to 9 days after swelling of the parotid gland appears. About 40 percent of susceptible individuals who are exposed develop subclinical infection but can transmit the disease.

Signs and Symptoms. The incubation period is about 18 days, but may be from 14 to 21 days. During this period there is usually no indication of illness. There may be a grippe-like sensation during the first stage of the disease, which may last from 12 to 24 hours. A slight rise in temperature may occur, with a mild sore throat and pain behind or below the ears. Pain, when chewing, may begin at this time, and some foods, such as lemon juice or pickles, will cause intense discomfort.

Swelling on both sides of the jaw follows, caused by inflammation of the parotid gland which usually lasts from 7 to 10 days (Fig. 14-1). During the acute stage of the disease, chewing and swallowing are very painful.

The patient is infectious from 24 hours before the appearance of the swelling until all evidence of the infection has subsided.

Since it is possible for adults, in whom it is more serious, to contract mumps, special precautions should always be taken to avoid contagion, for the disease may cause sterility or give rise to other complications.

○ TREATMENT

During the period of fever and swelling, treatment usually consists of bed rest. The diet should be soft or fluid and as bland as possible, since sour or seasoned foods stimulate the

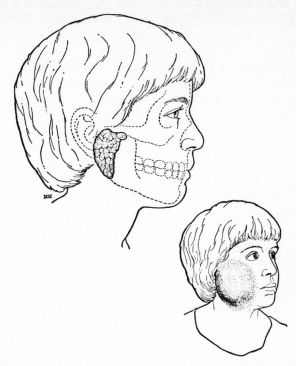

Fig. 14-1. Diagram of a normal parotid gland and its characteristic appearance in mumps. The submaxillary glands (below the jawbone) may be similarly involved in some cases.

flow of saliva, thus adding discomfort to the pain of chewing and swallowing caused by the swollen gland.

Either hot or cold compresses—whichever gives more comfort to the patient—may be applied over the infected gland, and aspirin may be given to alleviate the pain or fever.

Secondary involvement of the ovaries or testicles is the principal complication of mumps, the latter being by far the most common and the most likely to occur after puberty. An adequate period of bed rest is thought to minimize the likelihood of such an occurrence; in severe cases, mumps immune globulin was at one time suggested as a further defensive measure, but is no longer recommended.

A live attenuated mumps vaccine has been developed which has not caused clinical reactions and has given a good protective response in over 95 percent of susceptible individuals; it is also available combined with measles and rubella vaccines. Although the protective levels have not been as high as those attained from natural mumps infection, protection against mumps has been observed in children for as long as 2 years following vaccination. Just how long immunity does last has not yet been determined, and for that reason the vaccine is not recommended by the American Academy of Pediatrics at this time for use in infants and children. However, it is recommended for special groups of individuals who have not had mumps, including boys who are approaching puberty, adolescent and adult males, and children living in institutions such as summer camps or under other similar circumstances where contagion is likely. The older inactivated mumps vaccine is no longer recommended.

Whooping Cough (Pertussis). This highly contagious disease is characterized by paroxysms of coughing which end in an indrawn "whoop," frequently accompanied by vomiting. It is transmitted by direct contact with those suffering from whooping cough or with carriers and by indirect contact, as by toys, clothing, and the like. Most cases occur between 1 to 5 years of age, the highest number of fatalities being in the first year of life. It is caused by the germ *Bordetella (hemophilus) pertussis.*

Signs and Symptoms. The incubation period is from 5 to 21 days, but usually 10 days.

At first, the symptoms may be similar to those of an ordinary chest cold. However, in typical cases, the cough becomes increasingly frequent and severe and worse at night, when the characteristic paroxysms set in.

The paroxysm consists of a series of coughs which come in such rapid succession that the patient is unable to get his breath. At the end of the paroxysm the effort to draw in air is so great that it causes the characteristic inspiratory whoop. The child may vomit, especially if he has recently eaten. Attacks are aggravated by close rooms, drafts, tobacco smoke, and cold drinks. The duration of the disease may be prolonged, but on the average the paroxysmal stage of the cough lasts from 3 to 4 weeks.

The patient is infectious from 10 days before the appearance of the first symptoms until 1 week after the last paroxysm. Adults may also contract whooping cough and become quite ill, although, up to the time of the paroxysms, infection with the disease is often unsuspected.

○ TREATMENT

Extremely careful nursing care is needed for young infants, since at that early age whooping cough is a very serious disease. Older children, however, seem to do better when out of doors and in fresh air, especially during good weather. Needless to say, contact with other children and susceptible adults should be avoided.

Diet is important, especially if the paroxysms cause frequent vomiting. Small amounts of highly nourishing and easily digested food should be fed to the patient at frequent intervals, if possible shortly after an attack, so that some food will have a chance to be absorbed before the next paroxysm. Overeating and heavy, greasy foods should be avoided.

Steam inhalations are often helpful in severe cases. It may be necessary for the doctor to prescribe some form of sedative to control the attacks. Within recent years, injections of specific human hyperimmune serum, when available, has been found very useful in modifying the course and intensity of this disease. Sometimes a snug, flannel, abdominal binder helps to give needed support during paroxysms. Erythromycin or ampicillin may help shorten the course of the disease.

The condition may be prevented by active immunization. The first inoculation is given at the age of 2 months, using a combined vaccine containing antigens against diphtheria, tetanus, and pertussis. Subsequent injections of the same type vaccine are given at the ages of 4 months and 6 months. On this schedule, a high degree of protection against all three diseases is obtained.

Diphtheria. This acute, contagious disease is characterized by the formation of a false membrane on the lining of the throat. Severe general symptoms result from the body's absorbing the toxins of the bacteria that cause the disease. Infection occurs through contact with those ill with diphtheria or through droplet contamination by healthy carriers. There is also the possibility of milk-borne epidemics. The causative bacteria (*Corynebacterium diphtheriae*) may remain alive in ice for a long time.

Most infants are naturally immune during the first 6 months of life, but this protection rapidly disappears, so that by the end of their first year most infants are highly susceptible. The majority of adults, however, are immune to the disease, although at present there seems to be some increase in adult susceptibility.

Active immunity may be acquired through a previous attack or be induced artificially by the injection of a special, chemically modified preparation of diphtheria toxin. This product (now usually combined with whooping cough and tetanus toxoids in one injection) is widely used to protect infants and is one of the most effective preventive agents known.

Signs and Symptoms. The incubation period is usually 2 to 6 days, although it may be from 1 to 10 days. The disease may affect other areas (eyes, ears, or vagina), in addition to the throat.

Early symptoms may be slight, with a temperature from 99 to 102°F, accompanied by headache, lassitude, and sore throat. Chilly sensations, backache, and occasional vomiting may also be present. The throat appears at first reddened, and there is difficulty in swallowing.

Early in the course of the disease, the back of the mouth and tonsils become covered with a thin, grayish film which thickens until a dense gray membrane (the false membrane) covers most of the throat.

Coma or delirium is rarely seen except in fatal cases, but drowsiness is frequent. The temperature may be high at the onset of the coma and becomes progressively lower as the disease advances. Bleeding from the nose, throat, genitourinary tract, and, occasionally, from the gastrointestinal tract is sometimes an important complication.

Before the advent of antitoxin, the mortality rate from diphtheria varied from 30 to 80 percent. Fortunately, with modern forms of treatment this rate has been reduced to somewhat less than 5 percent.

Patients are infectious for about 24 hours prior to the appearance of symptoms and remain so for about 2 weeks.

○ TREATMENT

This disease is of a very serious nature and requires the closest medical supervision. The patient should be hospitalized because of the special facilities which are necessary for complete care, especially in the event of complications. Bed rest is essential for at least 2 weeks and often longer. During this period, complete nursing care and close observation are of paramount importance.

The diet should be soft to fluid, but high in caloric value. Saline throat irrigations may be given under the doctor's direction, and aspirin, together with other pain-relieving agents which must be prescribed, may be used to control fever and relieve pain and general discomfort.

Specific medical treatment consists of the administration of diphtheria antitoxin and certain antibiotics, especially erythromycin and penicillin. Generally, this treatment is strikingly effective, but there always exists the danger of complications, such as myocarditis and enlargement of the heart; to which patients with this disease are prone. Therefore, convalescence must *not* be hurried.

Acute Bacterial Meningitis. An acute infectious disease, meningitis is characterized by three specific stages: infection of the nasopharynx, invasion of the bloodstream, and inflammation of the coverings of the brain.

Transmission occurs by droplet infection either from patients with meningitis or from healthy carriers. The entry of infection is through the nose and throat, from which the bacteria invade the bloodstream and are carried to the brain.

The agents most commonly causing acute bacterial meningitis are *Hemophilus influenza* type B, *Neisseria meningitidis*— one group of which is responsible for the epidemic form of the disease, and the *Diplococcus pneumoniae* which at the present time seems to be causing a high percentage of the cases. In very young infants certain intestinal organisms are frequently incriminated.

Many more males than females are affected, and the disease is most common in late winter and early spring. The rate of infection and mortality is highest during the first year of life.

Signs and Symptoms. The incubation period is from 1 to 7 days.

Stage 1: Infection of the nasopharynx.

Symptoms may be negligible during the first, or carrier,

stage, or there may be evidence of an upper respiratory infection, with a bacteria-carrying nasal discharge.

Stage 2: Invasion of the bloodstream.

The patient may be apathetic or indifferent; he resists disturbance, his speech is monosyllabic, and he characteristically lies silent and immobile.   At first there may be only a slight temperature rise, but the skin is sore to the touch, and a bluish skin discoloration is not uncommon.   In this stage, too, a rash may develop, the patches varying greatly in size from mere pinpoints to large mottled blotches.   These are dusky red and fade after 4 to 5 days, leaving irregular brownish stains.

Stage 3: Inflammation of the leptomeninges (coverings) of the brain.

This stage of the disease begins with a severe headache, vomiting, muscle rigidity, and a sharp rise in temperature. Because of marked stiffness of the neck, the head may be held back rigidly, and the muscles of the spine may become so tense that the entire back is arched, causing the characteristic position associated with this disease (Fig. 14-2).   The pulse is slow and irregular, the veins of the forehead are swollen, and breathing is slow and labored.

Meningitis is contagious as long as the causative bacteria are present in the nasal secretions.   Isolation should be maintained for at least 2 weeks after its onset.   Susceptible children

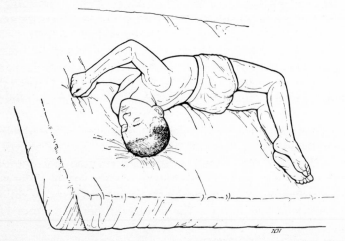

Fig. 14-2. The typical spasmodic arching of the back (opisthotonos), a characteristic of acute meningitis.

who have been exposed to infection should be isolated for 2 weeks from the date of exposure.

○ TREATMENT

This most serious disease is so demanding of every available modern clinical facility that hospitalization is essential as soon as the disease is recognized.

With the discovery of specific agents for the treatment of meningitis, fatalities from it have been lowered from a reported 50 to 90 percent of those stricken in 1908 to less than 10 percent today.

Both antibiotics (especially ampicillin, chloramphenicol or penicillin) and the sulfonamides are used in the treatment of meningitis, the specific agent or combination of agents depending upon the causative organism.   As soon as this has been identified by laboratory methods, the most effective agent available against that particular organism is given in maximum dosage.   In typical meningococcal and pneumococcal infection, penicillin is the drug of choice.

Poliomyelitis (Polio or Infantile Paralysis).   This acute infectious disease is caused by three serotypes of polio viruses that infect the central nervous system, especially the spinal cord.   Type I is the most frequent cause of the paralytic form of the disease; type II is the least liable to cause paralysis, and type III is intermediate.   Characteristically, the onset is acute and is followed in a small percentage of the cases by paralysis of various muscle groups, resulting from inflammation of the nerve cells of the spinal cord or the brain.

Polio occurs most frequently during the summer, the peak being usually in August or September.   It may be transmitted through droplet infection from secretions of the upper respiratory tract and undoubtedly can be transmitted through contaminated food, such as infected milk or ice cream, and by contamination from feces.   For these reasons, food control measures and a ban on swimming in potentially infected waters have proved to be at least partially effective against spread of the disease.

The greatest incidence occurs in children from 5 to 9 years of age, although there is a strongly increasing trend toward infection in the older age groups; the incidence during the first year of life is extremely low. Males are more susceptible than females. There is no obvious racial susceptibility.

Signs and Symptoms. The incubation period is probably from 5 to 35 days.

The first symptoms resemble those of a common cold or a severe gastrointestinal upset accompanied by diarrhea and vomiting. Irritability, with alternate periods of restlessness and sleeplessness, is quite common.

These symptoms may subside for a period of from several hours to 2 or 3 days. There then comes an acute flare-up, with severe headache, constipation, and the onset of paralysis, marked by flabbiness of the affected parts.

The fever accompanying infantile paralysis is deceptive, and one should be warned that it does not follow the typical course of many other diseases, for, at the onset, the temperature may rise to 102 or 103°F and then may rapidly subside in the next 24 to 48 hours.

The most characteristic early sign is the patient's inability to flex his spine. When raised in bed to a sitting position, he holds the back stiff, bracing himself with his hands and arms, and resists any attempt to bend his head forward toward his knees (Fig. 14-3).

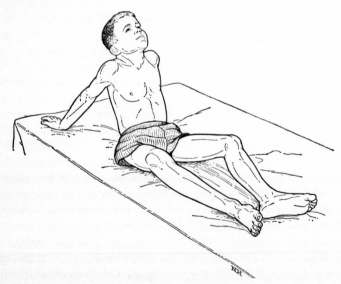

Fig. 14-3. The "tripod" position, a characteristic of early polio.

Forecasting the outcome of these cases is difficult, but there is one comforting fact: although this condition properly arouses great concern, less than 25 cases per 100,000 are fatal. About 20 to 30 percent of the cases occurring in later life develop paralysis, and of these, about 30 percent clear up within a year.

Contrary to popular superstition, polio causes no deterioration of the intellect.

While the period of infectiousness is now known, it is assumed that patients can infect others for several days prior to the onset of the symptoms and for at least the first 14 days after onset.

○ TREATMENT

Polio demands the best of medical care, and the doctor should be notified immediately if the condition is even *suspected,* especially if a child shows symptoms and there are cases of polio in the general vicinity.

Whether or not the patient should be hospitalized is not always an easy question to answer. Many general hospitals now admit polio cases, although in some localities they are still restricted to hospitals exclusively designated for the treatment of contagious diseases. Many cases can be successfully cared for at home, particularly those of the abortive type and even the more severe nonparalytic cases. While mild paralytic cases may be cared for at home, they are probably better off in an adequately equipped hospital because of the special facilities that may be required.

If a patient is nursed at home, certain considerations are of the utmost importance. For instance, because it is a contagious disease, special precautions must be taken to isolate the patient, to maintain separate personal belongings and eating utensils, and to exercise special contagious-disease nursing procedures, as outlined in Chapter 16. Special attention in this regard must be given to all discharges from the nose and throat and to the stools, which may be highly infectious.

The patient must be confined to bed, as absolute rest is of utmost importance. This is not only to facilitate recovery but to prevent paralysis, since it is considered possible that, if a child who should have *complete bed rest* is permitted out of bed too early or allowed too much activity, he may be predisposed to paralysis, which might not otherwise occur.

Victims of polio suffer quite severely from increased restlessness, irritability, and severe muscle pain as the result of muscle spasm. Aspirin in proper dosage often provides some relief, and hot fomentations applied directly to the affected muscles also seem to lessen the patient's discomfort by helping to counteract the muscle spasm.

In all cases it is extremely important that close and constant medical supervision be maintained, since many difficulties may arise which can only be dealt with as they occur. In the event of the slightest indication of bulbar (brain stem) involvement, with resulting respiratory paralysis, the immediate use of an iron lung is essential.

The successful treatment of polio depends on the most devoted, sympathetic, and understanding nursing care. It must be at all times under the most careful medical guidance, not only during the acute phase of the disease, but during the long periods of convalescence and of rehabilitation, as well as during the treatment and correction of any deformities that may have occurred. Many community facilities are available for this purpose, in addition to those of the National Foundation (previously called the National Foundation for Infantile Paralysis). These include equipment, nursing, and financial aid. Learn about these agencies and facilities in advance, so that in a crisis you will know those who can help you meet your needs.

Prophylaxis. Preventive injections of inactivated poliovirus vaccine, introduced in 1955, have brought polio largely into the category of preventable diseases, since the incidence of paralytic polio was reduced over 90 percent. In spite of this excellent record, however, certain technical problems became apparent with respect to duration of immunity and eradiction of virus from the intestinal tract. In 1961 and 1962 a trivalent oral polio vaccine known as TOPV became available and was found to have very definite advantages which are particularly useful in meeting special situations. For instance, the oral vaccine would be the protective measure of choice, on a community-wide basis, whenever an epidemic of poliomyelitis should strike or threaten an area.

The reason for this is that a single dose of the specific virus (type I, II, or III) causing a given epidemic induces a very prompt protective response and thus provides a very effective countermeasure. Of course, a full sequence of doses of all three types of virus is needed for full protection against all three types of polio which might be encountered over a long period of time.

In addition, the oral vaccine confers a definite degree of resistance within the gastrointestinal tract to reinfection with so-called "wild" polio viruses. This brings about what the immunologists call *herd immunity*, although the length of time that this type of protection will last has not yet been definitely determined.

Probably one of the most important advantages of the oral vaccine is the ease with which it can be administered (a few drops on the tongue, on a lump of sugar, or in a teaspoonful of syrup). Obviously this facilitates the immunizing of young children, who quite understandably, are horrified of an injection with a needle, and greatly simplifies its administration to very large numbers of people within a short period of time.

For these reasons, on the basis of the report of the Surgeon General's Special Advisory Committee, taken in conjunction with all available pertinent data, the American Academy of Pediatrics has stated that the use of oral poliovirus vaccine (TOPV) appears to be the optimum immunization procedure for the prevention of paralytic poliomyelitis in children. It is therefore the vaccine of choice for community-wide vaccination programs and for routine immunization in infancy and childhood. Administration is simple and pleasant for the child, since the vaccine is usually given to them on a lump of sugar or in formula, the first dose being given at the age of 2 months, the second dose at the age of 4 months, the third dose at about the age of 1½ years. Another repeat dose is given at 4-6 years of age.

The important thing is that all communities should continue to make certain that all infants are fully immunized by 1 year of age, and should have as an additional target the vaccination of the entire community population (excluding newborn infants and the acutely ill), at least up through the young-adult age group.

C-virus (Coxsackie Virus) Infection. Recently a series of viruses, consisting of two main groups (A and B) and some 30 subgroups, has been discovered which is immunologically different from polio virus, but which occurs very frequently in nature under the same conditions as the polio virus. In children these viruses may cause a type of illness which is very difficult to distinguish clinically from true nonparalytic polio. The name of the virus comes from its discovery in the feces of two ill children in Coxsackie, New York. It is now generally known simply as C-virus.

This organism provides three principal kinds of acute illness in children which resemble, respectively, nonparalytic polio with or without a rash, severe pains in the body muscles (epidemic myalgia), and acute intestinal "grippe." The peak incidence occurs in the summer and autumn, at the same time as the polio season, which gives a very serious aspect to the occurrence of such illness and makes its distinction from polio even more difficult.

The period of communicability is not known exactly but is probably greatest from 2 to 3 days to several days after onset. Virus may be present in the feces for several weeks.

Signs and Symptoms. The incubation period of C-virus infection may be from 2 to 10 days.

The signs and symptoms usually appear suddenly and include a fever, the temperature ranging from 100 to 105°F., accompanied by severe malaise lasting from 2 to 10 days. Headache is one of the chief symptoms, and nausea and vomiting often occur, especially when the disease resembles nonparalytic polio. In many cases there is severe abdominal pain, but the child may also suffer from severe chest pain. Sore throat occurs in about half the cases, and in many children, small circumscribed blisters or ulcers will be seen in the mouth. A sign which frequently causes confusion is that often the child's back and neck are stiff, an observation that immediately suggests the possibility of polio. Infection with C-virus does not, however, cause true paralysis, and fatalities—insofar as is known—are exceedingly rare, if indeed any occur.

Although its methods of transmission have not been fully worked out, it has been proved that the virus exists in the throat and the feces of patients, and apparently it persists in their stools for some time after the symptoms are gone. Presumably, therefore, contagion occurs through direct droplet infection and by fecal contamination of foodstuffs. There is also evidence that flies may be an important factor, since C-virus was isolated directly from flies in at least one large epidemic.

The disease occurs in the form of outbreaks involving whole family units, as well as large groups of children living together, as in summer camps, where apparently such outbreaks are becoming more frequent.

○ TREATMENT

There is no specific remedy for C-virus infection at present, but fortunately the disease is self-limiting, and, after it has run its course, recovery is complete.

Prophylaxis. The only means of prevention now known is to exercise stringent precautions against general contagion, with special emphasis on the avoidance of contaminated food and water, on strict personal cleanliness, as well as on careful sanitation of all eating utensils and toilet facilities.

15

Common Medical Emergencies and Conditions

There are various emergencies that may arise in the home or in a public place, which include many illnesses that are to a large extent unrelated, except for one common factor: whatever the condition may be, it has caused a person to become ill and require assistance. We have grouped these conditions under the very general classification of medical emergencies not primarily the result of some form of injury; the term *medical* is used in it broadest sense to include, as well, emergencies that are fundamentally of a surgical nature, such as acute appendicitis or gallstones.

MEDICAL CONDITIONS

Unconsciousness

One of the most baffling situations requiring emergency care is the unconscious person. As a rule, the first available person is called on for help after the stricken individual has become unconscious and, therefore, has not been able to observe the circumstances prior to the onset of unconsciousness. The important thing is to know what conditions might be responsible for the unconsciousness and, equally important, what conditions are *not*. With this knowledge, the first-aid worker will be better able to render proper emergency care, until the doctor arrives, and may well be instrumental in saving the person's life.

In other words, coma is a symptom of disease, not a disease in itself, and there are a great many conditions, ranging from brain disease to physical trauma, that may bring about loss of consciousness of various degrees. It may be a little misleading to attempt to list such conditions in order of frequency, but it is probable that under present-day conditions drug intoxication, particularly that due to alcohol or barbiturates, would rank first, with trauma, especially head injury, ranking second. Cerebral vascular disease is a common cause of coma, as are many types of poisons (aside from the barbiturates and alcohol). Diabetic coma due to either hypoglycemia or acidosis is not as frequent as formerly, but it still must be borne in mind in handling any case of coma.

The determination of the underlying cause of unconsciousness often requires a very careful physical examination and detailed laboratory work, but much can be learned on the spot from a history of what led up to the comatose condition: the patient's age, general medical background, and careful observation of the patient himself. Much of this book is devoted to the elucidation of conditions, with their signs and symptoms, which may give rise to coma, so that these need not be repeated here except to emphasize again certain cardinal signs which may well give a clue to diagnosis. These include a general inspection of the patient: is he flushed, pale or cyanotic; his position; such movements as he may be making; the presence of injury—particularly to the head. Has he recently had a convulsion or is he convulsing? Does the patient respond to external stimuli? The pupils of the eyes: are they dilated or pinpoint, even or uneven in size—especially important in head injury and drug intoxication cases. Breathing: is it rapid, shallow, slow, labored; the odor of the breath typical in diabetic acidosis and uremia, alcoholic intoxication, and other poisonings. The pulse rate: is it rapid, slow, weak or strong, regular or intermittent. Has the patient been incontinent of either urine or feces? These on-the-spot observations can be helpful as a guide to handling the case even before the hospital is reached, where more sophisticated observations and studies can be carried out.

The present-day drug scene should always be kept in mind, particularly in the younger age groups, and there are special signs (described in Chap. 12) which indicate this possibility. In addition, characteristic traumatic skin lesions following drug-induced coma have long been mentioned in the European literature and have been reported in this country by Mandy and Ackerman from the University of Miami School of Medicine.

The first manifestation is a dusky red patch that may either become indurated or hard or form large blisters. These lesions frequently arise on the wrists, palms, or fingers of patients resisting restraints, or the skin over the scapulae or sacrum of patients who have been lying on their backs for 24 hours or more (Fig. 15-1). Such lesions may also occur on other exposed areas of the extremities. Fully developed blisters may appear within a few minutes following pressure or friction and persist for from 10 to 14 days, after which they subside without leaving any scarring.

The phenomenon has been observed in patients who have become comatose as the result of carbon monoxide poisoning and many types of drug poisoning, including that due to barbiturates, the opium drugs and heroin, meprobamate, and others.

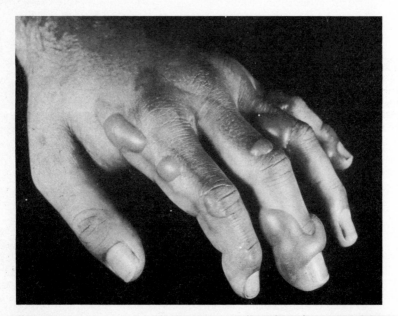

Fig. 15-1. In certain types of poisoning as well as drug abuse cases, large blisters may appear very shortly after frictional pressure such as may occur as the result of grappling with restraints. (Reproduced, with permission, from Mandy, S. and A. B. Ackerman: Characteristic Traumatic Skin Lesions in Drug-induced Coma, *J.A.M.A. 213:* 253–256, July 13, 1970.)

It has been suggested that the appearance of these lesions and their characteristic microscopic appearance may have important diagnostic significance with respect to drug-induced coma.

Emergency Measures. Whatever the cause of coma, it is often necessary to take certain life-support measures even before an exact diagnosis is made. Such measures include maintenance of an adequate airway coupled with assisted respiration if necessary and prevention of aspiration by turning the victim's head to one side; control of bleeding; prevention of shock by all suitable procedures; if there exists the possibility of hypoglycemic shock, glucose should be administered immediately as a potentially lifesaving measure.

Finally, physically handle the patient in such a way that if he *does* have serious injuries (such as cervical fracture), whatever manipulations are carried out, the damage will not be extended to vital structures such as the spinal cord.

Diabetic Coma. One of the causes of unconsciousness or semiconsciousness, for which the correct emergency care is of paramount importance, is diabetic coma. There are two forms. One results from the diabetic's inability to obtain the insulin he requires on schedule or from his eating improperly and *not* taking *enough* insulin. The other results from taking *too much* insulin or from not being able to get enough carbohydrate food to balance the amount of insulin he is accustomed to taking. Strictly speaking, the first condition is known as *diabetic coma* (or diabetic ketoacidosis), and the second as *insulin coma*.

The symptoms and appearance of a person in each of these two conditions are very different; therefore, it is usually not difficult to tell them apart.

Diabetic coma occurs when there is insufficient insulin in the body to fully metabolize carbohydrates and fats. Because the substances are only partially broken down chemically, they form various compounds that are acid in nature and seriously alter the body's chemistry. Consequently, the patient is thrown into a condition which is known medically as *acidosis*. If acidosis becomes severe enough, the individual gradually becomes confused, disoriented, and stuporous, and eventually lapses into coma.

Signs and Symptoms. The face is flushed, the lips are a

cherry-red color, the skin is very dry, the temperature is lowered although the patient looks as though he had a fever (a point of differentiation from heat stroke), and breathing is spasmodic. Characteristically, there is the sickly sweet odor of acetone (the odor of nail-polish remover) or spoiled fruit on the breath. This odor is a clue to the condition.

Do not confuse the odor of acetone with that of alcohol— an all too common mistake. People have been thrown into jail for being drunk when they were actually in diabetic coma.

This condition may have come on over a period of several hours, preceded by an intensification of all the characteristic symptoms of diabetes: excessive thirst; excessive urination; excessive appetite, followed by loss of appetite and increasing weakness, leading to drowsiness.

○ TREATMENT

Call for medical assistance immediately. From a strictly emergency care standpoint, there is little to be done until help arrives. However, if this is not available *quickly* and if insulin is at hand, it should be given by hypodermic injection, in doses of 50 units, repeated in 30 minutes. This action will save the person's life and will tide him over until medical aid arrives.

If neither medical aid nor insulin is available, treat the case as one of shock and administer fluids in large amounts by mouth. If the victim is unconscious, administer fluids by rectum, using a salt solution (1 teaspoonful to a quart of water) or bicarbonate of soda in the same concentration, in amounts up to 2 quarts or more.

Do *not* give sugar, carbohydrates, or fats *in any form.*

Many persons in diabetic coma tend to be nauseated, although there may be little in the stomach. Since the victim may be in a semistupor, he must be prevented, by turning the head to one side, from sucking vomited matter into the lungs, and it must be made certain that an adequate airway is maintained. These victims seem to do better in a semireclining position, particularly since a complicating heart condition may also be present.

Insulin Coma. In some ways, insulin coma presents just the opposite picture from diabetic coma. This condition is due to *too little* sugar in the blood as the result of *too much* insulin, which may be present for one reason or another.

Signs and Symptoms. The person presents an ashen-white countenance; the skin is moist and clammy and covered with a cold sweat; and he is obviously in a state of shock. The pulse is rapid, but the breathing is slow and shallow. There is *no odor* of acetone on the breath.

○ TREATMENT

Medical aid should, of course, be obtained immediately, but sometimes improvement can be brought about even before aid becomes available. What the victim needs is sugar, and this must be gotten into him very quickly, even if he is unconscious. To do this, keep placing a little granulated sugar under his tongue as rapidly as it is absorbed, until the victim regains consciousness. If this method is too slow, sugar solution should additionally be instilled by rectum, as a retention enema (q.v.).

Orange juice is an excellent source of carbohydrate (sugar) and, even if the victim is semiconscious, can be given in very small amounts, by teaspoon, until enough sugar has been absorbed to bring about a return of consciousness of sufficient degree to permit him to swallow larger amounts safely. From then on, recovery usually is rapid.

Sometimes it is impossible to get enough sugar into an unconscious person except by intravenous infusion of glucose in saline. In severe cases that do not respond quickly to other routes of administration, this should not be deferred, since the victim may go into convulsions if the blood sugar level becomes too low. This can be carried out en route by properly trained ambulance personnel and may prove to be a lifesaving procedure even if the case is not actually one of insulin coma.

Apoplexy (Stroke). This condition, which is also referred to as a *stroke* or, in New England particularly, as a *shock,* is caused by an interruption of the blood supply to a vital center within the brain. This interruption may be produced in three principal ways: (1) The most sudden, and the one which most frequently creates the most dangerous emergency situation, is produced by hemorrhage (spoken of as *cerebral hemorrhage*), which comes about, usually in an older person, when an artery within the brain substance ruptures as the result of arteriosclerosis or high blood pressure. (2) The condition may be produced by a gradual blocking, as by a blood clot or arteriosclerotic plaque, of an artery supplying an important center of the brain. This is spoken of technically as *cerebral thrombosis*. (3) Somewhat less frequently (about 10 percent of the cases), apoplexy is caused by blockage of an artery by an embolus coming from a distant part of the body. This is known technically as a *cerebral embolism*. Such an embolism may be a clot of blood or a bubble of air.

From a medical standpoint, it is important to try to differentiate between these conditions, as each requires different treatment, but such a differentiation and specialized treatment are not within the scope of first-aid care. It is important, however, to be able to recognize the nature and seriousness of the situation in order to carry out initial supportive procedures until medical aid can be procured.

Signs and Symptoms. The onset usually is sudden, and there is little specific warning. Previously, there may have been transient episodes of cerebral ischemia which produces periods of dizziness, mental confusion, or recurrent headache.

The victim may suddenly collapse, although not always completely losing consciousness. His face is red and congested; the veins of the neck may stand out; the eyes may appear to be unusually prominent, and often the pupils are not of equal size. His mouth may pull gradually to one side, and there is drooling of saliva. There may be vomiting or convulsions, or both.

The striking aspects of apoplexy are the signs which result from the interruption of the blood supply to a specific part of the brain. Very often, one whole side of the body will be paralyzed. This can be determined, even if the victim is unconscious, by carefully observing the looseness and limpness of an arm and leg on one side of the body as compared with those on the other side, although, if the victim is in profound coma, the differences may be very slight. The affected part of the brain will be on the side *opposite* the one that is paralyzed, since the left side of the brain controls the right side of the body, and vice versa. Speech may or may not be directly affected, depending upon which side of the brain was affected. In right-handed people, the speech center is on the left side of the brain, and in left-handed people it is usually on the right.

The degree of the symptoms will vary with the extent of the brain involvement. In the case of *cerebral thrombosis,* the onset will be slower, with perhaps mild symptoms and temporary recovery, before the acute attack. If only a small artery is involved, the symptoms will be mild, and recovery will be much more rapid.

Such a fortunate occurrence, however, must be taken as a warning, which, if unheeded, will ultimately and surely lead to a more severe and perhaps fatal recurrence.

In most cases that end fatally, death does not occur immediately, but may take place several hours or many days later, depending upon the degree of involvement and the effectiveness of the treatment.

○ TREATMENT

From the standpoint of emergency care, the most important need is to assure that the patient has a clear airway in order to minimize the effects of relative anoxia on an already damaged brain. Immediate medical aid should then be requested, since there are a number of specific procedures which, if undertaken quickly, may not only prove lifesaving but will greatly benefit the patient's ultimate prognosis. In the meantime:

1 Make the victim as comfortable as possible, in a *semireclining* position—do *not* use the shock position.
2 Loosen all clothing, and apply cool compresses to the forehead and face.
3 Keep curiosity seekers away; their presence may aggravate the condition in a semiconscious or conscious person.
4 If the victim vomits, prevent his aspirating the vomited matter, as the throat muscles may be partially paralyzed.
5 If he convulses, prevent the victim from injuring himself—particularly from biting his tongue. Place something soft but firm between his jaws to prevent this.

An apoplexy victim may go into shock later on, a condition requiring special medical treatment. If this occurs, the first-aider can only try to keep the victim warm and comfortable. Administration of sedatives should be left to the doctor; they may be dangerous—especially opiates—since these increase the pressure within the cranium and would make the condition worse. As a rule, sedatives should *not* be given, but in the convulsing patient diazepam or diphenylhydantoin USP, Dilantin® is sometimes used as a control measure by the physician.

Transport the victim to a hospital on a stretcher with a pillow under his head to elevate it slightly; any unnecessary joggling must be avoided.

Hypertensive Crisis. Another somewhat infrequent condition which may lead to coma is the so-called "hypertensive crisis," which may occur in a variety of serious medical situations, including renal disease, and in persons who are taking certain drugs—the so-called "monamine oxidase inhibitors" which include pargyline hydrochloride (Eutonyl®), pargyline hydrochloride and methyclothiazide (Eutron®), isocarboxazid (Marplan®), and tranylcypromine (Parnate®). If such individuals inadvertently eat certain foods such as strong cheeses, chianti wine or other alcoholic beverages, beans, and processed meats, or take "over-the-counter" cold preparations or antihistamines, an adverse reaction may occur which causes a very sharp rise in blood pressure, with the diastolic pressure going to 140 or more, extremely severe headache, and the threat of blindness, stupor, convulsions, and coma.

○ TREATMENT

This is an acute medical emergency, since the blood pressure must be quickly reduced by the intravenous administration of certain drugs such as trimethaphan camsylate (Arfonad®) or pentolinium (Ansolysen®), which temporarily lower the arterial pressure rapidly, thus avoiding a potentially fatal outcome. If a physician cannot be obtained quickly for a patient suffering a hypertensive crisis, he should be moved promptly, in a semi-sitting position, by ambulance to the nearest hospital emergency room.

Uremic Coma. Uremic coma is unlikely to be an emergency-care problem, since its onset is very gradual and usually occurs in a person who is known to have been ill for some time with a kidney or heart ailment. Nevertheless, because it may be of importance to be able to recognize the onset of symptoms so that medical aid may be summoned rapidly, uremic coma is mentioned here.

Signs and Symptoms. The victim usually complains of headache and appears drowsy and mentally confused. The skin is a sallow lemon color and is cold and dry; there is a generalized peculiar, stale odor emanating from his body, like that of old urine, although he may not be incontinent. Breathing is rapid, and there is a most unpleasant uriniferous odor on the breath. The pulse is rapid, full, and bounding. The drowsiness gradually increases and deepens into coma.

There are, of course, other conditions, which can bring about a temporary functional failure of the kidneys and produce a similar general picture. Therefore, if the person can be tided over by means of an artificial kidney (renal dialysis) or peritoneal dialysis, until his kidneys begin to function again, a miracle will have been achieved and he will survive.

Acute Heart Conditions

A *heart attack* is one of the most common major medical emergencies. It usually occurs in older persons, most frequently in men, who may have been known to have "heart trouble" or high blood pressure for some time. However, an attack can occur with calamitous suddenness in an individual supposedly in robust health. Depending upon its nature, a heart attack may or may not be characterized by agonizing pain, and it may or may not produce temporary unconsciousness. The majority of heart attacks do not produce instant death.

From the standpoint of emergency care, it is important to understand the general nature of the conditions which may produce symptoms of an acute heart attack.

Angina Pectoris. A very common form of heart disease is angina pectoris, characterized by severe gripping, oppressive pain in the chest, which may radiate to the neck, to the jaws, or, occasionally, down one arm.

Anginal attacks may be precipitated by stress, excitement, great emotion (particularly anger, hatred, or jealousy), heavy eating, or exertion. Because persons subject to anginal attacks are often heavy eaters, these attacks often are said to be "acute indigestion," and their real nature is not recognized. Anginal victims are confirmed users of bicarbonate of soda or of one of the many remedies for "acid indigestion" that beset the market.

As pointed out by Cohen, the clinical study of angina pectoris indicates that all cardiovascular signs relate to sympathetic overactivity, such as tachycardia, increase of blood pressure, arterial hypertonia, or increase of myocardial demands. The assumption of overactivity of the sympathetic system in angina pectoris would explain why such sympatholytic drugs as propranolol hydrochloride (Inderal®) and/or the stimulation of the carotid sinus are effective.

Signs and Symptoms. The person may experience semi-collapse but usually does not lose consciousness. Although the victim's face may turn gray, he may clutch his chest, have difficulty in breathing, and not move for fear of worsening his condition, there is not the degree of shock and overwhelming distress which often characterizes coronary thrombosis. The two conditions cannot always be easily differentiated, but as a rule an anginal attack is not as severe as a coronary attack.

After an interval of absolute quiet, the pain will begin to ease as the spasm relaxes. If it persists, death may result, but a fatal outcome is not frequent. It should be noted also that angina pectoris, coupled with general signs of failing health, may constitute premonitory symptoms of coronary thrombosis.

O TREATMENT

1 Place the victim in a sitting (not prone) position wherever he may be.

2 Protect him from exertion or emotional strain of any kind until the attack subsides.

3 Keep onlookers away, and give the victim as much of a feeling of understanding, protection, and security as possible.

4 Do not try to move him until the attack has passed; keep him warm and as comfortable as possible.

Look for an Emergency Medical Alert Symbol, or try to determine if this is the victim's first attack; if it is not, he may have nitroglycerine tablets or amyl nitrite ampuls with him. Administer either immediately. Place a nitroglycerine tablet under his tongue, where absorption takes place quickly, or break an amyl nitrite ampul and hold it under his nose, so that the vapor may be directly inhaled. Either drug usually brings prompt relief.

Upon recovery, it is important that the victim should not be subjected to any further nervous strain and that he avoid any exertion. He should see a doctor immediately, because with proper long-range treatment, both the incidence and the dangerous consequences of these attacks can be lessened.

Acute Coronary Thrombosis. This condition results from the plugging of one of the arteries or one of its branches which supply the muscle of the heart itself. The fate of the victim depends upon the rapidity with which he can be given definitive care and upon the size of the vessel that is plugged—he may survive the plugging of a small vessel, but if it is a large one, he may not. Plugging is due to the formation of a clot which gradually grows larger, until such a time as the blood can no longer flow to the starved muscle, and thus precipitates the agonizing attack.

Coronary thrombosis is a part of the process of general hardening of the arteries (atherosclerosis); while its manifestations may appear to be sudden, the processes which are responsible not only have been going on for a long time, but they might, to a large extent, have been both diagnosed and prevented.

The advent of intensive coronary care units in some 2,000 of the 7,000 hospitals in the United States has had a tremendous impact in reducing the mortality in those who survive long enough to reach the unit, as indicated by Table 15-1.

TABLE 15-1

EFFECTIVENESS OF INTENSIVE CORONARY CARE ON MORTALITY RATES

Time	I.C.C.	Non-I.C.C.
At 24 hours	8.4%	13.8%
At 96 hours	12.0%	20.8%
At discharge	19.9%	30.8%
Relative drop in mortality rate 35%		

The importance of prompt recognition, correct first-aid assistance, and rapid transportation to the coronary care unit, with sophisticated resuscitative procedures rendered en route by trained ambulance personnel, cannot be overemphasized.

It is significant to note that in spite of the wide availability of coronary care units, coronary artery disease remains the leading cause of death and accounts for more than 400,000 fatalities in the United States each year. Part of the answer lies in the fact that, as pointed out by Kuller et al., 60 percent of all deaths from arteriosclerotic heart disease occur outside of hospitals. Further, as underscored by an editorial in the Journal of the American Medical Association, "approximately 60 percent of all deaths from myocardial infarction occur within 1 hour of the onset of symptoms."

Signs and Symptoms. A victim of an attack of acute coronary thrombosis usually suffers with severe, agonizing, vise-like pain in the chest (may radiate down the left arm, into the fourth and fifth fingers, and up into the neck or through the back). He may collapse and lose consciousness; his face has an ashen pallor. There may be vomiting and urinary and fecal incontinence. Shock may be severe.

○ TREATMENT

1 Do not move the victim, except to get him out of the way of danger, until he is seen by a doctor. Keep him in a half-sitting position. Do not lay him down.

2 If nitroglycerine or amyl nitrite is available, use either, even before the doctor arrives.

3 Loosen all clothing; allow him to get as much air as possible; and if it is available, give him oxygen.

4 If the victim is conscious, do everything possible to reassure him and to allay his fear, for he will usually feel that he is very close to death.

5 If he should vomit, help him to do so with a minimum of effort, as further strain must be avoided at all costs.

Obtain medical help as quickly as possible. It may well be that no pulse can be felt. This will be because the heart either has gone into ventricular fibrillation, so that the effectiveness of its pumping action is almost completely abolished, or into actual cardiac arrest. This does not necessarily mean that the patient is dead, but it is an indication for the immediate institution of external cardiac massage (see pages 137–141).

If the patient has stopped breathing, mouth-to-mouth resuscitation should be started along with the cardiac massage, as it is sometimes possible to restore both cardiac and respiratory function pending the arrival of medical aid. Many cases, who otherwise certainly would have died, have been kept alive until the arrival of an ambulance and transportation to the acute coronary care unit of a modern hospital, where many highly sophisticated facilities are available for reviving and sustaining the victim of a coronary thrombosis through the critical period of his recovery.

More and more, these cases are being saved, largely as the result of two factors: (1) prompt and effective institution of resuscitative procedures within seconds or a minute or 2 after the attack takes place; and (2) improved coronary care procedures which, as has been indicated, many modern hospitals are now in a position to furnish.

With today's advanced technics the principal cause of death in acute myocardial infarction is left ventricular failure, which occurs in about 93 percent of fatal cases.

From this, it is apparent that the major problems in the intensive care of the coronary victim are the control of congestive heart failure and cardiogenic shock.

The most severe form of left ventricular failure is represented by cardiogenic shock. The most important index of cardiogenic shock is the profound drop in cardiac output, which is reflected in a weak, thready pulse, cold moist extremities, peripheral cyanosis, oliguria, and profound prostration.

The appropriate treatment of cardiogenic shock usually can be undertaken only by a physician or other especially trained person; it includes (1) whatever means may be necessary to prevent or overcome arrhythmias, such as the administration of propanolol (Inderol®), lidocaine, or, in an emergency, atropine, (2) administration of digitalis, and (3) some type of inotropic drug such as isoproterenol hydrochloride, USP (Isuprel® Hydrochloride), to improve cardiac output.

If you are responsible for aid to a victim of an acute heart attack where you are entirely on your own, as at sea aboard a small craft, and a doctor cannot reach him quickly, carry out such of the above instructions as you can. Also, give the victim an injection of ¼ grain morphine (if your doctor has seen fit to provide you with a small supply, in case of emergency). This may be repeated at 4-hour intervals until the acute pain has subsided and the victim is less apprehensive. Morphine should be used cautiously, however, because of possible undesired side effects, such as increasing the tendency to very slow heartbeat (bradycardia) and the development of irregular rhythm. In these respects, meperidine (Demerol®) is a preferable drug for the relief of severe cardiac pain.

Epinephrine, 0.5 cubic centimeter subcutaneously every 30 minutes to an hour, may be needed to combat cardiogenic shock until definitive medical aid becomes available. Isuprel® is the drug of choice but is not as likely to be available under isolated conditions as epinephrine.

If one of the small portable oxygen supply units is available, administer oxygen as freely as your supply will permit. Request immediate assistance and further instructions from the U.S. Coast Guard or other emergency service by radio.

Convulsions

There are many conditions that cause convulsions, some of which already have been discussed in relation to children. Convulsions are always alarming, but do not necessarily indicate a serious disease. However, their occurrence always requires a thorough search for the underlying cause.

Convulsions may involve the entire body or only a part, but whatever the extent of the seizure, there are involuntary twitchings of the muscle groups and usually unconsciousness.

Convulsions, in themselves, rarely produce death; the principal dangers are that the victim may injure himself; may be killed or injured by accident, as from falling out of a boat, off a subway platform, or into a piece of machinery or may die from the causative condition itself, such as a cerebral hemorrhage.

Convulsions are symptoms of some underlying disease or abnormal condition, the most common being of the brain. But many other conditions, as abnormal chemical changes in the body, various infectious diseases, injuries sustained at birth, and other accidents, may also produce convulsions.

Often, convulsions may occur in children as preliminary to, or in conjunction with, an acute illness. They may also accompany a fainting attack or be precipitated by a prolonged period of rapid breathing (hyperventilation), as may occur as the result of excitement in tense or nervous children or adults.

Epilepsy. Epilepsy is probably the most common cause of convulsions in most age groups. Of the many types of epilepsy, the forms known as *grand mal* and *petit mal* are most often encountered. Of these, grand mal is the more severe. Attacks of petit mal epilepsy are more often seen in children, but may occur in adults.

Signs and Symptoms. The victim of convulsions due to grand mal epilepsy has a premonition, or aura (realizes something is going to happen), loses consciousness, and falls. Sometimes he foams at the mouth; there are severe, convulsive spasms of the jaw muscles. He may vomit, urinate, or defecate. His face is livid; the veins in the neck are swollen; and breathing is loud and labored (hissing sound).

As a rule, the attack does not last for more than a few minutes, but sometimes, because one attack follows another with alarming frequency, a general anesthetic may be required to control the convulsions. Usually, however, the victim passes into a deep sleep after a single episode and awakens with little or no knowledge of what has happened, but sometimes he recovers without going to sleep and, after a period of mental confusion in which he appears to be "coming to," regains his composure and seems to be relatively normal. It should be borne in mind that epilepsy may simulate many other convulsive states and that some forms may be characterized by various psychotic disorders rather than convulsions *per se.*

Petit mal attacks are characterized by only a partial loss of consciousness, so that the patient remains aware of what is going on around him. The attacks may be accompanied by minor convulsive movements of the extremities, or eyes, but usually last for only a short time.

The victim seems to be perfectly normal just before and immediately after an attack, and there is not the characteristic premonition that precedes the grand mal attack.

○ TREATMENT

Those who are accustomed to handling epileptic seizures make little of the convulsions and do not become excited.

It is important to keep the victim of the attack from aspirating or choking on vomited matter, but since most attacks will terminate harmlessly by themselves, regardless of what you do or do not do, just protect the victim from injury and bide your time. When he recovers, do not be unduly sympathetic—you may only embarrass him. Give him a drink of water or tea, protect him from curious onlookers, and be sure that he is well enough to go on his way or that he is taken home. If the condition is more serious, see that he gets to a hospital.

Dizziness

Dizziness is a term commonly used to describe a great variety of sensations. The main characteristic of dizziness is the victim thinks he is going through some sort of movement when he really isn't; he may feel as if he were swaying, rocking, pitching, falling, whirling, drunk, or swimming, or that he is standing still and the room is going around him.

Dizziness is one of the most common medical symptoms, and may be caused by many different things. Severe dizziness can be most distressing and at times completely incapacitating. It is usually the result of some condition which affects the delicate organs of balance deep within the inner ear, or disrupts the nerve pathways which connect them to parts of the brain in the cerebellum, which correlate these with sensation coming in from the eyes, the muscles, and other parts of the body to achieve a normal sense of balance and orientation in space. Anything which interrupts or scrambles the orderly flow of these messages will produce some form of dizziness.

Dizziness becomes more common with advancing age because of the vascular changes seen in older people such as hardening of the arteries of the brain, heart disease, high blood pressure, menopause, and hardening of the brain tissue itself (cerebral sclerosis). It is somewhat more common in women than men.

Dizziness in older age groups may be brought on by sudden movement or changes in position of the head and is referred to, technically, as postural dizziness. It is not dangerous or particularly incapacitating except that the patient may fall and injure himself during brief moments of unsteadiness.

One quite common cause of dizziness is a condition known as Ménière's disease (see page 524).

Symptoms which may be confusingly like those of Ménière's disease are caused by transient infection (often due to a virus) of the internal ear, or a direct toxic effect by certain drugs and antibiotics such as streptomycin.

Infections of the middle ear, such as the common acute otitis media which becomes chronic, can also cause dizziness by indirect involvement of the middle ear.

Dizziness is also very common after head injuries, particularly concussions, and brain operations and operations on the middle ear or labyrinth to correct hearing disorders. Although it may last for a long time, it almost invariably clears up completely.

Such a simple thing as an accumulation of wax in the ear may cause severe fullness in the head, dizziness, and loss of hearing on one side, thus simulating some serious condition. Fortunately, this is very easy to relieve, and removal of the wax quickly results in a miraculous cure!

Another common condition, a prominent symptom of which is often dizziness, is motion sickness. This basically results from a scrambling of the various impulses coming to the control center in the brain from the eyes and the internal ear. The center thus receives a host of mixed-up messages as the result of sudden and rapid changes in direction, which it cannot sort out and balance properly, so that dizziness, among other symptoms of motion sickness, results.

○ TREATMENT

From the standpoint of emergency aid, about all that can be done is to help the victim lie down or put him in a semiprone position if you believe his condition may be due to high blood pressure, with his head held absolutely still on a pillow, folded coat or blanket. Dizziness is often accompanied by nausea or faintness. If the attack does not pass quickly, medical aid should be obtained. A subsequent medical checkup is imperative in order to correct the underlying causative condition. There are a number of prescription drugs that may provide prompt symptomatic relief.

Headache

The term *headache* is so much a part of our everyday vocabulary that it has become almost synonymous with any problem or unpleasant situation. But in a medical sense the term quite literally means an *aching head* or *head pain* and is a symptom rather than in itself an actual disease condition.

Hence, headache can suggest the possibility of a great many underlying conditions. Perhaps one of the better-known types is the throbbing, devastating headache that usually accompanies a hangover. This differs from the type, known as *tension headache,* associated with figuring out one's income tax, since they arise from different causes—the first, from dilated throbbing blood vessels, such as may be caused by a little too much alcohol; the second, from tense muscles at the back of the neck, constricted blood vessels, and the severe pain and distress caused by nervous tension, apprehension, and fatigue— a very common phenomenon!

Between these two extremes lies a vast range of underlying causes of many kinds of headache, as, for example, that due to a brain tumor, to another serious condition of structures within the cranium, to sinus congestion, eye strain, or high blood pressure.

But from the standpoint of everyday practicality, the two main types of headache which most often plague the average person are migraine and tension headache. As has already been suggested, they differ in their underlying mechanisms, and of the two, migraine is the more distressing and prostrating.

Migraine. Migraine affects between 5 and 10 percent of the population and is more common in women than in men; it usually begins between the ages of 15 and 35, but it may also affect children.

It is characterized by severe prostrating headache, at first affecting only one side of the head, often accompanied by nausea, dizziness, and sometimes symptoms resembling those of shock. Often, the person knows in advance that an attack is coming on because of spots before his eyes, sensitivity to light, and sometimes chills, flushing, and weakness. Often, because the body may retain fluid, the face will become puffy and bloated.

Then the severe throbbing headache sets in and becomes intense enough to completely prostrate the sufferer. The initial throbbing is eventually replaced by a steady ache which spreads to the entire face and neck.

The actual cause of this condition is not known, although much research has unearthed many contributing factors and explained the various body mechanisms which bring about the symptoms.

Migraine, for instance, is much more common in cities, especially among executives of both sexes, professional people, and active housewives. Heredity must play an important part, since about 65 percent of patients in one large clinic, specializing in the diagnosis and treatment of headache, stated that other members of their families also had migraine.

The onset of the condition is very often associated with the beginning of puberty, menstruation, or menopause, but it is a curious fact that about 80 percent of women who usually suffer with migraine become free of the condition when they become pregnant, and migraine usually does not recur until about 6 weeks after delivery.

Some investigators have implicated allergy as a causative factor, but, while allergy to foods or other substances may contribute, it does not seem to be a major force. (There is, of course, a typical headache due to allergy, but this is usually easily distinguishable from other kinds.)

The relationship, however, between migraine and the emotions seems so well established as to merit little argument. Persons who suffer from migraine usually are emotionally tense, have strong subconscious feelings of guilt, frustration or belligerence, and react abnormally to the many stress factors in their own particular environments because of the nature of their personality and specific genetic makeup. Hence, any situation which puts undue emotional strain on an individual subject to migraine may produce an attack.

However, it is difficult to say which comes first—the hen or the egg. As one eminent authority points out, the emotional storm begins only after body changes leading to the onset of the headache have taken place. Between attacks the person, who is often highly intellectual, is usually a calm, kindly, considerate individual. However, just prior to an attack, there is often a very marked change in mood, characterized by obvious hostility toward those with whom the victim is closely associated—particularly toward someone for whom the individual would be expected to have a high degree of love or respect.

Many authorities believe that feelings of hostility bear an important relationship to the onset of attacks. The histories of many such victims indicate that, in their childhood, the parents were not demonstrative in their affection for the child, but, on the contrary, were often unusually firm and strict disciplinarians. The resulting insecurity in childhood produced tensions which are manifested in later life. This, of course, is not true of all persons who have migraine, but, while there is probably no such thing as a personality that is a prototype for this condition, there can be little question that an understanding of the psychologic factors involved is extremely important from both the victim's standpoint and that of the physician.

Regardless of the kind of bizarre factors that bring about all this pain and discomfort, what actually *does* happen within the body to cause such distress?   The mechanics involved are now fairly well known and understood.

Signs and Symptoms.   During the preheadache period, when the victim first begins to have strange feelings and knows he is going to have an attack, certain blood vessels in the brain itself undergo a spasm, thus partially stopping the flow of blood to one area or another, as, for example, to an eye, and producing various symptoms, depending on the part or parts involved.   Some scientific investigators think this may be the result of a response of the nerves and blood vessels to certain substances circulating in the blood.

The second, or severe headache, phase comes about when the blood vessels in the skull (or more usually in the tissues overlying the skull) relax, as does a worn-out garden hose, and begin to pulse and throb furiously.   Sometimes this condition lasts so long and becomes so severe that the arteries become hard, rigid, and very tender.   The throbbing one-sided headache becomes a steady generalized torture, and there now usually develops tension and spasm of the neck muscles, which serves further to increase the misery.

○ TREATMENT

Much can be done by the family physician to help in preventing or minimizing the frequency of such attacks through sympathetic psychotherapy, education of the person in understanding his or her problem, and the use of certain drugs which act specifically on the blood vessels causing the difficulty.

As far as emergency treatment of an acute attack is concerned, those drugs which might be expected to have a specific effect can be obtained only on a doctor's prescription.   It is therefore very desirable, if you are subject to migraine attacks, to discuss a plan of treatment, in advance, with your doctor and to have the necessary remedies on hand.   Migraine attacks can be aborted, if medication is taken at the very first appearance of discomfort, much more easily than they can be relieved once they are in full swing.

Aside from specific medication, the migraine sufferer should lie flat on his back, with a low pillow under his head, in a dark, quiet room. Dizziness will be lessened if the head can be kept in this position, with as little movement as possible. An ice bag, applied at the base of the skull, and cold compresses, to the forehead, often give considerable relief. A cup of strong hot tea with plenty of sugar may also relieve nausea and weakness. Some individuals find that a dose of Epsom salts, or the equivalent, taken early in the attack helps to prevent the onset of severe symptoms, probably because it results in a moderate loss of fluid from the body.

If these measures do not produce relief in a reasonable time or if the symptoms become worse, a physician should be consulted both for relief of the acute attack and for subsequent treatment of the condition.

Learning to enjoy life, to obtain adequate relaxation, and to shed one's frustrations, animosities, and tensions and obtaining adequate exercise and sleep are of especial importance. Through proper treatment, life can be made much more pleasant and the victim is often freed of his difficulty.

Tension Headache. Somewhat less of a problem, but certainly no less common, is the tension-type headache.

This is almost a *sine qua non* of our modern high-pressure, tension-ridden existence. Physiologically, it is caused by prolonged tight contraction of the muscles of the head and neck, resulting in the typical symptoms which are known to almost everybody and are characteristic of this type of headache.

The condition is most common in those who are unduly responsive to pressure, anxiety, and apprehension and whose occupations or other circumstances keep them on a sort of high-pressure hot seat and laboring under a perpetual unconscious sense of insecurity or fear.

Signs and Symptoms. These headaches, while they may be severe, are nowhere near as prostrating as migraine; they are usually characterized by a steady ache in the front or back of the head, or in both. Sometimes they are accompanied by nausea and dizziness, and the scalp itself often is quite tender, the sufferer saying that he feels as if he has a tight band around his head.

○ TREATMENT

This type of headache provides a vast market for all kinds of pain relievers, tranquilizers, and sedatives which, when properly used, have their place in helping to relieve tension and provide symptomatic relief. In addition, for treating the acute attack, local heat and massage to the back of the head and neck muscles, as well as distraction from the underlying causative tensions, provide considerable relief.

From a long-range standpoint, the only means by which the sufferer can hope to avoid such recurrent discomfort is through a basic understanding of his reactions to life's stress and hence learning how to avoid, or really how not to develop, his tensions. The so-called "tranquilizer drugs," which enjoy such a vast sale, do this largely by blanketing the person's reaction to stress—he just doesn't care so much. However, such remedies are not and never can be the fundamental answer to the problems of modern living.

If headaches are recurrent, especially if they are increasing in intensity, see your doctor in order to make sure that there is no serious underlying cause.

In any event, there is much that he can do to help you. You can do much to help him help you by attaining serenity and understanding through the many channels open to you, and by following through on the old admonition "Know thyself."

Sleep Paralysis

Of all the disabilities that affect man, perhaps sleep paralysis is among the strangest and most baffling. It apparently is surprisingly common.

It occurs only when the victim is going to sleep or awakening from sleep. During the attack he is essentially conscious in that he is not truly asleep, and he is aware of his surroundings. Nevertheless, he is completely unable to move, is tormented by frightening anxieties, in most cases suffers from a sense of great oppression or weight on his chest, and feels as if he were going to suffocate.

The paralysis even extends to the speech apparatus so that

the victim is unable to speak and call out for help, although he may be able to groan and thus attract the attention of someone nearby to the fact that the sleeper is having "nightmares."

In addition to these distressing symptoms, there may be weird and frightening hallucinations, which have led to the association by some psychiatrists of sleep paralysis with narcolepsy and catalepsy. But it seems apparent from a study of a number of reported cases that sleep paralysis occurs without any association with these two conditions and is probably more common than generally suspected.

The paralysis in most cases lasts but a few seconds or, at most, a minute or two, but in rare cases the immobility may last for much longer periods of time.

A loud noise or the turning on of bright lights, which would ordinarily arouse a person under normal circumstances, does not bring an end to the attack, but it can be terminated quickly in most cases by the mere touch of another person or, at most, a mild shaking to dispel sleep. The attack may also terminate very quickly if the sleeper is able to move some part of his body, such as a finger or a toe.

Victims of sleep paralysis usually seek psychiatric or medical help as the result of some other complaint, and often the fact that the patient is a victim of sleep paralysis comes out as a secondary bit of information.

The condition is not infrequently seen by the family physician, who, unfortunately, does not have any very satisfactory or specific means at his command for alleviating the situation, since we have no clear understanding of the neurophysiologic mechanisms involved in producing the condition.

It seems probable that most individuals with this condition may simply be the victims of tension and distressing life situations to which no answer is readily apparent, and strong emotional tension during the day often seems to precede an attack that night. They therefore suffer emotional conflicts which can be manifested through sleep paralysis as well as other mechanisms.

It has been found that some cases have been benefited by periodic insulin treatments which are carefully regulated to produce a mild hypoglycemia without throwing the patient into insulin shock. Other forms of shock therapy also may be used.

Fortunately, most victims of sleep paralysis only experience attacks at relatively rare intervals and suffer no ill effects aside from having undergone a distressing mental experience.

Ménière's Disease

There is a group of conditions that can be classified, generally, under Ménière's syndrome, which has nothing whatever to do with convulsions, but which produces, at times, a picture that might be mistaken for a convulsion by an untrained person.

Signs and Symptoms. In various forms, Ménière's disease affects both the hearing and the equilibrium portion of the eighth nerve (the auditory nerve) and the labyrinth—the delicate semicircular canals in the inner ear that control balance and orientation in space. Certain conditions can affect and eventually abolish the functions of these organs so that the victim becomes subject to attacks of severe dizziness, nausea, and sometimes collapse to the point of simulating extreme shock. The disease usually affects only one side, and, when the victim falls to the ground, he does so as if he had been hit on the back of the head and falls toward the affected side.

Two signs help in diagnosis: (1) deafness on the affected side, which can readily be determined by asking the victim if he can hear a watch tick when it is held close to each ear; and (2) the eyes, which will be jerking rapidly back and forth, the most rapid jerk being in one direction with a somewhat slower return.

The victim will describe his dizziness by saying that the room is going around him, not—*and this is important*—that he is going around, which describes ordinary dizziness.

The important thing is that the symptoms produced can be quite severe and even dangerous, since the person may injure himself, or others as, for instance, when driving an automobile. Obviously, a person so afflicted should not drive an automobile. Unfortunately, the condition is much more common than is generally recognized, and many sufferers are attempting to carry on a normal daily existence, unaware of the nature of the malady which plagues them.

○ TREATMENT

The victim will be much more comfortable and his dizziness will be partially relieved if he can lie flat on his back, with his head held absolutely immobile.   These people feel and look as if they were seriousy ill, in acute shock, or even as if they were going to die, but death rarely, if ever, occurs.   The attack may last for an hour or more, but after the first collapse the victim lies quietly, except, possibly, for vomiting (he really is "seasick"), and does not want to be disturbed; however, a doctor should be called.

When the person recovers, he is perfectly normal, in full possession of his faculties, and, although he may feel a little unsteady, he is otherwise in good shape.   An ounce of whiskey is sometimes helpful during the recovery period.

Cases of this type are in need of highly competent care and should be referred to a specialist in diseases of the ear.   There are various treatments and several new drugs that offer great relief with respect to both the frequency and intensity of the attacks.   Once nerve degeneration has occurred, however, hearing loss is permanent, although tinnitus may be partially relieved.

There are many drugs which may be used in any particular case.   Most victims respond to diuretics, a low-salt diet, and nicotinic acid in sufficient doses to cause facial flushing, an action which helps dilate the vessels of the internal ear.   Tranquilizers are of considerable value in some cases, as are "sea-sickness" pills to help control the dizziness.   Although some specialists askew the use of alcohol, we have seen several cases in which alcohol proved a benefit both for its tranquilizing action as well as its blood vessel-dilating effect.

A treatment which was once popularized was surgical section of the vestibular portion of the eighth nerve.   In some cases this relieved the annoying tinnitus, but often left the person deaf.   Today, operation is found necessary in only the occasional severe case which has proven refractory to all medication.

Somewhat similar symptoms can be produced by blockage of the eustachian tubes, leading from the middle ear to the back of the throat, whose purpose it is to equalize the pressure in the middle ear.

It is partial blockage of these tubes that makes your ears "pop" in an elevator, or tunnel, or in going up or coming down in an airplane.   If chronic blockage occurs, pressure changes and inflammatory processes are set up in the middle ear which cause symptoms similar to those of Ménière's disease, with accompanying deafness that is different from that in true Ménière's disease. Such chronic cases must, of course, be treated by a specialist.

Motion Sickness

Motion sickness has always been a concomitant of travel, and may affect any susceptible person exposed to motion in any form, including travel by automobile, train, ship, or airplane. The majority of cases occur as the result of the motion, which produces strong stimuli upon the labyrinth of the ear, resulting in an effect akin to the end effects in Ménière's disease. Motion sickness under ordinary conditions of land travel used to be encountered more often than it is today, but it is quite possible for a person to become sick from a short ride in an automobile, from the gentle motion of a porch swing, or from a ride in an elevator.

Motion sickness is not, as many people believe, a neurotic trait, although it is true that if a person is apprehensive, he may be more disposed to such illness than if he were perfectly calm.

Most persons eventually become acclimated to rapid changes in motion, but even the most experienced may suffer. It has been stated that about 10 percent of all flight students are airsick during their first ten flights or so, but, after having completed their training, pilots and other crew members rarely become airsick, except in extremely turbulent air. The same individuals, however, are more susceptible when riding as passengers than when actively engaged in their duties.

Signs and Symptoms. Usually, the first indication of motion sickness is pallor, followed by drowsiness, yawning, cold clammy perspiration, and apprehension. There may be headache, dizziness, and vomiting. After vomiting, the victim may feel a little better temporarily, but this relief is short-lived, and he may continue to be nauseated. He may even think he is going to die, but, of course, he *never* does!

○ TREATMENT

Here are a few ways to combat the problem:

1 If you know you are subject to airsickness and the weather is obviously bad along the course of your proposed flight, be

sophisticated and wait a day or two for the weather to clear. If you must fly, the severity of these symptoms can be diminished by getting as much fresh air as possible from the overhead vent and by avoiding unpleasant sights and odors, such as from fellow passengers who are sick. With the high altitude commercial jets now in use, airsickness is often more a matter of apprehension on the part of the novice passenger than of motion.

2 It also helps to fix the eyes firmly on a given spot in the plane or boat in order to aid the balancing mechanism of the ear in maintaining a definite orientation in space.

3 Overindulgence in alcohol definitely predisposes a person to motion sickness. An overloaded stomach also is apt to give trouble, but going without food entirely is no sure preventive. A light meal 2 to 3 hours before taking off seems to offer the best assurance of comfort.

4 There are several motion-sickness remedies on the market which are effective and need only be taken in doses of one or two tablets a day. If you are planning a trip by air or sea, ask your doctor to recommend one of these remedies for you. The important point is to start taking the remedy a day or two before you leave so as to benefit from its full effect.

Another possible source of discomfort in flight is from blockage of the ears or sinuses as the result of pressure changes during ascent or descent. Usually, this difficulty is minor and easily overcome by swallowing, yawning, or chewing gum.

However, if you have a severe cold, the blockage cannot be so easily overcome because of the inflammation and congestion; severe pain or local damage may result. For that reason, persons with a severe cold should avoid traveling by air, if possible, during the acute phase. If you have to fly, consult your physician for medication, such as nose drops, which can be used before and during the flight to decrease the congestion and help nature maintain a normal pressure balance.

Illness and Flying

In these days of fast, pressurized ships which for the most part fly above the weather and the many special services provided when needed, there is very little reason for almost anyone not to fly. In fact, if the passenger can travel at all, he can cover long distances more quickly, safely, and comfortably by air than by any other means. A good rule of thumb (with a few exceptions) is that if a person looks normal, feels normal, and can walk up the steps of a ramp—stretcher cases can be easily carried up—he can fly without difficulty.

Obviously, however, certain restrictions are necessary regarding carrying ill passengers on commercial aircraft. Such restrictions are primarily related to the comfort of fellow passengers and to the relative lack of special medical equipment aboard the planes, rather than to any risk of air travel per se.

Those who should *not* fly without special precautions or services include: expectant mothers beyond the eighth month; heart patients whose conditions are so severe that they cannot comfortably walk up a flight of stairs, or those within 6 weeks of the onset of a severe heart attack; anyone with a contagious disease; anyone with an illness causing an objectionable odor, or who cannot take care of his own bodily needs; diabetics who cannot administer their own insulin or who are easily subject to reaction or coma; anyone liable to convulsions, as in epilepsy; and those with a very severe cold or upper respiratory infection.

There is an individual oxygen supply at each passenger's seat which automatically becomes available if pressure fails. This is in addition to a portable oxygen supply for anyone who might suffer a heart attack or other illness, as an emergency treatment measure. If all else fails, modern jets can safely descend in 2 to 3 minutes from altitudes of 40,000 to 10,000 feet, where most people can breathe easily.

And finally, most commercial flights over the U.S. are within 30 to 40 minutes of an emergency landing field and medical facilities in the event of a life or death emergency.

In spite of the safety and comfort of modern commercial flight, there are times when even a normal individual will experience some degree of emotional or physical discomfort. Apprehension arising through ignorance of what is happening can intensify almost any unpleasant situation that might arise during flight, especially motion sickness. This annoying condition is becoming rarer with the increasing confidence and sophistication of the traveling public, and bigger, more comfortable planes which largely fly in calm air *over* turbulent weather.

Flying is a wonderful way of getting places fast. The overall enjoyment of the trip can be greatly enhanced by following a few simple rules:

1 Get as much rest as possible before your trip, especially if your destination is in a distant time zone. This is important in order to compensate for the effect of time differences on your bodily habits, such as sleeping and eating.

2 Don't overindulge in either food or drink—neither will *really* cure apprehension.

3 If you are disposed to motion sickness or are afraid of being airsick, follow the simple rules mentioned under motion sickness. This makes it unlikely that you really *will* be airsick.

4 If you are pregnant, or have a serious medical condition, consult your physician as to the desirability of your flying.

5 If you are going into a foreign country, be sure you have complied with requirements relating to immunization against certain diseases, such as smallpox.

Circadian Rhythm

Another important factor that should be reckoned with in long-distance flying, particularly when passing through several time zones, is that man—like other creatures—has a built-in biologic clock or, to put it technically, is subject to an inherent circadian rhythm. This important physiological function governs many of man's physiological and psychological reactions at different times of the day, week, or month.

With the coming of the jet age and its swift transportation across many time zones in the space of a few hours, the importance of man's biologic clock has come to be of tremendous significance. It is a wonderful thing to be whisked from New York to London or to Honolulu, or somewhere else in the world, in a few hours' time, but it is very hard on the human body as far as the adjustment of the normal rhythm of its physiologic processes is concerned.

When one proceeds by surface transportation, the time changes occur so slowly that the body automatically is continually adjusting, so that one arrives at the final destination with his various biological functions working in normal time sequence. But when one moves rapidly across the same time zones in a relatively short period, there is no opportunity for such adjustment; the body which had been adjusted to one set of environmental circumstances just a few hours previously is quite suddenly faced with a whole new set, so that most normal functions are thrown out of their natural relationships. As a result, the bodily processes become disrupted, and even the mind itself may be subject to a degree of confusion, so that it is often difficult to think clearly and function with normal efficiency immediately upon arrival.

Aircraft passengers as well as crew members making long east-to-west or west-to-east flights are often subject to gastro-intestinal disturbances, including loss of appetite, diarrhea or constipation, menstrual irregularities, and undue fatigue, quite out of proportion to the physical effort exerted or the nervous strain involved in the trip itself. They may become depressed and find it difficult to orient to their new surroundings and, if on a business trip, to carry out their business efficiently and expeditiously without a period of adjustment.

That changes related to time are important in bringing about the condition is indicated by the fact that similar effects are not observed in those making equally long north-south runs, where possibly only one time change is involved, or no time change at all.

It is obvious that physiologic conflict arises when the rhythms triggered by the environment are out of step with the normal preset rhythms of the body. Until a sufficient time has elapsed for the biological clock to be reset and a period of adjustment to occur, annoying physiologic changes take place which impair both well-being and general effectiveness.

So far, no one really has an answer as to how to counteract the difficulty. At the present time, as far as east-west jet travel is concerned, it is best to simply recognize the situation for what it is and allow time in one's plans for a period of adjustment of 2 or 3 days after arrival for the bodily processes to return to normal. This is particularly applicable to those who must become involved in serious business negotiations.

Mountain Sickness (Altitude Sickness). Mountain sickness, more properly known as *altitude sickness,* has nothing to do with motion sickness, although many people seem to believe that it has. However, because altitude sickness can intensify the symptoms and total discomfort in a person with motion sickness, there is a relationship in that respect, at least.

Signs and Symptoms. Actually, this condition occurs because of the low concentration of oxygen in the rarefied air at high altitudes, which results in poorer oxygenation of the blood and produces the series of symptoms associated with mountain sickness (rapid breathing, anxiety, fatigue, lassitude, and occasionally, a marked exhilaration, with symptoms not unlike those of alcoholic intoxication). A potentially dangerous psychologic complication is the development of fixed ideas which may seriously warp an individual's judgment, leading him to commit acts that might jeopardize his safety and that of others with him. In many instances, also, a usually mild-mannered and pleasant person may become very ill-tempered, thus creating serious personality problems.

If a person is especially susceptible or if the altitude is sufficiently high, fainting or unconsciousness may result. It is a known fact that for every person there is an altitude beyond which he cannot go without losing consciousness; this ceiling varies from 15,000 to 30,000 feet, according to the individual. This factor also is influenced by the speed at which the ascent is made and the ability of the individual to compensate for the decreased oxygen concentration in the air.

○ TREATMENT

From a preventive standpoint, it has been suggested that a high carbohydrate diet may help to increase the altitude tolerance, but the *specific* treatment, of course, is the administration of pure oxygen. For that reason, oxygen is used in unpressurized planes on all flights above 10,000 feet. It should be available to those intending to ascend mountains above this level; susceptible individuals will be much more comfortable if they use oxygen at 5,000 to 8,000 feet until they become used to the altitude. Since expansion of intestinal gases is often a problem at higher altitudes, it is important that constipation or any other obstruction to the free passage of flatus be avoided. It is also helpful to wear an abdominal support to help avoid distention.

Glaucoma

A knowledge of the extremely delicate structures of the eye, particularly those immediately in front of and behind the iris, is particularly important in understanding the condition known as *glaucoma,* which may develop insidiously during middle age and, if unrecognized and untreated, will inevitably lead to blindness.

Glaucoma, which may occur in both acute and chronic forms, is probably the major cause of blindness in this country. It has been reliably estimated that almost 1,500,000 persons in this country have some degree of glaucoma without knowing it. Many will lose their sight if the condition is allowed to go untreated.

In its simplest terms, glaucoma is a disease caused by a buildup of pressure within the eyeball. This causes inflammatory changes which may be extremely painful and, if the condition is allowed to progress unchecked, degeneration of the optic nerve follows and results in blindness. The condition is present in 2 out of every 100 persons past the age of 40; the unfortunate part of it is that glaucoma may go unrecognized or unsuspected until considerable damage has been done.

As has been noted, glaucoma results from blockage to the free outflow of aqueous humor from the anterior chamber of the eye.

The tendency to blockage of the free outflow of fluid is increased by anything which will cause dilatation of the iris, since the fluid leaves the eye through the tissues in the tiny angle between the cornea and the iris. Hence, when the iris bunches up over this area, as it does when the pupil dilates, there is a more or less natural mechanical blockage to the outflow of fluid.

When the light is poor, the pupil, of course, dilates; many attacks of acute glaucoma therefore occur during darkness or at very low light levels, such as while one is watching moving pictures or television, or through the continual use of dark glasses when these are not required by excessive sunlight. Other things that may cause prolonged dilatation of the pupil, and hence "bunching" of the iris, are prolonged pain, constant tension, or any type of emotional disturbance which may create a perpetual state of nervousness, and any disease which causes chronic inflammation of the eyes.

Signs and Symptoms. Whatever the cause of the acute attack, the internal pressure in the eye increases sharply—so much that the eye actually feels hard to the touch, like a marble. The cornea takes on a steamy appearance, to the patient as well as to the examining doctor, and the patient sees rainbow-like halos around electric lights.

Also, because of the increased intraocular pressure, there may be extreme pain and headache, which in themselves cause further dilatation of the pupil, thus tending to make the condition worse. Sometimes the distress is so acute that nausea and vomiting occur.

If medical assistance is not sought promptly, enough damage may be caused to the eye ultimately to result in serious loss of sight, but, fortunately, there are a number of ways of relieving acute attacks.

○ TREATMENT

Certain drugs, when instilled into the eye, cause the pupil to constrict, thus helping to increase the drainage of aqueous humor through the angle between the iris and the cornea. Another drug, which may be taken by mouth simultaneously, cuts down on the rate of secretion of aqueous humor, thus further relieving the back pressure.

Once the first acute attack is over, further attacks must be guarded against by the regular use of certain drugs and whatever corrective measures may be required. In certain chronic cases, a tiny hole in the outside edge of the iris can be made surgically, to provide a channel for the fluid to escape from the posterior chamber directly into the anterior chamber without pursuing a circuitous route.

The chronic form of glaucoma in older people poses another great problem, because the development of the condition is so insidious that by the time actual symptoms occur of sufficient magnitude to cause the person to seek medical help, damage already may be extensive.

Anyone over 40, the age at which the disease is most likely to strike, should have regular examinations by a qualified physician specializing in diseases of the eye, at least once a year. If there is any undue discomfort or pain in one or both eyes, or if there is persistent headache without obvious explanation in between examinations, the eyes should be checked immediately.

In this way, early cases of glaucoma can be detected and

steps taken to at least minimize further development and prevent serious loss of vision in later years.

In addition to glaucoma, many other diseases can affect the eye, and there are many possible causes of blindness. In about 24 percent of the reported cases, blindness was caused by cataracts, which were the result of disease, injury, or changes due to advancing age. Most of these, of course, aside from injury, do not fall within the scope of this book, but it cannot be too strongly urged that, for any condition affecting the eyes, expert care be promptly sought. The value of regular eye checkups is of fundamental importance.

Tic Douloureux

Tic douloureux (trigeminal neuralgia) is a painful condition affecting the fifth or trigeminal nerve of the face. It may occur at any age but is much more likely after the age of 40; it is somewhat more common in women than in men. Tic douloureux gets its popular name from the fact that the brief but severe paroxysms of pain are often accompanied by contractions of the facial muscles, thus producing a so-called "tic." The "douloureux" part refers to the very painful nature of the condition.

The trigeminal, or fifth cranial, nerve is a so-called "mixed nerve" in that it has both sensory and motor functions, but it is the sensory function of the nerve which is concerned in tic douloureux.

Just exactly where the pain of tic douloureux originates, or what causes the condition, is unknown, although it is undoubtedly some type of involvement of the Gasserian ganglion—a sort of distribution point for all the ramifications of the fifth nerve itself. It is clear, however, that a painful reaction can be easily set off by the slightest stimulation of a so-called "trigger" point, which is usually on the lip or at the side of the nose. The slightest touch, or even a mere breeze, is capable of setting off the whole painful process. Even normal movement, such as chewing or talking, can set off a reaction. Hence, victims of tic douloureux have the greatest difficulty in shaving or even washing the face for fear of precipitating an attack of pain.

The pain itself is usually of short duration but occurs so frequently during the course of an attack that it appears to be almost constant. It is characteristically stabbing and lightning-like in nature, but typically involves only one side of the face, not progressing across the midline to the other side.

Sometimes the attacks occur spontaneously without any obvious reason, when the patient is at complete rest, and it is curious that sleep usually is not disturbed by pain except in severe cases after the condition has been in existence for some time. Attacks, however, are both more frequent and more severe under conditions of tension or when the individual is very tired.

There is no specific treatment, since the basic cause of the disease is unknown. Nugent and Berry have reported on a percutaneous radiofrequency desiccation technic, which, in their hands, seems to have given good results. In some cases the attacks may be greatly modified in both frequency and intensity by the administration of drugs which cause a dilatation of the blood vessels, such as histamine or nicotinic acid. The injection of alcohol directly into the Gasserian ganglion or an affected branch of the trigeminal nerve to produce temporary anesthesia was once widely used. However, the relief of pain afforded by this means is often not complete and is not necessarily permanent. Recently diphenylhydantoin, USP (Dilantin®) an older drug used successfully for years in the treatment of epilepsy, has been tried with apparently great success in suppressing both the frequency and the intensity of attacks.

Shingles

Shingles (herpes zoster) is an acute viral infection which involves the nerves carrying sensation between the skin and spinal cord, and which sometimes also causes inflammation within the spinal cord itself.

The disease is caused by the Varicella Zoster (V-Z) virus, the same virus which causes chickenpox (q.v.). Most, but not all, people who develop herpes zoster have had chickenpox in early childhood, and outbreaks of shingles have been linked with close contact with chickenpox cases (and vice versa). Herpes zoster is less communicable than chickenpox, but susceptibles exposed to a patient with vesicular zoster lesions may develop chickenpox.

In most cases, the virus probably lies dormant in the body

for long periods of time, until something activates it and shingles result. The triggering mechanism may be some form of injury to or around the spinal column, some chronic disease, or something so minor as not to be apparent at all.

Whatever sets the condition off, it usually starts with a chilly feeling, some fever, a general feeling of grippiness, and possibly a gastrointestinal upset. Three to five days later, the characteristic skin eruption appears, often preceded by sharp, burning pain along a band where the eruption eventually pops out. The lesions, which start near the spinal column and spread outward, consist of crops of vesicles on a reddened base, in a band which follows the course of the infected nerve. About 75 percent of the cases involve the chest, and almost invariably one side only.

The fluid in the vesicles is at first clear, and may contain quantities of the infecting virus. After 2 or 3 days, the fluid becomes cloudy and the lesions begin to crust, drying up in from 5 to 10 days. The continuing pain may be severe and difficult to relieve, particularly in older people.

Sometimes nerves other than those supplying the chest wall are involved; one such nerve serves the auditory canal. In this case, eruptions appear in and around the external auditory canal, the soft palate, and the area around the tonsils, which is also served by the same nerve. There also may be paralysis of the affected side of the face, which, fortunately, eventually clears up. Involvement of another nerve can cause a similar condition of the eye, where it produces ulcerations and opacities of the cornea. Eye involvement is extremely painful and may have serious complications.

Herpes Simplex. A somewhat similar but less generalized viral infection is known as herpes simplex. It consists simply of small local sores and is caused by an entirely different virus than herpes zoster. It would appear that most adults harbor this particular virus, which lies dormant until some minor triggering mechanism causes it to flare up and produce the lesions known commonly as fever blisters or cold sores. Both herpes simplex and shingles may be caused by several different viruses within a cytologic group and occasionally lead to serious complications. Factors which may commonly activate the condition are fatigue and severe sunburn.

O TREATMENT

There is no specific treatment for either herpes zoster (q.v.) or herpes simplex. A great many things have been tried to control the pain of herpes zoster, such as analgesic drugs, locally applied anesthetic ointments, and even deep x-ray therapy or the injection of local anesthetics near the spinal column. Gamma globulin and injections of protamine sulphate have been tried empirically, with dubious success. In older persons, corticosteroid drugs in larges doses administered early in the course of the disease may have a suppressive effect in relieving the inflammation and possibly shortening its duration. While no mode of treatment is really successful, when the pain and discomfort are as severe as they sometimes can be, both the doctor and the patient are willing to try almost anything.

Diffuse Esophageal Spasm

The esophagus is a soft, rather thin-walled muscular tube which passes the bolus of food along by means of reflex peristaltic movement which proceeds evenly in one direction from the mouth toward the stomach. When anything goes wrong with this system, interference with swallowing and other distressing symptoms, including severe chest pain, can result. It has been estimated that about one-sixth of cases of chest pain are due to disorders of the esophagus.

One of the most painful affections to which the esophagus is subject is known as diffuse esophageal spasm. This condition, a disturbance of motility of the esophageal musculature, was first described as long ago as 1889. Although it is a much more common occurrence than generally recognized, it has received relatively little medical attention.

Symptoms. The chief symptom is acute gripping substernal pain which may occur spontaneously at any time of the day or night; occasionally, it may only be precipitated by swallowing. The pain may radiate to the back, shoulders, neck, or ears, and it is severe enough to be confused at times with angina pectoris or myocardial infarction. In some cases, there is also profuse salivation, due apparently to excessive vagal stimulation. At times the spasm may become so severe that the patient can neither swallow nor eructate gas from the stomach. Apprehension and fear may be acute, and often the victim will walk about trying to gain relief.

There seems to be a strong underlying psychosomatic factor involved, as the attacks often occur during periods of great tension, anxiety, or other emotional pressures. Other precipitating factors may include rapid eating or excessive eating and the drinking of very cold, particularly carbonated, beverages as well as their overuse. It is important to recognize that although esophageal pain may be caused by many factors, diffuse esophageal spasm is a distinct clinical entity. There seems to be no special predilection for either sex or any particular adult age group.

○ TREATMENT

Depending on the nature of the individual case, medical measures may or may not prove helpful. In some cases, chlordiazepoxide (Librium®) or diazepam (Valium®) in sufficient doses relieves the anxiety and helps diminish muscle spasm. Atropine sulfate, 1/150 grain, placed beneath the tongue to aid rapid absorption, and repeated as necessary, works well in some but not all cases. From a long-range point of view, in those cases in which psychosomatic factors predominate, emotional guidance and support certainly should be of help in addition to suitable tranquilizers.

In the more severe and intractable cases, Ellis has reported encouraging results from a surgical procedure in which certain muscle fibers in the esophagus are cut to prevent spasm, and Rider et al. have recorded excellent results from simple esophageal dilatation, using an inflatable esophageal dilator. This essentially nonsurgical method has proved beneficial where ordinary methods have been relatively ineffective.

From an emergency standpoint, it is important to recognize diffuse esophageal spasm as an entity in order to differentiate it from potentially more serious conditions such as an acute heart attack.

Allergies

The treatment of most allergic conditions is not within the scope of emergency care. Occasionally, however, an acute condition, such as severe gastrointestinal allergy, arises which produces nausea, vomiting, diarrhea, collapse, migraine, acute asthma, or generalized giant hives.

Often the source of the allergy may not be obvious. For

instance, Wicher et al. point out that milk and milk products may contain significant quantities of penicillin and hence may prove dangerous when ingested by individuals sensitive to penicillin, of whom there are many. So-called "hidden" antibiotics, in addition to penicillin, which is the most common, may be contained in many products, especially milk products and meats. For this reason, the allergic reaction may not be due to the food itself, but to a foreign substance, as was true in a case described by Wicher et al., involving penicillin which the food (milk and ice cream) contained.

Gastrointestinal Allergy. Gastrointestinal allergy is common and the precipitating cause usually is known to the victim, but, occasionally, he may take food to which he is unknowingly allergic, and then the case may be serious.

Signs and Symptoms. Usually, there is prostration or collapse, vomiting, diarrhea, and, in severe cases, a profound state of shock which may come close to being fatal.

○ TREATMENT

These cases require prompt medical aid, but in the meantime the victim may be almost helpless and require assistance.

1 Vomiting and diarrhea may already be ridding the body of the offending substance; if not, an emetic and Epsom salts should be given to get rid of it.

2 Be sure that the victim is not suffering from some condition, such as appendicitis, in which a laxative would be dangerous. The clue indicating that this is an allergic condition is that abdominal tenderness and rigidity are not often present, although there may be a great deal of gas and distension; usually there is no fever. If the person's condition seems serious, call a doctor.

Hives (Urticaria). This condition is most likely to occur from eating food to which the person is allergic, but it can occur from reaction to such common things as wool, feathers, dog hairs, cat fur, etc., to pollens of various plants, or to heat or cold.

Signs and Symptoms. The person breaks out in large welts and is generally miserable, largely as the result of the severe itching and his unsightly appearance. The condition may become really dangerous if the swelling extends to the vocal cords.

○ TREATMENT

From the standpoint of emergency care, there is not a great deal that can be done.   Calamine lotion or rubbing alcohol, if applied directly to the welts, may offer a little relief.   Warm bicarbonate of soda applications have also been recommended.   A large dose of Epsom salts or other laxative helps to rid the body of the offending substance and reduce the swelling, but usually medical measures are required for any permanent relief.   The corticosteroids, antihistamines, and epinephrine in severe cases are very valuable in relieving the swelling and itching.

Asthma.   This condition constitutes a complicated medical problem, but is of emergency interest when breathing becomes so difficult that the person's life seems to be in danger.

Usually, an asthmatic attack does not come on without warning, but, when it does, a doctor should be summoned as quickly as possible.

○ TREATMENT

Little can be done without specific medical assistance or instruction, except to offer the victim such relief as is possible. Fresh air or oxygen is welcome; a sitting or upright position will facilitate breathing.   Occasionally, steam inhalations are helpful until a doctor can administer more specific remedies.

Infections

Asian Flu (Influenza).   Symptoms characteristic of influenza were described early in the twelfth century, being attributed by the astrologers of that time to the adverse influence of the planets.   The disease has puzzled scientists and confounded physicians ever since.

In spite of many huge and devastating epidemics throughout the centuries, the true cause of influenza was not fully known until the three related types of virus were discovered about the middle of this century.   The first to be identified, in 1933, was the type A influenza virus, which we now know to be the most frequent cause of Asian flu.   The other two types of virus which may cause influenza were discovered a few years later and are known, respectively, as types B and C.

Some believe a virus reservoir may exist somewhere in

central Asia. In fact, many of the great epidemics appear to have originated in that area, spreading to other countries through the normal channels of travel and commerce. But many authorities feel that there is still no solid evidence that a virus reservoir does, in fact, exist in any particular location. Nevertheless, under the conditions of today's high-speed travel, infection can be spread very rapidly from an epidemic area to any other part of the world and flare up into a new epidemic.

So-called Asian flu, as it exists at the present time, may be a severe or a relatively mild disease, although in any case it makes the victim feel very ill and may prostrate him for several days. Not all epidemics are mild, however, and, in some, the intensity of the disease and the mortality rate may be high because of complications and the affinity of the disease for certain age groups.

To understand how influenza vaccines work (or don't work), it is necessary to realize that the biology of the influenza virus is much more complex and changeable than that of other viruses. This is partly due to the fact that the coating of the influenza virus changes its characteristics periodically. As Gross has stated, "When one H or N of these surface antigens changes, it is likely that a mild epidemic will follow; when both H and N antigens change, then it is likely that a major pandemic will occur. The influenza virus that we have experienced since 1968 has technically been labeled a H_3N_2 type. The virus that appeared at Fort Dix in New Jersey in January, 1976 is called the A/New Jersey/76 virus; it is a type in which both H and N antigens have changed and therefore one would expect that if and when this virus became widespread, it [would] be responsible for a significant outbreak of influenza."

This virus is normally associated with influenza in swine but can be transmitted to man, particularly anyone who is exposed to infected hogs. In 1976, a number of severely ill cases turned up at the aforementioned military establishment without obvious reason, but no others were observed elsewhere in the world. Nevertheless, fears were aroused that a "swine flu epidemic" might occur and be similar to the Asian flu epidemic of 1957.

In 1957 there was a substantial epidemic caused by the so-called A/Victoria/75-type virus. In view of the possibility of a severe epidemic of both types occurring in 1977, a combination vaccine was prepared on a large scale, although for technical reasons each type is also available separately.

The combined vaccine gives a high rate of reactions and should be given only to the elderly and other high risk groups. But absolute protection with either vaccine cannot be guaranteed, although in some individuals the antibody level may remain high.

Signs and Symptoms. Often the symptoms of influenza are indistinguishable from acute sore throat, the common cold, and other similar upper respiratory infections. In fact, an outbreak of influenza may occur at the same time as an outbreak of common colds and may become apparent only by its more prolonged and prostrating effects. Also, it is considerably more contagious than an ordinary cold and hence can spread very rapidly and widely.

True Asian flu is usually characterized by an acute onset, severe prostration, headache aching muscles, sore throat, and a severe dry, hacking cough. In some cases the temperature may go as high as 104°F. Although the period of acute distress may not last much longer than 5 days, the victim usually feels dragged out and very weak for many days thereafter.

The commonest and most serious complication of influenza, particularly when it is severe, is pneumonia caused by secondary infection with one of several kinds of bacteria, most often by man's old enemy, the staphylococci. This complication greatly increases the fatalities from influenza.

Fortunately, we now have vaccines which provide some degree of protection, especially against type A, or Asian flu. A nationwide voluntary program of vaccination against this and related strains of influenza may go far in preventing the occurrence of any major epidemic and in minimizing the tremendous losses in time out from work which otherwise could occur.

○ TREATMENT

Prevention of influenza is of especial importance, as has been said, since there is no specific treatment once the disease has occurred. Those who do come down with it should remain in bed during the acute phase, particularly while the temperature is elevated, and consume as much fluid as possible. They should also be isolated from other people as much as possible, not so much to curb the spread of the disease, as to protect the victim from bacteria which might be in the noses and throats of the others—and which could cause a dangerous secondary infection, usually pneumonia.

Antibiotics are of no use in the treatment of viral influenza itself, but are valuable in meeting the threat of secondary bacterial infection if and when it occurs. The outlook indeed seems hopeful that, in view of the tools now available to the medical profession, we may never face again the devastating pandemics of 1918, 1957, 1968, and 1975.

Pleurodynia. *Pleurodynia* (Dabney's Grip; Bornholm disease) is an acute viral disease, characterized by severe paroxysmal chest pain which is aggravated by breathing and is accompanied by intermittent fever, headache, loss of appetite, and general grippe-like feelings. All of these symptoms can be severe and quite alarming, particularly since they may occur with frightening suddenness. Fortunately, however acute the distress, the disease itself is quite benign.

Group B Coxsackie viruses, which have some features in common with polio viruses, are the causative agents of pleurodynia as well as several other conditions. The Coxsackie organisms can be isolated from the throat secretions and bowel movements of infected cases.

Epidemics have been reported from Europe as well as various areas of the United States. The condition seems to appear only during the summer and early fall. Although it affects all age groups, it is most common in children and young adults.

Fortunately, the disease produces a long-lasting immunity, so that if you once have gone through its discomforts, it is unlikely that you will have to suffer through them again.

Pleurodynia apparently spreads by direct person-to-person contact and, as a result, several cases may crop up in a single household. As far as we know, the incubation period is from 3 to 5 days, the first symptoms are a sudden onset of pain in either the abdomen or chest, invariably accompanied by fever. Characteristically, the pain begins in the pit of the stomach and often shifts to the lower part of the chest on one side or the other. The pain is frequently so severe that the patient seems on the verge of collapse and may give all the appearance of having a "heart attack" or some acute abdominal catastrophe.

The breathing is rapid and shallow; the patient makes an effort to ease the pain by leaning forward and to one side while attempting to control the movements of his chest by holding one arm tightly around it. It is all too apparent that both movement and breathing aggravate the intense pain.

All of these symptoms give the appearance of an extremely acute crisis, and both the physician, who is excitedly called to the scene, and the family undertake hurried arrangements to move the patient to the hospital. While all this is being done, the symptoms often subside as fast as they come. The patient suddenly feels well, and the hospital arrangements are canceled—only to be put into effect again a short time later as the patient is seized with a recurrence of his severe chest or abdominal pain.

The pain often is so generalized that the victim has difficulty describing exactly where it is and usually says "I can't breathe" or complains of a feeling of severe pain and constriction in his chest—a symptom which probably led to the original name of "devil's grip."

The pain may be described as a dull ache—like that of a severe toothache, or sometimes a stabbing pain. Children, of course, react rather violently. They are restless, draw up their knees, and cry and sob with the severe pain. In younger children convulsions often accompany the high fever, which may exceed 104°F. but more commonly fluctuates between 101° and 103°. The fever is intermittent and usually reaches its highest peak during the bouts of pain.

Nausea may be severe, particularly in young children, but sometimes the pain is so severe as to limit vomiting.

A characteristic feature of the condition is that relapses tend to occur after the patient is apparently completely recovered, and may continue to occur over a period of a month or more.

○ TREATMENT

There is no specfic treatment, although back in 1888 Dr. Dabney prescribed bed rest, pain-killing drugs, and mustard plasters. Modern medicine seems not to have come up with anything better. But too early return to normal activity seems to lead to recurrence of the symptoms and possible complications.

Cystitis. Cystitis (inflammation of the urinary bladder) is much more common in women than in men, largely for anatomical reasons. It is due to local infection of the thick mucous membrane which lines the bladder. In itself, it is not usually serious since it is relatively amenable to various antibacterial agents such as certain sulfonamides and antibiotics, though treatment is sometimes prolonged. However, cystitis may frequently be secondary to some other more serious infection elsewhere in the urinary tract, such as the kidney, urethra, or, in men, the prostate.

It frequently is the result of a mechanical obstruction which blocks the complete emptying of urine from the bladder, thus permitting it to stagnate and become infected. Cystitis is also common after surgery or childbirth, particularly if it has been necessary to catheterize the patient due to temporary inability to void. It is also not uncommon following prolonged nonsurgical illnesses where the vital resistance of the body is lowered and the patient has had to lie abed for a long time.

The symptoms vary with the severity of the condition. In uncomplicated cystitis the usual complaint is of urinary urgency and frequency. There is burning pain during urination, accompanied by a feeling that the bladder has not been completely emptied, so that the patient is almost continually plagued with the urge to void. Aching pain low in the back is also characteristic, and frequently there may be low abdominal cramps not unlike those which accompany the menstrual period. Where the inflammation of the bladder is severe, blood may be present in the urine in sufficient quantities to be noted by the patient.

There is a strong tendency for the condition to become chronic or to reappear at more or less frequent intervals. It is for that reason that it is important to discover promptly any underlying difficulty, such as an urethral obstruction, that may be predisposing the bladder to become infected so easily. If the basic trouble is not eradicated, no amount of treatment will permanently clear up the bladder condition. As blood in the urine may also be indicative of some type of growth within the bladder, or some equally serious condition elsewhere in the urinary tract, it is extremely important to rule out these possibilities in order to avoid the dangers of malignancy later on. While the specific treatment of cystitis requires accurate diagnosis and exact therapy by a physician, considerable temporary relief can be obtained by the use of a hot-water bottle or heating pad to the lower part of the abdomen, the forcing of fluids to at least 3 quarts or more a day, avoidance of alcohol, and the use of some mild analgesic such as aspirin or a similar preparation.

Fortunately, there are specific prescription drugs which are quite effective in providing prompt relief of the symptoms until such time as the underlying cause can be found and cleared up.

Staphylococcal Infection. An aspect of infection which constitutes one of today's most important public health problems relates to infection by the staphylococcus germ.

It is amazing that one type of germ can cause so many diseases of greatly varying nature. For instance, just in the skin alone it causes carbuncles, boils, and impetigo and is partly responsible for acne. It is the most common cause of breast abscesses in nursing mothers. It produces inflammation of the eyes, pneumonia, abscesses of bones (osteomyelitis), and blood poisoning and is a vicious cause of food poisoning—particularly in summer. It is a common cause of bladder inflammation, particularly in hospital patients, and if it gets into the kidneys it can cause a very serious condition. Its presence makes a clean surgical wound "dirty" (badly infected), and it can add many unpleasant days to an otherwise normal and uneventful hospital stay. It has become the doctor's nightmare.

Solutions have been sought by the best medical and scientific minds in one of the greatest research efforts ever devoted to a single problem.

In essence, this is everybody's problem—in the hospital, in the home, and in the community as a whole. In other words, the hospital becomes seeded with germs from the people of the community using the hospital and from the staff of doctors, nurses, and general employees operating the hospital. The germs are carried *in* and spread from their noses and throats by coughing, sneezing, and talking; they are shed from their hair, from their skin, and from the dirt on their bodies.

As people come into the hospital for one reason or another, they leave their own quota of germs to be disseminated throughout the hospital by many pathways, and some carry the infection already present in the hospital back out with them to reseed the community itself. Thus there is a continuous and perpetually repeating cycle, in which the community, the home, and the hospital form the points of a dangerous triangle. Fortunately, we now know that the cycle can be broken. Meticulous care and all possible safeguards against hospital sepsis are already being taken by our best hospitals, and more and more are entering into preventive campaigns as they come to understand the problem. But this is not enough; basically, we must learn how to prevent home sepsis as well.

As one authority has pointed out, it is common for patients to go home (from hospitals) and infect their families and neighbors for years after, and to break the cycle, one must look to the home.

Not everyone, of course, has the problem in his own home, although his chances of sooner or later becoming exposed are great. When the problem does exist, it is a very personal one and there are many things which you yourself can do. Obviously, if you have an infectious illness of any type, the first thing to do is to see your doctor for specific treatment. Then the ground rules follow four general lines.

Perhaps more important than any other single factor is absolute cleanliness of the skin, because one of the main routes by which infection is transmitted is by direct contact. Pay special attention to the hands; wash them thoroughly after every toilet and always before eating or preparing food, using one of the several good antiseptic soaps on the market. Germs are easily carried into the food by dirty hands and can cause severe gastrointestinal upsets or other acute illness.

The second factor involves bedding and personal articles. These must be kept absolutely clean, as they can be a fertile source of germs. Blankets, particularly, easily harbor germ-laden dust, which is spread into the air every time the blanket is shaken. When bed linen and other personal articles are laundered, a chlorine bleach in the wash water provides good germ-killing power.

The third consideration is good general housekeeping, in order to keep dust and accumulated dirt on walls, woodwork, and furniture to an absolute minimum. Try to vacuum several times a week; a good cleaner traps better than 99 percent of the germs picked up.

Kitchen, playroom, and bathroom floors should be mopped

frequently with water containing a germicidal cleaner. Always use clean mop cloths—dirty ones just spread more germs around! If you follow the time-honored practice of shaking dust cloths either indoors or out, you'll only spread bacteria all over the place. Always leave dust cloths in a bucket of water containing a germicide overnight, and then wash them.

Toilet bowls should be cleaned daily, and the seat, wash basin, and bathtub should be wiped with a disinfectant solution at frequent intervals, particularly if a member of the household is suffering from a boil or other infection.

Many little, but nonetheless important, things can be done to make the home a medically safer and healthier place. For instance, cleanliness and correct food-handling practices in the kitchen are all-important. Needless to say, floors, working surfaces, and utensils should be absolutely clean.

If you have a cold, avoid sneezing in such a way that droplets might land on food, and always wash your hands after blowing your nose. Masks can be purchased at the corner drugstore which are cheap enough to throw away after use; they may save spreading infection to other members of the family.

Finally, don't forget about the hospital itself. When you plan to visit a sick friend, don't go if you have a cold or a skin infection, or if someone in your family has either. Your loved one and other patients may get well quicker if you stay home and send a good book, some ice cream, or flowers instead. If you do go, don't take the children; don't stay more than 15 minutes; and don't get close to the patient.

Through a systematic program—in the hospital and in the home—the germs in any environment can be controlled to the point where they are no longer troublesome.

ILLNESS CAUSED BY BACTERIALLY CONTAMINATED FOOD

Bacterially contaminated food causes several types of illness, commonly known as food poisoning. These conditions may be divided into those caused by foods which are rendered poisonous by certain natural conditions and those caused by foods that have been rendered toxic by bacterial action. Both categories are important; the first has already been discussed (see pp. 368–375 et seq.). The latter probably causes more widespread and serious illness.

Many bacteria can and do cause contamination of food, but three specific types of bacteria cause serious illness. Prevention of such contamination by proper methods of food handling, refrigeration, and canning is of paramount importance.

Staphylococcal Food Poisoning. One of the most common types is that due to contamination of the food by bacteria that are a species of *Staphylococcus,* which, when certain foods are stored at temperatures that are too warm, multiply rapidly, and secrete a very poisonous toxin that is not destroyed by heating or cooking and that, when eaten, produces violent gastrointestinal illness.

The foods which should be particularly suspect, especially in the summer, are all kinds of meats (particularly cold cuts and hamburger), dairy products, and certain baked goods, such as cream or custard pies (which should never be eaten during the summer unless freshly made and kept under good refrigeration). In fact, any food that has been left for some time in an open container, even if it has been in an icebox or refrigerator, should be considered a possible danger, since foods that have not been kept properly covered are easily contaminated by bacteria that can grow even at relatively cool temperatures.

Signs and Symptoms. The symptoms of staphylococcal poisoning come on a few hours after eating and consist of nausea, vomiting, abdominal pain, and diarrhea. Rarely is there fever. Often the victim feels as if he had the grippe, and, as a matter of fact, the condition is often erroneously referred to as "intestinal grippe," which misses completely the fact that the person probably has food poisoning.

○ TREATMENT
There is no specific treatment, but certain sulfonamides or antibiotics effectively hinder the growth of intestinal bacteria and may prove useful in shortening the course or relieving the severity of the disease. In severe cases the victim approaches a state of shock. Although a person suffering from this condition often fears he is going to die and even wishes he would, death rarely occurs. In severe cases medical care obviously is essential.

Salmonella Food Poisoning. Another type of bacterial infection of foods is caused by a group of bacteria known as the salmonellas, which consist of more than 600 species, all pathogenic for man and lower animals. Salmonellosis is probably the most common bacterial animal disease in the United States transmissible to man. It is undoubtedly far more widespread than the statistics show, since the vast majority of cases are not reported to health authorities. Salmonella organisms cause various manifestations in man, including the most common—acute gastroenteritis or food poisoning.

Salmonella organisms are widespread and contaminate a very high percentage of domestic food animals as well as household pets. Man almost always acquires the infection by eating contaminated food. Any item of food or drink may be tainted directly or indirectly by human or animal carriers of the disease-producing organisms.

Undoubtedly the greatest single source of human infection is poultry products, including chickens, ducks, turkeys, and eggs. These foods, in turn, can contaminate utensils, tables and various other items used in handling and food preparation. Other foods most likely to be contaminated are meats, cold cuts, frankfurters, fish, dairy products, especially soft cheeses, and many vegetables, both cooked and uncooked.

Contamination occurs from the handling of the food by a carrier of the bacteria, who himself may not show any symptoms, or from droppings of rats or mice; or the food may have been contaminated at its source, as in the case of meat from a diseased animal. Contamination of either cooked or uncooked food may occur as the result of unclean handling; if contamination *has* taken place, refrigeration will not help, since the organisms merely lie more or less dormant in the food and then come to life, so to speak, when they reach the intestinal tract. This type of poisoning often causes extensive epidemics, thus affecting whole groups of people at one time.

Signs and Symptoms. Symptoms come on after an incubation period of 8 or more hours, and are characterized by nausea, abdominal cramps, and severe watery diarrhea. The illness may start with a chill; or the victim may feel cold although his temperature may reach 102°F. The acute illness usually is over in 1 or 2 days, but the victim is left weak for some time. Often the condition can continue for as long as

2 weeks, during which time recontamination with the infecting organism is by no means impossible, particularly if the household is already contaminated.

In some cases, the nature of the disease may be much more severe, with an infection simulating typhoid fever, or an actual invasion of the bloodstream by the Salmonella organisms. When the bloodstream is invaded, about one fourth of the cases may develop many types of localized infection, including bronchial pneumonia, empyema, endocarditis or pericarditis, kidney infection, bone infection, or arthritis. In newborn infants and very young children, meningitis can occur.

Precise diagnosis of the disease rests upon running laboratory tests on the organisms obtained from the discharges of the intestinal tract or other site of infection, thus differentiating it from other diseases which may have similar manifestations.

○ TREATMENT

Treatment of acute salmonellosis is based essentially on correcting the dehydration which occurs as a result of the vomiting and diarrhea, and the use of certain antibiotics, particularly chloramphenicol—which, unfortunately, may have serious side-effects and must be used under carefully controlled conditions and under the direction of a physician. However, when only the intestinal tract itself is involved, it is questionable whether the use of antibiotics, even chloramphenicol, significantly reduces the duration of the illness. Some relief of the crampy pain and diarrhea can be obtained with paregoric or some similar intestinal antispasmodic and sedative. But to a certain extent the diarrhea serves a useful purpose in helping to rid the body of infective material.

It is much more important to avoid salmonellosis than to try to treat it after it has once been contracted. The safest course is to buy only products of the best grade and manufacture and to maintain scrupulous cleanliness about the home, particularly in the kitchen and in preparing foods.

Botulism. The most serious type of food poisoning, by far, is botulism, a preventable and treatable disease which, unfortunately, causes a distressingly high mortality. This condition is caused by contamination of food with a species of bacteria known as *Clostridium botulinum*, of which there are six types—A, B, C, D, E, and F. As pointed out by Smith and Holderman, however, food poisoning in any species of animal tends to be associated with certain specific types of this organism. Man, for instance, is mostly susceptible to types A, B, E, and F; birds are susceptible to A and C; ruminants to C and D.

Types A and B illness is the most common and is usually caused by contaminated meats (particularly in European countries) or vegetables, while illness caused by type E almost invariably is caused by contaminated fish. Botulinus organisms occur universally in garden soils and around any farm, and are present on all vegetables. When these are improperly washed and canned, ideal conditions are created for the growth and multiplication of the botulinus germs, which secrete an extremely potent toxin. For that reason, botulism is most often caused by improperly prepared *home-canned* vegetables, the most common offenders being string beans.

The botulinus toxin is heat-labile—can be destroyed by heat; if home-canned vegetables, or any other canned food which might be contaminated and favorable to the growth of the organism, are boiled for 20 minutes before being served, the toxin will be destroyed. This is a simple precaution and should *always* be taken if the slightest doubt exists.

The importance of adequate heating to destroy the toxin is emphasized by a report by Armstrong et al. of three cases of severe botulism poisoning, one of which was fatal, that occurred after eating home-canned gefilte fish prepared from Lake Superior whitefish, which had been stored in refrigerator for approximately 7 weeks.

In these cases, poisoning was due to *botulinum* type E, which is an inhabitant of fish intestines and is normally found in many other forms of aquatic life. While this type is easily killed by heat, at no time in the course of the home preparation of the poisoned gefilte fish was the temperature high enough to kill all spores, and a sufficient number proliferated during the 7-week storage period, even though refrigerated, to render the food highly toxic. Canning temperatures must be high enough and maintained over a long enough period of time to render home-preserved food safe.

So-called "cold" canning methods are unsafe. All food intended for canning should be cooked in a pressure cooker at 175°F. (80°C.) for at least 30 minutes. Foods prepared by other methods (drying, freezing, smoking, pickling) must be boiled or otherwise thoroughly cooked for at least 15 minutes to be safe.

Signs and Symptoms. Symptoms occur after about 2 days. There may be some gastrointestinal upset, but characteristic symptoms are dimness of vision, followed by double vision and drooping of the eyelids, difficulty in talking and swallowing, hoarseness, shortness of breath, falling blood pressure, and paralysis of the throat muscles, so that the victim may choke when he tries to swallow. There is no fever. These symptoms are a sign that medical aid is urgent. Death results from strangulation or heart failure and occurs in almost 75 percent of the untreated cases; it takes place in from 3 to 9 days after eating the contaminated food.

The diagnosis may be confirmed by various laboratory methods, but these require from 24 to 48 hours; when the disease is reasonably suspected on the basis of the above symptomatology, the urgency is so great that treatment should not be withheld pending laboratory confirmation.

Delay, resulting from possible confusion of the symptoms with other common conditions such as acute gastroenteritis, acute heart disease, drug poisoning, or other diseases which may give a somewhat similar clinical picture, may prove fatal. The clinical history of ingesting potentially contaminated food, together with the strongly suggestive symptoms and physical findings, are sufficient to warrant starting specific treatment immediately. The diagnosis can be confirmed later.

○ TREATMENT

Treatment is specific and is based on the prompt administration of antitoxin as soon as the disease is suspected. Early administration is important, because the antitoxin will fix circulating toxin and arrest or modify the course of the disease.

The National Communicable Disease Center in Atlanta, Georgia (telephone 404 633-3311), is able to provide antitoxin and other assistance on a 24-hour emergency basis. This center has on hand four types of antitoxin and makes the following recommendations:

> Trivalent A, B, and E toxin for all cases in which the toxin type has not been determined

Type E antitoxin for cases caused by fish and in which type E toxin has been identified

A supply of an antitoxin against four clinically important types (A, B, E, F), produced by the Serum Institute of Denmark, is also maintained and is recommended for cases in which type F toxin is suspected or known to be involved.

Lederle Laboratories, Pearl River, New York, also supply a bivalent antitoxin against types A and B.

With the availability of around-the-clock emergency service, there is little reason for delay in adequate treatment.

Recovery is prolonged, and expert medical and nursing care, including intensive supportive therapy, is of paramount importance.

SURGICAL CONDITIONS

Certain common acute surgical conditions may present emergency problems from the standpoint of caring for a person until competent medical assistance can be obtained, or recognizing that a serious situation exists and initiating steps to get the patient to a proper medical facility.

Acute Appendicitis.   This is by far the most important and common acute surgical illness to be borne in mind when faced with the problems of nausea, vomiting, and abdominal pain.

Appendicitis can occur at any age, but it is unusual in children younger than 4 years old, and when it occurs in this age group the symptoms usually are not typical.   It is the commonest and most important acute abdominal emergency in children of 5 years or older.   Fifty percent of the cases occur in this age group.   Acute appendicitis may also be seen in the elderly, where again the symptoms are not always typical and the condition, because of so many other possibilities, may be difficult to diagnose in this older age group.

Both the incidence and mortality are higher in males, particularly between the ages of 5 to 14 and after age 55.   Appendicitis is especially dangerous in the elderly because of the increased hazard of early perforation.

With early recognition and surgery, death rarely occurs, but with neglect or delay, the outcome may easily be fatal.

Appendicitis was recognized many years ago by McBurney, who issued the dictum which is still so true today: "The exploratory incision for the diseased appendix is much more free from danger than expectant treatment." What McBurney meant was very simple—it is safer to operate and find only a normal appendix than not to operate in the face of acute abdominal symptoms. Temporizing incurs the danger of perforation and peritonitis, with the possibility of many ensuing complications.

But appendicitis, when it does not occur in typical form, is not always easy to recognize and, conversely, it is quite possible for patients presenting perfectly typical symptoms not to have an inflamed appendix at all, although they may have some other form of intra-abdominal inflammation. On the other hand, those with symptoms not typical of appendicitis, or only mildly suggestive of the possibility of this condition, may turn out to have an acutely inflamed appendix.

Signs and Symptoms.   A characteristic attack begins with preliminary symptoms of tiredness, loss of appetite, nausea, and vomiting. Diarrhea is also a symptom in about 10 percent of the cases, although a far larger number suffer from constipation.

In the typical case the first definite symptom is usually a gripping, colicky pain in the pit of the stomach, followed in 2 to 4 hours by nausea and vomiting, which may be accompanied by a diarrhea-like feeling. After another 4 hours or so the pain shifts to the right lower side of the abdomen, which becomes acutely tender and spastic to touch. This latter symptom, following the above sequence of events, very strongly suggests the presence of acute appendicitis.

Fever is not always present and is the last symptom to appear, usually running around 99 to 102°F. Higher temperatures suggest either a complication such as rupture, with ensuing peritonitis, or some other condition which may simulate appendicitis, such as pneumonia.

It is important not to be lulled into a false sense of security that all is well if the abdominal pain suddenly stops after a period of up to 36 hours. This, in itself, is an ominous sign and suggests that the appendix has ruptured. Pain and increased signs of illness will occur shortly, as the result of abcess formation or when peritonitis caused by the rupture sets in.

Roughly a third of the patients who present the classical syndrome turn out not to have appendicitis, but have some other condition for which surgery may or may not have been indicated. The symptom of pain is particularly deceptive, since it can begin almost anywhere in the abdomen and radiate to any other part, rather than following the classical course from the pit of the stomach to the right lower quadrant.

The element of pain can be particularly confusing in young children. The only safe rule to follow is to suspect appendicitis in every child who complains of abdominal pain, even though the child at first may appear to have nothing more than a stomach ache, which often is not severe enough to interfere with the child's play. But if the pain increases in severity and is succeeded by the onset of nausea and vomiting, the child should be very closely observed, with the possibility of surgery in mind.

Often the appearance of the child alone will suggest the possibility of acute appendicitis. Most children with plain indigestion throw up at the drop of a hat and then appear quite all right. But the child with appendicitis usually looks and acts sick, tends to be apathetic with an anxious expression, and tends to protect his abdomen by avoiding all motion. He usually will lie quietly on one side, with the legs drawn up so as to keep the inflamed area in the lower right side as quiet as possible.

One of the greatest contributing factors to the mortality figures of appendicitis, particularly in children, is that so many parents still believe that the pain of appendicitis has to be severe and, if it is not, the child has only a stomach ache, and they do the worst of all possible things, which is to give a cathartic. Somewhere in every home there should be a sign pointing out a single fact—any abdominal pain may be serious, and the thoughtless use of laxatives can be fatal.

Another fallacy is the belief that anyone with appendicitis must have fever. This is by no means necessarily true, especially in children, and fever may not develop until the appendix has perforated, with the ensuing complication of peritonitis.

There is no single infallible test for diagnosing appendicitis, but probably the most dependable in the face of other presenting symptoms is acute right lower quadrant tenderness. When this sign is unquestionable, it may indeed be hazardous to overlook the strong possibility of the appendix being acutely inflamed and defer surgery.

○ TREATMENT

The treatment is *prompt* surgery.   Never give anyone suspected of having appendicitis anything to eat or drink, except possibly little sips of water.   Never give a laxative or any other medication.

The patient should be placed in a semireclining position, head and trunk raised about 30 degrees from horizontal, with a pillow under his knees to keep them flexed, and an ice bag, wrapped in a towel, applied to the lower right side of the abdomen.

The patient should be seen by a doctor as quickly as possible and arrangements should be made to get him into a hospital.

It is most important, when appendicitis is suspected, not to consider it casually as "indigestion" or a "bilious attack."   If appendicitis is suspected, something definitive *must* be done.

Gallstones (Gallbladder Attack).   Gallstones are common in certain types of persons in the middle-aged group, although they may also sometimes occur earlier or later in life.   On occasion, stones in the gallbladder or in the ducts leading from the gallbladder to the intestinal tract cause a severe spasm of the gallbladder in its attempt to expel them; this spasm is extremely painful and is the basis for what is called an *acute attack of gallstones*.   While this condition constitutes a surgical emergency, it is usually not as urgent or as serious as an attack of acute appendicitis, for the simple reason that, whereas the appendix, if neglected, may rupture, the gallbladder rarely does.   Moreover, many surgeons believe that it is better to operate after the acute phase of an attack has subsided.

Signs and Symptoms.   As a rule, a gallbladder attack does not come on without signs of gallbladder disease having existed for some time.   The victim has probably had a fondness for rich and fatty foods, which eventually become indigestible, and probably has been suffering from stomach distress, gas, and belching.   Usually, people so affected are short, squat, and overweight, but this is not always true.   The time comes when they are suddenly stricken with a severe viselike pain in the upper right side of the abdomen, feeling as if a tight band were being drawn around their middle.   The pain characteristically radiates to the right shoulder, although it may go straight through to the back, sometimes causing the person to double up in an attempt to relieve the cramp-like agony. There may or may not be nausea, accompanied by vomiting; when this does occur, it is repetitive, but is unproductive of anything but green bile and mucus.

○ TREATMENT

While surgery may not be required immediately, the person should be under the observation of a physician or surgeon in order to be prepared for any developments that would indicate an immediate operation. In the meantime, place him in a semireclining position. Heat, in the form of hot-water bags, is helpful. The severe pain will require heavy sedation, which can be given only by a doctor.

Perforated Ulcer of Stomach. When perforation of an ulcer of the stomach or of the first portion of the intestine (duodenum) occurs, it produces severe abdominal symptoms. *This is a potential surgical disaster.* It is most common in males who have previously had symptoms of ulcer and it usually occurs after a large meal or other dietary indiscretion.

Signs and Symptoms. The victim suffers excruciating general abdominal pain, severe prostration, and shock. There is board-like rigidity of the abominal muscles. Also, there is vomiting and a subnormal temperature.

Few other surgical emergencies cause such acute distress, and the victim is obviously in the gravest danger.

○ TREATMENT

The usual treatment is immediate surgery to close the perforation. In the meantime, give the victim nothing by mouth; keep him flat on his back, with the head of the bed raised slightly. Heavy sedation is indicated, but this can be given only by a doctor, except under extreme circumstances. The drugs of choice are morphine or meperidine (Demerol®) in large doses; only a physician can prescribe or administer drugs of this type.

These victims are either in shock or go into shock very quickly from the enormous peritoneal irritation by the stomach contents. This is one of the most urgent surgical emergencies, and no time whatever should be lost in temporizing; get the patient to a hospital as quickly as possible.   Notify the doctor in advance so that the operating room will be in readiness.

Incarcerated Hernia.   There are many kinds of hernias, some congenital, some traumatic as the result of attempting to lift too heavy an object without taking the proper position, or getting necessary help.   The types and anatomy of the many kinds of hernias which can occur are too numerous to discuss here.

The two most common are the inguinal hernia in which a segment of omentum or small intestine descends through the weakened, or almost closed, inguinal canal (more common in men, less so in women).   The second most common type is the femoral hernia where the same thing happens, but in the femoral canal, with the mass appearing in the upper leg, just below the crotch.   This type is more common in women.

In either case the obvious symptom is a bulge where there should not be one; this may disappear when the victim lies down, only to reappear when he stands up.   If the bulge does not disappear, such hernias are said to be "incarcerated."   If there is exquisite tenderness and redness over the area of the mass, which cannot be made to disappear, it is said to be strangulated; in this case the omentum or bowel may quickly become nonviable, due to the shutting off of its blood supply, and immediate surgery is indicated.

O TREATMENT

As a first-aid measure, a method to reduce the mass which may be tried is to place the victim in the knee-chest position (see Fig. 15-4, page 568), with the victim as relaxed as possible, and see if the mass does not spontaneously go back into the abdomen without any forceful pressure being applied.

A method which we have found to be effective under hospital conditions is to sedate the patient with diazepam (Valium®) and meperidine hydrochloride (Demerol®) and place him in a steep Trendelenburg position (see Fig. 6-1B; page 183). Very gentle slow pressure is then applied to the mass.   If it slips back into the abdomen, surgical correction can be postponed until the next day or two.   If the mass cannot be reduced without force, or becomes tender with redness of the overlying area, the hernia has become strangulated and immediate surery is imperative in order to avoid a gangrenous section of omentum or bowel.

Ectopic Pregnancy. This condition usually occurs when fertilization of the ovum takes place in a fallopian tube, or anywhere in the abdomen outside the uterus. The ovum, instead of passing on to the uterus and developing there, as is normal, becomes embedded in the tube. As the ovum grows, it reaches the point at which it breaks through or ruptures the tube, with profuse hemorrhage and profound shock to the victim.

Signs and Symptoms. The indications are one or two missed menstrual periods, spotting of blood from the uterus, followed by sudden acute abdominal pain, vomiting, and prostration bordering on collapse. The pulse is rapid and weak, and there is deepening shock.

○ TREATMENT

A doctor should be consulted at once, since this is another condition in which immediate surgery is the only means of averting a probable fatal outcome. In the meantime, the woman should be treated as for shock. Give nothing by mouth, in anticipation of an immediate operation.

MISCELLANEOUS CONDITIONS

Bursitis

Bursitis is inflammation, which may be acute or chronic, of a bursa, a smooth, glistening fibrous sac filled with a small amount of fluid which provides frictionless movement for tendons and muscles as they slide over bony prominences, joints, or ligaments. Because of these little sacs, the complex movements of the body's skeletal structures can be carried out smoothly and painlessly, almost as a wheel moves effortlessly on an axle because it turns on well-lubricated ball bearings.

When, as the resut of injury, irritation, or disease, inflammation develops within the sac itself, it becomes swollen and inflamed, and an excessive amount of fluid is secreted so that the sac may enlarge to several times its normal size. In older persons with long-standing inflammation, calcium accretions often develop within the bursal sac. This is the condition known as bursitis with all its painful symptoms.

Some bursae, of course, because of their location and the degree of use to which they may be exposed, are much more susceptible to inflammation than others. It is these which we most frequently hear about and to which common names have become attached.

For instance, a painful shoulder commonly results from inflammation of two important bursae which lie near the shoulder joint. One is just beneath the collarbone, between it and the shoulder joint itself, and the other lies beneath the big deltoid muscle in the shoulder, between it and the head of the humerus. This condition is spoken of as subacromial or subdeltoid bursitis, depending upon which bursa happens to be involved.

Inflammation of the bursa at the back of the elbow joint likewise is common and is known as olecranon bursitis. It often results from a fall or striking the elbow on a hard object. Pain and swelling may be severe. Another condition which affects the elbow joint is popularly referred to as "tennis elbow" or "golf elbow." Here the maximal amount of tenderness is to the outer side of the elbow and the pain is aggravated by extending the wrist backward and putting strain on the muscles of the forearm as one would do in holding and wielding a tennis racket.

Another well-known condition involving inflammation of a bursa is "housemaid's knee." This comes about as the result of repeated minor injury to the rather large bursa that lies between the kneecap and the skin, such as results from frequently repeated intervals of prolonged kneeling on some hard surface, as in washing floors or performing similar tasks.

Perhaps the most famous example is the well-known bunion which is simply a longstanding chronic inflammation of the bursa at the base of the great toe. There are also three bursae around the heel, any one of which can become acutely inflamed, as the result of a bony spur on the heel bone itself, or as the result of unaccustomed excessively long hikes.

○ TREATMENT

There are many forms of treatment, depending upon the location of the offending bursa and the nature of the underlying difficulty. Complete rest of the part and the application of warmth are often helpful. Sometimes the fluid can be removed by a hypodermic needle and syringe, and often a local anesthetic is injected to counteract the pain. Cortisone-like drugs often are specific in relieving the inflammation, and some physicians find x-ray treatments useful for the same purpose. Occasionally it is necessary to irrigate the bursa under local anesthesia or remove it surgically.

Nocturnal Leg Cramps

Nocturnal leg cramps are common, particularly in women, and because of the severe "charley horse" which they cause, are exceeding painful.

The basic cause of leg cramps is some metabolic abnormality within the muscle cells themselves, probably resulting from altered electrolyte metabolism. Many conditions can bring about the setting predisposing to leg cramps. Among the most common of these are stagnation of the blood which may be produced by varicose veins, prolonged standing or some other condition which slows down the flow of blood within the venous system itself; various foot deformities or the wearing of improper shoes—particularly abnormally high heels; pregnancy; osteoarthritis; and a rather rare condition known as Moenckeberg's sclerosis, which consists of extensive deposits of calcium in the walls of the arteries, thus impeding blood flow. A not uncommon cause is excessive potassium loss as the result of the improperly controlled use of certain types of diuretics.

There are, of course, other conditions such as neuritis and similar maladies which may produce leg pain at night and may sometimes be confused with true nocturnal leg cramps, but as a rule the type of pain is not as severe, is more or less steady, and is less acute.

The pain of nocturnal leg cramps appears to be triggered by stretching of the leg during sleep or semiwakefulness. Because of the abnormal reactivity of the muscle, a severe "charley horse" occurs and the large calf muscle (or gastrocnemius muscle, as it is known technically) becomes as hard as a rock as a result of the severe muscular contraction. This causes the foot to be pulled painfully downward and the victim leaps out of bed to counteract the strong pressure on the foot by standing on his toes in an attempt to stretch the muscle back to normal and return the foot to proper position. This does not always relieve the severe pain, which can persist for some time, in which case the use of hot compresses or a hot-water bottle and massage of the cramped-up muscle may be required to provide relief.

The tendency to such attacks is intensified by general fatigue and, particularly, prolonged standing without adequate moving around or exercise. Under such conditions there is a definite tendency for blood to pool or stagnate in the muscles of the lower leg, thus predisposing to nocturnal cramps.

Nocturnal cramps can, of course, occur in almost any set of muscles, as those of the arms, but the occurrence is by far most common in the legs.

○ TREATMENT

Basic treatment rests primarily on eradication of whatever may be the underlying cause. For instance, if venous stasis appears to be the underlying factor, and if this is associated with varicose veins, elimination of the varicosities may be helpful in relieving the muscle cramps. In addition, the wearing of elastic stockings or some other form of elastic support, particularly by those who have to stand on their feet for long periods of time, may be most helpful. The correction of any foot deformity that may be present, and the wearing of proper shoes, go without saying.

There are also two or three drugs which are quite helpful in many cases for which there does not appear to be any obvious cause. Quinine, which is widely used, acts by depressing the general reactivity of the muscle by slowing the conduction of nerve impulses within the muscle itself. However, quinine can cause severe ringing in the ears (tinnitus) and has many other potent actions; it may cause a severe reaction in sensitive individuals, so its use must be guarded; it is contraindicated in patients with any type of cardiac disease and in those who are pregnant. Aminophylline has also been used, and it has been claimed that the combination of aminophylline and quinine is much more effective than either drug alone. A preparation containing the two drugs is now on the market.

In some instances the administration of calcium is helpful, since a deficiency of calcium will in itself increase the excitability or reactivity of the nerves leading to the muscles as well as increase the irritability of the muscle itself. Just how calcium works in this connection, other than the fact that normally it is present in certain portions of the muscle, is not known. However, its administration in suitable doses is empirically known to be effective in many instances.

Arterial Occlusive Disease of the Lower Extremity

Not to be confused with noctural leg cramps is a severe constricting, cramping sensation of the muscles in the leg, especially those in the calf, sometimes described as a "charley horse," after walking a relatively short distance. This phenomenon is known medically as "claudication" and is one of the first signs of beginning obstruction of the femoral or popliteal arteries which supply the muscles of the leg (see page 14). In many cases it may be recognized in retrospect that the development of claudication had been preceded by increasing fatigability of the extremity on walking or other exercise. Cramping of the muscles is due to the diminished blood supply which is unable to meet the increased demands of exercise.

The most common causes of diminishing arterial flow are arteriosclerosis (hardening of the arteries) and diabetes. More infrequently, a severe attack of cramping may indicate sudden complete blocking of one of the leg arteries by an embolus from some distant site such as the heart in cases of subacute bacterial endocarditis.

In cases in which the blood supply is gradually shut off, claudication increases as the blood flow becomes less and less, and the distance the patient can walk without distress becomes shorter and shorter. In the course of time, two other symptoms develop—pain even when the leg is at rest and a dusky turgid redness of the foot and leg when it is held lower than the rest of the body.

If the blood supply becomes completely shut off, ulceration, followed by gangrene, develops in various areas—usually the toes or foot first. It should also be noted that any trauma to a vascularly deficient extremity may in itself result in a very slow healing ulceration or gangrene.

The concomitant presence of uncontrolled diabetes makes the situation much more serious and is in itself a predisposing cause of atherosclerosis and vascular insufficiency.

Peripheral arterial disease most frequently becomes symtomatic during the fifth and sixth decades but is not at all uncommon during earlier years, depending upon the predisposing life habits of the individual, including dietary habits, smoking, and the amount of regular exercise.

○ TREATMENT

In cases in which serious circulatory impairment eixsts, the treatment is surgical and is directed toward removing or bypassing the arterial obstruction. In cases in which several vital arteries of the leg have become extensively diseased, amputation may ultimately be required.

It is impossible to estimate the extent of arterial occlusive disease of the lower extremity among the general population, since many people with only mild claudication do not seek the advice of their physicians. However, it is safe to say that between 75,000 and 100,000 surgical procedures are undertaken each year in this country for the palliative treatment of this condition.

The moral is obvious: if a leg fatigues easily or tends to "cramp up" on walking, particularly if you are middle-aged or older, see your physician promptly.

Painful Menstruation (Dysmenorrhea)

Painful menstruation, while not strictly a medical emergency, often poses a problem of care and relief for the sufferer, usually younger girls and unmarried women whose menstrual cycles have not become fully established or regulated.

Painful menstruation is of two basic types: primary, when there is no discernible organic cause, and secondary, when the condition is definitely caused by, or is secondary to, some other factor, such as an abnormal ovarian condition, pelvic inflammation, or a badly placed or turned (retroverted or retroflexed) uterus. In the primary type, unless it is due to an endocrine disturbance or imbalance, treatment must be, for the most part, according to the symptoms at the time of the person's period, in addition to general health measures and exercises to improve her physical and emotional well-being. Only competent medical care will relieve the secondary type.

It has been found that the healthy, active, physically, and emotionally well-developed young woman is less prone to painful menstrual periods and that good posture also plays a great part.

A number of exercises have been worked out which are intended both to improve posture and develop the pelvic structure in such a way as to correct muscular imbalance that might predispose to dysmenorrhea. These exercises, *if performed regularly,* not only are of great preventive value, but will also help to improve the figure and general sense of well-being.

The exercises may be summarized as follows:

Exercise 1: Stand with feet together, right side of body about 18 inches from the wall. Place elbow against wall at shoulder level, with forearm and hand touching wall. Place heel of left hand on left side of lower back just below waist, fingers pointing downward. Keep abdominal muscles contracted.

Keeping knees straight, heels on floor, and using pressure from left hand, rotate hips forward as far as possible, then to right, then back, returning to starting position, in slow, continuous circular movement. (Fig. 15-2).

Exercise 2: Lie on back with legs together, knees raised, and feet on floor. Slip fingers of right hand (not whole hand) beneath body at waistline. Place left hand in hollow between abdomen and left hip. In three counts, tighten abdomen, push up pelvis, then relax. Try to breathe easily during the exercise (Fig. 15-3).

Exercise 3: Cross forearms on floor under side of head. Place knees slightly apart in a vertical position, feet together. In this position, contract and relax abdominal muscles slowly (Fig. 15-4).

Certain additional measures are of value in minimizing premenstrual tension and dysmenorrhea. These include avoiding nervous strain or apprehension, obtaining the required amount of sleep, and definitely restricting the amount of fluid and, especially, table salt for about 1 week prior to the expected onset of a period. Restriction of salt is especially important, since it tends to hold water in the body, and the gain in weight and the emotional tension experienced before a period are associated with this factor.

Many medications are used and prescribed for relieving the pain, tension, and discomfort of dysmenorrhea, but these should be employed only under the direction of the person's family doctor. In severe cases antispasmodic drugs may be

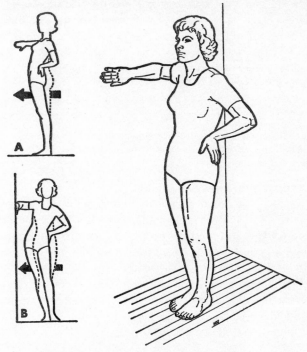

Fig. 15-2.   Exercises for strengthening the waist muscles.

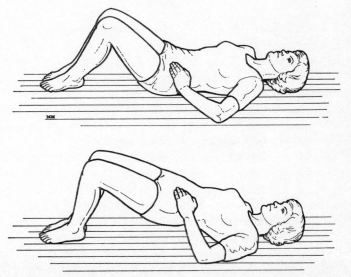

Fig. 15-3.   Exercise for strengthening the abdominal and pelvic muscles.

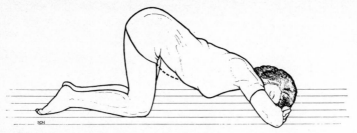

Fig. 15-4. The knee-chest position for helping to correct the position of the pelvic organs and to strengthen the abdominal muscles.

prescribed.   Often, however, immediate relief can be obtained if the person lies down and rests, using a hot-water bag, as warm as she can comfortably stand, over the lower abdomen. Avoiding fatigue and overexertion is also of great benefit, as a person who is overtired is likely to experience greater discomfort and perhaps even have a greater flow than normal.   Hot tea and coffee are also found to bring relief in some cases, and many women feel that an ounce or two of whiskey or brandy has a specific relaxing effect.   Aspirin should be avoided, in large amounts, as it may increase the flow.

DELIVERING A BABY

Sometimes, because of unforeseen circumstances, such as a severe storm that prevents the mother from getting to a hospital or a doctor from getting to her, an untrained person finds it necessary to attend a mother who is about to give birth to a baby.   Fortunately, if labor is progressing so rapidly that birth is imminent before medical aid can be procured, the process is usually normal and can proceed with little or no assistance.

Occasionally a birth may be so precipitous as to occur under difficult or unclean circumstances (as in a taxicab, for instance).   Under such conditions the best one can do is protect the mother and baby from contamination as effectively as possible and extemporize in her behalf with whatever useful materials may come to hand.   She should, of course, be shielded from public curiosity insofar as is feasible.

Under less stringent circumstances and time permitting, there are certain preparations which should be made, and certain simple steps to be taken after the baby arrives.   The whole procedure will, of course, be easier if the birth occurs at home rather than in a public place or conveyance.

The following articles will be required:

1 A large covered saucepan in which to sterilize articles by boiling.

2 A medium-sized pair of scissors for cutting the umbilical cord.

3 Three or four pieces of cloth tape for tying the cord before cutting, such as ordinary cotton binding tape found in almost every sewing basket, or strips torn from a sheet; even a pair of boiled shoe laces can be used, but *not* string, as it might cut through the umbilical cord.

    (Boil the articles listed above, covered for 10 minutes, and then *leave them covered* to cool until needed.)

4 A few sterile gauze pads or freshly laundered handkerchiefs.

5 Absorbent cotton balls.

6 Saline solution or lukewarm previously boiled water for sponging the baby's eyes.

7 Two sanitary napkins.

8 A medium-sized towel.

Prepare also a protective covering for the bed—rubber sheeting if you have it—and a warm, snug place for the newborn baby. A clothes basket lined with clean soft blankets is suitable.

If you have time for further preparations, put clean, freshly laundered sheets on the bed, and at the place where the mother's buttocks will be, cover the rubber sheeting with a clean sheet. Put a clean nightgown on the mother, and, if possible, thoroughly wash her genital area with a good lather of soap and hot water.

To facilitate your handling of the delivery, arrange the mother so that her buttocks will be near one side of the bed and so that she can brace her legs to aid her in bearing down and delivering the child (Fig. 15-5).

Do not try to delay the birth by having the mother cross her legs; if the process has reached this stage, you cannot stop it; furthermore, such attempts may result in injury or suffocation of the baby.

As labor progesses and the baby is forced down into the pelvis, preparatory to making its exit from the vulva, you will

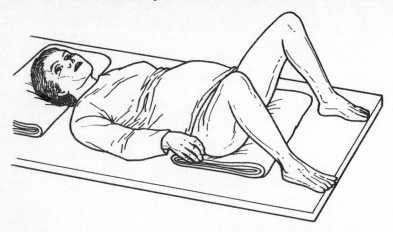

Fig. 15-5. Positioning the mother on a bed, table, or other surface for emergency delivery. A soft protective pad should be under her buttocks (a thick layer of newspapers if nothing better is available), as well as a soft support for her head.

see the hair on the top of its head, at the opening of the vulva (Fig. 15-6). By now the opening has stretched enough to permit the baby to slip through, but the skin around the vulva will be very tightly drawn. Usually, the baby's chin will be pointed downward just inside the lower part of the vulval opening. The problem at this time is that the baby will come so fast that the skin around the vulva will be torn before it can stretch enough to let it through. This often can be prevented by covering a hand with a freshly laundered towel and pressing in on the mother's skin in the midline between the opening of the anus and the opening of the vulva. At this point you will feel the baby's chin, and you can gently ease it up and through the vulval opening. If delivery is progressing very rapidly, gentle guidance of the head may be all that is required (Fig. 15-7).

The baby often will slip the rest of the way out spontaneously and will be bluish and covered with a whitish slippery substance known as the vernix caseosa.

In some cases it may be necessary to facilitate the delivery of the uppermost (anterior) shoulder by gently directing the baby's head in a downward direction without twisting or excessive pressure on the baby's head (Fig. 15-8). Then the opposite shoulder is delivered by gently directing the child's

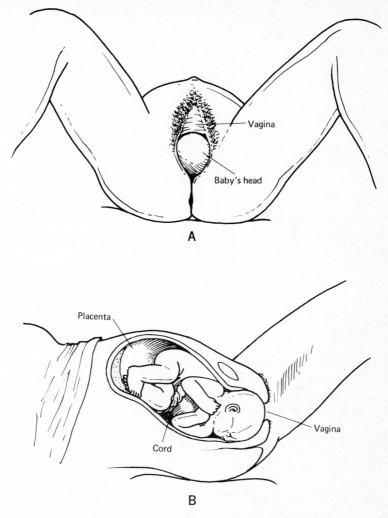

Fig. 15-6. The appearance of the top of the baby's head (caput) at the vulval opening (A) shows that actual delivery is beginning to take place. (B) Sagittal view showing position of the baby, inside the mother, at this stage.

head and body upward (Fig. 15-9).   Thereafter the child comes out easily.

Almost immediately the baby should give a lusty cry and start breathing.   To help him get started, pick him up by the ankles and hold him upside down in such a way that both

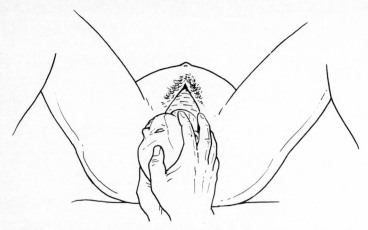

Fig. 15-7. Method of easing baby's head gently through the vulval opening so as to minimize the possibility of tearing the skin and deeper tissues between the vulva and anus.

ankles are firmly fixed and held in the grasp of your entire hand. To do this so that he will be facing you when he is upside down, grasp his right ankle between your thumb and first finger, and the left ankle between your index and third finger (Fig. 15-10). In this way the baby cannot slip (and he *is* slippery!). With your other hand, wipe out his mouth and nose with a sterile gauze pad or freshly laundered handkerchief, and then pat him gently but firmly between the shoulder blades. At this point he should start crying.

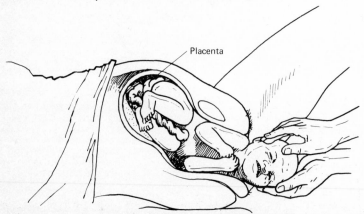

Placenta

Fig. 15-8. The baby's head is gently directed *downward* to help deliver the upper (anterior) shoulder, which usually is the first to emerge.

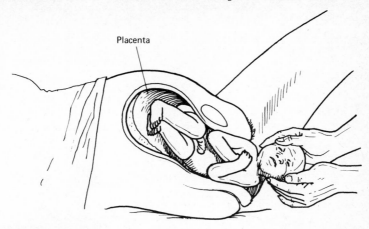

Placenta

Fig. 15-9. Then the lower (posterior) shoulder is delivered by very gently directing the axis of the baby's head and neck upward. Never pull hard in an attempt to drag the baby out; this could cause permanent damage to the baby or mother or both.

Now, lay the baby face downward across the mother's abdomen, with his head a little lower than the rest of his body to facilitate drainage of mucus, and proceed to tie off the umbilical cord. To do this, take one of the pieces of tape, and tie a good tight square knot 4 to 5 inches from where the umbilical cord joins the baby. Then, with another piece of tape tie another tight square knot about 2 inches further on toward the mother (Fig. 5-11 A and B).

Be sure that both knots are firm, will not slip, and are tight enough to control bleeding when the cord is cut.

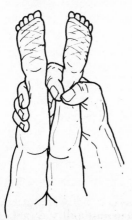

Fig. 15-10. Method of firmly holding the baby after delivery so that he cannot slip while cleansing his mouth and nose and initiating breathing.

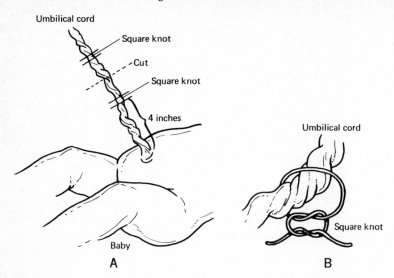

Fig. 15-11. The cord is firmly tied off (A) with two strips of tape (shoe laces will do in a pinch) and then cut between the two ties. The tie is made (B) using a square knot which will not slip.

When you are satisfied on this point—and there is no particular hurry—take the (sterilized) scissors and cut the cord between the ties. The baby is now freed from the mother and on its own.

Sponge the baby's eyes gently, using a fresh cotton ball dipped in lukewarm previously boiled water for each eye, wiping from the nose side out. Place him in his bassinet or equivalent, warmly wrapped in blankets that are arranged so that he cannot suffocate, and with his head a little lower than the rest of his body. Do *not* try to clean him. If you cannot keep him warm in any other way or if you have no other place for him, wrap him in a blanket and put him alongside his mother.

Now you can relax a little. It probably will be 10 to 20 minutes before the afterbirth (placenta) is delivered. When it is expelled from the vulva, probably with a gush of blood, catch it in a basin, and leave it for the doctor to examine, as he will have to determine whether the placenta is complete or a part of it remained in the womb, causing trouble later on. Do *not* pull the cord to hasten the delivery of the placenta, since doing this might tear a blood vessel and cause serious trouble. When the placenta is at the vulva, it can be brought out with a little gentle pressure.

The next step is important to prevent undue continued bleeding from the womb. Feel the mother's abdomen just below the umbilicus (navel) for a large firm mass. This is the enlarged womb, or uterus, which must contract to control the bleeding from its inside surface. To help the womb to contract, grasp it through the abdominal wall (which will be very relaxed, permitting you to do this easily) between your thumb and fingers and *gently* knead it (Fig. 15-12). You will feel it get almost stony hard in your fingers, and you should continue the kneading for about an hour, until the womb is firmly contracted and danger of hemorrhage is past.

In the meantime, cover the vulva with two sanitary napkins covered with a folded towel. Do not attempt to hold these in

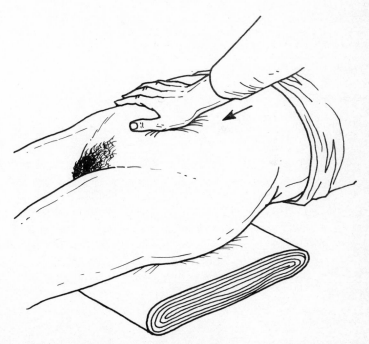

Fig. 15-12. Position of hand for compressing the uterus (which can easily be felt somewhat like a football) to stimulate contraction and thus help to control postpartum bleeding. In the absence of drugs to keep the uterus contracted, gentle manual kneading must be maintained for at least an hour, or until medical help becomes available.

place with the usual belt, as the pressure of the thighs is sufficient when the patient is lying down. Keep the mother warm and comfortable in bed, covering her with blankets and perhaps using a hot-water bag or two if she should have a slight chill. She may wish to have her face and hands sponged with cool water, and probably will enjoy a cup of hot tea or coffee.

Do *not* give whiskey or aspirin, as either might increase the tendency to bleed.

If the mother has bled a great deal or has had an unusual amount of pain, she may be in mild shock. If so, elevate the foot of the bed and treat her as for shock. Otherwise, just wait for the doctor to arrive, maintaining uterine massage to be sure that the womb remains contracted.

16

Home Care of the Ill

At the present time more sick people are cared for at home than in hospitals. There are many advantages to home care and only a few disadvantages. For example, people usually are more comfortable at home than in a hospital and feel a greater sense of security when near their families and loved ones. Having to go to a hospital frightens many people and makes them feel that their illness is more serious than it may in fact be, but if a person remains at home, he tends to minimize the seriousness of his condition and thus does not have an emotional handicap to overcome in getting well. And then there is, of course, the matter of expense. Many charges which a hospital must make for services can be avoided by being nursed at home.

On the other hand, there are many procedures and special nursing technics which cannot be carried out efficiently at home; when such services are required, a person is much better off in a hospital. Any major operation, of course, requires hospitalization, except under the most unusual circumstances, as does any illness requiring the constant and expert medical supervision that can be provided only by well-trained interns and nurses. In such an event, the patient should be given every assurance that he is going to the hospital to get *well* and that he will return home as soon as possible, to complete his convalescence there.

So much importance is now attached to proper home care of the ill that many services are available to help in this, and some modern hospitals offer home-nursing services which provide professional aid and an extension of many of the hospital's facilities.

UNDERSTANDING THE PATIENT

In caring for a sick person, it is important to realize that he may have an emotional as well as a physical hazard to overcome; the home nurse should make every effort to understand whatever problems seem to be preying on the patient's mind and attempt to clarify them to the patient's satisfaction. Maintain a firm but gentle and cheerful attitude at all times, and, even though you yourself may be worried and concerned for the patient's welfare, it will only make matters worse to show it.

It does not help, either, to be overly sympathetic toward the patient's aches and pains. However, this does not mean that one should be unfeeling, but, if a report of the patient's symptoms is accepted in a matter-of-fact manner and as a helpful record of the course of his illness, any overconcern of the patient for himself will be minimized. Many sick people, especially the elderly and those who in normal life may be nervous and high-strung, are understandably apprehensive about their condition and will subconsciously tend to exaggerate both the intensity and the importance of every little ache and pain. Also, many are unduly concerned over a high temperature, particularly if the nurse will not tell them what the thermometer reads or if she shows concern. In this connection, it often helps to explain that, in many instances, a fever is nature's way of fighting the disease and, for that reason, the doctor sometimes does not *want* to reduce the fever right away.

THE PATIENT'S ROOM

Important factors in the efficient care of the ill at home are the appearance, comfort, and equipment of the sickroom.

Whenever possible, it is advisable for the patient to have a room that can be devoted solely to his care and that will not be used by any other member of the family. It should be light and airy, but free of drafts, and should have heating arrangements that will permit the room temperature to be carefully controlled to suit the comfort of the patient. Try also to select a room that is quiet, away from the street but, if possible, with a view out of the window that will provide him with continuing interests. The room should be as near as possible to bathroom or toilet facilities.

A minimum amount of furniture should be kept in the sickroom in order to facilitate keeping it as neat and clean as possible. Such furniture as is used should be adapted to the nurse's requirements, as well as to the convenience and comfort of the patient. Some sort of cabinet stand should be provided, in which the various sickroom supplies can be kept—bulky utensils, such as bed pans, emesis basins, and hot-water bags, underneath; and articles that are small and frequently used, such as a clinical thermometer, disposable tissues, and drinking water, on top.

If it appears that the patient will be ill for a long time, it will be very helpful to the nurse if the bed is of the proper height. A special hospital bed, in which the head or foot can be raised by means of cranks, can be purchased or rented, but in many cases this is unnecessary. A hospital bed is about 33 inches high. A regular, single bed can easily be raised by using wooden blocks under each leg to bring it to the proper height. But be sure that whatever you use is firm and will not slip.

You may also need some sort of support, or cradle, to keep the bedclothes from weighing too heavily on the patient's body during a prolonged illness. These can be purchased or rented, but they can also be improvised with a little ingenuity, using rubber-insulated wire heavy enough to maintain its shape under the weight of bedclothes. Be sure that no rough or sharp ends are left that might injure the patient or tear the sheets. A simpler type, though it will probably not last as long as a wire cradle, can be made by cutting out a large cardboard carton and placing it under the bedcovers so as to hold them off the patient (Fig. 16-1).

Basic Sickroom Supplies

As soon as it becomes apparent that you are in for a spell of home nursing, get together the articles that will be required in the care of your patient, and arrange them neatly and con-

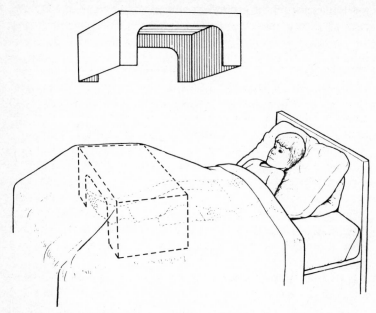

Fig. 16-1. A cradle to keep bedclothes off legs and feet, made from a cardboard carton.

veniently in the patient's room. The following articles should be included in a list of basic needs:

clinical thermometer	ice bag
paper and pencil	waterproof sheeting
rubbing alcohol	personal toilet articles
washcloth and towel	flashlight
hot-water bag	disposable tissues
bedpan and urinal	baby powder
absorbent cotton	hand lotion
tongue depressors	pitcher
drinking glass and straws	enema equipment
(or glass sipper)	toilet tissue
lubricating jelly	clean linen supply
antiseptic soap	bell (for patient's use)
hand basin	

It is important that each article be in an assigned place and that it be kept clean, dry, and always ready for use. This is a part of sickroom hygiene; scrupulous cleanliness and proper care of all equipment are of the highest importance.

Care of Sickroom Supplies

The clinical thermometer should be cleaned after each use, by rinsing it thoroughly under running *cold* water and then wiping it with a bit of gauze or cotton wet with rubbing alcohol. If you prefer, a special glass stand can be obtained which holds alcohol and into which the thermometer can be inserted and kept after each use. This is intended to stand on the supply table and is very handy. Be sure to shake the thermometer as soon as you have read it.

All rubber equipment should be cleaned and thoroughly dried after each use and stored where there is a good circulation of air. Rubber will keep better if it is lightly powdered with talc (baby powder), because it prevents the surfaces from sticking together.

To keep the bedpan in a sanitary condition, clean and disinfect it thoroughly after each use. This is easily done by steadying the bedpan on the toilet seat in such a way that the contents drain freely into the toilet and then washing the pan with a spray. The pan may be rinsed out with a small amount of creosote disinfectant and then dried. It will help to maintain the sanitary condition of the pan if a little water is put in it before each use, to prevent matter from sticking and to facilitate its cleaning.

INTEGRATING THE HOUSEHOLD AND NURSING SCHEDULES

To provide efficient nursing care without disrupting normal household activities too much, it is important to devise a schedule which not only will satisfy the requirements and convenience of the patient, but will fit in with household chores. If the patient is a child, the mother will probably be the logical one to decide upon necessary readjustments in the household, in accordance with the routine and scheduled requirements of the patient.

The Daily Nursing Routine

The two major duties of a nurse are (1) the accurate recording of information for the doctor and (2) the actual routine nursing care.

The records should include the following basic information:

1 Temperature, pulse, and respiration, taken at 4-hour intervals of very sick patients; of others, twice a day.

2 The total amount of fluid, including soups, beverages, and water, consumed by the patient in each 24-hour period.

3 The amount of urine excreted by the patient in a 24-hour period; in the case of very sick patients, this should be accurately measured. (A quart bottle makes an excellent measuring device.)

4 The number and nature of the bowel movements—note especially consistency, color, odor, and the presence of blood or mucus.

5 The amount and nature of the patient's sleep—sound, restless, fitful, or dozing.

6 General nature of patient's complaints, if any.

7 The time and nature of all medications or treatments. In this connection, be sure that the doctor leaves written orders, in addition to his verbal explanations, about any medications that are to be given, as well as how they are to be given. Be sure that you understand these instructions clearly.

With respect to routine care, the household schedule should be planned to accommodate the following basic program for the care of the patient.

Early morning care is one of the advantages, from the point of view of the patient, of being sick at home, because he doesn't have to be waked up before dawn to be given a bath and to clean his teeth—a most trying part of hospital routine. Give early morning care, so far as possible, according to the patient's wishes and your convenience, but it should be carried out at a regular time and should include the following procedures:

1 Let the patient use the bedpan. While you are disposing of the contents, give him a basin of water and soap so that he can wash his face and hands, comb his hair, and clean his teeth if he is able; if he is not, you will have to do this for him.

2 Freshen up the bed, get the patient into a comfortable position so that he can eat his breakfast, and make the necessary adjustments in the temperature of the room to meet daytime requirements.

3 Take and record his temperature, pulse, and respiration, and note the character and amount of urine and bowel movements, if any.

4 Give the patient his breakfast, and follow this with a sponge bath when you can fit it in.

During the day allow for these additional activities:

1 Give medications and other treatments as ordered by the doctor.

2 Set aside about an hour for visitors, so as not to upset your daily schedule. (If the patient has a contagious disease, allow no visitors.)

3 Arrange adequate rest periods for the patient, during which he can read or sleep as he wishes, and you also can have some free time.

Evening care, which may be divided by the evening meal, should include the following items:

1 Take and record temperature, pulse, and respiration.

2 Let the patient wash his face and hands and brush his teeth.

3 Give his entire body an alcohol rub.

4 Fix the bed for the night, and be sure to place needed articles within reach of patient.

5 Give evening medications, including a sedative, as ordered by the doctor.

NURSING PROCEDURES

None of the technics required in general nursing care is very difficult, but it helps to know some of the "tricks of the trade" so that it will be easier on you to provide the best possible care for the patient. General nursing procedures are very important and include several items.

Taking the Patient's Temperature. An accurate record of the patient's temperature, taken at regular intervals, provides a valuable guide to his condition and progress. The temperature may be taken either by mouth or by rectum; however, the thermometers used for these two methods are slightly different: the oral thermometer has a rather long, thin bulb, and the rectal thermometer, a short, blunt bulb. Do not confuse the two types of thermometer.

Either thermometer may be used to take the temperature by armpit if, for any reason, neither the oral nor rectal method is practical. The normal temperatures in degrees Fahrenheit by the three methods are as follows:

By mouth—98.6

By rectum—99.6

By armpit—97.4

In taking temperatures, leave the thermometer in the mouth or rectum for fully 1 minute, or even a little longer. If you are taking the temperature by armpit, leave the thermometer in place for at least 10 minutes, with the arm held close to the body. And according to Nichols, even an oral thermometer should stay in a child's mouth at least 10 minutes to register its maximum. The child should not be left alone during this period lest he or she bite the thermometer and suffer the danger of not only broken glass but mercury poisoning as well, as mentioned by Herrero.

To take the temperature by rectum, lubricate the rectal thermometer with a sterile lubricating jelly and gently insert it about 1½ inches into the anus. If the patient is a very young child, he should be held in order to avoid the possibility of breaking the thermometer. Hold the child's buttocks in the palm of your hand, with the thermometer protruding between the second and third or third or forth fingers; put your other arm arount the child to steady him (Fig. 16-2).

The temperature may vary a degree or so in a perfectly well person, depending on the time of day and other conditions. It is usually slightly higher in the late afternoon and lowest in the predawn hours.

A clinical thermometer is easy to read, since it has a red line or a heavy black one at the level indicating the normal temperature for the method for which the thermometer is intended. Each degree is divided into five equal parts, with each little line between the degree marks equaling two-tenths of a degree (Fig. 16-3). The temperature is determined by simply noting the level (to the nearest tenth) of the top of the column of mercury, as in any other thermometer.

A clinical thermometer is constructed in such a way that one side acts as its own magnifying glass. To read it, hold the thermometer at a convenient angle, and turn it to where the

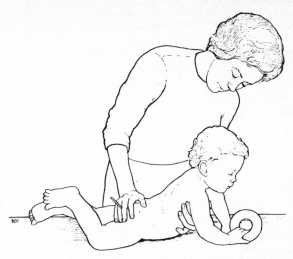

Fig. 16-2. Holding a baby while taking his temperature by rectum.

column of mercury is most readily seen.   It should be looked at in good daylight or in strong electric light.

Unlike other thermometers, the mercury in a clinical thermometer goes up, but it doesn't go down with the temperature.   Once it has been used, the mercury has to be shaken back to normal.   To do this, give the thermometer one or two sharp downward shakes with the wrist, being careful not to hit anything with it, for these thermometers break easily and are expensive.

Wash the thermometer in *cold* water, *not* hot, then wipe it with alcohol, dry it, and put it away in its case or in the thermometer stand if you are using one.

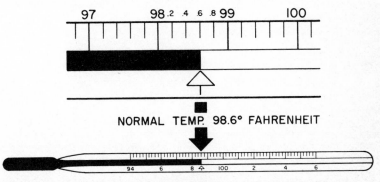

Fig. 16-3. How to read a clinical thermometer.

Taking the Patient's Pulse.   While you are taking the patient's temperature, you can save time by also counting the pulse beats and the respirations.   It is easiest to take the pulse at the wrist, where it can be felt against the bone on the thumb side, just above the wrist joint (Fig. 16-4).

It is felt by grasping the patient's wrist so that two or more of your fingers are over the pulse and your thumb is on the back of the wrist, thus holding the wrist steady and exerting pressure by a slight squeeze.

The pulse rate varies greatly under various conditions, but, at rest, the following number of pulse beats per minute are about normal:

Adult males—54 to 70

Adult females—75 to 80

Young children—82 to 180

As a general rule, there is usually an increase of about 10 beats per minute for each degree of rise in temperature, but this does not necessarily hold true, since in some diseases, there is a characteristic difference between the temperature and pulse which may be significant in diagnosis.   This is one reason that accurate records are important.   In taking the pulse, be sure to note its general character—full, bounding,

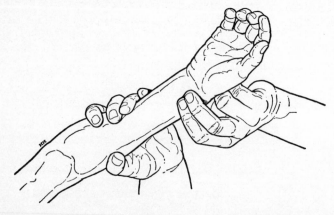

Fig. 16-4.   Of the many pulses in the body which are readily felt, one of the most convenient and commonly used is at the wrist and is obtained by gently compressing the radial artery against the bone (radius) of the forearm with two or more fingers.   Do not use your thumb to do this, as you may feel the pulse in your own thumb rather than the patient's pulse.

weak, or irregular—and make your observations a part of your record.

Counting the Patient's Respirations (Breathing Rate). As soon as you have finished counting the pulse beats, count the patient's respirations. This is easily done by holding the patient's arm in such a way that it lies slightly across his chest, and you can very easily feel the respiratory movements. You can also watch the rise and fall of the bedclothes, but in patients whose breathing is very shallow it is sometimes difficult to see this movement.

The respiratory rate may be increased by a great many factors, but in most normal individuals, under conditions of rest, it runs about 18 to 20 breaths per minute in adults, and about 40 to 45 per minute in young children.

Mouth Care

Mouth care should be carried out carefully in order to prevent food, secretions, and bacteria from accumulating. If the patient is able to care for his mouth himself, he should clean his teeth twice a day and follow this with a mouth rinse. Witch hazel, diluted half and half with water, is very satisfactory for this purpose, since it is soothing and leaves a clean taste in the mouth. Saline solution can be used, but it doesn't taste very good and has no special merit. Some commercial mouthwashes are pleasant tasting and are also good cleansers.

If the patient is incapable of performing this task, the nurse should make a careful inspection of the mouth each day, using a tongue depressor to hold the tongue and cheeks out of the way so that she can see all parts of the mouth.

1 Any sores or other abnormalities should be reported to the doctor.

2 All food particles should be carefully removed from between the teeth with a toothpick or dental floss, and then the teeth and gums should be gently cleaned, using a soft toothbrush moistened with a little water and a little dentifrice.

3 The tongue should also be carefully cleaned at this time, as it can accumulate decaying material and become offensive-smelling.

4 If possible, the patient should then rinse his mouth with witch hazel diluted with plain water or a mouthwash which he finds acceptable.

5   Careful attention should be given the lips, which may be very dry or chapped. Using a cotton ball or swab, clean and then anoint them with a little petrolatum, baby oil, or a good chapstick.

In addition to the regular mouth care twice a day, the patient should be allowed to rinse his mouth frequently with water.

Skin Care and Prevention of Bedsores

General skin care and cleanliness are of paramount importance, in order to keep the skin healthy and to prevent the development of bedsores, which, once they occur in a very ill person, are extremely difficult to cure. They can be prevented by keeping the skin scrupulously clean, well oiled, soft, and well nourished by gentle massage and by keeping pressure off bony prominences, such as the heels, hips, and buttocks.

Giving a Bed Bath.   Of the procedures mentioned, one of the most important is the daily bath.   Bathing the patient in bed is not difficult if you follow a simple routine.

1   Remove the top bedclothes and cover the patient with a bath blanket in such a way that only the part of the body you are washing is exposed.

2   Protect the bottom sheet with a heavy bath towel as you go along.

3   Using a basin of comfortably warm water and a mild high-grade soap (baby soap is excellent) proceed to wash the body a part at a time, from the head down.

4   When the upper half of the body has been washed, put a bed gown on the patient before proceeding with the rest of the body. (The bed gown may be turned back out of the way if it is long.)

5   Then wash the pelvic area, including the genitals. (The patient may do this for himself if he is able; otherwise, the nurse must do it, as cleanliness here is important.)

6   Wash the legs, giving special care to the feet. It is very important to see that they are not only washed but that they are thoroughly dried. In a very ill patient, especially one who may be diabetic, it is good practice to anoint each foot with oil, gently but thoroughly—baby oil is good for this—working it into the skin, especially the spaces between the toes; then

gently wipe off the excess oil and dust on a small amount of baby powder.

In caring for the feet, be very gentle; use a soft, *not* a harsh towel, as sores easily get started here and are hard to cure.

Avoiding Pressure.   If the patient is too ill to turn himself frequently or if he is paralyzed, the nurse must see to it that his position is changed often and that prolonged pressure on any of the bony prominences is avoided.   Avoiding pressure is sometimes difficult to do, but four basic nursing procedures, aside from the scrupulous care of the skin itself, will help to prevent pressure sores: (1) a properly made bed, (2) the frequent turning of the patient, (3) proper posture in bed so as to avoid undue pressures, and (4) the use of various devices for relieving pressure when it cannot otherwise be avoided.

Devices for Relieving Pressure.   One device for relieving pressure on the heels is a "doughnut" made by rolling up a tube of stockinet or an old stocking to make a ring thick enough to fit around the sides of the heel, preventing the back of the heel from rubbing on the bedclothes (Fig. 16-5).   Soft absorbent cotton may be placed in the bottom of the ring to provide a soft base in case the heel does actually touch.   Similar devices can be prepared to protect the elbows, ears, or any other spot which appears to give the patient the least bit of discomfort.

The buttocks require particular attention.   Here the bedclothes themselves may be a significant factor, particularly if they are at all rough or if a strong soap has been used in laundering.   Try to use bedclothes that are soft and smooth and that have been laundered with a mild soap and thoroughly rinsed.   It is important, also, to avoid wrinkles or food crumbs in the bed, as these can easily cause breaks and sores in the skin of very ill patients.

If there is any evidence at all of congestion in the skin of the buttocks which cannot be avoided by other means, the patient must use a soft rubber air ring covered with very soft absorbent cloth when he is in a position that brings weight to bear on his buttocks.   The same is true for the hipbones, which can be particularly bad trouble spots.

The bedclothes themselves may cause pressure that is very

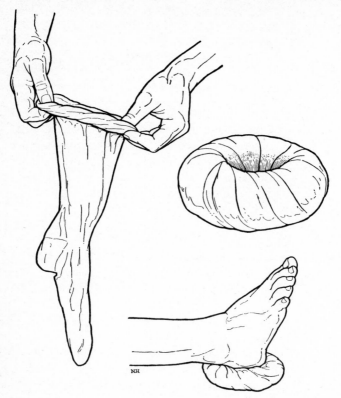

Fig. 16-5. Making a "doughnut" from a rolled-up stocking to prevent pressure on patient's heels.

annoying to the patient and in some cases actually harmful. This can be relieved by constructing a cradle to be placed over the patient so as to keep the bedclothes from touching him at all.

A cradle can easily be constructed by cutting a cardboard frame from a box of the proper size or by cutting barrel hoops in half and fastening them together with three strips of wooden lath that have been suitably smoothed. For certain special treatments requiring the application of heat or light, a small electric light bulb may be suspended inside such a device to supply both. Be careful to avoid burning!

Procedure for Making the Bed

A properly made bed is one of the greatest factors in the patient's general comfort and welfare and therefore has a great deal to do with his getting well quickly.   The bed must be made fresh once a day and straightened up frequently.   The reasons for this are that clean bed linen is very important in proper skin care, and there is nothing more uncomfortable than a mussy, wrinkled bed.   Keep the under bedclothes clean and tight, and avoid wrinkles at all costs.   You will soon develop the knack of making up a bed in such a way that the bottom sheet stays tight and smooth for a long time.   The top bedclothes should be warm enough to suit the comfort of the patient, but should be lightweight and not drawn so tightly that they produce an uncomfortable sense of constriction.

For the most part, you will probably have to make the bed with the patient in it; this is not a difficult procedure if you go about it in the right sequence, and it can be done without exposing the patient.

1   Loosen all the bedding from underneath the mattress, and then remove the top bedclothes, except for one blanket left over the patient; this is done by sliding the top sheet out from underneath the top blanket without exposing the patient.

2   Turn the patient on his side so that he is nearer one side of the bed; remove all but one pillow.

3   Starting with the outer edge, roll the soiled bottom sheet toward the patient's back until it is close up against him. Straighten the exposed half of the mattress and pull it tight.

4   Take a clean bottom sheet and, placing it lengthwise on the bed, make a roll of one half of it so that it is close up against the patient and underneath the rolled-up soiled sheet; tuck the edges in firmly under the mattress at the head and foot (Fig. 16-6).

5   Turn the patient toward the other side of the bed, helping him or lifting him over the little mound of soiled sheet and clean sheet in the middle of the bed.   Then, the rest is simple.

6   Pull off the soiled sheet, unroll the clean sheet and tuck it in under the mattress, pulling it as tight as possible and being sure to miter the corners.

Mitering the corners of the sheet helps to hold the entire sheet tight.   To do this, grasp the sheet at its free edge about 12 inches from the end, raise it up and let it fall on top of the bed.   The hanging part left at the corner is then tucked in, and the rest of the side is allowed to fall back in place.   The sheet is then tucked in all along the side of the bed, being

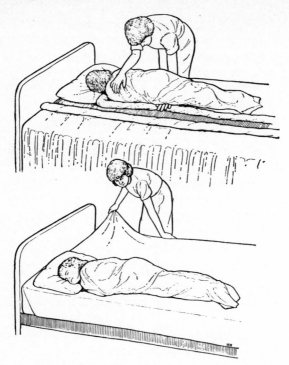

Fig. 16-6. Easy method of making bed with minimal disturbance to patient.

sure to leave no wrinkles. Then at the next corner the sheet is pulled diagonally as tightly as possible, and so on all around the mattress (Fig. 16-7).

7   Put on the clean top covers and tuck them in; change the pillow cases and replace the pillows for the patient, getting him settled back in a comfortable position.

Check to be sure there are no wrinkles in the bottom sheet. Pick up all the soiled linen and dispose of it in order to minimize any chance of spreading infection.

Procedure for Giving an Enema

The gentle and effective administration of an enema is often an important part of a nurse's duties, since this offers one of the safest and most satisfactory methods of eliminating waste from the lower intestinal tract. If done properly, it will cause little discomfort, and sufficient fluid can be instilled to effectively empty the rectum and lower colon.

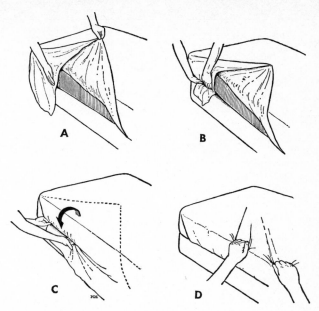

Fig. 16-7. Proper method of making bed to hold sheets tight and free of wrinkles by mitering corners.

1   Protect the sheet and mattress beneath the patient with waterproof sheeting or several layers of newspapers, covered by a sheet or towel that can be laundered or discarded.

2   Prepare the enema solution as ordered by the doctor in the amount specified (usually, about a quart or less for adults, and about a pint or less for children).

3   Assemble the enema apparatus by the bedside.   Make sure of three things: (a) do not hang the enema bag too high, since, if the fluid runs in too rapidly, it will cause great discomfort and bring about a reflex, resulting in the fluid being expelled before the right amount has run in; (b) do *not* use the standard hard-rubber enema tip if it can be avoided— use a soft-rubber enema tube, which will be more comfortable for the patient, will minimize the possibility of damaging the rectum, and, since it can be inserted further, is less likely to leak and will be more effective; and (c) make sure that the solution reaches the patient at approximately body temperature, since it is thus less likely to provoke an expulsive reflex.

4   Place the patient on his left side, with his knees partially drawn up in a comfortable position (Fig. 16-8).

5 Apply a good lubricating jelly to the first 3 or 4 inches of the enema tube.

6 Holding the tube in one hand, let a little fluid run from the tube to expel any air bubbles; then raise the buttocks with the other hand so as to expose the anus, and gently insert the tube for about 4 inches (less in children) or until you are sure that you have felt it slip well past the internal anal muscular ring.

7 Release the clamp and let the enema solution run in *slowly*. If the patient complains, slow down the rate of flow. Usually, if the bag is between 18 inches and 2 feet above the patient, the flow will be about right; but for children and for apprehensive adults it should be slower.

8 As soon as the proper amount has been given, take a piece of gauze or cotton, hold it about the tube so as to press gently against the anus, and slowly withdraw the tube, placing the free end in the enema bag until you have time to clean the apparatus.

The patient then is given the bedpan or permitted to go to the toilet if he is able, but it is desirable that the enema be

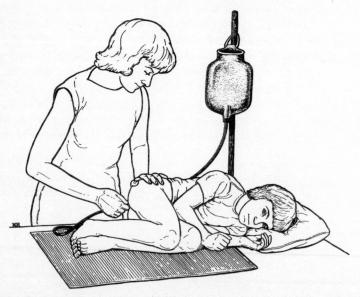

Fig. 16-8. In giving an enema, the patient lies on his left side with the knees drawn up in a comfortable position.

retained for a few minutes, if possible, in order to loosen up any matter that may be impacted in the rectum.

If a bedpan is used, it should be warmed slightly before being given to the patient.

If possible, leave the room while the patient is expelling the enema and let him call you when he is ready.

In the meantime, clean the enema apparatus and prepare it for storage. After washing it with soap and water, it is desirable to sterilize the whole outfit by boiling it for 6 minutes. Many nurses wear rubber gloves during this entire procedure, and it is to be highly recommended, for it saves almost unavoidable bacterial contamination of the hands. Be sure to freshen the air in the room.

Retention Enema. Enemas are used for many purposes other than for cleaning out the lower bowel. One of the most useful types of enema is known as a *retention enema,* which is used principally to get fluid into a patient when he is unable to take it by mouth or, for one reason or another, the fluid cannot be administered intravenously. Often, also, a retention enema is used as a vehicle for simple medications.

As has been suggested, this is a very useful route for administering salt in treating severe cases of heat exhaustion or heat stroke. When the enema is used in the treatment of heat stroke, it is given as cold as possible, often using ice water as a further aid to reducing the victim's very high temperature.

Whatever solution is used, it is given in a small amount and at a slow rate of flow in order not to stimulate the bowel into a reflex expulsion of the liquid. The object of the retention enema is to have the liquid retained until it is fully absorbed from the bowel. It is surprising how much fluid or medication can be gotten into a patient by this means.

Salt water (1 teaspoonful per quart) or ordinary lukewarm tap water is most commonly used. Sometimes an enema of oil is used and held in place to soften hard stools which may be blocking the passage through the lower rectum. This is a very common condition in elderly people.

The necessary equipment for giving a retention enema is simple and consists basically of a small soft-rubber tube, known as a *catheter,* and a small funnel. The fluid to be used should be slightly above body temperature, except when treating heat stroke.

1   Pour a small amount of fluid into the funnel and allow it to run into the catheter to expel air.

2   Then pinch the catheter to keep the fluid from running out onto the bed, and, after lubricating the catheter with a jelly, insert it well up into the rectum.

Be very gentle and explain to the patient what is going on and the reason for not yielding to the urge to expel the fluid as he feels it running in or experiences slight distention.

No more than 4 to 6 ounces should be given at any one time to an adult, and it is important that this be retained for as long as several hours in order to assure complete absorption.

In administering a retention enema, the patient is prepared and positioned in exactly the same way as for an ordinary enema. It is very important to explain to him just what is going to be done and the reason for it so that he will not be apprehensive and will cooperate in retaining the fluid.

If a funnel is not available, an ordinary enema bag and tube can be used, although the tip should be as small in diameter as possible in order not to stimulate the bowel into peristalsis. For that reason, a soft rubber catheter and funnel are best.

Another way to administer a retention enema is to use a bag or a can, containing substantial quantities of fluid, and to so regulate the flow of the liquid into the rectum that it runs in very slowly, drop by drop, over a period of many hours. In this way a great deal of fluid can be gotten into the patient, the actual rate of flow being determined by how much the patient can absorb in any given time without a feeling of discomfort or distention. The flow is regulated through the rubber tube by means of an adjustable screw clamp. Actually, if this technic had to be used at home under emergency conditions, a small "C-clamp," which is available in almost any home workshop, could be used for the purpose of constricting the tube sufficiently to slow down the flow.

Administering Medications

Another important duty of a home nurse is the administration of medications as ordered by the doctor. These will be of various types, to be administered by mouth or by some other route, such as by hypodermic injection. Usually, an untrained person would not be asked to give an injection, but under some circumstances it might be necessary for a member of the family, after proper instruction, to give such injections as insulin if for some reason professional assistance were not available.

In giving medications by mouth, be sure that you follow the doctor's instructions *exactly,* and that you have, *beyond any doubt,* the medicine that was ordered. Be sure that the label checks exactly with the doctor's instructions and that every time you give a medication you note, on a chart which you have prepared previously, exactly what it was you gave, how much, and at what time, as well as a note on the patient's immediate reactions, if any.

Another good point to remember is to keep all the patient's medications in one safe place, where they cannot get mixed up with other drugs if you should need them in a hurry and where they will be out of reach of children.

Do not give any medication that the doctor does not order —no matter who recommends it.

Throw old or unused medications away. Unless specifically advised by your doctor, do not "save" medicines for use at a later time.

Giving a Hypodermic Injection. Under some circumstances it may be necessary to give the patient a hypodermic injection when the drug is the kind that cannot be taken by mouth, is more effective when given as an injection, or when the patient for one reason or another is unable to take a medication by mouth. Also, drugs often act more rapidly when given by injection, and some drugs, such as insulin and epinephrine, are only effective when given by this route.

Administration of a drug by injection is a simple and painless procedure, provided certain easy steps are followed. Hypodermic syringes consist essentially of a glass cylinder with a plunger and a small needle attached to one end. They come in various sizes, but the one most likely to be used for the care of a patient at home is either 2- or 5-milliliter (cubic centimeters) capacity, and the amount of drug administered rarely exceeds 1 millileter (cubic centimeter) or about one-thirtieth of an ounce.

Unless you are using a prepackaged, presterilized disposable syringe and needle, you will probably have to sterlize the outfit before it can be used. This is very easily done by laying a square of gauze or cheesecloth on the bottom of a vegetable sieve, or strainer, and placing the separate parts of the syringe and the needle on it (Fig. 16-9). The entire assembly is then immersed in a pot of boiling water for 20 minutes (A). After the parts have cooled, they are reassembled *without* touching the shaft of the plunger or the shaft of the needle, because these two parts must be kept sterile, but once the syringe is put together, you can grip the handle without contaminating the needle itself.

Medications for injection are usually supplied in small rubber-capped vials or in glass ampuls, containing single doses of the particular medication.

To extract medication from a rubber-capped vial:

1 Wipe the rubber cap with a sponge soaked in rubbing alcohol in order to sterilize it (B).

2 Pull the plunger of the syringe out a distance approximating the amount of drug you wish to withdraw from the vial (C).

3 With the plunger in this position, plunge the needle through the rubber cap of the vial, push the plunger of the syringe all the way in (D), and invert the entire assembly so the vial is above the syringe (E).

4 Then pull out on the plunger to extract the amount of drug you actually wish to inject (F).

To extract medication from a single-dose ampul:

1 Wipe the neck thoroughly with alcohol.

2 Make a scratch mark at the constriction in the neck with the small file provided, and snap the neck off, using a piece of sterile gauze to protect your fingers and to prevent contaminating the neck of the ampul itself.

3 Extract the medication from the ampul in the same way as from the rubber-capped vial, but do *not* invert the ampul.

To give an injection:

1 Clean the skin with alcohol at the site where the medication will be injected. The best place to inject is the outer surface of an upper arm or the outer surface of a thigh or buttock.

2 After you have prepared the area, point the syringe straight up in the air and you will notice that there will be a small air bubble directly under the needle. Push in slightly on the plunger of the syringe in order to expel this air bubble before giving the injection (G).

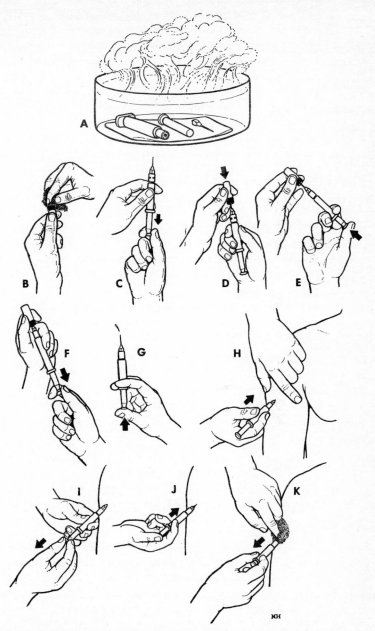

Fig. 16-9. Steps in giving a hypodermic injection. (See text for description of each maneuver.)

3 Pinch or stretch the skin where you are going to insert the needle in order to provide a firm surface and to minimize any sensation that the patient might have when the needle is inserted.

4 Insert the needle at a 45 to 60° angle, holding the syringe much as you would a dart. The needle is pushed through the skin with a firm, rapid movement, and, if the needle is sharp, the patient will scarcely feel the prick (*H*).

5 When the needle is all the way in, pull back a little on the plunger of the syringe to be sure that you have not entered a blood vessel (*I*). If you have, you will see a little bit of blood entering the syringe, in which case the needle should be withdrawn and reinserted. There should not be any blood in the syringe or anywhere else as the result of giving a hypodermic injection.

6 When you are sure that you have not entered a blood vessel, push down on the plunger gently and steadily until all the medication in the syringe has been deposited in the tissues (*J*).

7 When all the drug is in, place an alcohol-saturated sponge gently over the area where the needle entered the skin, and withdraw the needle and syringe (*K*).

The area may then be gently massaged with the sponge, to procure better distribution of the medication and to avoid the possibility of a lump at the site of injection.

Be careful to hold the needle still while you are giving the injection, to avoid injuring the tissues around the point of the needle.

Applying a Sterile Dressing

Sometimes a person who has undergone surgery is sent home early from the hospital and will require the dressing to be changed until healing becomes complete. This is not difficult to do and involves little danger of infection, provided certain simple rules are followed.

A prepared packaged dressing is sterile (uncontaminated with germs) only so long as it does not touch anything—and this includes your fingers—other than the inside of the package out of which it came.

In preparing to change a dressing:

1 Clear the bedside table, or prepare a tray that can be placed

on the bed, and cover it with a clean, freshly laundered towel.

2   Lay out on this the articles you will need (Fig. 16-10). These will include the special kinds or sizes of dressings required for the particular wound, scissors, adhesive tape, cotton

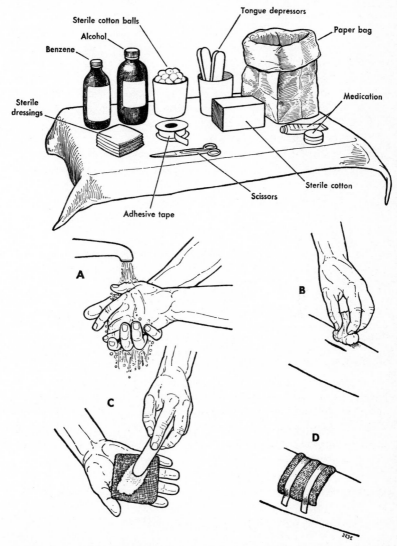

Fig. 16-10. Materials and steps in cleaning and dressing a wound.

balls, benzene or other suitable solvent for cleaning off any adhesive that may remain on the skin, and perhaps alcohol if the doctor wishes the skin around the wound cleaned with it at the time of the dressing. If an ointment is to be applied, boil a knife or tongue depressor with which to spread it on the wound. Also provide a paper bag into which the soiled dressings can be thrown for subsequent burning.

3 After thoroughly washing your hands, loosen the old dressings and gently work it off the wound *without touching* the wound with your fingers.

4 Clean the skin around the wound of any discharges and of bits of adhesive which may remain stuck, using benzene or other solvent on a large cotton ball, which you grasp with your fingers (or with a dressing forceps if you have it) on one side only.

5 When the skin is clean, dry it thoroughly with another cotton ball or, preferably, a folded gauze sponge, and then wipe it off with another cotton ball or sponge moistened with ethyl or rubbing alcohol.

6 Wipe away any excess alcohol, and allow the remainder to air-dry.

7 If ointment is to be applied, put the ointment on the dressing, using the boiled knife or tongue depressor, after thoroughly cleaning the wound. Do *not* apply the ointment directly to the wound and do *not* use too much ointment, as it will only soak into the dressings or tend to macerate the wound; use just enough to cover the surface lightly to prevent the dressings from sticking. If the ointment is in a jar, open it only long enough to take out what you need, and then put the cover back on.

8 If *no* ointment is to be applied, take the sterile dressings you will require from the packages in which they are provided, making sure that you touch only the edges, and apply the untouched parts to the wound itself. If a wound that is draining is to be dressed, it is better to fluff up each dressing as it is put on, as in this way more fluid is absorbed, the wound is kept drier, and there is better aeration.

9 When the dressings are in place, cover them with one or two flat gauze sponges for neatness. Then fasten the entire dressing in place with lengths of adhesive tape or bandage as required.

10 When you have completed the dressing, wash your hands thoroughly again, and get rid of the old dressing without

touching it—if possible, burn it, so that it cannot act as a further source of contamination.

Steam Inhalations

In patients with acute upper respiratory infection, it is often desirable to use steam inhalations to relieve inflammation and congestion in the bronchial tubes and to open up the sinuses and nasal passages; the inhalation may or may not contain medicated vapors.

This can be done easily by using materials readily available about the home.

1 Place an open umbrella or a large frame made from a cardboard carton at the head of the bed as a support for a blanket which is thrown over it to make a canopy.

2 Tuck the blanket in around the head of the bed, leaving a small opening at one side.

3 Set an electric plate and teakettle on a low chair of a stool beside the bed, near the opening in the blanket.

4 Make a funnel long enough to reach from the spout of the teakettle through the opening in the blanket, by rolling up heavy brown wrapping paper or newspaper into a cornucopia (Fig. 16-11).

5 Fill the teakettle about half full of water to which has been added any medication ordered by the doctor, and turn on the electric plate.

6 While the water is heating, anoint the patient's face and neck with cold cream, and cover his hair with a turban made out of a bath towel.

7 When the water is steaming, close the blanket around the paper funnel and let the treatment proceed for about 15 minutes. Because this may be too long for some, it is important not to leave a patient unattended, particularly if the patient is a child. The inhalations may be repeated every 2 hours or so. Make certain the whole apparatus cannot tip over and scald the patient!

Every precaution should, of course, be taken not to burn the patient with steam that is too dense, by upsetting the teakettle, or by letting the hot plate come in direct contact with the bedclothes; do not place the hot plate where the patient may accidentally step on it, should he climb out of bed. Be careful also that the water does not boil away while the treatment is in progress.

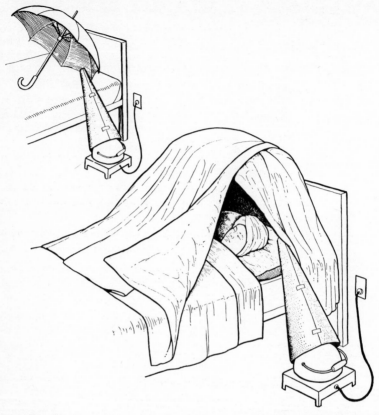

Fig. 16-11.   A tent for giving steam inhalations can easily be made by using an umbrella or from other gadgets and materials available in any household.

Hot Packs

It is sometimes desirable to apply hot packs to some area of the body, either to aid in combating inflammation or to relieve painful muscle spasm, as in cases of infantile paralysis.

For ordinary hot wet dressings, prolonged heat may be simply and easily applied by using a hot-water bag over the dressings which already been applied and saturated with whatever solution has been ordered or by using an electric heating pad, provided—*and this is important*—the wet dressing is first covered with a layer of oiled silk to prevent the electric pad from becoming wet.

Special apparatus is available for heating the large packs

required in treating infantile paralysis patients (which, fortunately, now are almost nonexistent), but, in an emergency and for the preparation of smaller packs, home equipment can be made to serve. To prepare these packs:

1 Sew together pieces of flannel or old clean blankets in the desired size.

2 Sew or pin a hem about 2 inches wide on each end of a bath towel so that pieces of broomstick, long enough to serve as handles, can be inserted in them (Fig. 16-12).

3 Anoint the skin surface to be treated with petrolatum or cold cream to minimize irritation.

4 Lay the flannel pack in the center of the towel and place it in a basin of boiling water just deep enough to cover the pack and heat it thoroughly.

5 When the pack is hot, pick up the towel, using the broomstick handles, and twist them so as to wring the excess water out of the pack.

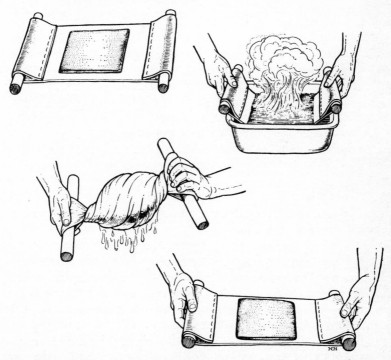

Fig. 16-12. Method of preparing and wringing out hot packs without burning the hands.

6 As soon as it is dry enough, carry it—still in the towel—to the patient and apply, making sure by feeling it yourself that the pack is not so hot that it will burn him.

7 When the pack is in place, cover it with a thick piece of flannel, blanket, or heavy bath towel, to conserve heat.

Alternative Method: A simpler method of preparation is to simply wrap the moistened pack material in heavy aluminum foil and place it in an oven with the temperature set at about 220°F. When heated, the packs are easily handled and require no particular manipulation other than making sure they are not hot enough to burn the patient.

Change the packs as often as necessary to maintain effective heat. In treating polio cases, packs are usually applied to the affected muscles three times a day and as required at night to relieve pain and spasms.

NURSING PATIENTS WITH CONTAGIOUS DISEASES

In caring for patients with contagious diseases, certain precautions are necessary to minimize the likelihood of contracting the disease yourself or spreading it to others when you leave the sickroom. The technic is not difficult.

First, wear a surgical mask when working about the patient, both to protect yourself and to protect him from contracting an outside infection. Also, wear a special gown over your regular clothes. This gown should be kept on a coatrack at the entrance to the patient's room and should be hanging in such a way that you can slip into it without getting the outside of it against your regular clothes (Fig. 16-13). In other words, think of the *inside* of the gown as being clean and the outside as contaminated.

When you leave the room, remove the gown without touching your clothes with the outside of the gown, and hang it up again so that it can be slipped into the next time you enter the room. Upon leaving the room, remove the mask and drop it into a paper bag prepared for that purpose, and put on a clean one the next time you go in.

Also, at the entrance to the room there should be a basin of water containing any reliable household antiseptic solution. When you have slipped off the gown and mask, rinse your

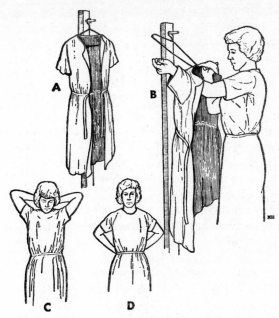

Fig. 16-13. How to put on a protective gown without contaminating the hands or clothes when nursing contagious disease cases.

hands thoroughly and dry them on a clean towel that is kept there for that purpose. Then go to a regular wash basin and wash your hands thoroughly, using a scrub brush and antiseptic soap for at least 1 minute.

Discarded masks and soiled gowns may be sterilized by boiling for 10 minutes in soapy water and then by putting them through whatever laundering procedure you are accustomed to using. Disposable masks are handy and are discarded after use.

Other points to be borne in mind in caring for patients with contagious diseases include the following:

1 The patient should have his own utensils, which are kept separate from the rest of the household's and thoroughly washed in scalding soapy water after each use.

2 Keep children and all pets out of the sickroom; allow adult visitors only if permitted by the doctor.

3 Disinfect all body discharges that may be infectious, as instructed by the doctor.

4 Do not lend or borrow books, toys, dolls, or other articles which, until they have been properly sterilized, may carry the germs of the disease. In some cases, such articles must be burned to prevent the spread of disease.

DIETS

Many different diets are used in the treatment of disease and are prescribed by doctors for various purposes. The concepts regarding nutrition in both health and disease have undergone considerable change in recent years, and much of what used to be accepted as true is no longer held to be so. For instance, the old adage, "Feed a cold and starve a fever," is no longer adhered to, since it is recognized that in fevers the basal metabolic rate of the patient is higher, and therefore the caloric intake must be greater to compensate for the increased consumption of the body's own tissues.

Any special diets required for the treatment of specific illness, as in diabetes for instance, would be prescribed in detail by the doctor, but for general home-nursing purposes it will suffice to understand the nature of a few basic types of diets which are commonly required.

Liquid Diet

A liquid diet is very often necessary for a while following certain operations and in the treatment of the acute phase of illness, such as in acute contagious diseases—including whooping cough, acute upper and lower respiratory infections, and certain gastrointestinal disturbances.

Starting with pure liquids, this diet can gradually be expanded by stages to include semisolid foods, preparatory to permitting the patient to have a more substantial menu.

In the early phases, only such things as orange juice or tea, clear meat broth, oatmeal gruel, eggnog (nonalcoholic), and ice cream are permitted. Sugar may be used as desired unless specifically forbidden.

Later, thickened broth, boiled rice, cornstarch puddings, tapioca, custard, jelly, creamed soups, junket, and a soft-boiled egg may be added.

Finally, the stage approximating a regular soft diet would permit such foods as bland cooked cereals like farina or Cream of Wheat®, buttered toast, creamed or boiled potatoes, puréed vegetables, and scraped meats. On such a diet, it is not difficult to maintain a daily intake of as much as 2500 to 3000 calories, depending upon the tolerance of the patient.

Soft (Low-residue) Diet

A diet of this type is often used during early convalescence from an acute illness and in the treatment of certain gastrointestinal disorders, including such diarrheal diseases as spastic colitis and dysentery. Generally speaking, roughage is avoided, and, with such modifications as may be required by a specific condition, the patient is limited to the following types of foods: fruit juices (if not forbidden because of diarrhea); cooked cereals with sugar and cream; boiled, poached or scrambled eggs; buttered white toast; creamed soups, meat broths, and puréed vegetables; rice; baked, boiled, creamed, or mashed potatoes; ice cream or sherbets; cream or cottage cheese; custards; chicken or other fowl (not fried); broiled or creamed fish; Jello; junket; simple puddings; and beverages, including tea, cocoa, or hot chocolate, but *not* coffee. Carbonated beverages may be used if they do not aggravate an existing case of diarrhea; sometimes ginger ale is particularly welcome, but alcoholic beverages should *not* be given.

On such a diet, more than 3000 calories a day may be consumed.

High-caloric, High-protein Diet

This type of diet is used to regain weight lost during a severe illness; to combat an illness that imposes a serious drain upon the body tissues, such as occurs in hyperthyroidism and in such wasting illnesses as cancer and tuberculosis; and to help an underweight or otherwise malnourished person to regain a normal weight.

In such a diet, the foods would include large quantities of milk and cream; butter; salad dressings and other fats; all meats and fish; high-carbohydrate fruits and vegetables, such as oranges, peaches, tangerines, grapes, cherries, bananas, figs, prunes, potatoes, beans, corn, peas, rice, beets, carrots, squash, and turnips; and various rich desserts. Foods that are known to be very high in protein are especially recommended; these include gelatin, all kinds of fowl, liver, eggs, veal, beef, lamb, and shellfish.

Such a diet easily provides an intake of 5000 to 6000 calories a day, which is sufficient to meet the most generous requirements.

ADDITIONAL NURSING INFORMATION AND HELP

Many special services exist in your community that are able and willing to be of help to you in caring for the sick at home. Look them up and get acquainted with them—before an emergency arises. The American Red Cross offers excellent home-nursing courses to give you basic training in the essentials of nursing. Public health nurses from the various visiting nurse associations will come to your home to help in the daily care of the patient and instruct you in special technics. In addition, you may find it helpful to utilize the services of a good practical nurse from a reputable nurses' agency, to relieve you and give you the needed time off which is absolutely essential for rest and relaxation.

Special services are also available from many organizations. such as the various National Foundations and welfare agencies. And special literature on the care of the sick can be procured from the Federal Security Agency, the American Red Cross, and your local and state health departments. All this is available for the asking; make use of it before needed so that you will be prepared if an emergency does arise.

Appendix

SCHEDULE FOR ACTIVE IMMUNIZATION OF INFANTS AND CHILDREN*

Age	Preparation
2 months	Diphtheria and tetanus toxoids combined with pertussis vaccine Trivalent oral polio virus vaccine for both breast-fed and bottle-fed infants.
4 months	A second administration of the above two preparations
6 months	A third administration of the above two preparations
1 year	Measles-Rubella or Measles-Mumps-Rubella combined vaccines Tuberculin test
1–12 years	Rubella and Mumps vaccines
1½ years	Diphtheria and tetanus toxoids combined with pertussis vaccine Trivalent oral polio vaccine
4–6 years	A repeat administration of the above two preparations
14–16 years	Combined tetanus and diphtheria vaccines (adult type) Note: For deep or severe wounds tetanus toxoid should always be given at the time of injury. For clean minor wounds no booster dose is required by a fully immunized child unless more than 10 years have elapsed since the last dose. For probably contaminated wounds, a booster dose should be given if more than 5 years have elapsed since the last dose.

* Revised schedule as approved by the American Academy of Pediatrics, Committee on Infectious Diseases, October 17, 1971.   Routine smallpox vaccination is no longer recommended.   Under special travel conditions it may, however, be required.

IMMUNIZATION RECORD

Surname:

Child's given name:	Dose No.	DPT Vaccine* (date)	Oral Poliomyelitis Vaccine (date)	Tuberculin Test (date)	Measles Vaccine (date)	Smallpox Vaccine (date)	Typhoid Vaccine† (date)
	1.						
	2.						
	3.						
Born:	4.						
	5.						
	6.						
	1.						
	2.						
	3.						
Born:	4.						
	5.						
	6.						
	1.						
	2.						
	3.						
Born:	4.						
	5.						
	6.						

* Diphtheria-Pertussis-Tetanus Vaccine
† Three injections at monthly intervals when required.

EMERGENCY TELEPHONE NUMBERS

Physicians:		Name	Phone
Family physician	Dr.		
	or Dr.		
Pediatrician	Dr.		
	or Dr.		
Surgeon	Dr.		
	or Dr.		
Eye Doctor	Dr.		
	or Dr.		
Nose and throat doctor	Dr.		
	or Dr.		
Obstetrician	Dr.		
	or Dr.		
Hospital			
	or		
Ambulance service			
	or		
First-aid rescue squad			
	or		
Dentist	Dr.		
	or Dr.		
Oculist	Dr.		
	or Dr.		

Poison Control Center* _____
Pharmacy _____
Nurses' registry _____
Visiting nurse association _____
Local department of health _____
Local police department _____
Fire department _____
Electric company _____
Gas company _____
Nearest state police _____
Auto towing service _____
Local radio station _____

* If you are unable to locate the Poison Control Center in your area, write to the U.S. Department of Health, Education, and Welfare, Public Health Service, Washington, D.C., for a copy of *Directory of Poison Control Centers*.

GLOSSARY

This glossary is not intended to serve as a medical dictionary. It was prepared with the thought of making available short, easily understood definitions of some thousand or so of the more common medical terms which might be encountered in medical parlance in connection with common illnesses and injuries.

In preparing this list, no set rules have been followed and there is no particular uniformity as to the type of words which have been included. For instance, names of anatomical parts or common diseases which it seemed obvious would be known to the average reader have been omitted, as have thousands of terms which it seemed likely would rarely, if ever, be encountered. On the other hand, some terms have been included for their possible general interest, or because they have been used in this book.

The definitions themselves have been made as simple as possible, and for the most part only the principal or most common meanings have been given.

A

abdomen   that portion of the trunk situated between the chest (thorax) and the pelvis.

abduct   to move a part outward, away from the midline of the body.

abortion   arrest of a disease or natural process before it has run its course, or termination of pregnancy before term.

abrasion   a superficial injury (scraping) of the skin.

abscess   a localized collection of pus; it is usually walled off by a protective tissue reaction.

absorption   the taking into the tissues of fluids or other substances; the term sometimes is used in connection with the healing of an inflammatory process.

accretions   most commonly used to indicate the accumulation of foreign matter in a part, such as the accumulation of foreign material in an artery as in arteriosclerosis.

acetabulum   the large cup-shaped depression in the hipbone into which the head of the thighbone (femur) fits.

Achilles' tendon   the large tendon at the back of the heel which moves the foot up and down on the ankle joint.

achlorhydria   lack of hydrochloric acid in the stomach.

acid-base balance   a term used to describe the normal ratio between the various acid and basic elements of the blood and tissue fluids, which normally are maintained in equilibrium but which may be distorted in disease.

acidosis   a term used to indicate a general acid condition of the body.

acromegaly   a disease of the pituitary gland which causes a marked enlargement of the bones of the face, hands, and feet.

Addison's disease   a disease of the adrenal gland which causes pigmentation of the skin.

adduct   to bring a part toward the midline of the body.

adenitis   inflammation and swelling of the lymph glands.

adenoids   lymphoid tissue located in the back portion of the nose and throat.

adenoma   a tumor, not necessarily cancerous, which resembles a gland in its cellular structure.

adenopathy   a general enlargement of the lymph glands of the body or any given area.

adhesion   a band of fibrous tissue between two parts which forms as the result of infection or injury.

adipose (tissue)   fat; fat tissue.

adnexa   the internal female genital organs aside from the uterus.

adrenal   an endocrine gland situated on the top of each kidney.

afebrile   without fever.

afterbirth   the placenta.

agranulocytosis   absence of the white cells of the blood which fight infection; often the result of a toxic reaction to drugs.

albuminuria   presence of albumin in the urine.

alimentary tract   the digestive tract as a whole.

alkaloid   an organic substance derived from plants; the term is usually used in connection with those substances having pharmacologic activity. Common examples are morphine and caffeine.

alkalosis   a condition which results when the body loses too much carbon dioxide or acid substances as the result of forced breathing or severe vomiting.

allergen   any substance that produces allergic symptoms in a patient.

allergy   an abnormal susceptibility to any substance which does not ordinarily cause adverse symptoms in the average person.

alopecia   baldness.

alpha-adrenergic   a drug which exerts its effect upon certain nerve receptors, known as "alpha receptors," within the sympathetic nervous system, which are stimulated by such sympathicomimetic amines as epinephrine. An alpha-adrenergic blocking agent, such as Dibenzyline (phenoxybenzamine hydrochloride), blocks such action and, in effect, produces a "chemical sympathectomy," thus causing, among other effects, a drop in blood pressure.

amebiasis   infection with the *Endamoeba histolytica,* i.e., amebic dysentery.

amenorrhea   absence of menstruation.

amnesia   loss of memory.

ampule   sealed glass container of sterile medication; ampoule.

anaerobe   a bacterium that can live only in the absence of oxygen.

analgesia   absence or suppression of the perception of pain; such an effect is produced by agents known as analgesics.

anaphylaxis   an exaggerated type of sensitivity to a protein substance; may be dangerous or even fatal.

anastomosis   joining together two tubelike structures, such as the intestine, blood vessels, or nerves.

anemia   lack of red blood corpuscles or hemoglobin, or both.

anesthesia   loss of sensation to the point that pain is totally abolished.

aneurysm   a sac or bulge formed by the weakening of the walls of an artery or vein.

angina   any disease marked by attacks of choking or suffocation, particularly with respect to a heart attack. Sometimes used in connection with severe throat or mouth infection.

angiography   the term is most commonly used to indicate the visualization of a part of the vascular system, such as an artery, through the use of a contrast medium and x-ray.

angioneurotic edema   a condition characterized by hives and swelling of the tissues as the result of allergy.

aniscoria   inequality the size of the pupils.

ankylosis   an abnormal fusing or joining together of the parts of a joint as the result of disease.

anomaly   any anatomical deviation from what is generally accepted as normal or average.

anorexia   lack of appetite.

anoxemia   a diminished or inadequate oxygen concentration in the blood.

anoxia   almost the same as anoxemia, but refers more specifically to lack of oxygen in the tissue cells themselves.

antacid   a substance used to counteract or neutralize gastric acidity.

antenatal   prior to birth.

ante partum   before delivery.

anterior   the front surface of any part of the body.

anthelmintic   a drug used to combat infestation with worms.

anthrax   a disease caused by the anthrax bacillus; commonly seen in wool handlers.

antibiotic   any agent derived from living sources which kills or inhibits the growth of bacteria.

antibody   a substance produced in the body as the result of allergy or an infectious agent.

anticholinergic   a drug which specifically blocks the passage of impulses through the parasympathetic nervous system.

anticoagulant   a substance which prevents the coagulation of blood.
antidote   any substance used to combat the effects of a poison.
antigen   any agent which, when taken into the body, stimulates the formation of specific protective substances known as antibodies.
antihistamine   any chemical compound which neutralizes or combats the physiologic effects of histamine, a chemical substance in the body which causes allergic reactions.
antipyretic   a drug which reduces fever.
antiseptic   any preparation that prevents the growth or multiplication of bacteria under conditions of use.
antiserum   a serum which contains specific antibodies against specific disease-producing substances such as tetanus or rabies antiserum.
antispasmodic   an agent that reduces spasm, particularly of the intestinal tract.
antitoxin   a substance injected into the body to combat or neutralize the effect of poisonous substances secreted by various disease-producing bacteria.
antivenin   a serum containing antibodies which are specific for a certain venom such as that of a snake or a spider.
antrum   the nasal sinus in the bone just below the eye, which very commonly becomes infected.
anuria   absence of urine formation.
anus   the outlet of the rectum and digestive tract.
aorta   the main and largest artery of the body.
aphagia   inability to swallow.
aphasia   inability to express one's self by any one of the usual means, or to comprehend expression.
aphonia   loss of voice from one of several possible causes.
aphrodisiac   a drug that arouses or stimulates the sexual instinct.
apnea   temporary cessation of breathing.
apoplexy   a stroke; cerebral hemorrhage.
appendectomy   removal of the appendix by surgical operation.
areola   the pigmented area around the nipple.
arrest   a stoppage of the heart or of respiration, due to the interruption of the nervous impulses controlling these functions.
arrythmia   any abnormal rhythm; usually used in connection with the heartbeat to refer to extra beats or skipped beats.
arteriole   a small arterial branch intermediate in size between the larger arteries and the capillaries.
arteriosclerosis   thickening and hardening of the arteries.
arteriosclerotic plaque   the formation of a mound of fatty debris within the lumen of an artery as the result of arteriosclerosis.   Such plaques may be the underlying cause of thrombus formation and the eventual occlusion of the artery.
arthralgia   pain in one or more joints.
arthritis   an inflammatory disease of the joints.
arthrodesis   the fusing of the surfaces of a joint by surgery.
arthroplasty   any operation designed to reconstruct a joint.
articulation   a joint between two bones; may be movable or immovable, but most commonly refers to the movable variety.
artificial kidney   a mechanical device so constructed that, when connected to a patient's circulation, impurities are dialyzed from the blood, thus temporarily substituting for the functions of the natural kidney.
ascariasis   infection with an intestinal worm known as *Ascaris lumbricoides*.
ascites   accumulation of fluid in the abdominal cavity.
ascorbic acid   vitamin C.

asepsis a technic having the objective of preventing bacterial contamination of a wound or instrument.

asphyxia suffocation.

aspirate to breathe in (to the lungs).

asthenia general weakness, and loss of strength, energy, and a healthy appearance.

asthma an allergic condition characterized by difficult breathing; caused by constriction and spasm of the bronchial tubes.

astigmatism uneven curvature of the refracting bodies of the eye so that an image is not sharply focused upon the retina.

astragalus the large bone of the ankle which joins with the two bones of the leg.

ataxia inability to coordinate the muscles properly; often used to describe a staggering gait.

atelectasis a collapse of the alveolar air spaces of the lungs.

atherosclerosis a type of arteriosclerosis.

atony the loss of tone or normal response in a muscle; i.e., partial paralysis of the muscle.

atresia absence of a body opening which normally should be present.

atrophy a wasting away of a specific tissue.

attenuation this term is usually applied to the decrease in virulence of an organism brought about by various means, so that it will not produce actual disease but will confer immunity.

audiogram a graph which shows the ability of the patient to hear tones of varying frequencies, from the lowest to the highest.

auditory (nerve) the eighth cranial nerve which has to do with both hearing and balance.

aura a premonition of impending illness—most commonly used in connection with epilepsy.

auricle a part of the heart which receives blood from the incoming veins and passes it to the ventricle.

auscultation a technic of listening for and interpreting sounds which occur within the body, particularly in the lungs.

autoclave a device used for sterilizing instruments and dressings by means of steam or heat.

autonomic usually used to refer to the involuntary or sympathetic nervous system.

avitaminosis any disease resulting from the lack of sufficient vitamin intake.

avulsion the tearing away of a part or tissue of the body.

axilla armpit.

B

bacillus a rod-shaped bacterium.

bacteremia the presence of bacteria in the bloodstream.

bactericide an agent that is capable of killing bacteria.

bacteriostatic agent any agent which is capable of preventing the growth of bacteria but not necessarily killing them.

balanitis inflammation, usually due to infection, of the head of the penis.

barbiturism addiction to, or poisoning by, any of the barbiturate drugs.

basal metabolic rate the rate at which the body converts food into energy; determined by ratio between the amount of oxygen taken in and carbon dioxide put out.

basilic vein the vein at the bend of the elbow commonly used for drawing blood.

belladonna   a drug derived from the plant *Atropa belladonna,* which is a powerful relaxing agent and blocks the activity of the parasympathetic nervous system.

bends   cramps in the abdomen and limbs due to bubbles of gas in the blood.

benign   noncancerous, nonmalignant, without danger.

beriberi   a disease arising from the lack of vitamin B_1 (thiamin) in the diet.

biceps   the large muscle of the front part of the arm which bends the forearm at the elbow.

bile   the secretion of the liver, which plays a most important role in digestion when it is mixed with the food in the intestinal tract.

biliary tract   the gall bladder and the ducts leading from the liver to the gall bladder and to the intestinal tract.

biopsy   the removal of a small piece of tissue for microscopic examination.

bleb   a blister.

bleeding time   time required for the bleeding from a small puncture wound of the finger to stop under carefully controlled conditions.

blepharitis   inflammation of the eyelids.

blind spot   the optic nerve area of the retina which itself does not have the power of vision.

block   an obstruction in any of the systems of the body, such as blood vessels or intestines.

blood count   a count made with a microscope and special counting chamber of the number of red and white cells in a cubic centimeter of blood.

blood type   one of the several groups into which all human blood can be divided.

bolus   a mass of food which has been chewed to the point of being ready to be swallowed, although frequently, due to the nature of the food itself or improper bite, chewing is often incomplete.

botulism   a type of food poisoning caused by the toxin of the *Clostridium botulinum,* as the result of improper canning methods.

bradycardia   slow heartbeat.

bronchiectasis   a disease caused by an accumulation of pus in the little pouches that are formed in the bronchi as the secondary result of some infection such as whooping cough.

bronchiole   a small subdivision of a bronchus.

bronchitis   an infection of the bronchial tubes.

bronchogenic   a type of lung cancer developing in the bronchi.

bronchopneumonia   inflammation of the smallest branches of the bronchial tubes, usually in both lungs.

bronchoscope   an instrument used for visually examining the internal surfaces of the larger bronchi.

bronchoscopy   examination of the bronchi through an instrument known as a bronchoscope.

bronchus   one of the main branches of the trachea carrying air into the various parts of a lung.

brucellosis   a disease of cattle commonly acquired by man from drinking milk, or eating cheese made from milk infected with the germ known as *Brucella melitensis.*

bruise   the leakage of blood into the tissues, giving a black-and-blue appearance, as the result of a blow.

bunion   an inflamed swelling of a joint of the big toe.

bursa   a little sac filled with clear fluid, overlying certain joints to prevent friction of tissues sliding over them.

bursitis   inflammation of any bursa; very common in the shoulder bursa.

C

cachexia severe malnutrition and poor health as result of a disease or lack of nourishment.

calcaneus the large heelbone at the back of the foot.

calcareous deposit any deposit of calcium or lime in a joint or tissue.

calcification the diffuse infiltration of a tissue with calcium; it occurs normally in the process of healing of a fractured bone.

calculus any abnormal concretion occurring in any of the various hollow organs or ducts of the body; i.e., kidney stones.

callus an overgrowth and thickening of the horny layers of the skin as the result of prolonged pressure or friction.

calorie a measurement of the energy value of foods; in food work, the *large calorie* is used; it is the amount of heat required to raise 1,000 grams of water 1° C.

cancer any growth in any tissue which has the power to invade other tissues and to spread to other parts of the body.

canker a lesion, chiefly of the mouth and lips, due to a virus or a vitamin deficiency.

capillary the smallest branch of an artery or vein.

capsule the fibrous covering of a joint; the term is also used to denote the covering of certain organs or of a growth in the tissues.

carbohydrate an element of food containing carbon, hydrogen, and oxygen; sugar and starch are both carbohydrates.

carbolic acid an acid derived from coal tar, also called phenol.

carbuncle a circumscribed deep infection of the skin and underlying tissue.

carcinogenic anything causing cancer.

carcinoma cancer.

cardiac pertaining to the heart; also may be used to refer to the upper portion of the stomach.

cardiogenic shock a condition which results from severe and sudden heart disease, most commonly following myocardial infarction caused by coronary thrombosis.

cardiopulmonary a term used to describe the heart and pulmonary circulation's function as a single unit.

cardiospasm spasm of the muscle which controls the entrance of food from the lower end of the esophagus into the stomach.

cardiovascular pertains to the heart and blood vessels throughout the body.

caries decay of bone or tooth.

carotid one of the main arteries of the neck supplying blood to the head.

carotid sinus a dilated area in the internal carotid artery, usually found just above the bifurcation of the common carotid artery; it contains very sensitive nerve endings which participate in the regulation of blood pressure.

carpal pertaining to the wrist.

carrier an individual who harbors the organisms of a given disease without himself showing symptoms, and is capable of transmitting the disease to others.

cartilage an elastic substance which covers the opposing surfaces of movable joints.

caruncle any small fleshy prominence; urethral caruncles are both common and painful.

cataract opacity of the crystalline lens of the eye, or its capsule.

catarrh any inflammation of a mucous membrane, a term most commonly used in connection with the nose and throat, as in a common cold.

cathartic a drug which produces evacuation of the intestinal tract.

catheter a tube used for withdrawing fluid from various structures of the body, or for irrigating various hollow organs such as the bladder.

caul an old term used for the amniotic sac which encloses the baby before birth and which usually ruptures at the time of delivery; if it does not, the baby is said to be born with a caul.

caustic a corrosive chemical which destroys tissue; usually one of an alkaline nature is implied.

cautery a hot instrument or corrosive chemical used to destroy tissue or to coagulate blood in controlling certain types of hemorrhage.

cavernous pertaining to large hollow cavities which may occur in various tissues normally or abnormally.

cecum the first portion of the large intestine, into which the small intestine empties; the vermiform appendix is attached to it.

cell the basic structural unit of all tissues.

cephalic pertaining to the head.

cercaria a free-swimming larval stage of a parasitic trematode worm, some species of which are capable of penetrating the human skin.

cerebellum that portion of the brain behind and below the cortex, the general function of which is the coordination of movement.

cerebral an adjective referring in a general way to the brain or cerebrum.

cerumen ear wax.

cervix lower portion of the uterus (womb), which opens into the vagina.

Cesarean section delivery of a baby by an operation which makes an opening directly into the uterus through an abdominal incision.

cheilosis sores of the lips, more specifically the corners of the lips, due to a vitamin B deficiency or a fungal or viral infection.

chemotherapy the treatment of disease by drugs, the latter being of such nature as to have a greater (adverse) effect on the disease-producing organism than on the patient.

chillblain mild frostbite of the hands and feet.

cholangitis inflammation of the bile ducts leading from the liver.

cholecystitis inflammation of the gall bladder.

cholelithiasis presence of stones in the gall bladder.

cholera a severe infectious disease caused by the *Vibrio comma* or cholera bacillus.

cholesterol a fat-like substance found in all animal fats and oils.

chorea a nervous disease commonly known as St. Vitus's dance.

choroid the dark pigmented inner lining of the eyeball.

choroiditis inflammation of the choroid; it is one of the more serious eye diseases.

chronic of long duration.

cicatrix a scar or heavy formation of fibrous tissue.

circadian (rhythm) refers to the period or time involved in the biological cycle, the duration of which may vary from 24 hours to much longer periods of time.

cirrhosis chronic progressive fibrosis of the liver.

claudication a set of symptoms, the principal one of which is pain arising on exercise of a given part of the body, often a leg, as the result of inadequate circulation.

clavicle collarbone.

cleft palate an opening in the midline of the palate as the result of failure of the two sides to fuse during embryonic development.

climacteric the menopause.

clitoris the small female external genital organ which is analogous to the male penis.

clonus neurologic sign characterized by rapid contraction and relaxation of a muscle or a group of muscles.

clubfoot any deformity of the foot which causes it to be twisted out of shape, usually toward the inner side.

coagulation time that time required for a sample of blood to clot under standard controlled conditions.

coalescence the blending or bringing together and fusion of various tissues or other aggregates.

coarctation a constriction of a vessel, commonly the aorta, which interferes with the flow of blood.

coccyx the lowermost bone of the spine.

cochlea a part of the inner ear which is an important part of the hearing apparatus.

colectomy removal of the colon.

colic spasm of the muscles of the intestinal tract, usually accompanied by severe abdominal pain.

colitis inflammation of the colon.

collyrium an eye lotion.

colon the longest division of the large intestine.

colostomy the establishment of an opening between the colon and the surface of the body for the purpose of providing drainage of the bowel.

colostrum the fluid which comes from the breast for a day or two following delivery, before the true milk is formed.

coma unconsciousness.

comatose partial or complete unconsciousness.

comedo pimple.

comminuted pertaining to a type of fracture in which the bone is broken into several small pieces.

communicable (disease) a disease which is readily transmissible from one person to another.

complex a group of symptoms or ideas.

compress a folded cloth or pad used for applying pressure to stop hemorrhage, or as a wet dressing.

concussion a condition of the brain resulting from a violent jar or shock.

condyloma a wartlike growth near or on the anus or genitals.

confluent the flowing together, or merging, of two or more parts.

congenital any condition which exists or was acquired before birth.

congestion the stagnation of blood in a given tissue.

conjunctivitis inflammation of the membrane of the eye.

contagion the transmission of disease by direct contact.

contagious a term used to describe a disease which is readily transmissible from one person to another.

contaminated often used in reference to a wound or other surface which has been infected with bacteria by artificial contact; may also refer to polluted water, foods, or drugs.

contraction a shortening of a part such as a muscle, as the result of the shortening effect of fibrous tissue formed by injury or inflammation.

contusion a bruise.

convalescence the period or process of recovery from a disease.

convulsion a series of violent involuntary muscular spasms; commonly referred to as a "fit."

cornea the transparent part of the sclera of the eye, overlying the pupil.

corpuscle a red or white cell of the blood.

cortex may be used to designate one of the main portions of the brain or the outer layers of one of the glands or organs of the body.

coryza common cold.

counterirritation an irritation of the skin which is deliberately induced to relieve pain or inflammation elsewhere by reflex action.

cradle cap a grayish-yellow crusting condition that sometimes appears in infants as the result of inadequate cleansing.

cramp a painful muscular spasm.

craniotomy an opening made into the skull for the purpose of obtaining surgical access to the brain.

cranium the skull; sometimes used to apply to the top of the skull.

cravat a special type of bandage made from a large triangular piece of cloth, usually muslin or cotton.

crepitation a grating sensation, felt betwen the ends of a broken bone.

cretinism a congenital condition caused by the poor functioning of the thyroid gland.

crisis the critical turning point of any disease.

crotalidae a large family of rattlesnakes comprising several genuses commonly found in this country.

croup a common disease of childhood, characterized by spasm of the larynx, which interferes with respiration.

cryotherapy the therapeutic use of cold in the alleviation of various disease processes.

cryptorchidism failure of the testicle to descend normally before birth from its original situation in the abdomen into the scrotal sac.

curettage the scraping of a cavity, such as the uterus, by a curet.

cutaneous pertaining to the skin.

cyanosis blueness of the skin due to insufficient oxygen in the blood.

cyst any growth which encloses a cavity; usually filled with fluid.

cystitis inflammation of the urinary bladder.

cystoscope an instrument used for visually examining the internal surface of the urinary bladder.

cystoscopy examination of the interior of the bladder by use of a cystoscope.

D

dacryocystitis inflammation of the tear sac of the eye.

debility weakness; general run-down condition.

debridement the surgical cleansing of a wound by removal of dead, injured, or infected tissue.

decalcification the absorption of calcium from a tissue or structure in which it is normally present.

decidua the lining of the uterus during pregnancy.

decompensation failure of the heart, as the result of disease, to maintain sufficient circulation of the blood to meet the demands of the body.

decubitus ulcers bedsores.

degeneration general deterioration, sometimes with loss of function or structure.

dehiscence the breaking down of a wound, especially of the abdomen.

dehydration loss of water from body or tissue, or the condition resulting from an inadequate supply of water.

delirium a disturbed mental condition usually resulting from fever or injury.

deltoid the large muscle of the shoulder.

delusion a belief or feeling which has no foundation in fact; a common symptom of various types of mental disturbances.

dementia a general name for all types of severe psychic disorders.

dentine the hard, living substance of a tooth immediately under the enamel and surrounding the tooth pulp.

depilate to remove hair.

dermatitis inflammation of the skin.

dermatology the study of the causes and treatment of diseases of the skin.

dermatophytosis a fungous infection of the skin commonly referred to as "athlete's foot."

dermatosis a general name covering any disease of the skin.

dermographia a highly reactive condition of the skin (common in certain types of allergy) which causes it to redden and swell wherever it is stroked with a finger.

desensitization process of rendering an individual clinically less sensitive to various proteins to which he would otherwise allergically react.

diabetes inability to metabolize carbohydrate as the result of failure of the pancreas to secrete insulin.

diaphragm the large muscle which is a major component in the act of respiration and which separates the chest cavity from the abdominal cavity.

diarrhea increased frequency of defecation, with discharge of watery or loose stools.

diastole the period in the pumping cycle of the heart during which the ventricles are relaxed and dilated and therefore are taking in blood.

diathermy treatment by a special apparatus that generates high-frequency radio waves which have the property of creating heat deep within the tissues.

Dick test skin test which measures sensitivity to scarlet fever toxins.

digitalization process of giving digitalis to the point where the maximum therapeutic effect is obtained without untoward side effects.

diphtheria an acute communicable disease.

diplegia paralysis of both arms or both legs.

diplopia double vision.

disinfectant an agent which destroys germ life, but which is too strong an irritant to use on the body.

disoriented to be confused as to one's relationship with either physical surroundings or with respect to a full grasp of a specific set of ideas.

distention the state of being inflated or enlarged, particularly of the abdomen.

diuresis increased urinary output.

diuretic an agent that stimulates the secretion of urine.

diverticulitis inflammation of diverticula in the walls of the colon.

diverticulum an outpouching of some hollow organ; often used to refer to a specific type of outpouching which occurs in the intestinal tract.

dorsal back or posterior side of the body.

douche the irrigation or washing out of any body cavity; frequently used in connection with the vagina or the external auditory canal.

dropsy the condition of waterlogging of the tissues which occurs in kidney or heart disease.

duct any tube which conveys the secretions of any gland from one point to another.

duodenal pertaining to or located in the duodenum.

duodenum the first portion of the small intestine immediately following the outlet of the stomach.

dura mater the tissue envelope which covers the brain.

dysarthria interference with the proper articulation of speech.

dyscrasia a general term used to refer to any disease of the blood.

dysentery a diarrheal type of disease which occurs in two forms, one caused by *Shigella dysenteriae,* and the other by an amoeba *Endamoeba histolytica.*

dysfunction lack of function or abnormal function of a given part or organ.

dysmenorrhea painful menstruation.

dysphagia interference with the act of swallowing.

dyspnea difficult breathing.

dystocia any abnormality of the normal process of birth.

dystrophy an abnormality of the metabolism of muscles; most commonly used to refer to the disease known as progressive muscular dystrophy.

dysuria painful urination.

E

ecchymosis diffusion of blood into the tissue spaces.

eclampsia a toxic condition which may occur during pregnancy, characterized by acute uremia-like symptoms and convulsions.

ectopic out of normal place, as in ectopic pregnancy.

ectropion a contraction of the eyelid, usually the lower, so that it is turned outward and becomes easily irritated.

eczema an inflammatory skin disease, very often of an allergic origin.

edema retention of excess fluid in the tissues.

effusion the leakage of fluid from the tissues into a cavity, such as fluid in the pleural cavity.

electrocardiogram a tracing obtained electronically which accurately shows the functional condition of the heart.

electroencephalogram a graph of the brain waves, obtained by electrical apparatus; abnormalities provide a useful diagnostic aid in determining many types of cerebral disease.

electrolyte a term used in medicine to refer to a variety of soluble inorganic chemicals in the tissues and blood.

elephantiasis a chronic tropical disease, or enlargement of a part due to lymphatic blockage.

embolism the blocking of a blood vessel by a clot, called an embolus, which has broken off from a distant site and blocks the vessel at the point at which it cannot pass.

embryo the child in the womb in the earliest stages of development.

emetic an agent which will produce vomiting.

emollient any substance which possesses softening and soothing properties.

emphysema the infiltration of any tissue by air or gas.

empyema the accumulation of pus in the pleural cavity; sometimes used to indicate pus in a hollow organ such as the gall bladder.

encephalitis inflammation of the brain tissue.

encephalogram the injection of air into the spaces of the ventricles of the brain for diagnostic purposes.

endemic a term referring to the origin or existence of a disease in a general geograhpic area.

endocarditis inflammation of the lining of the heart; common as a result of rheumatic fever.

endocrine glands glands whose secretions are absorbed directly into the bloodstream.

endometrium the lining of the uterus.

endotoxin a disease-producing toxin which is wholly within the bacterial cell itself, as opposed to *exotoxin,* which is excreted by the organism.

endotracheal within the trachea; usually used in reference to a tube which is placed into the trachea through the oropharynx to facilitate respiration during illness or anesthesia.

enteritis inflammation of the small intestine.

enuresis bed wetting.

eosinophiles one of the types of white cells of the blood which are increased in number in allergic conditions and certain infections.

epidemic the occurrence of a disease in many people, over a large area.

epidemiology the study of the occurrence and spread of infectious diseases.

epidermis the superficial layers of the skin.

epidermophytosis infection of the skin by a specific fungus.

epididymis the duct which carries the sperm cells from the testes.

epidural outside or above the dura, the heavy sheath which covers the brain.

epiglottis the lidlike structure which automatically covers the opening to the larynx during the act of swallowing, to prevent food going into the larynx.

epilation pulling hair out by the roots.

epilepsy a functional disease of the central nervous system, of which convulsions are the most striking feature.

epileptiform convulsive seizures similar to those observed in true epilepsy.

epistaxis nosebleed.

epithelization healing over a wound by the growing epithelial cells of the skin.

epulis a type of tumor of the gums or jaw.

erosion ulceration, or eating away of a structure.

eructation belching.

erysipelas an acute infectious disease of the skin caused by streptococci.

erythema reddening of the skin (as in sunburn) in response to some type of injury or inflammation.

erythrocytes the red cells of the blood.

eschar the dead slough covering a severe burn wound.

esophagus the tube leading from the pharynx to the stomach.

estrogen one of the classes of female sex hormones.

ethmoid one of the nasal sinuses located behind the nose in the ethmoid bone.

etiology the causative agent of a disease.

euphoria an unusual sense of well-being and mental happiness.

eustachian tube the tube leading from the back of the throat to the middle ear, the purpose of which is to equalize pressure in the middle ear.

evert to turn a part, such as a foot, outward.

exacerbation a flare-up or a worsening of a disease condition.

exanthem any contagious disease characterized by skin eruption.

excision the cutting out of a part or growth.

excoriation irritation of the superficial layers of the skin, usually by some irritant substance such as sweat or urine; may also refer to scratching.

exfoliation the falling off of superficial layers of the skin, as in some of the childhood diseases.

exophthalmos exaggerated protrusion of the eyeballs, as in hyperthyroidism.

exostosis an outgrowth of bone.

expectorant a drug which loosens the mucous secretions of the bronchial tubes and facilitates their removal.

exsanguinating a term often applied to severe hemorrhage, which may be serious enough for the victim to lose a substantial part or all of his blood volume.

extirpation the complete removal of a part, usually an internal organ.

extrasystole extra heartbeat.

extravasation the spreading out of blood or other fluid into the tissue spaces.

exudate fluid containing white cells and other cellular elements given off by the tissues in response to infection or severe chemical irritation; pus.

F

facies the expression or appearance of the face, which may be characteristic of various disease conditions.

fallopian tube a tube extending from uterus to ovary.

fang the front teeth of poisonous snakes through which the venom is injected into the wound.

fascia the fibrous tissue sheaths which invest many muscles and organs of the body.

fat embolism an embolism of fat which has entered the circulation as the result of some operative procedure or, commonly, extensive fractures.

fauces the passageway between the mouth itself and the pharynx.

febrile a condition accompanied by fever, with the implication that the temperature is considerably elevated.

feces bowel movements; the stools.

felon a severe infection of the soft tissues of the end of a finger; sometimes called a whitlow.

femoral a term used to refer to the femur itself, or to the thigh and its various structures such as the femoral artery or vein.

femur the bone of the thigh; the largest bone of the body.

fetus the embryo after the second month of pregnancy.

fibrillation rapid twitching of a muscle due to independent action of its fibers.

fibrin a substance in the blood which is essential for clot formation and which constitutes the network about which the clot forms.

fibroma a benign type of growth composed of fibrous tissue.

fibula the smaller and less important of the two bones of the lower leg.

fistula an abnormal tract or tubelike channel of fibrous tissue leading from any hollow organ to the surface.

flatulence gas in the intestines.

fluoroscope an instrument similar to an x-ray machine which is used to observe directly various structures of the body, without actually taking a picture.

fomentations hot wet dressings.

fontanels the openings between the bones of the skull in very young children before the bones fuse together as the child grows older.

foramen any natural opening through a bone or other structure of the body.

fracture broken bone.

frontal pertains to the region of the forehead.

frostbite damage to the tissues as the result of prolonged exposure to extreme cold.

fulguration the burning away of a growth by means of a cautery.

fulminating an adjective describing any condition which occurs suddenly and with great severity.

fundus a term which is used to apply to the retina of the eye and its related structures, or the body of the uterus.

fungus a microscopic vegetable organism; several are able to cause disease in a variety of ways.

furuncle a form of small skin abscess involving a sebaceous gland.

furunculosis generalized acne or pimples.

fusion joining together; commonly used in connection with spinal fusion.

G

gait used technically to refer to the way a person walks.

gall bladder the sac located just beneath the liver which stores bile until needed.

ganglion a small, hard tumor in a tendon sheath, or a small swelling in the covering of a joint.

gangrene local tissue death as the result of injury, or cutting off of its blood supply.

gastritis inflammation of the lining of the stomach due to irritant substances.

gastrocnemius the large muscle which forms the calf of the leg.

gastroenteritis a generalized infection of the gastrointestinal tract.

gastroenterology the study of diseases of the digestive system.

gavage feeding a patient by means of a tube placed in the stomach through the mouth or nose.

genitals the genitalia, or external sexual organs.

genitourinary the organs composing the urinary and genital systems.

geriatrics medical treatment of the aged.

germ any microorganism; sometimes used to mean a very early stage of an embryo.

germicide any agent capable of killing all microorganisms under conditions of use.

gestation pregnancy.

gingivitis inflammation of the gums.

gland any group of cells or organ that produces any type of secretion.

glaucoma a disease which produces increased pressure within the eyeball; if unrelieved, it may cause blindness.

globulin an important group of proteins in the blood, some of which confer protection against disease.

glomerulonephritis a type of kidney disease in which the glomeruli themselves are specifically damaged.

glomerulus a little coil of capillaries around each tubule in the kidney; the basic units in the secretion of urine.

glossitis inflammation of the tongue.

glycosuria sugar in the urine; characteristic of diabetes.

goiter an enlargement of the thyroid gland.

gonads either the ovaries or the testicles.

gonococcus the bacterium which is the cause of gonorrhea.

gout an hereditary disturbance of metalobism in which uric acid is retained in the body and deposited about the joints.

graft the repair of a tissue defect by placement of similar tissue from elsewhere in the same patient or from a donor; i.e., skin grafts.

granulation tissue "proud flesh," a growth of young capillaries and fibrous tissue cells which is the basis for healing in some wounds.

granuloma a type of tumor produced by chronic or low-grade infection, composed of granulation-like tissue.

gravid pregnant.

groin the inguinal region; the junction of the abdomen with the thigh.

gynecomastia abnormal enlargement of one or both breasts, either in the male or female.

H

hallucination an apparent perception of one of the senses which a patient thinks he experiences, but which has no factual basis.

hallucinogenic any agent or drug which has the capacity to stimulate hallucinations of any type—visual, olfactory, or auditory.

harelip congenital failure of the upper lip to fuse in the midline during embryonic life; it must be corrected by surgery.

hay fever allergy to various pollens.

heart block a short circuit in the conducting mechanisms of the heart, so that the auricles and ventricles beat independently of each other.

heliotherapy treatment of disease by exposure to the sun; formerly an important part of the treatment of tuberculosis.

helminthiasis infestation of the intestinal tract with worms.

hemangioma a tumor composed of blood vessels or large spaces containing blood; may or may not be malignant.

hemarthrosis accumulation of blood in a joint.

hematemesis vomiting of blood.

hematinic any drug which increases the hemoglobin and red cell count of the blood.

hematology the study of the blood and its diseases.

hematoma the localized collection of blood in the tissues as the result of injury, or a broken blood vessel.

hematuria blood in the urine.

hemianopsia absence of vision in one half of the visual field in one or both eyes.

hemiplegia paralysis of one side of the body.

hemodialysis the process of removing certain noxious agents from the blood by a process of diffusion through a semipermeable membrane. The procedure is lifesaving in certain types of poisoning and in renal failure.

hemoglobin the oxygen- and carbon dioxide-carrying pigment in the red blood cells.

hemoglobinuria the presence of hemoglobin in the urine, as in blackwater fever.

hemolysis the disintegration of the red corpuscles of the blood due to some adverse factor, as in a transfusion reaction.

hemophilia an inherited blood disease of males only, but inherited through the mother; characterized by inability of the blood to clot.

hemoptysis coughing up blood from the lungs, as in advanced cases of tuberculosis.

hemorrhage bleeding, particularly if it is of excessive degree.

hemorrhoidectomy the surgical removal of piles (hemorrhoids).

hemostasis stopping hemorrhage.

hemothorax blood in the pleural or thoracic cavity.

hepatitis inflammation of the liver; *viral* hepatitis is common and sometimes fatal.

hermaphrodism the presence of the reproductive organs of both sexes in a single individual.

hernia literally, the protrusion of any organ through an opening into another body cavity where it doesn't belong, as the result of a congenital or traumatic defect; most common is an inguinal hernia where a loop of intestine descends into the inguinal canal in the groin.

herpes zoster shingles, the result of infection by the V-Z virus of the sensory roots of the spinal nerves.

hiatus any opening in the normal anatomical structures through which other structures pass.

hirsutism excessive hairiness.

Hodgkin's disease serious disease characterized by gradual enlargement of lymph nodes.

hookworm a worm of the genus *Necator americanus*, which may become parasitic in the human intestine and cause great disability. It is common in the southern states.

hordeolum a sty.

hormone a substance secreted by an endocrine gland which has effects upon other glands or systems of the body.

humerus the bone of the upper arm.

hydrated used technically to indicate that the patient is in a satisfactory state of water balance; he is not losing more water than he is taking in.

hydrocele a collection of fluid in the sac which surrounds a testicle; treatment is a simple surgical procedure.

hydrocephaly blockage of an outlet of the ventricles of the brain, which interferes with the drainage of the cerebrospinal fluid; the increased pressure thus created causes a great enlargement of the skull.

hydrophobia rabies; a virus disease which affects the brain and causes the animal to become "mad." In humans, death is inevitable unless the Pasteur treatment is instituted early.

hydrotherapy treatment by massage and exercise under water; a key part of the treatment of paralytic polio.

hymen the membrane which partially closes over the vaginal opening prior to the first intercourse.

hyoid bone a bone in the throat just above the voice box at the base of the tongue.

hyperemia increased blood flow to a part or tissue.

hyperesthesia increased susceptibility of the skin to sensation, such as to the prick of a pin; of diagnostic significance in certain neurologic diseases.

hyperglycemia increased amounts of sugar in the blood.

hyperidrosis excessive sweating.

hyperimmune serum a serum which is extremely rich in protective antibodies and which has been artificially produced in animals or in humans by the injection of a specific disease antigen.

hyperinsulinism too much insulin in the blood, which lowers the blood sugar level and produces insulin shock; often used therapeutically in the treatment of nervous disorders.

hyperkeratosis an overdevelopment of the hard horny layer of the skin; or, a disease of the cornea of the eye.

hyperkinesis an increased level of general bodily activity often seen in some types of thyroid disease.

hypernephroma a malignant growth of the kidneys.

hyperperistalsis increased activity of the musculature of a hollow tube; more specifically of the intestine.

hyperpituitarism a disease due to overactivity of the pituitary gland which characteristically produces a gigantic individual with typically deformed bones.

hyperplasia an increase in the number of cells composing a given tissue.

hyperpnea increase in the rate and amplitude of respiration.

hyperpyrexia high fever.

hyperreflexia overactive reflexes.

hypersensitivity increased sensitivity to some foreign physical or chemical agent.

hypertension high blood pressure.

hyperthyroidism increased activity of the thyroid gland—Grave's disease.

hypertonic being in a state of increased tension.

hypertrichosis excessive growth of hair.

hypertrophy increase in size of a part or structure.

hyperventilation a condition in which there is prolonged rapid, deep breathing, with lowering of the amount of carbon dioxide in the blood; this may result in a convulsive-like disorder sometimes referred to as respiratory or hyperventilation tetany.

hypodermic injection of a medicament beneath the skin.

hypoglycemia too low a level of sugar in the blood.

hypophysis the pituitary gland.

hypopituitarism inactivity of the pituitary gland, characterized by the persistence of childlike characteristics and excessive fat.

hypospadias opening of the urethra on the under surface of the penis rather than at the tip where it belongs.

hypotension low blood pressure.

hypothyroidism too little activity of the thyroid gland, giving rise to sluggish activity, cold clammy skin, and excess weight.

hypoxia an abnormally low content of oxygen in the inspired air. This is in contrast to the term *hypoxemia,* which refers to deficient oxygenation of the blood itself.

hysterectomy excision of the uterus.

hysteria a psychic disturbance characterized by lack of control over one's emotions or physical acts.

I

iatrogenic a term referring to any condition of an abnormal or undesirable nature which is brought about as the result of treatment.

icterus jaundice; the yellow appearance of the skin and other tissues due to an excessive appearance of bile pigments.

idiosyncrasy a peculiar susceptibility to some foreign substance or physical agent.

idiot a feeble-minded adult person having a mental age below two years.

ileitis an infection of the portions of the small intestine near the cecum.

ileocolostomy a short-circuiting operation which establishes a connection between the ileum and some part of the colon.

ileum the portion of the small intestine between the jejenum and the cecum.

ileus intestinal obstruction.

imbecility feeble-mindedness.

immobilization holding a part firmly in place, as by means of splints.

immunity resistance to the effects of a disease agent, poison, or allergen.

immunization the process of protection against disease by stimulating the formation of specific antibodies.

impacted stuck in something so as to be hard to remove.

impetigo an infectious skin disease characterized by a diffuse pustular eruption, due to staphylococcal or streptococcal infection.

inanition the result of starvation.

incarceration the imprisonment of a tissue by surrounding bands or adhesions, such as may happen when a loop of bowel becomes incarcerated in an inguinal hernia.

incision a wound usually made deliberately, in connection with surgery, by a clean cut as opposed to a laceration.

incontinence inability to prevent the flow of urine or feces.

incubation period the time between infection and the first appearance of the symptoms of a disease.

indolent slow in healing.

induration hardening or firming of a tissue as the result of cellular infiltration due to infection, inflammation, or trauma.

infantilism the persistence of childlike characteristics into adult life.

infarction death of a localized area of tissue due to the cutting off of its blood supply.

infection the creation of disease processes within the tissues by microorganisms.

inflammation tissue reaction to chemical or physical injury or bacterial infection.

influenza an acute infectious disease involving the respiratory tract and other systems. It may be due to a virus or to infection with the *Hemophilus influenza bacillus.*

infusion the slow injection of fluid into a vein.

ingestion the taking in of food or other substances.

inguinal region the groin.

inhibition interference with, or slowing down of, some body activity; in a psychiatric sense, a mental block with respect to specific thoughts and activities.

innervation the nerve or group of nerves which controls the activity of a muscle or other organ.

innocuous not harmful or poisonous.

inoculation injection of any biological substance intended to confer protection against disease.

intracranial any lesion that occurs within the cranium or skull itself.

ipecac a powder prepared from the plant *Cephaëlis ipecacuanha*; it is widely used in the form of a fluid extract or syrup as an emetic and, in smaller doses, as an expectorant agent.

iritis inflammation of the iris.

ischemia a deficiency in the blood supply or a lack of blood supply in any given area or part.

ischium one of the bones of the pelvis.

isodynamic equality in strength or power, particularly applied to opposing sets of muscles.

isolation separation of those ill with a transmissible disease from others.

isotonic equal osmotic pressure between two solutions; as an example, a good eye wash is isotonic with tears.

J

Jacksonian epilepsy convulsions due to a localized lesion in the brain resulting from pressure or injury.

jaundice the presence of excessive bile pigments in the bloodstream which give to the skin, mucous membrane, and eyes a distinct yellow color.

jejenum the final portion of the small intestine immediately following the duodenum.

joint-mouse any loose calcareous deposit in a joint.

jugular veins the main blood vessels collecting the blood from the head and neck.

K

keloid an overgrowth of fibrous tissue in a scar.

keratin a horny protein-like substance in the upper layers of the skin, and which is the principal constituent of the hair and nails.

keratitis inflammation of the cornea due to infection or injury.

keratoconjunctivitis inflammation of both the cornea and the overlying conjunctiva, giving a diffuse inflamed appearance to the eye.

keratosis any horny growth of the skin, such as the little raised plaques seen on the skin of many elderly individuals.

kleptomania pathologic stealing by an individual who has an uncontrollable compulsion to steal.

Koplik's spots tiny bluish-white spots that appear in the mouth before the rash appears in measles.

kyphosis humpback.

L

labia the folds of skin and mucous membrane which compose the vulva.

labyrinth the internal ear.

laceration any wound made by a tearing and cutting action upon the tissues.

lacrimation the formation and discharge of tears.

lactation secretion of milk.

laminectomy the surgical removal of a portion of a vertebra.

lanugo soft, fuzzy; infantile type of hair.

laparotomy a surgical opening into the abdominal cavity for the purpose of operating upon any of the abdominal organs.

laryngectomy removal of the larynx or voice box (Adam's apple).

laryngitis inflammation of the larynx.

laryngoscope an instrument for directly visualizing the larynx and its related structures.

larynx the voice box, which contains the vocal cords and also the special sphincter which prevents the aspiration of food or liquid into the trachea.

latent concealed or hidden injection or disease.

lateral to one side; away from the midline of the body.

lavage a washing out of a hollow organ such as the stomach.

lesion any abnormal pathologic condition of any tissue or part.

lethargy lack of ambition to do anything, coupled with a feeling of sleepiness.

leukemia a disease of the blood characterized by an increase in the number of white cells and pathological changes in the bone marrow and other organs.

leukocyte a white blood cell.

leukocytosis an increase in the number of white cells per cubic millimeter of blood.

leukopenia a decrease below normal of the number of white cells in the blood.

leukorrhea any abnormal vaginal discharge.

ligament a tough band of fibrous tissue which joins bones about a joint, or supports any organ.

ligature a string made from any material such as catgut, silk, or cotton that is used for the purpose of controlling bleeding, to tie shut blood vessels which have been cut.

lipoma any tumor composed principally of fat; not malignant as a rule.

lithiasis the presence of a stone in any organ or duct.

livid suffused with blood to give a bright, congested appearance; usually applied to the face.

lobe any anatomically well-defined part of a large organ, separated from the rest of the organ by clefts; i.e., the lobes of the lungs.

lobectomy a surgical removal of one part of an organ, such as one lobe of a lung.

lockjaw tetanus, caused by the *Clostridium tetani*; characterized by acute spasm of the jaw muscles which prevents the mouth from being opened.

lordosis a deformity of the spine which throws the chest out and the lower spine in, giving a "sway" back.

lumbago backache in the lumbar region.

lumbar the region of the spine and surrounding trunk between the thorax and the brim of the pelvis.

lupus tuberculous infection of the skin.

lymph the almost colorless, slightly yellow, nutrient fluid which circulates in the lymphatic vessels.

lymphadenitis inflammation of the lymph glands.

lymphadenopathy enlargement of the lymph glands, either generally or of a specific area.

lymphatic the tiny vessels which carry lymph from the tissues to the bloodstream or the lymph glands.

lymphoma malignant disease of a lymph node.

lysis the gradual fall in temperature, improvement of a disease, or the subsidence of an infection.

M

maceration softening, reddening, and superficial ulceration of the skin due to prolonged exposure to moisture.

macula any lesion of the skin which is not raised above the surface; the area on the retina, near the optic nerve, which is the area of most sensitive vision.

malacia softening of a part or tissues; see ostiomalacia.

malaise a generalized feeling of vague bodily discomfort.

malaria a disease caused by infection of the red blood cells with one of several types of protozoan parasites of the genus *Plasmodium*.

malignant cancerous.

malleolus the large rounded bony protruberances on either side of the ankle joint.
malleus one of the little bones or ossicles in the middle ear.
malunion improper healing or lack of healing of a fracture.
mammary gland a breast.
mandible the jaw.
maniacal a psychic state in which the patient is in a state of uncontrollable excitement.
manic-depression a major emotional illness.
manubrium the main section of the sternum or breastbone.
marasmus an extreme state of emaciation in children.
masochism a morbid pleasure, often accompanied by sexual gratification, derived from physically painful experiences.
mastectomy an operation by which one breast is surgically removed.
mastitis inflammation or infection of the tissues of the breast.
mastoid the large bone behind the ear; it contains large air spaces which may become severely infected as the result of untreated middle-ear infection; this condition is known as mastoiditis.
maxilla the upper jaw.
meatus the opening of any tube or duct on the surface of the body, such as the urinary meatus.
meconium the material in the intestinal tracts of newborn infants before true feces are formed.
mediastinum the space between the lungs containing the heart, great vessels, nerves, trachea, and esophagus.
medulla oblongata that portion of the brain between the cerebellum and the spinal cord.
melancholia mental depression characterized by marked apathy.
melanoma a highly malignant type of cancer characterized by the presence of large numbers of cells containing the pigment known as melanin.
menarche the onset of menstruation about the time of puberty.
meninges the coverings of the brain and spinal cord.
meningitis infection and inflammation of the coverings of the brain and spinal cord, as in cerebrospinal meningitis; often due to the organism known as the meningococcus.
meniscus a cartilage which acts as a cushion between the opposing surfaces of the knee joint.
menopause the period when menstruation normally ceases.
menorrhagia excessive flow during a menstrual period.
menses the monthly menstrual period; more specifically, the actual vaginal discharge which occurs at this time.
mesentery the tissue by which the intestines are attached to the back surface of the abdominal cavity and which contains the blood vessels, lymphatics, and nerves supplying the intestines.
metabolism the conversion of food into energy and waste products.
metacarpal bones the bones between the wrist and the fingers; the bones of the palm of the hand.
metastasis the implanation of cancer cells or an infection in some organ or site other than the point at which the disease first occurred.
metrorrhagia bleeding from the uterus between menstrual periods.
migraine very severe headache, often accompanied by dizziness, nausea, and prostration.
miliaria heat rash; a diffuse pimple-like eruption of the skin common in infants, but which may occur in adults as the result of excessive heat and the inability to perspire freely.

miosis   contracted pupils.
mitral valve   the valve in the heart between the left auricle and the left ventricle.
molar bone   the cheekbone.
moniliasis   infection of practically any tissue of the body with a mold known as *Candida albicans.*
monocyte   a large white cell of the blood having a single nucleus.
mononucleosis   an acute infectious disease characterized by increased numbers of monocytes in the blood, fever, sore throat, prostration, and enlargement of the lymph nodes of the neck.
morbid   any disease condition; or an abnormal interest in the sad or unpleasant.
morbidity   more or less a synonym for *illness,* generally used to refer to the rate of a given illness in a population.
morphology   the configuration of the cells which make up the structure of tissues; often used to apply to diseased tissues.
mortality   a term usually used in connection with the death rate for a specific disease in a specific population, based on the total number of deaths in relation to the total number of individuals in the rated population.
mucosa   any mucous membrane; often used to refer to the lining of the intestines.
mucous membrane   a membrane which lines many organs of the body and contains little glands which secrete mucus.
mucus   a viscid, watery-like secretion elaborated by the mucous membranes of the body, which serves as a lubricant and has mild antibacterial properties.
multigravida   a woman who has had more than one child.
murmur   a sound which may be detected in the heart when one of the valves is either leaking or is partially closed shut as the result of disease or congenital malformation.
myalgia   pain in muscles.
myasthenia gravis   a progressive, fatal disease of the muscles characterized by slow paralysis of various muscle groups.
mycology   the study of diseases due to fungous infection.
mycosis   a disease due to infection by any fungus.
mydriasis   enlargement or dilatation of the pupils of the eye.
myelin   the fatty protective substance that forms a sheath around many nerves; diseases which cause damage of this sheath are known as the demyelinating diseases.
myelitis   inflammation or infection of the nerves of the spinal cord; less frequently used to indicate inflammation of the bone marrow.
myocarditis   disease of the heart muscle itself.
myopia   nearsightedness.
myositis ossificans   a chronic progressive disease in which the muscles of the body are slowly converted into bony-like tissue.
myringotomy   incision of the eardrum to establish drainage in infection of the middle ear.
myxedema   a disease due to too little thyroid activity; characterized by swelling of the tissues, general sluggishness, and many other symptoms.

N

Nabothian glands   little glands in the cervix that may form cysts and require treatment.

narcissism sexual attraction to one's self; self-love.

narcolepsy a pathologic and uncontrollable desire to sleep, or abnormal periods of sleep.

narcosis drug-induced sleep.

narcotic any drug which produces sleep and relieves pain; most are habit-forming.

nasal pertaining to the nose.

nasopharynx the internal portions of the nose and throat.

necropsy autopsy; examination of a dead body by dissection.

necrosis tissue death from any cause.

Neisserian infection gonorrhea.

neonatal newborn.

neoplasm any new growth in the tissues; not necessarily malignant, but often implies malignancy.

nephrectomy removal of a kidney by surgical operation.

nephritis disease of the kidney due to infection or irritation.

nephrosis any disease of the kidney, particularly that type involving the tubules.

neuralgia pain along the course of a nerve; usually spasmodic and of an aching character.

neurasthenia nervous exhaustion.

neuritis inflammation of a nerve due to infection or the toxic effects of some foreign agent such as alcohol.

neurodermatitis an itching eruption of the skin which is due to some nervous disorder.

neurological pertaining to the diagnosis and treatment of disease of the nervous system.

neurosis a minor emotional disorder.

neurotic a person whose emotions have an undue influence over his physical being.

neutrophil a type of white cell in the blood, otherwise known as a poly-morphonuclear leukocyte, which is of great importance in combatting infection.

nevus a mole or birthmark.

nidation the embedding of the ovum in the lining of the uterus so that it can obtain nourishment to grow.

nocturia the necessity to get up at night to urinate.

nodule any small lump.

nucleus the central and vital portion of any cell.

nullipara a woman who has not yet had her first baby.

nystagmus uncontrolltable movement of the eyeballs in a to-and-fro motion due to disease of the internal ear or central nervous system.

O

obsession a morbid preoccupation with a fixed idea or set of ideas.

occipital the region of the back part of the head.

occlusion stoppage as a of a blood vessel due to a clot or embolus.

occult obscure, unknown, not obvious.

ocular pertaining to the eyes.

oleocranon the back of the elbow; formed by a tip of the ulna which curves around the lower end of the humerus.

olfactory pertaining to the organs or sense of smell.

oliguria too little output of urine.

omentum   the apron of fatty tissue which hangs down from the stomach to cover most of the front surface of the abdominal organs.

omphalitis   inflammation or infection of the naval, or "belly button."

onychectomy   surgical removal of a finger or toe nail.

onychomycosis   fungous infection of the nails.

oophorectomy   surgical removal of one or both ovaries.

opacity   obscuring of the normal transparency of the cornea or lens of the eye.

ophthalmia   generalized inflammation of the eye.

ophthalmology   the study of the diseases of the eye and their treatment.

opiates   technically, various alkaloids derived from the opium or poppy plant; sometimes used in a general way to refer to any drug which produces sleep.

opisthotonus   a convulsive rigid arching of the back which is characteristically seen in severe meningitis.

orchiectomy   surgical removal of one or both testicles; same as orchidectomy.

orchitis   inflammation or infection of the testicles.

orthopedics   the surgical specialty concerned with the treatment of injuries, deformities, and diseases of the bones.

orthoptics   the science of treating visual defects of a mechanical nature.

ossicle   any small bone, particularly the little bones of the internal ear, consisting of the malleus, incus, and stapes.

ossification   the process of forming bone, either normal or abnormal.

osteitis   inflammation of a bone.

osteoarthritis   a degenerative disease which may involve many joints at one time.

osteoarthropathy   any disease involving the bones and joints.

osteochondritis   an inflammatory process of bone and cartilage about a joint.

osteomyelitis   infection of a bone; this may be a severe and difficult-to-cure condition.

otitis   inflammation of the ear; otitis external: inflammation of the external auditory canal; otitis media: inflammation of the middle ear; otitis interna: inflammation of the internal ear or labyrinth.

otolaryngological   pertaining to diseases of the ear and respiratory passages.

otosclerosis   a disease of the ear which produces deafness by the abnormal development of bone tissue in the internal ear.

ovariectomy   removal of an ovary.

ovulation   the act of ripening and extrusion of an ovum from the ovary.

ovum   the female germ cell or egg.

oxyuriasis   intestinal infestation with pinworms (seat worms).

P

palate   the roof of the mouth.

palliative   any agent which affords relief but does not cure a disease condition.

pallor   paleness.

palpable   feelable.

palpation   the act of discerning a mass or organ by feeling with the fingers.

palpitation   abnormally rapid beating of the heart, often accompanied by a sensation of suffocation.

palsy   paralysis; "shaking palsy," paralysis agitans.

pancreas an intra-abdominal gland which secretes insulin in addition to important digestive enzymes.

pancreatitis infection of the pancreas.

pandemic an epidemic of disease originating or existing over a very large geographic area.

panophthalmitis a generalized severe inflammation of all the ocular structures.

pansinusitis infection of all the sinuses.

papilledema swelling of the head of the optic nerve, usually due to increased intracranial pressure, as from a tumor.

papilloma any wart-like growth of the skin or mucous membrane.

papule a small, solid, circumscribed eruption of the skin; a maculopapular type of rash is common in many disease conditions and consists of a mixture of macules and papules on the skin surface.

paracentesis drainage of fluid from the peritoneal cavity by means of a large needle inserted through the abdominal wall.

paralysis abolition of muscle function due to interference with its nerve supply at any point.

paranoia a mental disease characterized by abnormal suspicions or other delusions which often are so logical as to be accepted as factual by unsuspecting observers.

paraplegia paralysis of the entire lower part of the body, including both legs.

parasympathetic nervous system a subdivision of the autonomic nervous system composed of nerves coming from the cervical and sacral regions of the spinal cord.

parathyroid little glands, usually four in number, situated on the back of the thyroid gland, which regulate calcium metabolism.

paratyphoid an infectious intestinal disease similar to typhoid fever, caused by the *Salmonella paratyphi.*

parenchyma the substance of a gland or solid organ.

parenteral administration of any medication by any route other than the internal tract.

paresis mild paralysis.

paresthesia any abnormality of sensation.

Parkinson's disease a form of paralysis agitans.

paronychia an infection of the tissues at one side of a fingernail or a toenail.

parotid gland the salivary gland situated just below and in front of the ear.

parotitis inflammation and infection of the parotid gland.

parous having had at least one child.

paroxysm a sudden and intense recurrence of symptoms, such as the pain in colic.

parturition the act of giving birth.

passive immunization transient protection, produced by the administration of the serum of animals which have already been rendered immune through the injection of specific antigens, against a specific disease. Tetanus antiserum is a common example.

patella the kneecap.

patent open, unobstructed.

pathogenic capable of causing a disease process.

pathognomonic a symptom or physical sign which is sufficiently characteristic of a disease as to make possible a diagnosis on the basis of the symptom alone.

pathology the study of manifestations of disease in the various tissues of the body.

patulous being spread wide open; loose; easily entered.

pectoral muscles the large muscles of the front of the chest.

pediatrics the medical specialty devoted to the diagnosis and treatment of diseases of children.

pediculosis infestation of the body or scalp with lice.

pellagra a severe deficiency disease caused by insufficient dietary intake of niacin, one of the B complex vitamins.

pemphigus a generalized, sometimes fatal, skin disease characterized by recurring crops of large blisters.

peptic ulcer an ulcer produced by acid gastric juice in the stomach.

percussion a method of creating sounds having diagnostic significance, by tapping the fingers of one hand laid on an area, as the chest, with a finger on the other hand.

pericarditis inflammation of the tissues composing the sac about the heart known as the pericardium.

periosteum the dense, fibrous, tissue-like sheath covering a bone.

periostitis acute inflammation or infection of the periosteum.

peristalsis successive waves of muscular contraction and relaxation proceeding uniformly along a hollow tube such as the esophagus or intestines.

peritoneal dialysis a technic for removing impurities from the blood in cases of renal failure, using the patient's own peritoneum as the dialyzing membrane. A suitable electrolyte solution is introduced into the peritoneal cavity and removed after a period of time, bringing with it various impurities which accumulated as the result of renal failure. The technic is also used in certain types of poisoning.

peritoneum the glistening fibrous tissue sac which invests the inner walls of the abdominal cavity and the organs which it contains.

peritonitis inflammation or infection of the peritoneum.

pernicious intractable to the point of eventually being fatal.

peroneal a term referring to the fibula or anatomical structures immediately surrounding it, such as the peroneal artery or nerve, or the outside of the lower leg.

pertussis whooping cough.

petechia tiny diffuse ecchymotic (black-and-blue) areas in the skin seen in certain severe diseases.

phagocyte a type of cell found in the blood and tissues which has the power of engulfing bacteria or particles of foreign material.

phalanx any bone of a finger or toe.

pharmacodynamic the pharmacologic or metabolic effects of drugs or medicine on the body.

pharynx the space between the mouth, the posterior portion of the nasal passages, and the esophagus. Pharyngitis is a common infectious inflammation of the pharynx.

phimosis tightness of the prepuce (foreskin) of the penis, so that it cannot be drawn back of the glans (head).

phlebitis infection of the walls and lining of a vein.

phobia an abnormal dread of some specific thing.

photomicrograph a photograph of the minute characteristics of a specimen made through a microscope.

photophobia abnormal sensitivity to light, such as is seen in measles.

phrenetic a highly excited state of mind and physical activity, which may at times border on the maniacal.

phrenic nerve the nerve which activates the diaphragm. It is sometimes desirable to put one lung partially at rest as in treating tuberculosis; this is done by cutting this nerve, an operation known as phrenicotomy.

phthisis tuberculosis.

pigmentation the deposition of pigment in the skin as the result of physical or metabolic causes. Suntanning is one common form of pigmentation of physical origin.

pinkeye an acute infection of the conjunctiva which is highly contagious.

pinworms seat worms; intestinal infestation with *Enterobius vermicularis*.

pituitary gland often called the master gland of the body since it influences the functions of many other glands and organs; located in the brain, behind the eyes.

placenta the afterbirth.

plague an acute infectious disease characterized by severe prostration, delirium, and diarrhea; caused by the *Pasteurella pestis*.

plantar the sole of the foot.

plasma the fluid portion of the blood from which the red and white cells have been removed; for therapeutic use it contains an anticoagulant to prevent clotting.

platelet a small cellular element in the blood which plays an important role in the clotting process.

pleura the glistening fibrous tissue sheath which lines the inner surface of the chest wall and envelops the lungs.

pleurisy an infection of the pleura, characterized by acute pain on breathing.

plumbism lead poisoning.

pneumonectomy surgical removal of a lung.

pneumonia an acute infectious disease of the lungs commonly caused by a germ called the pneumococcus.

pneumothorax air in the pleural cavity.

poliomyelitis infantile paralysis; an acute viral infection of the motor nerves controlling muscle function in the spinal cord.

pollinosis hay fever; allergy to pollens.

polyarthritis arthritis in many joints at one time; usually acute.

polydipsia excessive thirst; a symptom of diabetes.

polyp any stalklike growth arising from mucous membrane.

polyphagia excessive craving for food; hunger; a second symptom of diabetes.

polyuria excessive output of urine; a third symptom of diabetes.

popliteal the area or space behind the knee joint.

portal vein the large vein that collects the blood from the spleen and intestinal tract and carries it to the liver.

posterior the back or dorsal surface of the body or part.

postmortem examination of a body after death; autopsy; necropsy.

postnasal the region behind the nose, toward the back part of the throat.

postoperative following operation.

post partum after childbirth.

postvaccinal following vaccination; usually refers to some type of reaction.

precocious unusually developed, or unusually brilliant.

precordial refers to the general area over the heart and lower part of the thorax.

premenstrual immediately before menstruation.

prenatal before birth.

prepuce the foreskin of the penis.

primipara   a woman who is about to deliver a baby for the first time.
procititis   inflammation and infection of the rectum.
proctectomy   excision of the rectum.
proctoscopy   direct visual examination of the rectum with an instrument known as a proctoscope.
prodromal   preliminary symptoms which occur prior to the actual onset of a disease.
prognosis   the probable outlook as to recovery from disease.
prolapse   the dropping downward of an internal organ from its normal position.
proliferate   the increase in growth of a given tissue by reproduction of the same type of cell composing that particular tissue.
prone   lying flat with the face downward.
prophylaxis   taking measures to prevent the occurrence of a given disease.
prostate   gland at the base of the male bladder which often becomes enlarged in later life and is often subject to cancer.
prostatectomy   removal of the prostate.
prostatitis   inflammation of the prostate.
prosthesis   an artificial part made to replace a natural one.
prostration   collapse.
pruritus   itching.
psittacosis   virus disease of birds transmissible to man.
psoriasis   a chronic skin disease of unknown cause, characterized by large red patches.
psychiatry   the study and treatment of diseases of the mind.
psychopathic   pertains to a patient suffering from any disorder of the mind.
psychosis   any deep-seated, usually serious mental disorder.
psychosomatic   pertaining to bodily manifestations of any disorder of the mind.
psychotherapy   treatment based on the use of mental relationships and procedures, rather than on physical procedures or the use of drugs; sometimes drugs are used to supplement psychotherapeutic technics.
ptomaine poisoning   poisoning from toxins in putrefied food.
puberty   technically, the period between the establishment of secondary sex characteristics and the completion of physical growth.
puerperium   the convalescent period following the birth of a baby.
pulmonary   referring to the lungs or related structures, particularly with respect to physiologic function.
purpura   a blood disease characterized by a marked tendency to bleed.
purulent   pertaining to pus.
pustule   a small bleb containing pus.
pyelitis   infection of the kidney at the point at which it empties into the ureter.
pyemia   generalized severe blood poisoning.
pylorus   the opening at the outlet of the stomach into the duodenum or first portion of the small intestine.

Q

quadrant   a term used to designate a specific area of the abdominal wall.
quadriplegia   paralysis of both arms and both legs.
Q.I.D.   a Latin abbreviation meaning four times a day.
quinidine   a drug made from cinchona bark which is useful in treating irregularities of the heartbeat.

quinine   a drug made from cinchona bark which is very useful in the treatment and suppression of malaria.

quinsy   a severe type of sore throat with abscess formation in the tissues around a tonsil.

R

rabies   hydrophobia. An animal or human suffering from this condition is said to be rabid, or "mad."

rachitic   suffering from rickets, a condition due to vitamin D deficiency in the diet and lack of sunlight.

radiation   treatment with various types of radioactive energy, either from radium or similar sources, or x-rays.

radiologist   a doctor specializing in the diagnosis and treatment of disease by means of x-ray.

radius   the bone in the forearm on the side towards the thumb.

rale   an abnormal type of sound which is produced in the lungs by various types of disease.

recrudescence   the reoccurrence of symptoms following a period when the disease seemed to have been improving; practically the same as relapse.

rectum   the muscular reservoir lying between the last portion of the colon and the anus.

reflex   involuntary muscular action in response to some stimulation.

refraction   the process of determining and then counteracting the optical error in the eye with glasses.

regenerative process   any process which tends to restore the natural function of an organ or part.

regression   improvement in the symptoms of a disease, or the subsidence of a disease process.

regurgitation   spitting up undigested food; or the flow of blood in the heart in a reverse direction due to a leaky valve.

remission   an abatement in the symptoms of a disease.

remittent   alternately decreasing and increasing.

renal   referring to the kidney, particularly with respect to function.

resect   the surgical cutting away of a part or tissue.

resolution   the subsidence of an inflammatory process.

respiration   the act of breathing; the exchange of oxygen and carbon dioxide in the tissues.

resuscitation   the act of reviving an unconscious person by any means, including artificial respiration.

retention   inability to void urine or feces.

retina   the lining of the back of the eye which receives visual images and transmits them, through the optic nerve, to the brain.

retinitis   inflammation of the retina.

retractor   an instrument used for holding the tissues apart during a surgical operation.

retroflexed   the bending backward of an organ; most commonly used in connection with the uterus when it is turned backward in any degree upon itself, a common gynecologic condition.

retrosternal   refers to the area immediately beneath the sternum, where there are located, of course, many vital organs.

retroversion   a position of the uterus in which it is bent backward in the pelvis.

Rh factor a group of substances, the presence of which in human red blood corpuscles determines whether the blood is Rh positive or negative. Those with negative blood cannot be repeatedly transfused with Rh-positive blood because of resulting destruction of blood cells and severe reaction.

rhinitis inflammation of the nasal mucous membrane.

rickets a condition of abnormal calcium and phosphorous metabolism caused by insufficient vitamin D or insufficient exposure to ultraviolet rays.

rigidity extreme muscle tenseness.

rigor a chill.

ringworm a fungous infection of the skin, characterized by red, scaly ring-shaped patches which seem to heal in the center as they spread.

roentgenologist another term for radiologist.

Romberg test swaying of the body when standing erect with the feet close together and the eyes closed; it is often indicative of a serious disturbance of equilibrium caused by underlying disease. It may be observed in alcoholism and other drug-induced conditions.

rubefacient an agent used for the production of counterirritation of the skin.

rubella German measles.

rubeola regular measles.

ruminants animals having a stomach with four parts: rumen, reticulum, omasum, abomasum. The cow is the best-known example.

rupture a hernia; also means the tearing apart of a tissue such as a muscle.

S

sacroiliac pertaining to the joint and ligaments between the sacrum and the ilium; a common site of low back pain.

sadism sexual satisfaction derived from inflicting pain upon others.

saline water containing ordinary table salt in such concentration that it is soothing rather than irritating to the tissues.

Salmonella a group of bacteria which may cause a severe type of food poisoning.

salmonellosis a disease condition caused by any one of the large group of salmonella bacteria; it includes such gastrointestinal disorders as paratyphoid fever and food poisoning.

salpingitis inflammation and infection of the fallopian tubes.

saphenous vein the long vein near the inner surface of the thigh, which is often tied off in the treatment of varicose veins.

sarcoma a malignant growth arising from connective tissue.

scabicide any drug which destroys the *Sarcoptes scabei,* the cause of scabies.

scabies a severely itching skin disease caused by the itch mite, which burrows beneath the skin and is very difficult to get rid of.

scapula the shoulder blade.

scarlatina scarlet fever.

Schick test a test used to determine an individual's susceptibility to diphtheria.

schizophrenia dementia praecox, a mental disease in which the mind appears to be split into two parts.

sciatica inflammation of the sciatic nerve.

sclera   the white opaque portion of the eyeball.

sclerosis   hardening of any tissue; multiple sclerosis is hardening of small areas throughout various portions of the nervous system.

scoliosis   a bending or curving of the spinal column to one side or the other.

scotoma   a blind spot in one of the visual fields; or dancing specks before the eyes (scintillating scotomata).

scrotum   the sac between the thighs in the male containing the testicles.

scurvy   a disease due to insufficient intake of vitamin C in the diet.

sebaceous glands   the little glands of the skin which secrete the oily substance known as sebum.

seborrheic dermatitis   a skin disease characterized by large reddened patches covered with greasy scales.

sepsis   generalized body poisoning by the products of bacterial infection.

septicemia   blood poisoning.

septum   a wall of tissue separating two cavities.

sequelae   the complications which may follow a disease.

sequestrum   a fragment of bone which separates as the result of infection or injury.

serum   the fluid portion of the blood after the cells and clotting elements have been removed; also wrongly used for antiserum.

shingles   herpes zoster.

sigmoid   the S-shaped terminal portion of the descending colon.

sinus   an infected fibrous tissue tract leading into a tissue but not connected with any organ; also used to designate one of the nasal sinuses, or the blood sinuses of the skull.

slough   dead tissue which may form in a wound, particularly one which is infected; *sloughing* refers to the formation or separation of this dead material.

smallpox   an acute, severe contagious disease characterized by a typical foul-smelling skin eruption; caused by a virus.

somatic   pertaining to the body.

soporific   a drug which produces deep sleep.

spasm   strong involuntary contraction of a muscle or group of muscles.

spasticity   a general tightness of a muscle, or mild unrelaxing spasm.

speculum   an instrument to expand, and thus facilitate looking into, the superficial body openings such as the nose, ears, or vagina.

sphincter   a circularly arranged muscle which acts as a valve to control the retention or release of fluids or semisolid materials in the body.

splenectomy   removal of the spleen.

splenomegaly   enlargement of the spleen.

sprain   the stretching or partial tearing of the capsule or ligaments of a joint.

stapes   one of the three small bones of the middle ear.

staphylococcus   one of the most common pus-producing germs.

stasis   stagnation or congestion of blood in a part.

stenosis   partial block of a duct or blood vessel by narrowing of its lumen.

sterilization   the process of rendering any substance or material completely free of any germ life.

sternocleidomastoid muscle   the large muscle which is easily felt at the side of the neck.

sternum   the breastbone.

stimulant   any agent that increases the level of a normal or depressed bodily process.

stomatitis   infection or inflammation of the lining of the mouth.

strain   an overstretching or tearing of a muscle or its tendon.

strangulation   choking; also used technically to indicate cutting off circulation to an organ or tissue by compression, as in a strangulated hernia.

streptococcicosis   a general term applying to all diseases caused by streptococci.

streptococcus   a very common and important germ that causes many types of infection and disease in man.

stricture   the narrowing of a duct or any natural passage by an inflammatory process, as in urethral stricture.

stridor   noisy, labored breathing.

stroke   a cerebral hemorrhage or thrombosis.

sty, stye   acute inflammation of a sebaceous gland on the edge of an eyelid.

subacute bacterial endocarditis   a chronic form of inflammation of the lining of the heart, caued by a variety of bacteria, most commonly a nonhemolytic streptococcus viridans.

subclavian artery   the large artery just under the collarbone, which supplies blood to the main artery of the arm, and to the head, neck, and axilla through its branches.

subcutaneous   just beneath the skin.

subdural   any lesion in the brain which occurs beneath the dura or heavy sheath-like covering of the brain; often used in connection with the subdural hematoma following a blow to the head.

substernal   the area beneath the sternum; substantially synonymous with *retrosternal*.

sunstroke   a condition due to prolonged exposure to the sun, characterized by coma and a high body temperature.

supinate   to turn the forearm so that the palm faces upward.

suppuration   the formation of pus in a wound.

suture   a thread composed of catgut, silk, cotton, or other material used for sewing any two structures together in the course of a surgical operation.

sympathectomy   the surgical excision of a portion of the sympathetic nervous system to attain beneficial effects in certain disease conditions.

sympatholytic   a drug which prevents the passage of impulses along the fibers of the sympathetic nervous system.

syncope   fainting.

syndrome   a group of symptoms which are suggestive of a certain disease.

synergism   the interaction of two drugs, which produces a greater effect than the sum of their individual effects.

synovitis   inflammation of the membrane lining a joint.

systemic   referring to anything that affects the body as a whole.

systole   the period during which the heart contracts to force blood out into the circulation.

T

tachycardia   very rapid heart beat.

tachyphylaxis   the development of a state in which a given drug has less and less effect.

tachypnea   technically means an excessively rapid rate of respiration; it also refers to a neurotic condition characterized by excessively rapid, shallow breathing.

tapeworm   a large worm which becomes parasitic in the intestinal tract and causes physical wasting of the victim.

tarsus   the ankle joint.

temporal   the region of the forehead.

tendinous   a term usually used in connection with that portion of a muscle, having tendon-like structure, which connects to a bone.

tenesmus   ineffectual and painful straining to urinate or defecate.

tenosynovitis   infection of the sheaths covering the tendons.

tetanus   lockjaw.

therapeutics   the treatment of disease.

thoracic   a term which pertains to the chest, usually in reference to the rib cage, or to the vertebrae in the chest area.

thoracotomy   surgical opening of the chest wall.

thrombocytopenia   lack of platelets in the blood.

thrombosis   the formation of a thrombus in a blood vessel.

thrombus   a blood clot which forms inside a blood vessel.

thrush   an infection of the lining of the mouth due to a fungus.

thyroidectomy   partial or total excision of the thyroid gland.

tibia   the larger of the two bones of the leg.

tic   a spasmodic twitching of a face muscle.

tick   a blood-sucking parasite that may carry disease to both man and animals.

tick paralysis   a progressive paralysis which sometimes follows the bites of certain ticks, particularly if the bite occurs about the neck or head and the tick is not removed promptly.

T.I.D.   a Latin abbreviation meaning three times a day.

tinnitus   buzzing or roaring in the ears.

torticollis   wry neck.

toxemia   general poisoning of the system due to absorption from some local site of infection.

toxic psychosis   a psychosis brought about by various toxic agents such as alcohol or other abused drugs, or infection.

toxin   any poisonous substance formed by bacteria.

toxoid   a chemically modified toxin which, when injected, stimulates the body to form protective substances against a specific disease, but which itself is not harmful.

tracheotomy   an opening made surgically in the trachea to create an airway in cases of respiratory obstruction.

trachoma   an acute infectious disease of the conjunctiva and cornea of the eye, which produces severe and painful symptoms.

trauma   injury.

trichinella   a parasite which occurs in pigs and infects man through the eating of inadequately cooked pork.

trichinosis   a disease caused by the trichinella spiralis which is ingested in insufficiently cooked pork containing encysted larvae.

trimester   a period of three months; the normal nine-month term of pregnancy in the human is conveniently divided into the first, second, and third trimesters.

trismus   spasm of the muscles of the jaw; commonly seen in tetanus (lockjaw).

trocar   a sharp, pointed, tube-like instrument which is used for draining off fluid from a cavity, as from the chest cavity or the abdominal cavity; in the first instance, the procedure is known as thoracentesis, and in the second as paracentesis.

tularemia   a disease of rodents, especially rabbits, which often is transmitted to man; caused by the *Pasteurella tularensis*.

tumescence swelling.

tumor any localized enlargement of a tissue; the term does not necessarily imply malignancy.

turgid a synonym for a swollen, congested, often discolored area.

typhoid . an acute infectious intestinal disease with marked systemic symptoms caused by *Salmonella typhosa.*

typhus a severe systemic disease characterized by prostration and a skin eruption; caused by an organism belonging to the Rickettsia; transmitted in one form by body lice and in another by rat fleas.

U

ulcer an open lesion on the skin or mucous membrane, as of the stomach.

ulna the larger of the two bones of the forearm.

umbilicus navel; "belly button."

uremia the toxic condition produced by the accumulation of nitrogenous waste substances in the blood due to failure of kidney function.

ureter the tube connecting the kidney to the bladder.

urethra the tube leading from the bladder to the outside of the body.

urethritis inflammation and infection of the urethra.

urticaria hives; usually due to some form of allergy or hypersensitivity.

uterus the womb.

uvula the small cylinder-like mass which hangs down from the center of the soft palate.

V

vaccination protection against smallpox by inoculation with the virus of cowpox (vaccinia).

vaccine a preparation which, when injected into the body, will stimulate the formation of protective substances against a specific disease.

vaccinia a virus disease of cattle, known as cowpox; the virus which causes this disease is used to prepare the vaccine, for use in humans, which protects against smallpox.

vagal a term usually used to describe the effects produced by stimulation or inhibition of the vagus nerve.

vaginitis an inflammation or infection of the vagina.

varicella chickenpox.

varicose vein, varicosity a vein that has become stretched, dilated and tortuous due to failure of the valves that control the flow of blood.

variola smallpox.

vascular usually used to indicate the degree of blood supply of a given part, or to refer to the system which distributes blood throughout the body.

vasoconstrictor any drug which causes a constriction of the blood vessels and raises blood pressure, or "shrinks" tissues by local application.

vasopressor any agent which raises the blood pressure by causing contraction of the capillaries or smaller arteries.

vector refers to the carrier of a disease, whether it be an insect, animal, or other agent.

venom a poison, the term usually being used in connection with the poisonous substances derived from snakes, spiders, bees, wasps, or other insects.

ventricles   the large chambers of the heart which pump blood outward from the heart.

ventricular   referring to one of the ventricles of the heart; often used in connection with describing some condition such as the contractions or absence of contractions, or a particular type of lesion.

verruca   a wart.

vertebra   one of the bones making up the spinal column.

vertigo   dizziness.

vesicle   a small blister.

vesicular   usually used to designate small blisters or blebs on the skin.

virulence   the potency of a germ in its ability to infect or produce disease.

virus   a parasitic infectious microorganism which is capable of living and multiplying only within the substance of a living cell. It is so small that it will pass through the very finest filters.

viscus   an organ of the body.

vulva   the external genital organs of the female.

vulvovaginitis   inflammation of the vulva and vagina; a condition which is not uncommon in young infants.

W

whooping cough   pertussis.

womb   the uterus.

wry neck   torticollis; a pulling of the neck to one side by spasm of the muscles.

X

xanthoma   small yellow plaque in the skin due to a fat deposit.

xerophthalmia   severe conjunctivitis due to insufficient intake of vitamin A.

xiphoid   the smallest and most dependent portion of the breastbone.

x-ray   a special, penetrating type of gamma radiation emitted by a high-voltage electronic tube which is used to make photographic pictures of the bones and other internal organs of the body; roentgen rays.

Y

yaws   a severe skin disease seen in the tropics; caused by an organism similar to that of syphilis, the *Treponema pertenue.*

Z

zygoma   the cheekbone.

REFERENCES

Aaron, H. et al. (eds.): Mumps Virus Vaccine, *Med. Lett. Drug Ther. 10*(4): 14–15, Feb. 23, 1968.
————: LSD, *Med. Lett. Drug Ther. 9*(1): 1–2, Jan. 13, 1967.
Aaron, H. et al. (eds.): Methadone in the Management of Opiate Addiction, *Med. Lett. Drug Ther. 11*(24): 97–99, Nov. 28, 1969.
Aaron, H. et al. (eds.): Treatment of Hypertensive Crisis, *Med. Lett. Drug Ther. 12*(7): 31–32, Apr. 3, 1970.
Aaron, H. et al. (eds.): Marijuana, *Med. Lett. Drug Ther. 12*(8): 33–35, Apr. 17, 1970.
Aaron, H. et al. (eds.): Diagnosis and Management of Reactions to Drug Abuse, *Med. Lett. Drug Ther. 12*(16): 65–68, Aug. 7, 1970.
Ad Hoc Committee on Cardiopulmonary Resuscitation of the Division of Medical Sciences, National Academy of Sciences-National Research Council; Cardiopulmonary Resuscitation, *JAMA 198:* 372–379, Oct. 24, 1966.
Adams, J. P. and F. D. Fowler: Wringer Injuries of the Upper Extremity: A Clinical, Pathological and Experimental Study, *Southern Med. J. 52:* 798–803 (July) 1959.
Ager, E. A., K. E. Nelson, M. M. Galton, J. R. Boring, III, and J. Jernigan: Two Outbreaks of Egg-Borne Salmonellosis and Implications for Their Prevention, *JAMA 199*(6): 122–128, Feb. 6, 1967.
Alexander, F., T. M. French et al.: "Studies in Psychosomatic Medicine: An Approach to the Cause and Treatment of Vegetative Disturbances," The Ronald Press Company, New York, 1948.
Alexander, J. O.: Scabies in Children, *Clin. Pediat. 8:* 73–85, 1969.
American Academy of Pediatrics, Report of the Subcommittee on Accidental Poisoning: Evaluation of Gastric Lavage and Other Factors in the Treatment of Accidental Ingestion of Petroleum Distillate Products, *Pediatrics 29*(4): 648–674, Apr., 1962.
————, Report of the Committee on the Control of Infectious Diseases: Measles, 1964.

————, Report of the Committee on the Control of Infectious Diseases, 15th ed., 1966.

————, Committee on Accident Prevention: Accidental Poisoning in Childhood, 1956.

————, Committee on Control of Infectious Diseases: Measles Immunization and Tuberculin Testing, *Newsletter Supplement,* June 1, 1967.

————, Committee on Control of Infectious Diseases: Inactivated Measles Vaccine, Discontinuance of Use, *Newsletter Supplement,* Nov. 15, 1967.

————, Committee on Control of Infectious Diseases: Mumps Virus Vaccine, *Newsletter Supplement,* Dec. 15, 1967.

————, Subcommittee on Accidental Poisoning: New Hazards of Chemicals and Drugs to Children, *Newletter Supplement,* Jan. 15, 1968.

————, Subcommittee on Accidental Poisoning: Recommendation: For the Use of Syrup of Ipecac and Activated Charcoal, *Newsletter,* p. 4, Jan. 15, 1966.

————, Report of the Committee on Infectious Diseases, 16th ed., 1970.

————, Penalty for Possessing Marijuana Should Be a Dismeanor, News Release, Dec. 2, 1970.

————, Warning on Hazards of Laundry Products Used in Newborn Nursery, News Release, Aug. 4, 1971.

————, Lead-based Paint, News Release, November 30, 1971.

————, Report of the Committee on Control of Infectious Diseases, 17th ed., 1974.

————, Committee on Accident Prevention: Auto Safety for the Infant and Young Child, statement, Oct., 1974.

————, Committee on the Pediatric Aspects of Physical Fitness, Recreation and Sports: Snowmobile Safety, Dec., 1974.

American College of Surgeons, Committee on Trauma, R. H. Kennedy (ed.): "Emergency Care of the Sick and Injured," W. B. Saunders Company, Philadelphia, 1966.

————, Committee on Trauma: Standards for Emergency Ambulance Services, *Bulletin,* American College of Surgeons, May–June, 1967.

————, Committee on Trauma: Essential Equipment for Ambulances, *Bulletin,* American College of Surgeons, May, 1970.

————, Committee on Trauma: A Guide to the Evaluation of Serious Head Injuries, *Bulletin,* American College of Surgeons, Feb., 1974, pp. 21–23.

American Heart Association, Committee on Cardiopulmonary Resuscitation, Subcommittee on Training of Ambulance Personnel. "Discussion Guide for the Slide-Set on Training of Ambulance Personnel in Cardiopulmonary Resuscitation," American Heart Association, 1965.

————: *Instructors Manual of Basic Cardiac Life Support,* by permission of the American Heart Association, 1974.

American Medical Association, Committee on Medical Aspects of Automotive Safety: Automobile Safety Belts during Pregnancy, *JAMA 221* (1): 20–21, July 3, 1972.

American Social Health Association: "A Guide to Some Drugs Which Are Subject to Abuse," September, 1970.

Apfelberg, D. B. et al.: High-pressure Silicone Injection Injury of the Hand, *J. Trauma 15*:922–925, 1975.

Appelbaum, E.: The Problem of Fever of Unknown Origin, *Bull. N.Y. Acad. Med. 43*(10): 889–898, Oct., 1967.

Arena, J. M.: Diagnosis and Treatment—Two Current Poisonings: Tricyclic Drugs and Methadone, *Pediatrics 51*(5): 919–922, May, 1973.

————: Poisoning—General Treatment and Prevention, Part I, *JAMA* 232(12): 1271–1275, June 23, 1975.

————: Poisoning—General Treatment and Prevention, Part II, *JAMA* 233(4): 358–363, July 28, 1975.

Armstrong, R. W., F. Stenn, V. R. Dowell, Jr., G. Ammerman, and H. M. Sommers: Type E Botulism from Home-canned Gefilte Fish—Report of Three Cases, *JAMA* 210(2): 303–305, Oct. 13, 1969.

Artz, C. P. and D. R. Yarbrough: Present Status of the Treatment of Burns, *Bull. N.Y. Acad. Med.* 43(8): 627–635, Aug., 1967.

Barnard, J. H.: Cutaneous Response to Insects, *JAMA* 196: 259–262, Apr. 18, 1966.

Barnett, J. A. and J. P. Sanford: Bacterial Shock, *JAMA* 209(10): 1514–1517, Sept. 8, 1969.

Bass, M.: Sudden Sniffing Death, *JAMA* 212(12): 2075–2079, June 22, 1970.

Beeson, P. B. and W. McDermott (eds.): "Cecil-Loeb Textbook of Medicine," 11th ed., W. B. Saunders Company, Philadelphia, 1963.

Behnke, R. S.: The Use of Cryotherapy in the Training Room (Revised), Prepared for Faculty, Staff, Coaches and Athletes of the Illinois State University Athletic Department, Personal Communication, 1966–1967.

Berdjis, C. C. and J. A. Vick: Endotoxin and Traumatic Shock, *JAMA* 204(3): 99–102, Apr. 15, 1968.

Berenberg, W.: Roseola Infantum (Exanthem Subitum), *Postgrad. Med.*, Sept., 1963, pp. 234–237.

Berens, J. J.: Thermal Contact Burns from Streets and Highways, *JAMA* 214 (11): 2025–2027, Dec. 14, 1970.

Berger, R. S.: The Unremarkable Brown Recluse Spider Bite, *JAMA* 225(9): 1109–1011, Aug. 27, 1973.

Berlin, B. S. and T. Campbell: Hospital-Acquired Herpes Zoster Following Exposure to Chickenpox, *JAMA* 211(11): 1831–1833, Mar. 16, 1970.

Birdwood, G.: A Pill for the Maladies of Society?, *Wld. Med. J.* 2: 26–31, 1970.

Block, J. B.: Angiosarcoma of the Liver Following Vinyl Chloride Exposure, *JAMA* 229(1): 53–54, July 1, 1974.

Bloomfield, D. K.: Fainting: When Is It Ominous? *Consultant*, pp. 5–7, May, 1966.

Bouzarth, W. F.: Management of Head Injury by Industrial Nurses, *Ind. Med.* 39(1): 21–22, Jan., 1970.

————: The ABC's of Emergency Care of Serious Head Injuries in Industry, *Ind. Med.* 39(1): 25–29, Jan., 1970.

————: Management of Head Injury Is a Vital First-Aid Measure, *Ind. Med. & Surg.* 42: 28–29, 1973.

Brody, J. A., E. R. Alexander, and M. L. Hanson: Measles Vaccine Field Trials in Alaska. Two-Year Follow-up of Inactivated Vaccine Followed by Live, Attenuated Vaccine, and of Immune Globulin with Live, Attenuated Vaccine, *JAMA* 196(9): 757–760, May 30, 1966.

Brown, A. W. A.: The Attraction of Mosquitoes to Hosts, *JAMA* 196: 249–252, Apr. 18, 1966.

Buckley, E. E. and N. Porges, (eds.): "Venoms," Publication No. 44 of the American Association for the Advancement of Science, Washington, D.C., 1956.

Burch, G. E. and T. D. Giles: The Burden of a Hot and Humid Environment on the Heart, *Modern Concepts of Cardiovascular Disease*, Vol. XXXIX(8): 115–120, Aug., 1970.

Burks, J. S. et al.: Tricyclic Antidepressant Poisoning—Reversal of Coma, Choreoathetosis, and Myoclonus by Physostigmine, *JAMA 230*(10): 1405–1407, Dec. 9, 1974.

Burrington, J. D.: Aluminum "Pop Tops," *JAMA 235*(24): 2614–2617, June 14, 1976.

Byers, R. K.: Lead Poisoning (Review Article), *Pediatrics 23:* 585–603, March, 1959.

Cantarow, A. and Max Trumper: "Lead Poisoning," The Williams and Wilkins Co., Baltimore, Md., 1944.

Chism, S. E. and A. B. Soule: Snowmobile Injuries—Hazards from a Popular New Winter Sport, *JAMA 209*(11): 1672–1674, Sept. 15, 1969.

Christensen, N. A.: Current Treatment of Potential Tetanus: An Ongoing Problem of Universal Importance, *Mod. Treat. 8:* 629–640, Aug., 1971.

Citron, B. P., M. Halpern, M. McCarron, G. D. Lundberg, R. McCormick, I. J. Pincus, D. Tatter, and B. J. Haverback: Necrotizing Angiitis Associated with Drug Abuse, *New Eng. J. Med. 283*(19): 1003–1011, Nov. 5, 1970.

Cohen, E. J.: Letter to the editor on Angina Pectoris—Mechanism and Treatment, *JAMA 212*(12): 2122, June 22, 1970.

Cohen, S.: Cocaine, *JAMA 231*(1): 74–75, Jan. 6, 1975.

———, Amphetamine Abuse, *JAMA 231*(4): 414–415, Jan. 27, 1975.

———, Marihuana Ingredient Has Various Medical Uses, *JAMA 235*(12): 1199, 1201, March 22, 1976.

Cole, Jonathan O. and Martin B. Katz: The Psychotomimetic Drugs: An Overview, *JAMA 187*(10): 182–185, March 7, 1964.

Coleman, Allan B.: Accidental Poisoning, *New Eng. J. Med. 277*(21): 1135–1137, Nov. 23, 1967.

Collier's Encyclopedia, vol. 21, 1963.

Cort, W. W.: Studies on Schistosome Dermatitis. Status of Knowledge after More than Twenty Years, *Amer. J. Hyg. 52:* 251–307, Nov., 1950.

Craft, A. W., D. A. Shaw, and N. E. F. Cartlidge: Head Injuries in Children, *Br. Med. J.* 4: 200–203, 1972.

Craig, A. B., Jr.: Underwater Swimming and Loss of Consciousness, *JAMA 176*(4): 255–258, Apr. 29, 1961.

Czapek, E. E.: Editorial—Aspirin, Acetaminophen, and Bleeding, *JAMA 235* (6): 636, Feb. 9, 1976.

Davidson, R. H. and L. M. Peairs: "Insect Pests of Farm, Garden, and Orchard," page 648, 6th ed., John Wiley & Sons, Inc., New York, 1966.

DePalma, A. E., D. S. Kwalick, and N. Zukerberg: Pesticide Poisoning in Children, *JAMA 211*(12): 1979–1981, Mar. 23, 1970.

Dillaha, C. J. et al.: North American Loxoscelism, *JAMA 188*(1): 153–156, Apr. 6, 1964.

Dille, J. M. and R. P. Ahlquist: The Synergism of Ethyl Alcohol and Sodium Pentothal, *J. Pharmacol. Exp. Ther. 61*(4): 385–392 (1937).

Doenicke, A.: Beeinträchtigung der Verkehrssicherheit durch Barbiturat-Medikation und durch die Kombination Barbiturat/Alkohol, *Arznei-mittel-Forsch. 12:* 1053, Nov., 1962.

Doty, D. B., A. E. Anderson, E. F. Rose, R. T. Go, C. L. Chiu, and J. L. Ehrenhaft: Cardiac Trauma—Clinical Correlations of Myocardial Contusion, *Annals of Surgery 180:* 452–460, Oct., 1974.

Dranov, J.: Questions and Answers—Forced Diuresis in Treatment of Barbiturate Intoxication, *JAMA 234*(4): 429, Oct. 27, 1975.

Drapanas, T., A. J. Yates, R. Brickman, and M. Wholey: The Syndrome of Occult Rupture of the Spleen, *Arch. Surg. 99:* 298–306, Sept., 1969.

DuPont, J. R.: Current Concepts in Human Rabies, *Clin. Med.*, pp. 37, 40–41, Dec. 1966.

Dyer, R. F. and V. H. Esch: Polyvinyl Chloride Toxicity in Fires—Hydrogen Chloride Toxicity in Fire Fighters, *JAMA 235*(4): 393–397, Jan. 26, 1976.

Ecker, A. and T. Perl: Management of Major Trigeminal Neuralgia (Tic Douloureux) by Precise Alcoholic Injection of the Gasserian Ganglion, *Clin. Med.*, pp. 831–836, May, 1965.

Eddy, N. B., H. Halbach, H. Isbell, and M. H. Seevers: Drug Dependence: its Significance and Characteristics, *Bull. Wld. Hlth. Org. 32:* 721–733, 1965.

Editorial: Botulism: Still a Tragedy, *JAMA 210*(2): 338, Oct. 13, 1969.

Editorial: Early Care for the Heart Attack Suspects, *JAMA 209*(1): 105–106, July 7, 1969.

Editorial: Rum Fits and DT's, *JAMA 212*(12): 2112–2113, June 22, 1970.

Ellis, F. H., Jr., et al.: Surgical Treatment of Esophageal Hypermotility Disturbances, *JAMA 188:* 862–866, June 8, 1964.

Ellison, A. E.: Editorial—Skiing Injuries, *JAMA 223*(8): 917–919, Feb. 19, 1973.

Epilepsy Foundation: "Epilepsy. Answers to Some of the Most Frequently Asked Questions about Epilepsy," The Epilepsy Foundation, Washington, D.C.

Espelin, D. E. and A. K. Done: Amphetamine Poisoning—Effectiveness of Chlorpromazine, *New Eng. J. Med. 278*(25): 1361–1365, June 20, 1968.

Falk, H., J. L. Creech, Jr., C. W. Heath, Jr., M. N. Johnson, and M. M. Key: Hepatic Disease among Workers at a Vinyl Chloride Polymerization Plant, *JAMA 230*(1): 59–63, Oct. 7, 1974.

Farbman, A. A.: Neck Sprain—Associated Factors, *JAMA 223*(9): 1010–1015, Feb. 26, 1973.

Fardon, D. W., C. W. Wingo, D. W. Robinson, and F. W. Masters: The Treatment of Brown Spider Bite, *Plastic and Reconstructive Surgery 40*(5): 482–488, Nov., 1967.

Farrington, J. D.: Death in a Ditch, *Bulletin, American College of Surgeons 52*(3): 121–130, May–June, 1967.

Fischer, D. S., R. Parkman, and S. C. Finch: Acute Iron Poisoning in Children, *JAMA 218:* 1179–1184, 1971.

Fitts, W. T., Jr.: Men for the Care of the Injured: A Crisis Facing the 70s, *Bulletin, American College of Surgeons 55*(10): 9–17, Dec., 1970.

Foley, W. J., M. E. McGinn, and S. M. Lindenauer: Automobile Drivers and Cerebrovascular Insufficiency, *JAMA 207*(4): 749–751, Jan. 27, 1969.

Fowler, J. M. (ed.): "Fallout: A Study of Superbombs, Strontium 90, and Survival," Basic Books, Inc., New York, 1960.

Frahm, Von M., K. Löbkens, and K. Soehring: Der Einfluss subchronischer Alkoholgaben auf die Barbiturat-Narkose von Meerschweinchen, *Arzneimittel-Forsch*, 12: 1055–1056, Nov., 1962.

Fraser, H. F.: Letter to the Editor—Propoxyphene Antidotes, *JAMA 204*(6): 229, May 6, 1968.

Freeze Urged on Snakebite Cryotherapy, *Medical World News*, p. 89, Sept. 15, 1967.

Frey, C. F., D. F. Huelke, and P. W. Gikas: Resuscitation and Survival in Motor Vehicle Accidents, *J. Trauma 9*(4): 292–310, 1969.

Friedman, A. P.: How to Prevent Tension Headache, *Consultant*, p. 16, Jan., 1967.

Froimson, A. I.: Tennis Leg, *JAMA 209*(3): 415–416, July 21, 1969.

Gass, G. Z.: Hardcore Personality and Industrial Illness and Accidents, *Ind. Med. 39*(4): 33–37, April, 1970.

Gelberman, R. H., J. M. Jurist, and J. L. Posch: High-pressure Injection Injuries of the Hand, *J. Bone & Joint Surg. (Amer.) 57:* 935–937, 1975.

Gellis, S. S. (ed.): "Year Book of Pediatrics," Chicago, Year Book Publishers, Inc., 1955–1956, page 638.

Gertsch, W. J.: "American Spiders," D. Van Nostrand, New York, 1949.

Gettler, A. O. and J. O. Baine: The Toxicology of Cyanide, *Am. J. Med. Sci. 195:* 182–198, 1938.

Gettler, A. O. and A. V. St. George: Cyanide Poisoning, *Am. J. Clin. Pathol. 4:* 429–437, 1934.

Gilbert, I. H.: Evaluation and Use of Mosquito Repellents, *JAMA 196:* 253–255, Apr. 18, 1966.

Gill, R. J., and F. MacD. Richardson: Diagnosis and Treatment of Coma, *Medical Science,* pp. 44–52, Aug., 1966.

Glass, T. G., Jr.: Early Debridement in Pit Viper Bites, *JAMA 235*(23): 2513–2516, June 7, 1976.

Gleason, M. N., R. E. Gosselin, et al.: Clinical Toxicology of Commercial Products—Acute Poisoning, Williams & Wilkins, Baltimore, Maryland, 1969.

Glenn, Frank: Priority Evaluation and Management of Multiple Injuries, *American Journal of Surgery,* pp. 461–467, Mar., 1953.

Goldstein, D. H.: Benzene Poisoning, pp. 1776–1777, Beeson, P. B. and W. McDermott, Cecil-Loeb Textbook of Medicine, W. B. Saunders Co., Philadelphia, 1963.

Gonzales, T. A., M. Vance, M. Helpern, and C. J. Umberger: "Legal Medicine: Pathology and Toxicology," 2d ed., Appleton-Century-Crofts, Inc., New York, 1954.

Goodman, J. M., P. W. Wagers, B. H. Barbour, and M. D. Bischel: Barbiturate Intoxication, *West. J. Med. 24:* 179–186, 1976.

Goodman, L. S., and A. Gilman (eds.): "The Pharmacological Basis of Therapeutics," 3d ed., The Macmillan Company, New York, 1965.

Goss, C. M. (ed.): "Gray's Anatomy of the Human Body," 28th ed., Lea & Febiger, Philadelphia, 1966.

Gould, L. et al.: Hemodynamic Effects of Ethanol in Patients with Cardiac Disease, *Quart. J. Stud. Alcohol 33:* 714–721, 1972.

Goulding, Roy: Acetaminophen Poisoning, *Pediatrics 52*(6): 883–885, Dec., 1973.

Greenberg, L. A.: "What the Body Does with Alcohol," Popular Pamphlets on Alcohol Problems, No. 4, Rutgers University, Center of Alcohol Studies, New Brunswick, New Jersey, 1955.

Gregory, C. F.: Synovitis and Bursitis, *The Medical Clinics of North America,* W. B. Saunders Company, Philadelphia, Nov., 1959.

Grollman, A.: "Pharmacology and Therapeutics," Lea & Febiger, Philadelphia, 1962.

Grosfeld, J. L., T. S. Morse, and E. J. Eyring: Lawn Mower Injuries in Children, *Arch. Surg. 100:* 582–583, May, 1970.

Gross, P. A.: Swine Influenza Program—A Special Letter to the Medical Profession, *Membership Newsletter, No. 249,* The Medical Society of New Jersey, June–July, 1976.

Gueron, M. and R. Yaron: Cardiovascular Manifestations of Severe Scorpion Sting, *Chest 57:* 156–162, 1970.

Hall, G. E.: When Death Occurs: Some Practical Aspects, *JAMA 197*(12): 329–330, Sept. 19, 1966.

Haller, J. Alex, Jr.: Newer Concepts in Emergency Care of Children with Major Injuries, *Pediatrics 52*(4): 485–487, Oct., 1973.

Halstead, B. W.: "Dangerous Marine Animals," Cornell Maritime Press, Cambridge, Md., 1959.

Hanes, W. J.: Tic Douloureux: A New Theory of Etiology and Treatment. Report of 40 Cases, *J. Oral Surg. 20:* 222–232, May, 1962.

————: Further Observations on the Treatment of Tic Douloureux on an Allergic Basis, *Headache*, pp. 134–137, Jan. 1964.

Hanson, James W., K. L. Jones, and D. W. Smith: Fetal Alcoholic Syndrome, *JAMA* 235(14): 1458–1460, Apr. 5, 1976.

Harrel, G. T.: Rocky Mountain Spotted Fever, *Medicine 28:* 333–370, 1949.

Harrison, T. R., R. D. Adams, I. L. Bennett, Jr., W. H. Resnik, G. W. Thorn, and M. M. Wintrobe, (eds.): "Principles of Internal Medicine," 5th ed., McGraw-Hill Book Co., New York, 1966.

Haugen, R. K.: The Café Coronary, *JAMA 186:* 142–143, Oct. 12, 1963.

Heimlich, H. J.: A Life-Saving Maneuver to Prevent Food-Choking, *JAMA 234:* 398–401, Oct. 27, 1975.

Herrero, F. A.: Letter to the Editor—Broken Mercury Thermometers, *JAMA 224*(3): 401, Apr. 16, 1973.

Hershey, Falls B. and C. E. Aulenbacher: Surgical Treatment of Brown Spider Bites, *Annals of Surgery 170:* 300–308, Aug., 1969.

Hirschfeld, A. and R. Behan: The Accident Process, *JAMA 186:* Oct. 19, 1963.

Hodgson, T. A., Jr.: Pollution Levels Linked to Daily Mortality Rates, *Environmental Science and Technology*, July, 1970.

Howlett, L. and R. J. Shephard: Carbon Monoxide As a Hazard in Aviation, *Journal of Occupational Medicine 15*(11): 874–877, Nov., 1973.

Huang, T. T., J. B. Lynch, D. L. Larson, and S. R. Lewis: The Use of Excisional Therapy in the Management of Snakebite, *Annals of Surgery 179:* 598–607, May, 1974.

Hyman, M. M.: The Social Characteristics of Persons Arrested for Driving While Intoxicated, *Quart. J. Stud. Alc.*, Suppl. No. 4, pp. 138–177, 1968.

Inaba, D. S., G. R. Gay, J. A. Newmeyer, and C. Whitehead: Methaqualone Abuse—"Luding Out," *JAMA 224*(11): 1505–1509, June 11, 1973.

International Comments: When Is a Patient Dead? *JAMA 197*(8): 153, Aug. 22, 1966.

Iskrant, A. P.: Statistics and Epidemiology of Burns, *Bull. N.Y. Acad. Med. 43*(8): 636–645, Aug., 1967.

Jaffe, M. E.: Treatment of the Acute Stroke, *J. Med. Soc. N.J. 67*(9): 535–537, Sept., 1970.

Jansen, G. Thomas: Treatment of Basal Cell Epitheliomas and Actinic Keratoses, *JAMA 235*(11): 1152–1154, March 15, 1976.

Johnson, D. M.: Fatal Tetanus after Prophylaxis with Human Tetanus Immune Globulin, *JAMA 207:* 1519, Feb. 24, 1969.

Johnson & Johnson: "Therapeutic Uses of Adhesive Tape," 2d. ed., Johnson & Johnson, New Brunswick, N.J., 1958.

Joshi, V. V.: Effects of Burns on the Heart—A Clinicopathological Study in Children, *JAMA 211*(13): 2130–2134, Mar. 30, 1970.

Jude, James R.: The Physician's Role in Sudden Death, *The Heart Bulletin 11*(5): 81–83, Sept.–Oct., 1962.

Juillerat, E. E., Jr.: Survey of Fatal Clothing Fires, *Bull. N.Y. Acad. Med. 43*(8): 646–648, Aug., 1967.

Keller, Mark: Personal communication, Feb. 11, 1971.

Kelly, A. P., Jr. and J. I. Fox: Pneumatic Splinting of Hand Injuries, *Archives of Environmental Health 7:* 282–285, Sept., 1963.

Keyvan-Larijarni, H. and A. M. Tannenberg: Methanol Intoxication: Comparison of Peritoneal Dialysis and Hemodialysis Treatment, *Arch. Intern. Med. 134:* 293–296, 1974.

Knochel, J. P.: Dog Days and Siriasis: How to Kill a Football Player, *JAMA 233*(6): 513–515, Aug. 11, 1975.

Kwalick, D. S. and B. Surowiec: Parathion Poisoning in a Family, *J. Med. Soc. N.J. 67*(10): 603–607, Oct., 1970.

Lampe, K. F.: Systemic Plant Poisoning in Children, *Pediatrics 54*(3): 347–351, Sept., 1974.

Lane, C. E.: Stingers In Season, *Sea Secrets 15*(4): 10–11 (Fourth Series), July–August, 1971.

Langfit, T. W. and F. MacD. Richardson: Intervertebral Disc Disease, *Medical Science*, pp. 66–76, Sept., 1966.

Lawrence, J. W. (Director, Lee County Health Dept., Fort Myers, Fla.): Personal communication, Sept. 21, 1970.

Lee, W. R.: Deaths from Electric Shock in 1962 and 1963, *Brit. Med. J.*, pp. 616–619, Sept., 1965.

Lerman, S.: Glaucoma, *Sci. Amer. 201*(2): 110–117, Aug., 1959.

Levy, G. and J. B. Houston: Effect of Activated Charcoal on Acetaminophen Absorption, *Pediatrics 58*(3): 432, Sept., 1976.

Lewin, Philip: "Backache and Sciatic Neuritis," Lea & Febiger, Philadelphia, 1943.

Lichtenstein, B. W. and A. H. Rosenblum: Sleep Paralysis, *J. Nerv. & Ment. Dis.* 95: 153–155, Feb., 1942.

Liden, C. B., F. H. Lovejoy, and C. E. Costello: Phencyclidine—Nine Cases of Poisoning, *JAMA 234*(5): 513–516, Nov. 3, 1975.

Liebowitz, D. and H. Schwartz: Cyanide Poisoning. Report of a Case with Recovery. *Am. J. Clin. Pathol. 18:* 965–970, 1948.

Linden, M. E.: Some Psychological Aspects of Rescue Breathing, *Amer. J. Nursing 60*(7): 971–974, July, 1960.

Linnoila, M. and S. Hakkinen: Effects of Diazepam and Codeine, Alone, and in Combination with Alcohol, on Simulated Driving, *Clin. Pharmacol. Ther. 15:* 368–373, Apr., 1974.

Linton, A. L., R. G. Luke, and J. D. Briggs: Methods of Forced Diuresis and Its Application in Barbiturate Poisoning, *Lancet 2:* 377, Aug. 19, 1967.

Livingston, S.: Breathholding Spells in Children—Differentiation from Epileptic Attacks, *JAMA 212*(13): 2231–2235, June 29, 1970.

Lockhart, W. E.: Treatment of Snakebite, *JAMA 193*(5): 336–338, Aug. 2, 1965.

————: Letter to the editor on Snakebite Cryotherapy, *Medical World News*, p. 19, Oct. 13, 1967.

Louria, D. B.: The Current Heroin Situation in the United States, *Wld. Med. J. 2:* 33–35, 1970.

Ludwig, A. M. and J. Levine: Patterns of Hallucinogenic Drug Abuse, *JAMA 191*(2): 104–108, Jan. 11, 1965.

Luisada, A. A. and L. M. Rosa, "Treatment of Cardiovascular Emergencies," McGraw-Hill Book Company, New York, 1960.

Lynn, H. B.: Wringer Injuries, *JAMA 174:* 500–502, Oct. 1, 1960.

McLaughlin, Harrison L.: "Trauma," W. B. Saunders Company, Philadelphia, 1959.

Maibach, H. I., W. A. Skinner, W. G. Strauss and A. A. Khan: Factors That Attract and Repel Mosquitoes in Human Skin, *JAMA 196:* 263–266, Apr. 18, 1966.

Mandy, S. and A. B. Ackerman: Characteristic Traumatic Skin Lesions in Drug-induced Coma, *JAMA 213*(2): 253–256, July 13, 1970.

Marr, J. J.: Portuguese Man-of-War Envenomization: A Personal Experience, *JAMA 199*(5): 337–338, Jan. 30, 1967.

Martin, E. W. et al. (eds.): "Remington's Pharmaceutical Sciences," 13th ed., Mack Publishing Company, Easton, Pa., 1965.

Masco, H. L.: Letter to the editor on Scorpion Bite Treatment With Chlorpromazine, *JAMA 212:* 2122, June 22, 1970.

May, W.: Eye Injuries: Emergency Treatment, *Appl. Ther. 8(7):* 611–613, July, 1966.

Medical News Report 2(19): May 11, 1970, "Injury, One of the Nation's Greatest Health Problems."

Meltzer, L. E.: "Current Concepts of the Coronary Care Unit," lecture given at Postgraduate Course, Middlesex General Hospital, New Brunswick, N.J., Oct. 22, 1969.

Meyer, J. A., J. F. Neville, Jr., and W. G. Hansen: Traumatic Rupture of the Aorta in a Child, *JAMA 208(3):* 527–529, April 21, 1969.

Milby, Thomas H.: Prevention and Management of Organophosphate Poisoning, *JAMA 216(13):* 2131–2133, June 28, 1971.

Miller, M. H. and T. C. Toups: "Acute Cyanide Poisoning; Recovery with Sodium Thiosulfate Therapy," *J. Ind. Med. Assoc. 44:*1164, 1954.

Mongé, J. J. and N. F. Reuter, Snowmobiling Injuries, *Arch. Surg. 105:* 188–191, Aug., 1972.

Most, H. and Levine, D.: Schistosomiasis in American Tourists, *JAMA 186:* 453–457, Nov. 2, 1963.

Moyer, C. A., J. E. Rhoads, J. G. Allen, and H. N. Harkins (eds.): "Surgery: Principles and Practice," 3d ed., J. B. Lippincott Company, Philadelphia, 1965.

Muller, G. P.: "Davis' Applied Anatomy," 8th ed., J. B. Lippincott Company, Philadelphia, 1929.

Murray, R.: Electric Shock, *New Eng. J. Med. 268(20):* 1127–1128, May 16, 1963.

National Communicable Disease Center: Reported Incidence of Notifiable Diseases in the United States, 1970, *Morbid. & Mortal. Week. Rep. 19:* 1–60, 1971.

———: Surveillance Summary: Tetanus—United States, 1968 and 1969, *Morbid. & Mortal. Week. Rep. 19:* 162–163, 1970.

National Safety Council, Statistics Division: *Accident Facts,* 1967 ed., National Safety Council, Chicago.

New Jersey, Chapter 195 Laws of, approved Sept. 4, 1970: An Act Concerning Reporting of Epileptiform Seizures.

Newkirk, H. M., A. E. Downe, and J. B. Simon: Fate of Ingested Hepatitis B Antigen in Blood-Sucking Insects, *Gastroenterology 69(4):* 982–987, Oct., 1975.

Nichols, G. A.: Measurements of Oral Temperature in Children, *J. Pediat. 72:* 253–255, 1968.

Nodine, J. H., and J. H. Moyer (eds.): "Psychosomatic Medicine. The First Hahnemann Symposium," Lea & Febiger, Philadelphia, 1962.

Nugent, G. R. and B. Berry: Trigeminal Neuralgia Treated by Differential Percutaneous Radiofrequency Coagulation of the Gasserian Ganglion, *J. Neurosurg. 40:* 517–523, Apr. 1974.

Ochsner, A. and M. E. DeBakey (eds.): "Christopher's Minor Surgery," 8th ed., W. B. Saunders Company, Philadelphia, 1959.

Ommaya, A. K., F. Faas, and P. Yarnell: Whiplash Injury and Brain Damage—An Experimental Study, *JAMA 204(4):* 285–289, Apr. 22, 1968.

Overgaard, J., S. Christensen, et al.: Prognosis after Head Injury Based on Early Clinical Examination, *Lancet 2:* 631–635, 1973.

Parish, L. C.: Nobody Gets Scabies Anymore, *Consultant,* pp. 24–26, May-June, 1970.

Parker, Brent M.: The Effects of Ethyl Alcohol on the Heart, *JAMA 228(6):* 741–742, May 6, 1974.

Parker, R. R.: Rocky Mountain Spotted Fever, *JAMA 110:* 1273–1278, 1938.
Patty, F. A. (ed.), Industrial Hygiene and Toxicology, 2d revised ed., Interscience Publishers, New York, 1963.
Paul, N. W.: Ganglions: Conservative Treatment, *Western Med. 3:* 378–382, 1962.
Perchuk, E.: The Diagnosis and Treatment of Nocturnal Leg Cramps, *Clin. Med.,* pp. 1167–1174, July, 1964.
Peters, Allen H.: Tick-borne Typhus (Rocky Mountain Spotted Fever)—Epidemiologic Trends, with particular Reference to Virginia, *JAMA 216*(6): 1003–1007, May 10, 1971.
Pillsbury, D. M., W. B. Shelley, and A. M. Kligman: "Dermatology," W. B. Saunders Company, Philadelphia, 1956.
Pless, I. B., K. Roghmann, and P. Algranati: The Prevention of Injuries to Children in Automobiles, *Pediatrics 49*(3): 420–427, March, 1972.
Prindle, R. A.: Why Are We Here? Conference on Burns and Flame-Retardant Fabrics, *Bull. N.Y. Acad. Med. 43*(8): 618–626, Aug., 1967.

Rawls, W. B., W. L. Evans, Jr., C. V. Mistretta, and F. M. D'Alessandro: Nocturnal or Recumbency Muscle Cramps: A New Method of Treatment, reprinted from *Medical Times,* June, 1959.
Ray, J. F., III, W. O. Myers, and R. D. Sautter: Letter to the Editor—Lye Ingestion, *JAMA 229*(7): 766, Aug. 12, 1974.
Redding, J. S., R. A. Cozine, G. C. Voight, and P. Safar: Resuscitation from Drowning, *JAMA 178*(12): 1136–1139, Dec. 23, 1961.
Regan, T. J.: Ethyl Alcohol and the Heart, *Circulation 44:* 957–963, 1971.
Richardson, J. D., R. P. Belin, and W. O. Griffin, Jr.: Blunt Abdominal Trauma in Children, *Annals of Surgery 176*(2): 213–216, Aug., 1972.
Rider, J. A., H. C. Moeller, E. J. Puletti, and D. C. Desai: Diagnosis and Treatment of Diffuse Esophageal Spasm, *Arch. Surg. 99:* 435–440, Oct., 1969.
Roberts, K. B. and E. C. Roberts: The Automobile and Heat Stress, *Pediatrics 58*(1): 101–104, July, 1976.
Roden, V. J.: Aspirin: A Dangerous Pulmonary Foreign Body, *J. Pediatr. 83*(2): 266–268, Aug., 1973.
Rogers, F. L. and J. P. Igini: Beverage Can Pull Tabs, *JAMA 233*(4): 345–348, July 28, 1975.
Rubbo, S. D.: Prophylaxis against Tetanus, in L. Eckmann (ed.), "Principles on Tetanus," *Proceedings of the International Conference on Tetanus,* Hans Huber, Bern, Switzerland, 1967, pp. 341–354.
Rubsamen, D. S.: Head Injury with Unsuspected Cervical Fracture: A Malpractice Trap for the Unwary Physician, *JAMA 229*(5): 576–577, July 29, 1974.
Rushton, J. G.: Sleep Paralysis, *Med. Clin. N. Amer. 28:* 945–949, July, 1944.
Ryan, A. J.: "Medical Care of the Athlete," McGraw-Hill Book Company, New York, 1962.

Salisbury, R. E., J. L. Hunt, G. D. Warden, and B. A. Pruitt, Jr.: Management of Electrical Burns of the Upper Extremity, *Plast. Reconstr. Surg. 51:* 648–652, June, 1973.
Sargent, E. N. and A. F. Turner: Emergency Treatment of Pneumothorax, *Am. J. Roentgenol. 109:* 531–535, 1970.
Sargent, E. N. and A. F. Turner: Emergency Treatment of Pneumothorax. ICU—A Review of the Literature on Intensive Care, Number 23 of a series, The Upjohn Company, 1971.
Sauer, G. C.: "Manual of Skin Diseases," 2d ed., J. B. Lippincott Company, Philadelphia, 1966.

Schneck, J. M.: Sleep Paralysis: Psychodynamics, *Psychiat. Quart. 22:* 462–469, July, 1948.
———: Sleep Paralysis, *Amer. J. Psychiat. 108:* 921–923, June, 1952.
———: Sleep Paralysis: A New Evaluation, Diseases of the Nervous System *18:* 144–146, April, 1957.
———: Sleep Paralysis without Narcolepsy or Cataplexy. Report of a Case, *JAMA 173:* 1129–1130, July 9, 1960.
———: Disguised Representation of Sleep Paralysis in Ernest Hemingway's "The Snows of Kilimanjaro," *JAMA 182*(4): 318, 320, Oct. 27, 1962.
Scudese, V. A., K. Hamada, and A. Awitan: Fat Embolism—A Problem of Increasing Importance in Traumatic Surgery, *J. Med. Soc. N.J. 67*(5): 211–214, May, 1970.
Shaffer, L. L.: Letter to the Editor—Ketamine, *JAMA 229*(7): 764, Aug. 12, 1974.
Sharpe, J. C. and F. W. Marx, Jr. (eds.): "Management of Medical Emergencies," 2d ed., McGraw-Hill Book Company, New York, 1969.
Shelness, A. and S. Charles: Children As Passengers in Automobiles: The Neglected Minority on the Nation's Highways, *Pediatrics 56*(2): 271–284, Aug., 1975.
Sherwin, D. and B. Mead: Delirium Tremens in a Nine-Year-Old Child, *Amer. J. Psychiatry 132*(11): 1210–1212, Nov., 1975.
Shires, G. T. (ed.): "Care of the Trauma Patient," McGraw-Hill Book Company, New York, 1966.
Shirkey, H. C. (ed.): Pediatric Therapy, 3d ed., The C. V. Mosby Co., St. Louis, 1968.
Shubin, Herbert and M. H. Weil: Shock Associated with Barbiturate Intoxication, *JAMA 215*(2): 263–268, Jan. 11, 1971.
———: Bacterial Shock, *JAMA 235*(4): 421–424, Jan. 26, 1976.
Shulman, B. H. and G. D. Reddy: "Purse Poisons," *Pediatrics 51:* 126, Jan., 1973.
Simon, F. A. and L. K. Pickering: Acute Yellow Phosphorus Poisoning—"Smoking Stool Syndrome," *JAMA 235*(13): 1343–1344, March 29, 1976.
Simpson, K.: Current Medico-Legal Problems: The Moment of Death, *Guy's Hosp. Gaz.* (London), pp. 601–606, Nov. 11, 1967.
Sladen, A. and H. L. Zauder: Methylprednisolone Therapy for Pulmonary Edema Following Near Drowning, *JAMA 215*(11): 1793–1795, Mar. 15, 1971.
Sleath, G. W. and L. T. Archer: Demonstration: 4 Minutes To Save a Life, *Appl. Ther. 9*(11): 910–911, Nov., 1967.
Smith, C. N.: Personal Protection from Blood-Sucking Arthropods, *JAMA 196:* 236–239, Apr. 18, 1966.
Smith, L. D. S. and L. V. Holderman: "The Pathogenic Anaerobic Bacteria," Charles C. Thomas, Publisher, Springfield, Illinois, 1968.
Smith, M. E., R. L. Evans, E. J. Newman, and H. W. Newman: Psychotherapeutic Agents and Ethyl Alcohol, *Quart. J. Stud. Alcohol 22:* 241–249, 1961.
Sorenson, W. R.: Letter to the Editor—Polyvinyl Chloride in Fires, *JAMA 236*(13): 1449, Sept. 27, 1976.
Sparger, C. F.: Problems in the Management of Rattlesnake Bites, *Arch. Surg. 98:* 13–18, Jan., 1969.
Spencer, F. J.: The Devil and William Dabney: An Epidemiological Postscript, *JAMA 195*(8): 133–136, Feb. 21, 1966.
Stahnke, H. L.: The L-C Treatment of Venomous Bites or Stings, *The First Aider*, Vol. XXXV #13, Cramer's, Gardner, Kansas, March 1, 1966.

Starzl, T. E.: Treatment of Frostbite Today, *Consultant*, pp. 44–47, Jan., 1967.

Steckler, R. M., J. A. Epstein, and B. S. Epstein: Letter to the editor on Seat Belt Trauma to the Lumbar Spine, *JAMA 207*(4): 758–759, Jan. 27, 1969.

Stewart, R. D.: Methyl Chloroform Intoxication—Diagnosis and Treatment, *JAMA 215*(11): 1789–1792, March 15, 1971.

Stewart, W. W. (ed.): Symposium, May 18–19, 1970, Philadelphia, Pa., "Drug Abuse in Industry," Halos and Associates, Inc., Miami, Florida, 1970.

Stimson, P. M. and H. L. Hodes: *"A Manual of the Common Contagious Diseases,"* 5th ed., Lea & Febiger, Philadelphia, 1956.

Sturner, W. Q. and J. C. Garriott: Deaths Involving Propoxyphene—A Study of 41 Cases over a Two-Year Period, *JAMA 223*(10): 1125–1130, March 5, 1973.

Tabershaw, I. R. and W. R. Gaffey: Mortality of Workers in the Manufacture of Vinyl Chloride and Its Polymers, *Journal of Occupational Medicine 16*(8): 509–510, Aug., 1974.

Talbott, J. A. and J. W. Teague: Marihuana Psychosis—Acute Toxic Psychosis Associated With the Use of *Cannabis* Derivatives, *JAMA 210*(2): 299–302, Oct. 13, 1969.

Taylor, R. L., J. I. Maurer, and J. R. Tinklenberg: Management of "Bad Trips" in an Evolving Drug Scene, *JAMA 213*(3): 422–425, July 20, 1970.

Tennant, F. S., Jr., B. A. Russell, S. K. Casas, and R. N. Bleich: Heroin Detoxification—A Comparison of Propoxyphene and Methadone, *JAMA 232*(10): 1019–1022, June 9, 1975.

Thorndike, A.: *"Athletic Injuries: Prevention, Diagnosis and Treatment,"* 5th ed., Lea & Febiger, Philadelphia, 1962.

Tipton, D. L., Jr., V. C. Sutherland, T. N. Burbridge, and A. Simon: Effect of Chlorpromazine on Blood Level of Alcohol in Rabbits, *Amer. J. Physiol. 200:* 1007–1010 (1961).

Tong, T. G., N. L. Benowitz, C. E. Becker, P. J. Forni, and U. Boerner: Phencyclidine Poisoning, *JAMA 234*(5): 512–513, Nov. 3, 1975.

Tylden, E.: Cannabis and Hallucinogens, *Wld. Med. J. 2:* 36–38, 1970.

Ullman, K. C. and R. H. Groh: Identification and Treatment of Acute Psychotic States Secondary to the Usage of OTC Sleeping Preparations, *Amer. J. Psychiatry 128:* 1244–1248, Apr., 1972.

Ungerleider, J. T., D. D. Fisher, and M. Fuller: The Dangers of LSD: Analysis of Seven Months' Experience in a University Hospital's Psychiatric Service, *JAMA 197*(6): 109–112, Aug. 8, 1966.

United States Department of Agriculture: Home and Garden Bulletin No. 137, "Controlllng Chiggers," issued Dec., 1967.

United States Department of Defense: "NATO Handbook: Emergency War Surgery," United States Government Printing Office, Washington, D.C., 1958.

————, Samuel Glasstone (ed.): "The Effects of Nuclear Weapons," rev. ed., United States Atomic Energy Commission, Washington, D.C., April, 1962.

United States Department of Health, Education, and Welfare, Health Services and Mental Health Administration, National Institute of Mental Health: "LSD—Some Questions and Answers," Public Health Service Publication No. 1828, United States Government Printing Office, Washington, D.C., 1969.

————, "Marihuana: Some Questions and Answers," Public Health Service Publication No. 1829, United States Government Printing Office, Washington, D.C., 1969.

————, "Narcotics: Some Questions and Answers," Public Health Service Publication No. 1827, United States Government Printing Office, Washington, D.C., 1969.

United States Department of Health, Education, and Welfare, Public Health Service, Health Services and Mental Health Administration: "The Up and Down Drugs: Amphetamines and Barbiturates," Public Health Service Publication No. 1830, United States Government Printing Office, Washington, D.C., 1969.

United States Department of Health, Education and Welfare, Public Health Service: "Botulism in the United States: Review of Cases 1899–1967 and Handbook for Epidemiologists, Clinicians, and Laboratory Workers," Atlanta, Nov., 1968.

Van der Heide, C. and J. Weinberg: Sleep Paralysis and Combat Fatigue, *Psychosom. Med. 7:* 330–334, Nov., 1945.

Van Dusen, W. and H. B. Brooks: Treatment of Youthful Drug Abusers, *Mod. Med.,* pp. 74–76, July 27, 1970.

Waller, J. A.: Control of Accidents in Rural Areas, *JAMA 201:* 176–181, 1967.

————, Medical Impairment and Highway Crashes, *JAMA 208*(12): 2293–2296, June 23, 1969.

1953.

Weider, A. (ed.): "Contributions Toward Medical Psychology: Theory and Psychodiagnostic Methods," The Ronald Press Company, New York, 1953.

Weitzner, H. A.: Sleep Paralysis Successfully Treated with Insulin Hypoglycemia, *AMA Arch. Neurol. & Psychiat. 68:* 835–841, Dec., 1952.

Welsh, A. L.: "Psychotherapeutic Drugs," Charles C. Thomas, Publisher, Springfield, Illinois, 1958.

Wenger, D. R.: Avulsion of the Profundus Tendon Insertion in Football Players, *Arch. Surg. 106:* 145–149, Feb., 1973.

Wertzberger, J. J. and L. F. Peltier: Fat Embolism: The Importance of Arterial Hypoxia, *Surgery 63:* 626–629, 1968.

Whittlesey, R. H.: Postscript on Appendicitis, *Consultant,* pp. 5–7, Nov.–Dec., 1966.

Wicher, K., R. E. Reisman, and C. E. Arbesman: Allergic Reaction to Penicillin Present in Milk, *JAMA 208*(1): 143–145, Apr. 7, 1969.

Wilder, R. J., J. R. Jude, W. B. Kouwenhoven, and M. C. McMahon: Cardiopulmonary Resuscitations by Trained Ambulance Personnel, *JAMA 190:* 531–534, Nov. 9, 1964.

Wilentz, W. C. et al.: Rupture of the Aorta in Medical Examiner Cases—Report of Nine Cases and a Review of the Literature, *J. Med. Soc. N.J. 68*(1): 29–32 (Jan.) 1971.

Williams, P. C.: "The Lumbosacral Spine: Emphasizing Conservative Management," McGraw-Hill Book Company, New York, 1965.

Winick, C.: "The Narcotic Addiction Problem," American Social Health Association, New York, 1968.

Wisconsin School Health Council: "School Health Emergencies: A Plan for Meeting Them," Wisconsin State Board of Health, Madison, Wisconsin, 1960.

Witt, Paul: Personal communication, Apr. 28, 1971.

Wolfson, E. A.: Drug Abuse: The Doctor's Role, *J. Med. Soc. N. J. 67*(8): 465–471, Aug., 1970.

Wong, F. M. and W. J. Grace: Sudden Death after Near-Drowning, *JAMA 186*(7): 724–726, Nov. 16, 1963.

Zimmerman, L. M. and R. Levine, (eds.): "Physiological Principles of Surgery," W. B. Saunders Company, Philadelphia, 1957.

Zinsser, H. F. and G. S. Thind: Right Bundle Branch Block After Nonpenetrating Injury to the Chest Wall, *JAMA 207*(10): 1913–1915, Mar. 10,
1969.

Index